Skeletal Muscle Physiology: Role of Nutrition

Skeletal Muscle Physiology: Role of Nutrition

Editor: Niki Doyle

AMERICAN
MEDICAL PUBLISHERS
www.americanmedicalpublishers.com

AMERICAN
MEDICAL PUBLISHERS
www.americanmedicalpublishers.com

Cataloging-in-Publication Data

Skeletal muscle physiology : role of nutrition / edited by Niki Doyle.
p. cm.
Includes bibliographical references and index.
ISBN 979-8-88740-456-1
1. Musculoskeletal system--Physiology. 2. Muscles--Physiology. 3. Nutrition.
4. Musculoskeletal system--Diseases--Nutritional aspects.
5. Musculoskeletal system--Diseases--Diet therapy.
6. Musculoskeletal system--Wounds and injuries--Nutritional aspects.
7. Musculoskeletal system--Wounds and injuries--Diet therapy. I. Doyle, Niki.
QP321 .S54 2023

American Medical Publishers,
41 Flatbush Avenue,
1st Floor, New York,
NY 11217, USA

ISBN 979-8-88740-456-1 (Hardback)

Contents

Preface

Skeletal muscle is one of the three major muscle tissues found in humans. It is made up of thousands of muscle fibers encased by connective tissue sheaths. It is present throughout the body and responds to stimuli by contracting. It serves many functions including maintenance of body position and posture, joint stabilization, storage of nutrients, production of movement and regulation of body temperature. Insufficient dietary protein can cause muscle damage through a variety of mechanisms. Furthermore, intense training can lead to skeletal muscle breakdown which can be worsened by a lack of protein in the diet. Insufficient hydration can reduce blood flow to working muscles that makes them more vulnerable to injury. This book explores all the important aspects of skeletal muscle physiology in the present day scenario. It also provides significant information to help develop a good understanding of the role of nutrition. Those in search of information to further their knowledge will be greatly assisted by this book.

This book is a result of research of several months to collate the most relevant data in the field.

When I was approached with the idea of this book and the proposal to edit it, I was overwhelmed. It gave me an opportunity to reach out to all those who share a common interest with me in this field. I had 3 main parameters for editing this text:

1. Accuracy – The data and information provided in this book should be up-to-date and valuable to the readers.

2. Structure – The data must be presented in a structured format for easy understanding and better grasping of the readers.

3. Universal Approach – This book not only targets students but also experts and innovators in the field, thus my aim was to present topics which are of use to all.

Thus, it took me a couple of months to finish the editing of this book.

I would like to make a special mention of my publisher who considered me worthy of this opportunity and also supported me throughout the editing process. I would also like to thank the editing team at the back-end who extended their help whenever required.

Editor

1

Higher Protein Density Diets are Associated with Greater Diet Quality and Micronutrient Intake in Healthy Young Adults

Jess A. Gwin[1,2], J. Philip Karl[2], Laura J. Lutz[3], Erin Gaffney-Stomberg[3], James P. McClung[2] and Stefan M. Pasiakos[2]*

[1] Oak Ridge Institute for Science and Education Supporting the Military Nutrition Division of the US Army Research Institute of Environmental Medicine, Natick, MA, United States,
[2] Military Nutrition Division of the US Army Research Institute of Environmental Medicine, Natick, MA, United States, [3] Military Performance Division of the US Army Research Institute of Environmental Medicine, Natick, MA, United States

Correspondence:
Stefan M. Pasiakos
stefan.m.pasiakos.civ@mail.mil

Objective: This study characterized habitual dietary protein intake in healthy young adults entering military service and explored whether diet protein density is associated with diet quality and micronutrient intake.

Methods: An FFQ was used to estimate habitual dietary intake and calculate HEI scores in 276 males [mean(SD), age:21.1y(3.8)] and 254 females [age:21.2y(3.7)]. Multivariate-adjusted MANCOVA and ANCOVA models were used to identify associations between protein density quartiles and HEI scores and micronutrient intake. Higher HEI components scores for sodium, refined grains, and empty calories indicate lower intake; higher scores for all other components indicate higher intakes.

Results: Mean(SD) energy-adjusted protein intakes were 29.3(3.2), 36.0(1.4), 40.8(1.3), and 47.9(3.9) g/1,000 kcal for protein density quartiles 1–4, respectively. For males, empty calorie scores as well as dark green and orange vegetable scores were higher in quartiles 3 and 4 than 1 and 2 (all, $p < 0.05$). Scores for total vegetable, dairy, and total protein foods were lower in quartile 1 vs. quartiles 2, 3, and 4 (all, $p < 0.05$). Sodium scores decreased as quartiles increased ($p < 0.001$). Total HEI, fruit, whole grains, seafood and plant protein, fatty acids, and refined grain scores did not differ. For females, total HEI, vegetable, and total protein foods scores were higher in quartiles 3 and 4 than 1 and 2 (all, $p < 0.05$). Empty calorie scores increased as quartile increased ($p < 0.05$). Dairy scores were higher in quartiles 2, 3, and 4 than 1 ($p < 0.05$). Whole fruit scores were lowest in quartile 1 ($p < 0.05$). Whole grain as well as seafood and plant protein scores were higher in quartile 4 vs. 1 (both, $p < 0.05$). Sodium scores decreased as quartile increased ($p < 0.001$). Fatty acids scores did not differ. For males and females, micronutrient intakes progressively increased across quartiles with the exception of calcium and vitamin C, (all, $p < 0.05$). Intakes remained nearly the same when controlled for fruit and vegetable intake.

Conclusion: These cross-sectional data suggest that habitually consuming a higher protein density diet is associated with better scores for some, but not all, diet quality components in males, better overall diet quality scores in females, and greater intakes of micronutrients in both male and female healthy, young adults entering military service.

Keywords: protein, diet quality, micronutrients, shortfall nutrients, healthy eating index

INTRODUCTION

Dietary protein recommendations are established as the minimum amount of dietary protein intake necessary to maintain nitrogen balance (1). However, accumulating evidence demonstrates that protein intakes above the Recommended Dietary Allowance (RDA; 0.8 g • kg^{-1} • d^{-1} for healthy adults) are metabolically advantageous and may reduce chronic disease risk (2), enhance satiety (3), and body composition during weight loss (4) and exercise training (5). Protein-containing foods are comprised of more than their constituent amino acids; they also contain a high ratio of micronutrients to energy and are therefore nutrient-dense (1). As a result, consuming a higher protein-dense diet, defined as consuming more energy from protein-containing whole foods without increasing total energy intake, may enhance diet quality and improve micronutrient intake (1, 6).

Diet quality is considered a primary modifiable risk factor associated with preventable health complications and chronic disease development (7, 8). Ensuring dietary micronutrient intakes meet minimum requirements is one strategy to optimize diet quality. Optimizing diet quality is particularly important for populations whose health and physical performance are critical to occupational success and resilience to injury and stressors associated with unaccustomed physical training, including healthy young adults entering initial military training (9–11). The Dietary Guidelines for Americans 2015–2020 recently identified several micronutrients that are often underconsumed and are therefore considered shortfall nutrients (12). These include potassium, choline, magnesium, calcium, vitamins A, D, E, and C (12), which serve critical roles in bone health, blood pressure regulation, cancer, and cardiovascular disease prevention (13–16). Suboptimal intakes of iron, folate, zinc, and vitamins B1, B2, B3, and B12 may diminish physical performance and limit beneficial adaptations to physical training (5, 17, 18). Nutrient-dense, protein-containing whole-foods are excellent sources of the aforementioned micronutrients (19, 20). It is also possible that increasing the protein density of the diet may be related to better overall food choices that contribute to better diet quality and micronutrient intake. In contrast it is conceivable that consuming more protein-containing foods may negatively impact diet quality if these foods are higher in saturated-fat and sodium (i.e., processed and non-lean meats). However, whether consuming higher amounts of total energy as protein-containing foods improves or diminishes diet quality and micronutrient intakes is not well-described (1).

This cross-sectional study characterized habitual dietary protein intake in healthy young adults entering military service and explored whether the protein density of the diet was associated with diet quality, as indicated by Healthy Eating Index (HEI) scores and micronutrient intake. We hypothesized that when controlling for energy density and total energy intake, diet quality, and micronutrient intakes would be greater in those consuming higher quantities of dietary protein.

METHODS

This research was carried out in accordance with US Army Regulation 70–25 and the provisions of Title 32 Code of Federal Regulations Part 219 Protection of Human Subjects. This research was approved by the Institutional Review Board at the US Army Research Institute of Environmental Medicine.

Participants

The study sample included 890 healthy adults (ages 17–42 y) entering initial military training. Data collection occurred over four study iterations which took place as follows: February, 2010 at Fort Jackson, SC ($n = 223$); June 2012 and February 2013 at Fort Sill, OK ($n = 492$); and April 2015 at Fort Jackson, SC ($n = 175$). All data were collected as part of primary studies designed to assess the effects of calcium and vitamin D supplementation on bone health (11, 21, 22). All participants provided informed, written consent.

Dietary Intake

The 3-month 2005 Block Food Frequency Questionnaire (FFQ) was used to assess dietary intake prior to initial military training accession. This semi-quantitative FFQ captures usual intakes of food groups and nutrients for 3 months prior to administration using a food item list (23). Respondents select the frequency (i.e., never to every day) and quantity of foods they consumed from the food item list, and are asked to specify if foods were modified or standard items (i.e., low-fat vs. full-fat foods). The FFQ is commonly used to assess dietary intakes and is validated for use in the general US population and has been used to assess dietary intake in military populations (24–27). Charts of photographed foods denoting portion sizes were provided to assist in portion size estimation, and registered Dietitians were available to answer participant questions regarding the FFQ. Questionnaires were analyzed by Nutrition Quest (Berkeley, CA, USA) using the US Department of Agriculture Food and Nutrient Database for Studies version 1.0. Analysis included computation macro- and

Abbreviations: DGOVL, Dark green and orange vegetables and legumes; FFQ, food frequency questionnaire; HEI, Healthy Eating Index; RDA, recommended dietary allowance.

micronutrient intakes in addition to HEI total and component scores. Participants were excluded from analyses if they had missing data or indicated implausible energy intakes (males < 800 or > 5,000 kcal/d; females < 300 or > 4,500 kcal/d) (8, 9). Those that reported consuming supplements at least once per week were also excluded. Demographic information was collected through self-report. Dietary intakes from 276 males [mean (SD), age: 21.1 y (3.8), body mass index: 25.8 kg/m^2 (3.7)] and 254 females [age: 21.2 y (3.7), BMI: 24.2 kg/m^2 (2.9)] were included in the final statistical analyses.

Healthy Eating Index Components

HEI is a diet quality measure that reflects conformance to the Dietary Guidelines for Americans (28). HEI total scores are the composite of 12 component scores and range from 0 to 100; with 100 denoting perfect compliance with the Dietary Guidelines for Americans. HEI component scores are categorized as indicators of adequacy and moderation. Adequacy components included: total fruit, whole fruit, total vegetables, dark green and orange vegetables and legumes (DGOVL), dairy, total protein foods, seafood and plant protein, whole grains, and fatty acids. Higher adequacy component scores indicate higher consumption. Moderation components included: sodium, refined grains, and empty calories (i.e., calories from solid fats, alcohol, and added sugars). Higher moderation component scores indicate lower consumption of these categories. Collectively, higher total and component scores suggest better dietary quality vs. lower scores. HEI 2010 was used for the current analyses to maintain consistency within the data set since a majority of the data had been analyzed by Nutrition Quest (Berkeley, CA, USA) prior to the release of HEI 2015.

Statistical Analyses

A multivariate-adjusted ANCOVA model was used to identify associations between quartiles of protein intake and means of energy adjusted protein intake as well as means of relative protein intake. A multivariate-adjusted ANCOVA model was used to identify associations between quartiles of protein intake and total HEI score. Multivariate-adjusted MANCOVA models were used to identify associations between quartiles of protein intake and HEI component scores (i.e., total fruit, whole fruit, total vegetables, dark green and orange vegetables and legumes (DGOVL), dairy, total protein foods, seafood and plant protein, whole grains, fatty acids, sodium, refined grains, and empty calories) as well as micronutrients of interest. A sex-by-protein density quartile interaction was detected for the Total HEI and HEI component scores. Therefore, these data was analyzed for each sex separately (i.e., Model 1). Model 1 was adjusted for study iteration, age, ethnicity, race, physical activity, smoking status, energy density (kcal/g of food consumed) and total energy intake. No sex-by-protein density quartile interaction was detected for micronutrient intakes. Thus, sex was added to Model 2 as a covariate. For Model 3, fruit and vegetable intakes were added to Model 2 as covariates. Race was categorized as white, black, or other. Ethnicity was categorized as Hispanic or non-Hispanic. Habitual physical activity was categorized as yes (i.e., at least one time per week) or no (i.e., never or rarely). Smoking habits were categorized as yes (i.e., current smoker) or no (i.e., non-smoker or former smoker). Data were analyzed using the Statistical Package for the Social Sciences (version 24.0; IBM SPSS). A Bonferroni correction was applied to correct for multiple comparisons. All results are presented as mean (SD) as appropriate. Adherence to model assumptions was verified and statistical significance was set at $p < 0.05$.

RESULTS

Protein Density Quartiles

Mean ± SD energy-adjusted protein intakes increased across protein density quartiles [29.3 (3.2), 36.1 (1.4), 40.9 (1.3), and 47.9 (3.9) g/1,000 kcal, respectively; all, $p < 0.05$; **Table 1**)]. Protein intakes expressed as percent of total energy intake increased across protein density quartiles (11.7 (1.3), 14.4 (0.6), 16.4 (0.5), and 19.2 (1.6) percent, respectively; all, $p < 0.05$). Relative protein intakes across protein density quartiles were lower in quartile 1 [0.9 (0.5)] than quartiles 2, 3, and 4 (1.2 (0.6), 1.3 (0.6), and 1.3 (0.5) g • kg^{-1} • d^{-1}, respectively; all, $p < 0.05$.

HEI Total and Component Scores

For males empty calorie and DGOVL component scores were higher in protein density quartiles 3 and 4 than 1 and 2 (all, $p < 0.05$; **Table 2**). Component scores for total vegetable, dairy, and total protein food consumption were lower in protein density quartile 1 compared to quartiles 2, 3, and 4 (all, $p < 0.05$). Sodium component scores decreased progressively as protein density quartile increased ($p < 0.001$). Total HEI, total fruit, whole fruit, whole grains, seafood and plant protein, fatty acids, and refined grain scores did not differ across protein density quartiles.

For females total HEI, total vegetables, DGOVL, and total protein foods were higher in protein density quartiles 3 and 4 than quartiles 1 and 2 (all, $p < 0.05$; **Table 3**). Empty calorie component scores increased as protein density quartile increased ($p < 0.05$). Dairy component scores were higher in quartiles 2, 3, and 4 than quartile 1 ($p < 0.05$). Refined grain component scores

TABLE 1 | Habitual estimated protein intake by protein density quartile in healthy young adults[1].

Protein intake	Protein density quartile			
	1 (n = 135)	2 (n = 134)	3 (n = 134)	4 (n = 127)
g/1,000 kcal[2]	29.3 ± 3.2^a	36.1 ± 1.4^b	40.9 ± 1.3^c	47.9 ± 3.9^d
Percent total energy[3]	11.7 ± 1.3^a	14.4 ± 0.6^b	16.4 ± 0.5^c	19.2 ± 1.6^d
g/kg body weight[3]	0.9 ± 0.5^a	1.2 ± 0.6^b	1.3 ± 0.6^b	1.3 ± 0.5^b

[1] *Values are means (SD).*
[2] *Data are analyzed using ANCOVA adjusted for age, ethnicity, race, physical activity, smoking status, and total energy intake, within a row, values not sharing superscript letters are different at the univariate level, $p < 0.05$.*
[3] *Data are analyzed using ANCOVA adjusted for age, ethnicity, race, physical activity, smoking status, and energy density within a row, values not sharing superscript letters are different at the univariate level, $p < 0.05$.*

TABLE 2 | Healthy Eating Index (HEI) scores based on habitual protein intake in healthy young males[1, 2].

HEI score	Protein density quartile				*P*-value[4]
	1 (*n* = 54)	2 (*n* = 70)	3 (*n* = 78)	4 (*n* = 74)	
Total HEI score[3]	51.3 ± 12.1	53.5 ± 12.6	54.7 ± 10.2	56.1 ± 9.7	$P = 0.22$
Total fruit	3.3 ± 1.6	3.2 ± 1.6	2.8 ± 1.5	2.8 ± 1.4	$P = 0.03$
Whole fruit	2.9 ± 1.5	2.9 ± 1.7	2.6 ± 1.7	2.9 ± 1.6	$P = 0.85$
Total vegetables	2.7 ± 1.0[a]	3.0 ± 1.2[a,b]	3.3 ± 1.1[b]	3.5 ± 1.2[b]	$P = 0.003$
DGOVL[5]	1.9 ± 1.8[a]	2.5 ± 1.8[a]	3.3 ± 1.7[b]	3.3 ± 1.7[b]	$P = 0.001$
Whole grains	2.2 ± 1.8	2.8 ± 2.3	3.2 ± 2.5	3.2 ± 2.6	$P = 0.12$
Dairy	4.8 ± 2.1[a]	6.1 ± 2.3[b]	6.3 ± 2.4[b]	5.7 ± 2.7[b]	$P = 0.001$
Total protein foods	4.2 ± 0.8[a]	4.7 ± 0.5[b]	4.9 ± 0.3[b,c]	5.0 ± 0.3[c]	$P = 0.001$
Seafood and plant protein	3.1 ± 1.5	3.2 ± 1.5	3.0 ± 1.6	3.4 ± 1.6	$P = 0.45$
Fatty acids	5.1 ± 2.8	4.3 ± 2.6	4.7 ± 2.2	4.5 ± 2.3	$P = 0.14$
Sodium[6]	6.3 ± 1.7[a]	4.6 ± 1.9[b]	3.1 ± 1.9[c]	2.2 ± 1.8[d]	$P = 0.001$
Refined grains[6]	8.0 ± 2.4	7.6 ± 2.2	7.1 ± 2.3	7.8 ± 2.1	$P = 0.08$
Empty calories[6]	6.9 ± 5.9[a]	8.4 ± 5.1[a]	10.5 ± 3.7[b]	11.9 ± 3.6[b]	$P = 0.001$

[1]*Values are mean ± SD.*
[2]*Data are analyzed using MANCOVA are adjusted for age, ethnicity, race, physical activity, smoking status, energy density, and total energy intake, within a row, values not sharing superscript letters are different at the univariate level, $p < 0.05$.*
[3]*Data are analyzed using ANCOVA adjusted for age, ethnicity, race, physical activity, smoking status, energy density, and total energy intake, within a row, values not sharing superscript letters are different at the univariate level, $p < 0.05$.*
[4]*P-value < 0.05 indicates a main effect of protein density quartile.*
[5]*Dark green and orange vegetables and legumes (DGOVL).*
[6]*Moderation components higher scores reflect lower intakes.*

were lowest in protein density quartile 2 and whole fruit scores were lowest in quartile 1 (both, $p < 0.05$). Seafood and plant protein as well as whole grain consumption were only higher in protein density quartile 4 compared to quartile 1 (both, $p < 0.05$). Sodium component scores decreased progressively as protein density quartile increased ($p < 0.001$). Fatty acids component scores did not differ across protein density quartiles.

Micronutrient Intakes

Composite micronutrient intake differed ($p < 0.001$) by protein density quartile in both model 2 and 3. For model 2, individual micronutrient intakes, except calcium and vitamin C, progressively increased (all, $p < 0.05$) with increasing protein density quartiles (**Table 4**). Calcium intakes in protein density quartile 1 were lower than quartiles 2, 3, and 4 ($p < 0.001$). Vitamin C intakes were not different across protein density quartiles. Model 3 indicated that independent of fruit and vegetable intake, all micronutrients progressively increased across protein density quartiles except vitamins A, E, C, and folate (all, $p < 0.05$) (**Table 5**). Vitamin A and C intakes in protein density quartile 1 were lower than quartiles 2, 3, and 4 (all, $p < 0.001$). Vitamin E intakes were not different across protein density quartiles. There was not a protein density quartile-by-sex interaction indicated by model 3, ($p = 0.13$).

DISCUSSION

This cross-sectional study assessed whether consuming greater amounts of dietary protein, resulting in higher diet protein density, was associated with diet quality and dietary micronutrient intakes in healthy young adults. We demonstrate that habitually consuming high protein density diets, independent of energy density and total energy intake, was associated with better scores for select diet quality components in males, better overall diet quality scores in females, and greater micronutrient intakes for both males and females. We also demonstrate that the relationship between protein density and intake of several micronutrients was independent of fruit and vegetable intake. These associative data suggest that consuming a high proportion of total energy derived from protein-containing whole foods supports healthy dietary intake patterns that align with current nutrition guidelines for Americans.

To our knowledge, only one other study (29) has addressed whether consuming greater amounts of protein-containing foods was associated with diet quality in healthy adults. In that study total protein intake was negatively associated with diet quality in males but positively associated with diet quality in females. In addition, animal-based protein intake was negatively associated with diet quality in males, whereas animal-based protein intake was positively associated with diet quality in females. Regardless of sex, plant-based protein intake was positively associated with better diet quality. Similarly, we demonstrate that consuming a higher protein-dense diet was associated with consuming more protein from seafood and plants than lower protein-dense diets, but only in females. It is possible that, in this population, males may consume more of their protein from animal sources, whereas in females there may be a larger contribution from plant-based sources. The remaining divergent

TABLE 3 | Healthy Eating Index (HEI) scores based on habitual protein intake in healthy young females[1, 2].

HEI score	Protein density quartile				*P*-value[4]
	1 ($n = 81$)	2 ($n = 64$)	3 ($n = 56$)	4 ($n = 53$)	
Total HEI score[3]	51.7 ± 11.2^{a}	54.1 ± 10.9^{a}	61.7 ± 11.9^{b}	66.4 ± 12.3^{b}	$P = 0.001$
Total fruit	3.1 ± 1.7	3.4 ± 1.7	3.8 ± 1.4	3.9 ± 1.4	$P = 0.05$
Whole fruit	2.9 ± 1.7^{a}	$3.1 \pm 1.6^{a,b}$	3.8 ± 1.3^{b}	4.0 ± 1.4^{b}	$P = 0.001$
Total vegetables	2.8 ± 1.3^{a}	3.0 ± 1.2^{a}	3.8 ± 1.1^{b}	4.1 ± 1.1^{b}	$P = 0.001$
DGOVL[5]	2.3 ± 1.8^{a}	2.6 ± 1.7^{a}	4.0 ± 1.5^{b}	4.3 ± 1.3^{b}	$P = 0.001$
Whole grains	2.4 ± 1.9^{a}	$3.0 \pm 2.4^{a,b}$	$3.1 \pm 2.6^{a,b}$	3.6 ± 2.6^{b}	$P = 0.03$
Dairy	3.9 ± 1.9^{a}	6.2 ± 2.5^{b}	6.2 ± 2.8^{b}	7.0 ± 2.8^{b}	$P = 0.001$
Total protein foods	3.9 ± 0.9^{a}	4.4 ± 0.8^{b}	4.8 ± 0.5^{c}	5.0 ± 0.2^{c}	$P = 0.001$
Seafood and plant protein	2.9 ± 1.5^{a}	$3.2 \pm 1.5^{a,b}$	$3.6 \pm 1.5^{a,b}$	3.9 ± 1.4^{b}	$P = 0.006$
Fatty acids	5.5 ± 2.9	4.5 ± 2.6	5.4 ± 2.9	5.6 ± 2.8	$P = 0.13$
Sodium[6]	6.6 ± 2.5^{a}	4.3 ± 2.0^{b}	$3.5 \pm 2.1^{b,c}$	2.5 ± 2.0^{c}	$P = 0.001$
Refined grains[6]	$8.0 \pm 2.6^{a,b}$	6.8 ± 2.9^{a}	8.3 ± 2.2^{b}	8.5 ± 2.1^{b}	$P = 0.01$
Empty calories[6]	7.2 ± 5.4^{a}	9.5 ± 3.9^{b}	11.5 ± 4.1^{c}	14.0 ± 4.0^{d}	$P = 0.001$

[1] *Values are mean ± SD.*
[2] *Data are analyzed using MANCOVA are adjusted for age, ethnicity, race, physical activity, smoking status, energy density, and total energy intake, within a row, values not sharing superscript letters are different at the univariate level, $p < 0.05$.*
[3] *Data are analyzed using ANCOVA adjusted for age, ethnicity, race, physical activity, smoking status, energy density, and total energy intake, within a row, values not sharing superscript letters are different at the univariate level, $p < 0.05$.*
[4] *P-value < 0.05 indicates a main effect of protein density quartile.*
[5] *Dark green and orange vegetables and legumes (DGOVL).*
[6] *Moderation components higher scores reflect lower intakes.*

associations between diet quality, protein quantity, and intakes of animal- and plant-based protein foods (i.e., without including seafood proteins) in the Camilleri study are difficult to reconcile with our findings, which may be largely a function of the diet scoring methodologies used. HEI estimates dietary conformance to the Dietary Guidelines for Americans, whereas the PANDiet index used by Camilleri et al. estimates the probability that usual dietary intakes meet French and or European Union nutritional recommendations (28, 29). Nevertheless, the data from Camilleri et al. highlight an important analytical limitation of the HEI, which does not provide specific examination of all protein food sources or the characteristics of these food items (i.e., lean meats or low-fat dairy). As such, the potential for animal- and plant-based protein foods to be differentially related to diet quality in healthy young adults entering military service cannot be discerned. We were also unable to identify which food sources were responsible for the increasing sodium intakes across protein density quartile. It is possible that the individuals in the highest protein density quartile consumed more processed protein-containing foods, which are typically higher in sodium (30). Lastly, at the time of data analysis, the HEI 2010 was the current method for assessing diet quality and conformance to the Dietary Guidelines for Americans. Future analyses in similar cross-sectional studies using the HEI 2015 would allow for differentiation of added sugars and saturated fats that is unattainable within the empty calories component score of the HEI 2010.

The Dietary Guidelines for Americans recommend a shift toward consuming nutrient-dense foods at the expense of limiting empty calorie intake (i.e., energy from solid fats, added sugars, and alcohol) (12). In the current study, we demonstrate that those in the highest dietary protein density quartile also habitually consumed more total vegetables, including nutrient-dense dark greens, orange vegetables, and legumes, more whole grains (females only), more dairy, and less empty calories. The apparent protein-related increases in dietary nutrient-density and diet quality were not a function of simply consuming more food (i.e., total energy), but rather a combination of consuming more nutrient-dense foods, and fewer nutrient-poor foods that contain empty calories. These findings are comparable to those derived from NHANES 2003–2004, which suggest that those consuming greater amounts of nutrient-dense foods, not protein *per se*, limited empty calorie intake (31). These findings may be particularly beneficial in the context of healthy weight management and are corroborated by data from other prospective, cross-sectional studies demonstrating lower central adiposity and body mass index in American adults habitually consuming more protein, independent of total energy intake (32, 33).

Individuals in the highest dietary protein density quartile also consumed more non-protein, nutrient-rich foods. This could suggest that the relationship between protein density of the diet and diet quality was mediated by those non-protein foods and general eating habits rather than solely the protein density of the diet. However, when controlling for fruit and vegetable intake, micronutrient intakes across protein density quartiles remained nearly the same. This suggests that food sources of protein within a protein-dense diet are related to nutrient intakes. However,

TABLE 4 | Estimated daily micronutrient intakes across protein density quartile in healthy young adults[1, 2].

Micronutrients of interest	Protein density quartile				*P*-value[3]
	1 (*n* = 135)	2 (*n* = 134)	3 (*n* = 134)	4 (*n* = 127)	
Potassium (mg)	1092.0 ± 316.7[a]	1207.6 ± 291.9[b]	1304.2 ± 292.9[c]	1442.7 ± 334.8[d]	*P* = 0.001
Calcium (mg)	356.6 ± 110.1[a]	438.1 ± 114.0[b]	449.2 ± 123.8[b]	482.8 ± 178.2[b]	*P* = 0.001
Magnesium (mg)	117.8 ± 27.4[a]	134.2 ± 32.5[b]	150.1 ± 39.6[c]	163.0 ± 41.5[c]	*P* = 0.001
Folate (mg)	101.0 ± 45.6[a]	112.9 ± 47.6[a]	132.5 ± 54.4[b]	148.1 ± 73.7[b]	*P* = 0.001
Choline (mg)	123.5 ± 30.0[a]	150.0 ± 34.0[b]	173.9 ± 39.5[c]	205.6 ± 58.1[d]	*P* = 0.001
Iron (mg)	6.1 ± 1.5[a]	6.8 ± 1.3[b]	7.3 ± 1.7[b]	8.0 ± 2.0[c]	*P* = 0.001
Zinc (mg)	4.5 ± 1.0[a]	5.4 ± 0.7[b]	6.2 ± 1.2[c]	7.2 ± 2.1[d]	*P* = 0.001
Vitamin A (retinol activity eq., mcg)	283.2 ± 118.0[a]	346.2 ± 147.0[b]	419.0 ± 245.6[c]	446.1 ± 216.4[c]	*P* = 0.001
Vitamin C (mg)	68.1 ± 44.5	58.5 ± 34.6	58.1 ± 31.3	62.3 ± 34.3	*P* = 0.56
Vitamin D (IU)	50.0 ± 37.1[a]	73.7 ± 43.7[b]	84.7 ± 61.1[b]	103.3 ± 58.6[c]	*P* = 0.001
Vitamin E (alpha-tocopherol, mg)	3.5 ± 1.1[a]	3.4 ± 1.0[a,b]	3.8 ± 1.2[a]	3.9 ± 1.5[a,c]	*P* = 0.001
Vitamin B1 (mg)	0.7 ± 0.2[a]	0.8 ± 0.2[b]	0.8 ± 0.2[b]	0.9 ± 0.2[c]	*P* = 0.001
Vitamin B2 (mg)	0.8 ± 0.2[a]	1.0 ± 0.3[b]	1.1 ± 0.3[b]	1.2 ± 0.3[c]	*P* = 0.001
Vitamin B3 (mg)	8.8 ± 2.1[a]	10.3 ± 2.1[b]	11.2 ± 2.3[c]	13.1 ± 2.8[d]	*P* = 0.001
Vitamin B12 (mcg)	1.9 ± 0.7[a]	2.5 ± 0.6[b]	2.9 ± 1.0[c]	3.7 ± 1.2[d]	*P* = 0.001

[1] *Values are mean ± SD.*
[2] *Data are analyzed using MANCOVA adjusted for age, sex, ethnicity, race, physical activity, smoking status, energy density, and total energy intake, within a row, values not sharing superscript letters are different at the univariate level,* $p < 0.05$.
[3] *P-value* < 0.05 *indicates a main effect of protein density quartile.*

we did not examine whether individuals who consumed a diet with a higher protein density were doing so as part of a strategy to eat an overall healthier diet. Thus, future prospective studies are required to determine causation and identify which food sources of protein may drive this relationship. Additionally, relative protein intakes in the current study were above the RDA, but within the Acceptable Macronutrient Distribution Range for protein (10–35% of total calories) (34). These findings align with our previous observations that protein intakes are generally higher than the RDA in similar military populations (35) and free-living Americans (36).

The potential impact of inadequate micronutrient intake cannot be delineated in the current study, although the biological functions of micronutrients suggest suboptimal intakes may hinder physiologic adaptations and performance during strenuous, unaccustomed physical training (9). Specifically, suboptimal intakes of vitamin D and iron have been recognized to have detrimental effects on health and performance in those entering the military (9–11, 37). Intakes of these nutrients progressively increased as protein density quartile increased suggesting consuming more protein may be beneficial. While the effects of folate and vitamin E on performance are not well-studied, in general suboptimal intakes of folate and vitamin E raise concern as folate is vital for cellular synthesis, growth, and repair (38) and vitamin E is a key antioxidant and contributes to anti-inflammatory processes (39). Similarly, low magnesium intake would suggest a potential greater risk of inefficient energy metabolism and suboptimal neuro-muscular function (40). Although it would be helpful to understand how the estimated micronutrient intakes across protein density quartiles compares to recommended intakes, we cannot directly compare micronutrient intake adequacies to the DRIs due to limitations of the FFQ (41, 42). For example, FFQs rely on single time-point data collection to estimate food intake. Multiple days of direct dietary intake assessment are required when determining adequacy of nutrient intakes (41, 42). However, these data do suggest that increasing the protein density of the diet does seem to relate to better overall diet quality, in this population of healthy young people.

While we were not able to directly address the effects of dietary protein on muscle and performance in the current study, it is reasonable to speculate that higher quality, higher protein diet patterns positively influence skeletal muscle mass, adaptations to exercise, and physical performance. Higher protein intakes offset protein catabolism and support nitrogen balance in individuals exposed to aerobic exercise training (43, 44). Dietary protein, and its constituent amino acids, are also a primary determinant of skeletal muscle protein turnover. Thus, dietary patterns that support routine high-quality protein ingestion, particularly following exercise, should promote beneficial adaptations to training, and facilitate repair and remodeling of existing muscle protein, and accretion of new muscle protein mass (45). The well-established effects of dietary protein on muscle integrity would support shifting dietary patterns in favor of protein dense foods and such a shift would not reduce diet quality since consuming a higher protein density diet appears possible without displacing other nutrient rich, non-protein foods that contribute an overall healthy diet.

TABLE 5 | Estimated daily micronutrient intakes across protein density quartile when adjusted for fruit and vegetable intake in healthy young adults[1, 2].

Micronutrients of interest	Protein density quartile				P-value[3]
	1 (n = 135)	2 (n = 134)	3 (n = 134)	4 (n = 127)	
Potassium (mg)	1092.0 ± 316.7[a]	1207.6 ± 291.9[b]	1304.2 ± 292.9[b]	1442.7 ± 334.8[c]	P = 0.001
Calcium (mg)	356.6 ± 110.1[a]	438.1 ± 114.0[b]	449.2 ± 123.8[b,c]	482.8 ± 178.2[c]	P = 0.001
Magnesium (mg)	117.8 ± 27.4[a]	134.2 ± 32.5[b]	150.1 ± 39.6[b]	163.0 ± 41.5[c]	P = 0.001
Folate (mg)	101.0 ± 45.6[a]	112.9 ± 47.6[a,b]	132.5 ± 54.4[a,b]	148.1 ± 73.7[b]	P = 0.001
Choline (mg)	123.5 ± 30.0[a]	150.0 ± 34.0[b]	173.9 ± 39.5[c]	205.6 ± 58.1[d]	P = 0.001
Iron (mg)	6.1 ± 1.5[a]	6.8 ± 1.3[b]	7.3 ± 1.7[b]	8.0 ± 2.0[c]	P = 0.001
Zinc (mg)	4.5 ± 1.0[a]	5.4 ± 0.7[b]	6.2 ± 1.2[c]	7.2 ± 2.1[d]	P = 0.001
Vitamin A (retinol activity eq., mcg)	283.2 ± 118.0[a]	346.2 ± 147.0[b]	419.0 ± 245.6[b]	446.1 ± 216.4[b]	P = 0.001
Vitamin C (mg)	68.1 ± 44.5[a]	58.5 ± 34.6[b]	58.1 ± 31.3[b]	62.3 ± 34.3[b]	P = 0.02
Vitamin D (IU)	50.0 ± 37.1[a]	73.7 ± 43.7[b]	84.7 ± 61.1[c]	103.3 ± 58.6[d]	P = 0.001
Vitamin E (alpha-tocopherol, mg)	3.5 ± 1.1	3.4 ± 1.0	3.8 ± 1.2	3.9 ± 1.5	P = 0.25
Vitamin B1 (mg)	0.7 ± 0.2[a]	0.8 ± 0.2[b]	0.8 ± 0.2[b]	0.9 ± 0.2[c]	P = 0.001
Vitamin B2 (mg)	0.8 ± 0.2[a]	1.0 ± 0.3[b]	1.1 ± 0.3[b]	1.2 ± 0.3[c]	P = 0.001
Vitamin B3 (mg)	8.8 ± 2.1[a]	10.3 ± 2.1[b]	11.2 ± 2.3[b]	13.1 ± 2.8[c]	P = 0.001
Vitamin B12 (mcg)	1.9 ± 0.7[a]	2.5 ± 0.6[b]	2.9 ± 1.0[c]	3.7 ± 1.2[d]	P = 0.001

[1] *Values are means (SD).*
[2] *Data are analyzed using MANCOVA adjusted for age, sex, ethnicity, race, physical activity, smoking status, energy density, total energy intake, fruit intake, and vegetable intake, within a row, values not sharing superscript letters are different at the univariate level, $p < 0.05$.*
[3] *P-value < 0.05 indicates a main effect of protein density quartile.*

CONCLUSION

This study demonstrated that habitually consuming more protein resulting in a diet with a higher protein density is associated with better scores for some, but not all, diet quality components in males, better overall diet quality scores in females, and greater intakes of micronutrients in both young male and female adults prior to reporting for military service.

DISCLOSURE

of Army, Department of Defense, or the US Government. Any citations of commercial organizations and trade names in this report do not constitute an official Department of the Army endorsement of approval of the products or services of these organizations.

The views and assertions expressed herein are those of the authors and do not reflect the official policy of the Department

AUTHOR CONTRIBUTIONS

JG and SP had primary responsibility for the final content and wrote the manuscript. JG and JK analyzed the data. JG, PK, LL, EG-S, JM, and SP designed the research and approved the final paper.

FUNDING

This project was funded by US Army Medical Research and Materiel Command. The study sponsor had no role in study design, collection, analysis, and interpretation of data; writing the report, nor the decision to submit the report for publication.

ACKNOWLEDGMENTS

We acknowledge the Soldier volunteers that participated in this study and the command staff at Fort Jackson, SC, and Fort Sill, OK who provided access to potential volunteers. We also thank Susan McGraw for assisting with data management and Katelyn Guerriere assisting for with study coordination.

REFERENCES

1. Phillips SM, Fulgoni VL III, Heaney RP, Nicklas TA, Slavin JL, Weaver CM. Commonly consumed protein foods contribute to nutrient intake, diet quality, and nutrient adequacy. *Am J Clin Nutr.* (2015) 101:1346S–2S. doi: 10.3945/ajcn.114.084079
2. Rodriguez NR. Introduction to Protein Summit 2.0: continued exploration of the impact of high-quality protein on optimal health. *Am J Clin Nutr.* (2015). 101:1317S–9S. doi: 10.3945/ajcn.114.083980
3. Leidy HJ, Clifton PM, Astrup A, Wycherley TP, Westerterp-Plantenga MS, Luscombe-Marsh ND, et al. The role of protein in weight loss and maintenance. *Am J Clin Nutr.* (2015) 101:1320S–9S. doi: 10.3945/ajcn.114.084038
4. Carbone JW, McClung JP, Pasiakos SM. Recent advances in the characterization of skeletal muscle and whole-body protein responses to dietary protein and exercise during negative energy balance. *Adv Nutr.* (2018) 10:70–9. doi: 10.1093/advances/nmy087
5. Thomas DT, Erdman KA, Burke LM. American college of sports medicine joint position statement. Nutrition and athletic performance. *Med Sci Sports Exerc.* (2016) 48:543–68. doi: 10.1249/MSS.0000000000000852
6. Alkerwi A. Diet quality concept. *Nutrition.* (2014) 30:613–8. doi: 10.1016/j.nut.2013.10.001
7. World Health Organization. *Preventing Chronic Diseases: A Vital Investment.* Geneva: World Health Organization (2005).
8. Sotos-Prieto M, Bhupathiraju SN, Mattei J, Fung TT, Li Y, Pan A, et al. Association of changes in diet quality with total and cause-specific mortality. *N Engl J Med.* (2017) 377:143–53. doi: 10.1056/NEJMoa1613502
9. McClung JP, Karl JP, Cable SJ, Williams KW, Nindl BC, Young AJ, et al. Randomized, double-blind, placebo-controlled trial of iron supplementation in female soldiers during military training: effects on iron status, physical performance, and mood. *Am J Clin Nutr.* (2009) 90:124–31. doi: 10.3945/ajcn.2009.27774
10. Karl JP, Lieberman HR, Cable SJ, Williams KW, Young AJ, McClung JP. Randomized, double-blind, placebo-controlled trial of an iron-fortified food product in female soldiers during military training: relations between iron status, serum hepcidin, and inflammation. *Am J Clin Nutr.* (2010) 92:93–100. doi: 10.3945/ajcn.2010.29185
11. Gaffney-Stomberg E, Lutz LJ, Rood JC, Cable SJ, Pasiakos SM, Young AJ, et al. Calcium and vitamin D supplementation maintains parathyroid hormone and improves bone density during initial military training: a randomized, double-blind, placebo controlled trial. *Bone.* (2014) 68:46–56. doi: 10.1016/j.bone.2014.08.002
12. U.S. Department of Health and Human Services, U.S. Department of Agriculture. *2015–2020 Dietary Guidelines for Americans.* 8th ed. (2015). Available online at: http://health.gov/dietaryguidelines/2015/guidelines/ (accessed October 19, 2019).
13. Omenn GS, Goodman GE, Thornquist MD, Balmes J, Cullen MR, Glass A, et al. Effects of a combination of beta carotene and vitamin A on lung cancer and cardiovascular disease. *N Engl J Med.* (1996) 334:1150–5. doi: 10.1056/NEJM199605023341802
14. Zeisel SH, Da Costa K-A. Choline: an essential nutrient for public health. *Nutr Rev.* (2009) 67:615–23. doi: 10.1111/j.1753-4887.2009.00246.x
15. Weaver CM. Potassium and health. *Adv Nutr.* (2013) 4:368S–77S. doi: 10.3945/an.112.003533
16. Baaij JH, Hoenderop JG, Bindels RJ. Magnesium in man: implications for health and disease. *Physiol Rev.* (2015) 95:1–46. doi: 10.1152/physrev.00012.2014
17. Lukaski HC. Vitamin and mineral status: effects on physical performance. *Nutrition.* (2004) 20:632–44. doi: 10.1016/j.nut.2004.04.001
18. McClung JP, Gaffney-Stomberg E. Optimizing performance, health, and well-being: nutritional factors. *Mil Med.* (2016) 181(Suppl. 1):86–91. doi: 10.7205/milmed-d-15-00202
19. O'Neil CE, Keast DR, Fulgoni VL, Nicklas TA. Food sources of energy and nutrients among adults in the US: NHANES 2003–2006. *Nutrients.* (2012) 4:2097–120. doi: 10.3390/nu4122097
20. Huth PJ, Fulgoni VL, Keast DR, Park K, Auestad N. Major food sources of calories, added sugars, and saturated fat and their contribution to essential nutrient intakes in the U.S. diet: data from the national health and nutrition examination survey (2003–2006). *Nutr J.* (2013) 12:116. doi: 10.1186/1475-2891-12-116
21. Lutz LJ, Karl JP, Rood JC, Cable SJ, Williams KW, Young AJ, et al. Vitamin D status, dietary intake, and bone turnover in female soldiers during military training: a longitudinal study. *J Int Soc Sports Nutr.* (2012) 9:38. doi: 10.1186/1550-2783-9-38
22. Hughes JM, Gaffney-Stomberg E, Guerriere KI, Taylor KM, Popp KL, Xu C, et al. Changes in tibial bone microarchitecture in female recruits in response to 8 weeks of US Army Basic Combat Training. *Bone.* (2018) 113:9–16. doi: 10.1016/j.bone.2018.04.021
23. Block G, Subar AF. Estimates of nutrient intake from a food frequency questionnaire: the 1987 National Health Interview Survey. *J Am Diet Assoc.* (1992) 92:969–77.
24. Lutz LJ, Gaffney-Stomberg E, Scisco JL, Cable SJ, Karl JP, Young AJ, et al. Assessment of dietary intake using the healthy eating index during military training. *US Army Med Dep J.* (2013) 91, 91–8.
25. Lutz LJ, Gaffney-Stomberg E, Williams KW, McGraw SM, Niro PJ, Karl JP, et al. Adherence to the dietary guidelines for americans is associated with psychological resilience in young adults: a cross-sectional study. *J Acad Nutr Diet.* (2017) 117:396–403. doi: 10.1016/j.jand.2016.09.018
26. Lutz LJ, Gaffney-Stomberg E, Karl JP, Hughes JM, Guerriere KI, McClung JP. Dietary intake in relation to military dietary reference values during army basic combat training; a multi-center, cross-sectional study. *Mil Med.* (2018a) 184:usy153. doi: 10.1093/milmed/usy153
27. Lutz LJ, Nakayama AT, Karl JP, McClung JP, Gaffney-Stomberg E. Serum and erythrocyte biomarkers of nutrient status correlate with short-term ?-carotene, ?-carotene, folate, and vegetable intakes estimated by food frequency questionnaire in military recruits. *J Am Coll Nutr.* (2018b) 38:171–8. doi: 10.1080/07315724.2018.1490215
28. Guenther PM, Casavale KO, Reedy J, Kirkpatrick SI, Hiza HA, Kuczynski KJ, et al. Update of the healthy eating index: HEI-2010. *J Acad Nutr Diet.* (2013) 113:569–80. doi: 10.1016/j.jand.2012.12.016
29. Camilleri GM, Verger EO, Huneau JF, Carpentier F, Dubuisson C, Mariotti F. Plant and animal protein intakes are differently associated with nutrient adequacy of the diet of French adults. *J Nutr.* (2013) 143:1466–73. doi: 10.3945/jn.113.177113
30. Poti JM, Mendez MA, Ng SW, Popkin BM. Is the degree of food processing and convenience linked with the nutritional quality of foods purchased by US households? *Am J Clin Nutr.* (2015) 101:1251–62. doi: 10.3945/ajcn.114.100925
31. Britten P, Cleveland LE, Koegel KL, Kuczynski KJ, Nickols-Richardson SM. Impact of typical rather than nutrient-dense food choices in the US Department of Agriculture Food Patterns. *J Acad Nutr Diet.* (2012) 112:1560–9. doi: 10.1016/j.jand.2012.06.360
32. Pasiakos SM, Lieberman HR, Fulgoni IIIVL. Higher-protein diets are associated with higher HDL cholesterol and lower BMI and waist circumference in US adults. *J Nutr.* (2015) 145:605–14. doi: 10.3945/jn.114.205203
33. Berryman CE, Agarwal S, Lieberman HR, Fulgoni VL III, Pasiakos SM. Diets higher in animal and plant protein are associated with lower adiposity and do not impair kidney function in US adults. *Am J Clin Nutr.* (2016) 104:743–49. doi: 10.3945/ajcn.116.133819
34. Trumbo P, Schlicker S, Yates AA, Poos M. Dietary reference intakes for energy, carbohdrate, fiber, fat, fatty acids, cholesterol, protein and amino acids. *J Acad Nutr Diet.* (2002) 102:1621–30. doi: 10.1016/S0002-8223(02)90346-9
35. Pasiakos SM, Karl JP, Lutz LJ, Murphy NE, Margolis LM, Rood JC, et al. Cardiometabolic risk in US Army recruits and the effects of basic combat training. *PLoS ONE.* (2012) 7:e31222. doi: 10.1371/journal.pone.0031222
36. Berryman CE, Lieberman HR, Fulgoni VL, Pasiakos SM. Protein intake trends and conformity with the Dietary Reference Intakes in the United States: analysis of the National Health and Nutrition Examination Survey, 2001–2014. *Am J Clin Nutr.* (2018) 108:405–13. doi: 10.1093/ajcn/nqy088
37. Richards T, Wright C. British Army recruits with low serum vitamin D take longer to recover from stress fractures. *J R Army Med Corps.* (2018) jramc-2018-000983. doi: 10.1136/jramc-2018-000983
38. Woolf K, Manore MM. B-vitamins and exercise: does exercise alter requirements? *Int J Sport Nutr Exerc Metab.* (2006) 16:453–84. doi: 10.1123/ijsnem.16.5.453

39. Traber MG. Vitamin E inadequacy in humans: causes and consequences. *Adv Nutr.* (2014) 5:503–14. doi: 10.3945/an.114.006254

40. Zhang Y, Xun P, Wang R, Mao L, He K. Can magnesium enhance exercise performance? *Nutrients.* (2017) 9:946. doi: 10.3390/nu9090946

41. Otten JJ, Hellwig JP, Meyers LD. *Dietary Reference Intakes: The Essential Guide to Nutrient Requirements.* Washington, DC: National Academies Press (2006).

42. Subar AF, Freedman LS, Tooze JA, Kirkpatrick SI, Boushey C, Neuhouser ML, et al. Addressing current criticism regarding the value of self-report dietary data. *J Nutr.* (2015) 145:2639–45. doi: 10.3945/jn.115.219634

43. Moore DR, Camera DM, Areta JL, Hawley JA. Beyond muscle hypertrophy: why dietary protein is important for endurance athletes. *Appl Physiol Nutr Metab.* (2014) 39:987–97. doi: 10.1139/apnm-2013-0591

44. Kato H, Suzuki K, Bannai M, Moore DR. Protein requirements are elevated in endurance athletes after exercise as determined by the indicator amino acid oxidation method. *PLoS ONE.* (2016) 11:e0157406. doi: 10.1371/journal.pone.0157406

45. Burd NA, De Lisio M. Skeletal muscle remodeling: interconnections between stem cells and protein turnover. *Exerc Sport Sci Rev.* (2017) 45:187–91. doi: 10.1249/JES.0000000000000117

2

Asian Indians with Prediabetes have Similar Skeletal Muscle Mass and Function to those with Type 2 Diabetes

Sucharita Sambashivaiah[1], Stephen D. R. Harridge[2†], Nidhi Sharma[3], Sumithra Selvam[4], Priyanka Rohatgi[5] and Anura V. Kurpad[1,3]*

[1] Department of Physiology, St. John's Medical College, Bengaluru, India, [2] Centre for Human and Applied Physiological Sciences, King's College London, London, United Kingdom, [3] Division of Nutrition, St. John's Research Institute, Bengaluru, India, [4] Division of Epidemiology and Biostatistics, St. John's Research Institute, Bengaluru, India, [5] Apollo Hospitals, Bengaluru, India

***Correspondence:**
Sucharita Sambashivaiah
sucharita.dr@gmail.com

†ORCID:
Stephen D. R. Harridge
orcid.org/0000-0002-8203-0769

Background: Type 2 Diabetes (T2D) is a major concern among Asian Indians, not least because many develop T2D at despite having a normal BMI (body mass index), and with relatively low body fat. Asian Indians are also generally considered to have relatively low skeletal muscle mass and strength, this has not been explored in the context of T2D.

Aim: The present study aimed to compare skeletal muscle mass, function and contractile quality (strength/mass) between healthy controls, those with prediabetes (PD) as well as T2D middle-aged non-obese Asian Indians.

Methods: Adult males between the age of 20–50 years, consisting of healthy controls ($n = 44$), PD ($n = 125$) and T2D ($n = 55$) were studied. Skeletal muscle mass was measured using Dual X-ray Absorptiometry (DXA). Isometric and dynamic muscle function was measured using an isokinetic dynamometer (at 0, 60, 120, 180 degree/s). Muscle contractile quality was derived by dividing the peak muscle torque with the respective LMM (lower limb muscle mass). Fasting blood glucose (FBG) and insulin were used to derive insulin resistance (HOMA-IR).

Results: The control group was on average 10 years younger than the other two groups ($p < 0.01$). The LMM was similar across the three study groups. However, the age-adjusted mean muscle torque was significantly lower in both absolute and normalized isometric and isokinetic strength in PD and T2D groups compared to controls ($p \leq 0.01$), with the difference persisting even after adjusting for age and other covariates. However, there was no difference in muscle strength and contractile quality between the PD and T2D study groups.

Conclusions: Muscle strength and contractile quality would appear to be sensitive and early indices of the trajectory toward diabetes in Asian Indians and more so than skeletal muscle mass. It is thus important to recognize the importance of functional measurements among this population when considering the role of muscle in diabetes. The data also would suggest that specific muscle conditioning (e.g., resistance training) might have efficacy in improving function as well as muscle mass, and thus aiding in the prevention of the trajectory toward the development of T2D.

Keywords: skeletal muscle, muscle mass, muscle function, body fat, diabetes mellitus, prediabetes

INTRODUCTION

Both contractile and metabolic signals play integral roles in regulating muscle homeostasis (1). The interrelationships between metabolic and mechanical signals help maintain contractile function (strength), metabolic health, physical well-being, and quality of life (2). Ideally, muscle bulk (mass) along with function should reflect an optimum balance between metabolic and contractile function (3). Therefore, skeletal muscle mass alone has been used as a reflection of nutritional and physical activity status in both health and disease (4). However, muscle mass is a static measure, depending on its composition of contractile and cytoskeletal proteins, as well as intra and intermyocellular fat (5). Recent evidence suggests that there is excessive intramyocellular fat in Indians with PD (6), and therefore it is likely that muscle mass may not be altered in such subjects. In such circumstances, it is likely that skeletal muscle contractile function may provide more sensitive diagnostic information, particularly in chronic disease. An example of this is the finding of a relation between all-cause mortality or morbidity and reduced forearm muscle strength (7).

A further dimension of muscle function is contractile quality. Whilst this reflects force per unit area or mass, it can also be considered relevant to an array of muscle characteristics, including glucose metabolism, intramuscular adipose tissue, capillary density, structural composition, and fatigability (8, 9). Currently, there is a lack of literature exploring the role of skeletal muscle mass, function, and contractile quality in chronic disease. This is important, since, for example, muscle function, or greater muscle contractility, has been linked to upregulation of glucose transporters (10). Therefore, it is critical to evaluate muscle function, skeletal muscle mass as well as contractile quality in populations who are considered to have low muscle mass (10), and who have a predisposition for T2D (11).

T2D is now a major concern among Asian Indians, particularly in the subcontinent, where the number has increased markedly from 26 million in 1990 to 65 million in 2016, with an increase in crude prevalence from 5.5 to 7.7% in the same time period (12). Increasing modernization and adoption of a more sedentary lifestyle that not only results in a positive energy balance and fat deposition, but also less skeletal muscle use, could contribute to the marked increase in T2D among Asian Indians (13). This occurs at a normal BMI and has led to the terms "metabolic obesity" and "the thin-fat Indian" (13). While age-related loss in muscle mass and function among T2D has been studied extensively in western populations (14, 15), there are no studies in young and middle-aged Asian Indians who constitute a major proportion of the population in India. There are also no studies that compare skeletal muscle mass and function in healthy Asian Indians with those with PD and T2D. The aim of the present study was thus to compare skeletal muscle mass, function and contractile quality of the major limb muscle (quadriceps) between healthy males, PD and T2D middle-aged non-obese Asian Indians.

MATERIALS AND METHODS

Participants

The study population consisted of healthy controls ($n = 44$), prediabetes ($n = 125$) and T2D ($n = 55$). Adult males between the age of 20–50 years were recruited in and around St. John's Medical College and Hospital and through advertisements. The participants were reviewed for inclusion criteria at the first point of contact including their preexisting medical records. All participants were having either fasting blood sugar or HbA1C data already available at the first point of contact. This information was used to shortlist the eligible candidates. They were then invited to undergo a 75-g oral glucose tolerance test (OGTT) and HbA1C. The eligible participants were investigated for plasma glucose obtained by the GOD POD method (Beckman Coulter AU480, Japan), and glycosylated hemoglobin (HbA1c, HPLC, BioRad, Variant Turbo II, India). The previous day of the OGTT clear instructions were given to the participant to fast for 8–10 h before the testing. The American Diabetes Association Expert Committee criteria (16) were used for the diagnosis of PD. For the control group, the following criteria were used FBG, $\leq$100 mg/dL, postprandial plasma glucose, $\leq$140 mg/dL, or HbA1c $\leq$ 5.6%. If dysglycemia was detected by either fasting pl glucose (101–125 mg/dL), postprandial plasma glucose (141–199 mg/dL) or HbA1c (5.7–6.4%) the subject was characterized as PD. For T2D, those diagnosed earlier, with duration of $<$5 years, and on treatment with oral hypoglycaemic agents were recruited. The purpose of the study and the potential risks involved were explained to each subject and written informed consent was obtained. All were in good health as determined by medical history and physical examination. Those with conditions such as anemia, joint injuries, hypertension, cardiovascular disease, tuberculosis, cancer, and thyroid disorders were excluded. All participants underwent serum lipid profiling, including serum cholesterol, high-density lipoprotein (HDL), low-density lipoprotein (LDL) and triglyceride estimations using a Chemiluminescence Immunoassay (Siemens, Model EXL with LM 1 & 2, Germany). Plasma insulin was measured by electrochemiluminescence (ADVIA Centaur CP, Siemen's Healthineers, India). Insulin resistance and beta-cell function (HOMA-IR and HOMA-%B) were assessed by the homeostatic method using standard formulae for calculation (17). Physical activity levels (PAL) were calculated based on a physical activity questionnaire (18). All protocols were approved by the

Institutional Ethics Committee, St. John's National Academy of Health Sciences, Bengaluru, India (IEC reference number 66-2014/112-2014 /116-2015).

Body Composition

All participants underwent anthropometric assessment. This included weight recorded in minimal clothing to the nearest 0.1 kg, using a digital scale (Salter digital scale, 9069 PK3R, Tonbridge, UK) and height to the nearest 0.1 cm, using a Stadiometer (Holtain, Crymych, UK). Their waist and hip circumferences were measured using a standard non-stretchable tape at the narrowest point between the iliac crest and ribcage (waist) and at the level of the greater trochanter (hip). Body composition was assessed using DXA (Model DPXMD 7254, Lunar Corporation, Madison, WI). The mass of lean soft tissue, fat, and bone mineral for both the whole body and specific regions were measured. The defined central adiposity included fat (kg) in the trunk, including the android region. The trunk region included the neck, chest, abdominal, and pelvic areas. Its upper perimeter was the inferior edge of the chin and the lower borders intersected the middle of the femoral necks without touching the brim of the pelvis. The android region was the area between the ribs and the pelvis and was totally enclosed by the trunk region. Appendicular muscle index (AMI) an indicator of sarcopenia status was derived using appendicular muscle mass (AMM) which is equivalent to the sum of lean soft tissue in both the right and left arms and legs (19). Equation used for AMI was, $AMI = AMM/Ht^2$ (20).

Muscle Strength and Contractile Quality

Skeletal muscle strength of the knee extensors (quadriceps) of the dominant leg was assessed using an isokinetic dynamometer (Kin Com AP1, Chattanooga Group, Tennessee, USA). All participants underwent familiarization session before the actual protocol. For majority of the participants, familiarization was performed on the previous day of the experiment. If participants could not come on 2 days, we performed the familiarization session on the experimental day. However, adequate rest period (1–2 h) was given before the actual skeletal muscle strength assessment. Participants were instructed to perform a standardized 5-min warm-up indoor brisk walk, following which they were seated in the dynamometer in an upright position. Stabilization straps were placed across the chest and the hip to prevent the involvement of upper limb and trunk muscles during the test. The thigh was stabilized by placing support over the distal third of the thigh. The axis of dynamometer was aligned with the axis of rotation of knee (lateral condyle) and the distal support pad was placed proximal to the malleoli. The lever arm between the center of rotation of the dynamometer and the point of application of force-length was recorded. Maximal isometric torque (0 degree/s) was measured with the lever arm locked at the position of 30 degrees of knee joint extension from the knee flexed (90 degree) position. Peak isokinetic strength for knee extensor was assessed at 3 angular velocities 60, 120, 180 degree/s. A slow angular velocity of 60 degrees/s was used as the main dynamic measure for relation to the metabolic data as this angular velocity allows sufficient time for force development and complete muscle activation to have occurred at the point of the measurement (21). The best of three maximal voluntary contractions for knee extension was used for the analysis. For majority of the participant's right leg was used for the assessment, however if there was any history of pain or injury to the right leg, left leg was used for the assessment. The corresponding lower limb muscle mass (LMM) was considered for the contractile quality calculation. Subjects were provided with a rest interval of 2–3 min between each contraction and 5 min rest between each velocity. Muscle contractile quality was derived by dividing the peak torque (Nm) at each angular velocity by the appropriate lower limb muscle mass (Nm/kg) (22).

Statistical Analyses

Descriptive statistics are reported as mean and SD/SE for normally distributed continuous variables, else median with 25 and 75th percentiles, and number and percentage for the categorical variables. The comparison of specific characteristics between the three groups was performed using analysis of variance for normally distributed data. *Post-hoc* multiple comparisons were performed using the Bonferroni correction. For the non-normally distributed data, the Kruskal-Wallis test was used to compare between the three groups and the Mann–Whitney U-test for two group comparisons. Age-adjusted analyses for between-group differences in muscle strength and contractile quality at various angular velocities were performed using ANCOVA. Multivariate linear regression analysis was performed to find the association between muscle strength and contractile quality for isokinetic strength (60 degree/s) in T2D, PD compared to controls, adjusted for age, percent fat and PAL. The relationships between LMM, strength and contractile quality with FBG, HbA1c, HOMA-IR were assessed using correlation coefficient analyses. Partial correlations were adjusted for age. In all analyses, $P < 5\%$ was considered statistically significant. All analyses were performed using SPSS version 24.0.

RESULTS

Among 224 participants enrolled in the study, 24.5, 55.8, and 19.6% belonged to the T2D, PD and healthy control groups, respectively. The average self-reported duration of T2D was 3.0 ± 1.5 years. Overall, the mean age of the study subjects was 39.2 ± 10.8 years. Descriptive statistics for the characteristics of study subjects by study groups are presented in **Table 1**. The mean age of the study subjects was significantly different across the study groups with controls being the youngest.

There was no significant difference in the mean BMI, percent fat and total lean mass between the groups (**Table 1**). The mean android fat and muscle to fat ratio were significantly different between PD and control groups with no significant difference between T2D and prediabetes groups. The AMI was similar across the study groups. The reported levels of physical activity were significantly different between the PD and T2D groups. The AMI for T2D and PD study groups were not ≤ 2 SD of the young control mean values.

Basal plasma insulin levels were not significantly different between the groups. Mean FBG, HbA1c, and HOMA -IR were

TABLE 1 | Descriptive statistics of the study groups.

Variable	Diabetes (n = 55)	Pre-diabetes (n = 125)	Control (n = 44)
Age (yr)	48.0 ± 8.7[a,c]	37.6 ± 9.3[b]	32.6 ± 11.4
Height (m)	1.68 ± 0.07	1.68 ± 0.06	1.66 ± 0.06
Weight (kg)	68.5 ± 11.0[c]	72.5 ± 9.2	70.6 ± 9.3
Body mass index (kg/m^2)	24.7 ± 3.9	25.5 ± 2.7	24.8 ± 3.1
Percent fat (%)	29.3 ± 6.6	31.8 ± 5.7	29.2 ± 7.5
Android fat (kg)	2.2 ± 0.8	2.3 ± 0.8[b]	2.0 ± 0.8
Total lean mass (kg)	46.1 ± 4.8	46.6 ± 4.6	47.1 ± 5.3
Muscle to fat ratio*	2.4 (1.9, 2.9)	2.1 (1.8, 2.5)[b]	2.3 (1.9, 2.8)
AMI index (kg/m^2)	9.2 ± 6.8	9.9 ± 4.2	10.4 ± 0.9
Waist hip ratio	0.93 ± 0.06[a,c]	0.89 ± 0.06	0.90 ± 0.06
FBG (mg/dl)	167.4 ± 64.8[a,c]	100.3 ± 9.4	90.3 ± 5.7
HbA1c (%)	8.6 ± 2.2[a,c]	5.7 ± 0.4	5.3 ± 0.2
Basal Insulin (μU/ml)*	11.9 (6.9, 18.2)	11.3 (7.4, 15.5)	9.8 (6.9, 13.7)
Total cholesterol (mg/dl)	176.6 ± 47.9	183.0 ± 36.6	177.3 ± 44.2
Triglycerides (mg/dl)*	169 (115, 242)[a,c]	126 (89, 169)	125 (81, 161)
HOMA-IR*	1.8 (1.2, 2.8)[c]	1.5 (1.0, 2.1)	1.3 (0.9, 1.8)
HOMA-β*	55.2 (35.8,83.9)[a,c]	66.5 (48.2, 97.9)	78.5 (55.9, 112.7)
Physical activity level	1.6 ± 0.16[c]	1.5 ± 0.13	1.5 ± 0.21

[a]*Indicates diabetic group significantly different from control group.*
[b]*Indicates pre-diabetes group significantly different from control group.*
[c]*Indicates diabetic group significantly different from pre-diabetes group.*
kg, Kilogram; m, meter; AMI, Appendicular muscle index; FBG, Fasting blood glucose; mg, milligram; dl, decilitre; HOMA, Homeostatic model assessment; IR, insulin resistance; β, Beta cell function.
Reported as Mean ± SD, median (25 and 75th percentile).

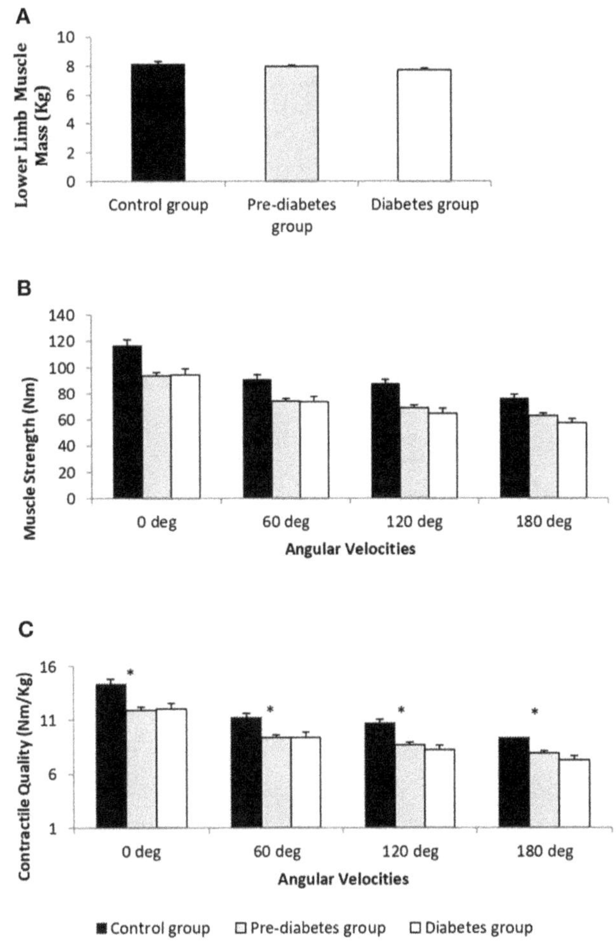

FIGURE 1 | Comparison of lower limb muscle mass (kg) **(A)**, absolute muscle strength (Torque, Nm) **(B)**, and muscle contractile quality (Nm/kg limb muscle mass) **(C)** in the diabetes (n = 55), pre-diabetes (n = 125), and control (n = 44) groups. *T2DM and PD groups are significantly different from control group $p < 0.01$; age adjusted data represented as mean ± SE.

significantly higher in T2D compared to PD and control groups, with no significant difference between PD and control groups. Mean HOMA β was significantly lower in T2D compared to PD and control groups.

The comparison of LMM between the study groups is represented in **Figure 1A**. Mean LMM was not significantly different between the groups ($p = 0.07$). The comparison of muscle strength and contractile quality between the study groups at the different angular velocities is shown in **Figures 1B,C**, respectively. There was no significant association between age with muscle strength, and contractile quality ($\rho = -0.11$, $P = 0.11$; $\rho = -0.12$, $P = 0.08$). However, age was significantly different between the study groups. When an age-adjusted analysis was performed the data still showed significant differences in absolute muscle strength (torque) and strength normalized for muscle mass (contractie quality) between the study groups ($p \leq 0.01$) across all angular velocities. Age-adjusted results revealed that both maximal muscle strength and contractile quality were significantly lower in T2D and PD groups compared to the control group ($p \leq 0.01$). However, there were no significant differences between the T2D and PD groups in any of the functional measurements. Muscle strength and contractile quality derived from isometric (0 degree) and isokinetic (60 degree) were compared between the three groups using multiple linear regression adjusting for different covariates (**Table 2**). After adjusting for age, percent fat and PAL as co-variates, muscle strength ($\beta = -24.6$, 95% CI −35.9 to −13.2 for isometric; $\beta = -17.2$, 95% CI −26.5 to −8.0 for isokinetic) and contractile quality ($\beta = -2.75$; 95% CI −4.02 to −1.47 for isometric; $\beta = -2.04$; 95% CI −3.12 to −0.95; for isokinetic) were significantly lower in PD compared to controls with no significant difference between PD and T2D or Control and T2D. There was a significant correlation between skeletal muscle strength and contractile quality with the duration of type 2 diabetes ($\rho = -0.33$, $P = 0.04$; $\rho = -0.34$, $P = 0.03$). After adjusting the same with age, body fat and PAL in regression analysis the significance disappears ($\beta = -4.18$, $p = 0.06$; $\beta = -0.10$, $p = 0.17$).

A pooled analysis was performed to explore the relationship between LMM, muscle strength and contractile quality with HOMA-IR (**Figure 2**). After adjusting for age, there was a

TABLE 2 | Multivariate regression models for muscle mass, strength, and contractile quality across the study groups.

	Leg lean mass			Muscle strength			Muscle contractile quality		
	β	95% C.I.	*P*-value	β	95% C.I.	*P*-value	β	95% C.I.	*P*-value
Control vs. PD									
Model	−0.09	−0.44 to 0.25	0.60	−17.2	−26.5 to −8.00	<0.001	−2.04	−3.12 to −0.95	<0.001
PD vs. T2D									
Model	−0.18	−0.56 to 0.20	0.35	−0.59	−9.88 to 8.69	0.90	0.13	−0.97 to 0.23	0.82
Control vs. T2D									
Model	−0.37	−0.91 to 0.18	0.18	−9.49	−23.6 to 4.64	0.18	−0.62	−2.30 to −1.6	0.46

Adjusted for age, percent fat, PAL; CI, confidence interval; PD, prediabetes; T2D, Type 2 Diabetes.

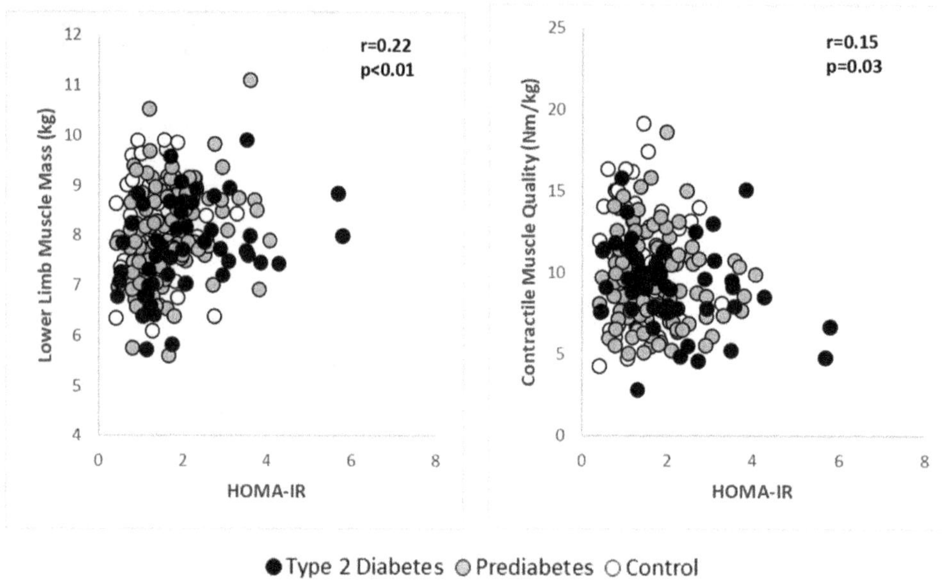

FIGURE 2 | Age adjusted relationships between lower limb muscle mass and contractile muscle quality with HOMA-IR in the pooled study groups.

significant positive association between LMM and HOMA-IR ($r = 0.22$, $p < 0.01$). Skeletal muscle strength was not associated with HOMA-IR, however, there was a significant, inverse relationship between muscle contractile quality (Isokinetic 60 degree) and HOMA-IR ($r = -0.15$, $p = 0.03$). It was noted that for every unit increase in HOMA-IR, muscle contractile quality decreased by 0.54 Nm/kg (β = −0.54; 95% C.I. −0.97 to −0.09). Age-adjusted associations between FBG, HbA1c with LMM, muscle strength and contractile quality were not significant.

DISCUSSION

This data is the first to examine skeletal muscle mass and function in major limb muscles in regard to metabolic disease in an Indian population. The data from the present study shows that quadriceps function when measured both in absolute (Nm) and relative (Nm/kg muscle mass) terms, and for both isometric and dynamic contractions, was similar between individuals with PD and T2D. However, the contractile function was lower in both of these groups compared with healthy controls, even when allowing for the younger age of the controls. Interestingly however, muscle mass (LMM) did not differ between the three study groups when corrected for age. The study also revealed a significant positive association between insulin resistance (HOMA-IR) and muscle mass for pooled data, whilst muscle contractile quality was inversely and significantly associated with insulin resistance.

A loss of muscle mass and function has been reported among T2D individuals particularly in the lower extremities compared to healthy individuals (23). The majority of these reports come from European (24) or American (25) or East Asian elderly population (26) with T2D, in whom age-related changes cannot be separated from the changes due to their diabetes status (27, 28). One possible explanation for the lower force per unit mass in the PD and T2D individuals in the present study concerns the level of neural drive to the muscle during the voluntary contractions. The assumption was that this would be similar in the three groups, but it cannot be excluded that PD and T2D individuals were less able to activate their knee extensor muscles during contractions. For activations to be determined, the twitch interpolation technique (29) would need to be utilized, which was not possible in the present study.

The proposed mechanisms by which T2D/PD could by themselves induce changes in skeletal muscle, beyond aging, could be the independent effect of insulin resistance on mitochondrial dysfunction, protein degradation, and autophagy pathways in the skeletal muscle (30–32). One of the potential mechanisms by which insulin resistance could induce mitochondrial dysfunction and negatively impacting muscle mass and function could be lipid accumulation or the lipotoxicity hypothesis. Excessive lipid accumulation due to defective muscle lipid oxidation could cause impaired mitochondrial number or function (reduced oxidative enzyme capacity) (33). However, Nair et al. demonstrated that Indians irrespective of their diabetes status had higher OXPHOS capacity than Northern European Americans indicating a dissociation between mitochondrial dysfunction and insulin resistance (34). However, this study was performed on a small sample of migrant Indians in the USA. With environmental factors and lifestyle habits differing across native compared to migrant Indians, extrapolation of the data needs further exploration.

There was a significant positive association between lower limb muscle mass and insulin resistance in the present study. This finding has not been reported earlier in Asian Indians. The majority of studies have demonstrated an inverse association between insulin resistance and muscle mass. For instance, the third National Health and Nutrition Examination Survey demonstrated that relative muscle mass, as estimated by bioelectrical impedance, was inversely associated with insulin resistance and PD (35). Similarly, a 10-year longitudinal study demonstrated that there was an independent inverse association between insulin resistance and muscle mass among middle-aged and older healthy Americans of Japanese origin (36). However, the Baltimore Longitudinal Study of Aging (2003–2011) reported hyperglycemia was not related to decreased skeletal muscle mass over time among multiracial Americans (37). The fact that muscle mass was related to insulin resistance positively in the current study even after adjusting for age needs further exploration, but maybe explained, in part, by inter- and intramyocellular lipid accumulation, contributing to the muscle bulk. A recently published analysis of muscle biopsy samples from our group showed evidence of excessive intramyocellular fat among Asian Indians with PD compared to healthy controls (6).

Contractile quality was shown to be inversely associated with HOMA-IR in the present study. This finding was similar to The Health ABC elderly cohort (70–79 years), with muscle mass and contractile quality demonstrating similar association, but not with strength (38). The current study population being younger with an average age of 39 years and included PD and T2D compared to the elderly population from the Health ABC elderly cohort. With every unit increase in HOMA-IR, there was a 0.54 Nm/kg decrement in contractile quality in the present study. In a similar study performed on Japanese population with Type 2 Diabetes, it was noted that knee extensor contractile quality decreased by 0.40 Nm/kg (body weight) with every unit increase in HOMA IR (39). The Korea National and Health Examination Survey (KNHANES) VI on Type 2 Diabetes population demonstrated that the hand grip strength normalized for body weight demonstrated a decrease of 3.70 kg/kg with every unit increase in HOMA IR (40).The fact that the current study group might have changes in skeletal muscle earlier than other population emphasizes the need for early evaluation of skeletal muscle mass and function including planning of preventive strategies.

Based on a recent systematic review and meta-analysis, the role of insulin on the human skeletal muscle anabolism through increased muscle protein synthesis (MPS) has been shown to be influenced by amino acid delivery (41). The branched chain amino acid leucine is known to play vital role in the MPS (42, 43). However, the leucine requirement in normal, well-nourished Western and Indian men has been determined to be 2.5 times higher than the 1985 FAO/WHO/UNU recommendation. On the contrary, lysine has been shown to be the most limiting in cereal protein and at a much lower concentration with relatively poor digestibility and utilization (44, 45). With majority of Asian Indians consuming a cereal based diet they pose a risk of a deficiency of quality protein, in terms of indispensable amino acid (particularly lysine). This is due to the fact that 60% of their protein are from cereals with relatively low quality and digestibility (46). Whether high-quality protein intake could harness the positive effects of insulin on muscle metabolism needs to be explored particularly among Asian Indians. However, the role of insulin in reducing muscle protein breakdown (MPB) is independent of amino acid availability (37). It is suggested that impaired insulin signaling leading to insulin resistance could have an effect on muscle metabolism (MPS and MPB) and endothelial dysfunction beyond glucose intolerance (47). Further, Mesinovic et al. suggested that there could be a bidirectional link between T2D and skeletal muscle changes, and the existence of one condition may increase the risk of developing the other. Physical inactivity, insulin resistance, inflammation, increased advanced glycation end-products accumulation, increased oxidative stress, and vascular complications can all affect various components of muscle health (muscle mass, strength, and contractile quality) and impaired muscle health could further contribute toward the development and progression of T2D (48). Therefore, it is important to explore, through a multipronged approach, the different mechanisms that could regulate skeletal muscle mass, strength, and contractile quality in Asian Indians.

While muscle function among PD and T2D was reduced in comparison with healthy controls, the PD and T2D groups were comparable in both muscle mass, absolute strength, and contractile quality. We had expected a graded response between the control, PD and T2D study groups as the metabolic disease progressed, even though this was a cross-sectional study. The reasons for this lack of difference between PD and T2D remain to be elucidated, but these findings suggest that in a population where reported prevalence rates of T2D are high, a simple functional evaluation of muscle strength may not only act as an early prognostic tool but also may act as a positive feedback mechanism for participants trying to increase their levels of activity and physical fitness. After adjusting for age, percent fat and PAL there was no significant difference in muscle strength and contractile quality between T2D and control groups. This was surprising and could suggest that there are factors beyond those which been explored as part of the study. The fact that the T2D individuals were on oral hypoglycemic agents (OHA) and which might have had an independent effect on muscle strength and contractile quality cannot be ruled out. With a body of literature suggesting that OHA could cause muscle atrophy and rest demonstrating no effect (49). It is nearly impossible to differentiate the effect of OHA from that of a disease process in diabetes mellitus. With the small sample size and lack of detailed pharmacological profiling available as part of the study, we could only speculate at this stage and could form the basis of future studies.

CONCLUSION

Skeletal muscle mass, strength, and contractile quality were similar between PD and T2D Asian Indians, but lower compared to healthy controls, with the findings persisting even after adjusting for the age differences between the groups. This would suggest that the measurement of skeletal muscle function, as well as mass, among Asian Indians is important in order to detect early deterioration in metabolic health. The data also suggest the need to evaluate the role of resistance exercise in improving muscle strength and quality through well-designed clinical studies in Asian Indians.

AUTHOR CONTRIBUTIONS

SSa was part of the conception and design, the performance of the measurements and analyses, interpretation of the data, and drafted the manuscript. AK and SH were part of conception and design, interpretation of data, writing of manuscript, and final approval of manuscript. NS was involved in the performance of measurements and analyses. PR involved in screening and recruitment of subjects. SSe was involved in statistical analyses.

FUNDING

The major support for this study came from the Wellcome Trust/DBT India Alliance Fellowship [grant number IA/I/13/1/500907] awarded to SSa. The study was also supported partially by funding received by the Rajiv Gandhi University of Health Sciences, Bangalore, India and The Physiological Society's International Senior Research Grant, UK.

ACKNOWLEDGMENTS

Authors would like to acknowledge Ms. Ammu Anna Kurien, Mr. Sreejith B, Mrs. Princiya Rufus, and Dr. Pranathi Racha for their support during the data collection. We would also like to thank Dr. Tinku Thomas and Dr. Ronald J. Bosch for constant input during the designing of the study. Dr. Ganapathi Bantwal and Dr. Vageesh Ayyar for helping with the recruitment of the participants.

REFERENCES

1. Lai N, Gladden LB, Carlier PG, Cabrera ME. Models of muscle contraction and energetics. *Drug Discov Today Dis Models.* (2008) 5:273–88. doi: 10.1016/j.ddmod.2009.07.001
2. Correa-de-Araujo R, Harris-Love MO, Miljkovic I, Fragala MS, Anthony BW, Manini TM. The need for standardized assessment of muscle quality in skeletal muscle function deficit and other aging-related muscle dysfunctions: a symposium report. *Front Physiol.* (2017) 8:87. doi: 10.3389/fphys.2017.00087
3. McLeod M, Breen L, Hamilton DL, Philp A. Live strong and prosper: the importance of skeletal muscle strength for healthy ageing. *Biogerontology.* (2016) 17:497–510. doi: 10.1007/s10522-015-9631-7
4. Wolfe RR. The underappreciated role of muscle in health and disease. *Am J Clin Nutr.* (2006) 84:475–82. doi: 10.1093/ajcn/84.3.475
5. Schrauwen-Hinderling VB, Hesselink MK, Schrauwen P, Kooi ME. Intramyocellular lipid content in human skeletal muscle. *Obesity.* (2006) 14:357–67. doi: 10.1038/oby.2006.47
6. Sucharita S, Pranathi R, Correa M, Keerthana P, Ramesh LJ, Bantwal G, et al. Evidence of higher intramyocellular fat among normal and overweight Indians with prediabetes. *Eur J Clin Nutr.* (2019) 73:1373–81. doi: 10.1038/s41430-019-0402-4
7. Li R, Xia J, Zhang XI, Gathirua-Mwangi WG, Guo J, Li Y, et al. Associations of muscle mass and strength with all-cause mortality among US older adults. *Med Sci Sports Exerc.* (2018) 50:458–67. doi: 10.1249/MSS.0000000000001448
8. Hazzard WR, Halter JB. *Hazzard's Geriatric Medicine and Gerontology.* 6th ed. New York, NY: McGraw-Hill Medical Pub. Division (2009).
9. Cawthon PM, Fox KM, Gandra SR, Delmonico MJ, Chiou CF, Anthony MS, et al. Do muscle mass, muscle density, strength, and physical function similarly influence risk of hospitalization in older adults? *J Am Geriatr Soc.* (2009) 57:1411–9. doi: 10.1111/j.1532-5415.2009.02366.x
10. Bryant NJ, Govers R, James DE. Regulated transport of the glucose transporter GLUT4. *Nat Rev Mol Cell Biol.* (2002) 3:267–77. doi: 10.1038/nrm782
11. Mohan V. Why are Indians more prone to diabetes? *J Assoc Physicians India.* (2004) 52:468–74. Available online at: http://www.japi.org/june2004/R-468.pdf
12. India State-Level Disease Burden Initiative Diabetes Collaborators. The increasing burden of diabetes and variations among the states of India: the Global Burden of Disease Study 1990-2016. *Lancet Glob Health.* (2018) 6:e1352–62. doi: 10.1016/S2214-109X(18)30387-5
13. Kurpad AV, Varadharajan KS, Aeberli I. The thin-fat phenotype and global metabolic disease risk. *Curr Opin Clin Nutr Metab Care.* (2011) 14:542–7. doi: 10.1097/MCO.0b013e32834b6e5e
14. Umegaki H. Sarcopenia and diabetes: hyperglycemia is a risk factor for age-associated muscle mass and functional reduction. *J Diabetes Investig.* (2015) 6:623–4. doi: 10.1111/jdi.12365
15. Kim TN, Park MS, Yang SJ, Yoo HJ, Kang HJ, Song W, et al. Prevalence and determinant factors of sarcopenia in patients with type 2 diabetes: the Korean Sarcopenic Obesity Study (KSOS). *Diabetes Care.* (2010) 33:1497–9. doi: 10.2337/dc09-2310

16. ChamberlainJJ, Rhinehart AS, Shaefer CF Jr, Neuman A. Diagnosis and management of diabetes: synopsis of the 2016 American Diabetes Association Standards of Medical Care in Diabetes. *Ann Intern Med.* (2016) 164:542–52. doi: 10.7326/M15-3016
17. Matthews DR, Hosker JP, Rudenski AS, Naylor BA, Treacher DF, Turner RC. Homeostasis model assessment: insulin resistance and β-cell function from fasting plasma glucose and insulin concentrations in man. *Diabetologia.* (1985) 28:412–9. doi: 10.1007/BF00280883
18. Vaz M, Bharathi AV, Thomas T, Yusuf S, Kurpad AV. The repeatability of self-reported physical activity patterns in rural South India. *Asia Pac J Clin Nutr.* (2009) 18:71–5. Available online at: http://apjcn.nhri.org.tw/server/APJCN/18/1/71.pdf
19. Kuriyan R, Thomas T, Ashok S, Jayakumar J, Kurpad AV. A 4-compartment model based validation of air displacement plethysmography, dual energy X-ray absorptiometry, skinfold technique & bio-electrical impedance for measuring body fat in Indian adults. *Indian J Med Res.* (2014) 139:700–7. Available online at: http://www.ijmr.org.in/article.asp?issn=0971-5916;year=2014;volume=139;issue=5;spage=700;epage=707;aulast=Kuriyan
20. Kwon HJ, Ha YC, Park HM. The reference value of skeletal muscle mass index for defining the sarcopenia of women in Korea. *J Bone Miner Metab.* (2015) 22:71–5. doi: 10.11005/jbm.2015.22.2.71
21. Jones DA, Rutherford OM, Parker DF. Physiological changes in skeletal muscle as a result of strength training. *Q J Exp Physiol.* (1989) 74:233–56. doi: 10.1113/expphysiol.1989.sp003268
22. Metter EJ, Lynch N, Conwit R, Lindle R, Tobin J, Hurley B. Muscle quality and age: cross-sectional and longitudinal comparisons. *J Gerontol A Biol Sci Med Sci.* (1999) 54:B207–18. doi: 10.1093/gerona/54.5.B207
23. Guerrero N, Bunout D, Hirsch S, Barrera G, Leiva L, Henriquez S, et al. Premature loss of muscle mass and function in type 2 diabetes. *Diabetes Res Clin Pract.* (2016) 117:32–8. doi: 10.1016/j.diabres.2016.04.011
24. Cruz-Jentoft AJ, Baeyens JP, Bauer JM, Boirie Y, Cederholm T, Landi F, et al. Sarcopenia: European consensus on definition and diagnosis: report of the European working group on sarcopenia in older people. *Age Ageing.* (2010) 39:412–23. doi: 10.1093/ageing/afq034
25. Kalyani RR, Tra Y, Yeh HC, Egan JM, Ferrucci L, Brancati FL. Quadriceps strength, quadriceps power, and gait speed in older U.S. adults with diabetes mellitus: results from the National Health and Nutrition Examination Survey, 1999-2002. *J Am Geriatr Soc.* (2013) 61:769–75. doi: 10.1111/jgs.12204
26. Chen LK, Liu LK, Woo J, Assantachai P, Auyeung TW, Bahyah KS, et al. Sarcopenia in Asia: consensus report of the Asian Working Group for Sarcopenia. *J Am Med Dir Assoc.* (2014) 15:95–101. doi: 10.1016/j.jamda.2013.11.025
27. Kirkman MS, Briscoe VJ, Clark N, Florez H, Haas LB, Halter JB, et al. Consensus development conference on diabetes and older adults. Diabetes in older adults: a consensus report. *J Am Geriatr Soc.* (2012) 60:2342–56. doi: 10.1111/jgs.12035
28. Abdelhafiz AH, Sinclair AJ. Management of type 2 diabetes in older people. *Diabetes Ther.* (2013) 4:13–26. doi: 10.1007/s13300-013-0020-4
29. Herbert RD, Gandevia SC. Twitch interpolation in human muscles: mechanisms and implications for measurement of voluntary activation. *J Neurophysiol.* (1999) 82:2271–83. doi: 10.1152/jn.1999.82.5.2271
30. Wang X, Hu Z, Hu J, Du J, Mitch WE. Insulin resistance accelerates muscle protein degradation: activation of the ubiquitin-proteasome pathway by defects in muscle cell signaling. *Endocrinology.* (2006) 147:4160–8. doi: 10.1210/en.2006-0251
31. Wada J, Nakatsuka A. Mitochondrial dynamics and mitochondrial dysfunction in diabetes. *Acta Med Okayama.* (2016) 70:151–8. Available online at: http://www.lib.okayama-u.ac.jp/www/acta/pdf/70_3_151.pdf
32. Sarparanta J, García-Macia M, Singh R. Autophagy and mitochondria in obesity and type 2 diabetes. *Curr Diabetes Rev.* (2017) 13:352–69. doi: 10.2174/1573399812666160217122530
33. He J, Watkins S, Kelley DE. Skeletal muscle lipid content and oxidative enzyme activity in relation to muscle fiber type in type 2 diabetes and obesity. *Diabetes.* (2001) 50:817–23. doi: 10.2337/diabetes.50.4.817
34. Nair KS, Bigelow ML, Asmann YW, Chow LS, Coenen-Schimke JM, Klaus KA, et al. Asian Indians have enhanced skeletal muscle mitochondrial capacity to produce ATP in association with severe insulin resistance. *Diabetes.* (2008) 57:1166–75. doi: 10.2337/db07-1556
35. Srikanthan P, Karlamangla AS. Relative muscle mass is inversely associated with insulin resistance and prediabetes. findings from the third national health and nutrition examination survey. *J Clin Endocrinol Metab.* (2011) 96:2898–903. doi: 10.1210/jc.2011-0435
36. Han SJ, Boyko EJ, Kim SK, Fujimoto WY, Kahn SE, Leonetti DL. Association of thigh muscle mass with insulin resistance and incident type 2 diabetes mellitus in Japanese Americans. *Diabetes Metab J.* (2018) 42:488–95. doi: 10.4093/dmj.2018.0022
37. Kalyani RR, Metter EJ, Egan J, Golden SH, Ferrucci L. Hyperglycemia predicts persistently lower muscle strength with aging. *Diabetes Care.* (2015) 38:82–90. doi: 10.2337/dc14-1166
38. Barzilay JI, Cotsonis GA, Walston J, Schwartz AV, Satterfield S, Miljkovic I, et al. Insulin resistance is associated with decreased quadriceps muscle strength in nondiabetic adults aged >=70 years. *Diabetes Care.* (2009) 32:736–8. doi: 10.2337/dc08-1781
39. Nomura T, Ikeda Y, Nakao S, Ito K, Ishida K, Suehiro T, et al. Muscle strength is a marker of insulin resistance in patients with type 2 diabetes: a pilot study. *Endocr J.* (2007) 54:791–6. doi: 10.1507/endocrj.K07-055
40. Lee MR, Jung SM, Bang H, Kim HS, Kim YB. Association between muscle strength and type 2 diabetes mellitus in adults in Korea: data from the Korea national health and nutrition examination survey (KNHANES) VI. *Medicine.* (2018) 97:e10984. doi: 10.1097/MD.0000000000010984
41. Abdulla H, Smith K, Atherton PJ, Idris I. Role of insulin in the regulation of human skeletal muscle protein synthesis and breakdown: a systematic review and meta-analysis. *Diabetologia.* (2016) 59:44–55. doi: 10.1007/s00125-015-3751-0
42. Breen L, Churchward-Venne TA. Leucine: a nutrient 'trigger' for muscle anabolism, but what more? *J Physiol.* (2012) 590:2065–6. doi: 10.1113/jphysiol.2012.230631
43. Jackman SR, Witard OC, Philp A, Wallis GA, Baar K, Tipton KD. Branched-chain amino acid ingestion stimulates muscle myofibrillar protein synthesis following resistance exercise in humans. *Front Physiol.* (2017) 8:390. doi: 10.3389/fphys.2017.00390
44. Kurpad AV, Regan MM, Raj T, Vasudevan J, Kuriyan R, Gnanou J, et al. Lysine requirements of chronically undernourished adult Indian men, measured by a 24-h indicator amino acid oxidation and balance technique. *Am J Clin Nutr.* (2003) 77:101–8. doi: 10.1093/ajcn/77.1.101
45. Kurpad AV, Regan MM, Raj T, Varalakshmi S, Gnanou J, Thankachan P, et al. Leucine requirement and splanchnic uptake of leucine in chronically undernourished adult Indian subjects. *Am J Clin Nutr.* (2003) 77:861–7. doi: 10.1093/ajcn/77.4.861
46. Minocha S, Thomas T, Kurpad AV. Dietary protein and the health–nutrition–agriculture connection in India. *J Nutr.* (2017) 147:1243–50. doi: 10.3945/jn.116.243980
47. Muniyappa R, Sowers JR. Role of insulin resistance in endothelial dysfunction. *Rev Endocr Metab Disord.* (2013) 14:5–12. doi: 10.1007/s11154-012-9229-1
48. Mesinovic J, Zengin A, De Courten B, Ebeling PR, Scott D. Sarcopenia and type 2 diabetes mellitus: a bidirectional relationship. *Diabetes Metab Syndr Obes.* (2019) 12:1057–72. doi: 10.2147/DMSO.S186600
49. Campins L, Camps M, Riera A, Pleguezuelos E, Yebenes JC, Serra-Prat M. Oral drugs related with muscle wasting and sarcopenia. *Rev Pharmacol.* (2017) 99:1–8. doi: 10.1159/000448247

3

Variables Influencing the Effectiveness of Creatine Supplementation as a Therapeutic Intervention for Sarcopenia

Darren G. Candow[1]*, Scott C. Forbes[2], Philip D. Chilibeck[3], Stephen M. Cornish[4], Jose Antonio[5] and Richard B. Kreider[6]

[1] Faculty of Kinesiology and Health Studies, University of Regina, Regina, SK, Canada, [2] Department of Physical Education, Brandon University, Brandon, MB, Canada, [3] College of Kinesiology, University of Saskatchewan, Saskatoon, SK, Canada, [4] Faculty of Kinesiology and Recreation Management, University of Manitoba, Winnipeg, MB, Canada, [5] Department of Health and Human Performance, Nova Southeastern University, Davie, FL, United States, [6] Department of Health and Kinesiology, Texas A&M University, College Station, TX, United States

***Correspondence:**
Darren G. Candow
Darren.Candow@uregina.ca

Sarcopenia is an age-related muscle condition characterized by a reduction in muscle quantity, force generating capacity and physical performance. Sarcopenia occurs in 8–13% of adults $\geq$ 60 years of age and can lead to disability, frailty, and various other diseases. Over the past few decades, several leading research groups have focused their efforts on developing strategies and recommendations for attenuating sarcopenia. One potential nutritional intervention for sarcopenia is creatine supplementation. However, research is inconsistent regarding the effectiveness of creatine on aging muscle. The purpose of this perspective paper is to: (1) propose possible reasons for the inconsistent responsiveness to creatine in aging adults, (2) discuss the potential mechanistic actions of creatine on muscle biology, (3) determine whether the timing of creatine supplementation influences aging muscle, (4) evaluate the evidence investigating the effects of creatine with other compounds (protein, conjugated linoleic acid) in aging adults, and (5) provide insight regarding the safety of creatine for aging adults.

Keywords: muscle, strength, resistance training, mechanisms, safety

INTRODUCTION

The original criteria for determining sarcopenia focused on muscle quantity (1); however, over the past few decades, numerous groups (International Working Group on Sarcopenia, Special Interest Group, European Working Group on Sarcopenia in Older People, Foundation for the National Institutes of Health, Asian Working Group on Sarcopenia, European Society of Clinical Nutrition and Metabolism, and International Sarcopenia Initiative) have expanded this criterion to include muscle strength and physical performance measures (2). Sarcopenia, now identified with an ICD-10-CM code by the World Health Organization (3) occurs in 8–13% of adults $\geq$ 60 years of age (4). The European Working Group on Sarcopenia in Older People classifies aging adults with low muscle strength (Grip strength test: <27 kg for males, <16 for females; Chair stand test: >15 s for five stands) as being pre-sarcopenic; those with low muscle strength and low muscle quantity (Appendicular skeletal muscle mass: <20 kg for males, <15 kg for females; Appendicular skeletal muscle mass/height^2: <7.0 kg/m^2 for males, <6.0 kg/m^2 for females) as being sarcopenic, and those with low muscle strength, low muscle quantity and low physical performance (Gait speed: ≤0.8 m/s; Short Physical Performance Battery test: ≤ 8 point score; Timed Up-and Go test: ≥20 s; 400 m walk test: non-completion or ≥6 min for completion) as having severe sarcopenia (5). Sarcopenia is associated with disability, frailty, cachexia, morbidity, and various diseases (6, 7). Contributing factors of sarcopenia include changes in neuromuscular function, skeletal muscle morphology, protein kinetics, hormonal regulation, oxidative and inflammatory stress, physical inactivity, and nutrition [for reviews see (8, 9)].

The European Society for Clinical and Economic Aspects of Osteoporosis, Osteoarthritis and Musculoskeletal Diseases [ESCEO; (10)] and International Conference on Sarcopenia and Frailty Research task force (11) recommends that nutritional interventions be emphasized to help overcome sarcopenia. We propose that creatine supplementation has the potential to be an anti-sarcopenic intervention. Three meta-analyses have been performed involving creatine supplementation and resistance training. In the first meta-analysis, Candow et al. (12) found a greater effect from creatine supplementation during resistance training on muscle mass (+0.94 kg) and upper-body maximal strength compared to placebo during resistance training in over 300 participants (>50 years of age). Expanding on these findings, Devries and Phillips (13) showed that creatine supplementation during resistance training resulted in greater gains in muscle mass (+1.33 kg) and upper- and lower-body maximal strength, and physical performance (30-s chair stand test) compared to placebo during training in over 200 aging adults (>45 years of age). In the most recent meta-analysis, Chilibeck et al. (14) showed that creatine supplementation during resistance training significantly increased muscle mass (+1.37 kg), and upper- and lower-body maximal strength compared to placebo during resistance training in over 700 aging adults (>57 years of age). Collectively, these meta-analyses indicate that the addition of creatine to resistance training significantly increases muscle mass (1.21 kg), maximum strength and has promise for improving tasks of physical performance in aging adults. However, variability in the responsiveness to creatine supplementation is typically high in aging adults and several factors determine whether an individual experiences greater gains in muscle mass and muscle/physical performance from creatine supplementation and resistance training. Therefore, the purpose of this perspective paper is to: (1) propose possible reasons for the inconsistent responsiveness to creatine in aging adults, (2) discuss the potential mechanistic actions of creatine on muscle biology, (3) determine whether the timing of creatine supplementation influences aging muscle, (4) evaluate the evidence investigating the effects of creatine with other compounds (protein, conjugated linoleic acid) in aging adults, and (5) provide insight regarding the safety of creatine for aging adults.

Creatine

Creatine (methylguanidine-acetic acid) is a naturally occurring nitrogenous organic acid (15). Ninety-five percent of creatine is stored in skeletal muscle while the remainder is found in brain, liver, kidneys, and testes (16). In skeletal muscle, approximately two-thirds of creatine is bound to phosphate and stored as phosphocreatine (PCr), the remaining one-third of creatine is unbound and stored as free creatine (15). An average 70-kg individual maintains a total creatine pool (PCr + free Cr = total creatine) of ~120 mmol/kg of dry muscle mass (17). Approximately 2 g/day (1–2%) of intramuscular creatine stores are broken down and excreted in the urine as creatinine (15). Both exogenous dietary intake and endogenous *de novo* synthesis are used to replace lost creatine. Dietary sources of creatine include meat, fish, and poultry with trace amounts in plants (18, 19). For example, one pound of uncooked salmon and beef contains about 2 g of creatine (18). Since plants only contain trace amounts, strict vegetarians and vegans typically have lower skeletal muscle total creatine stores (20). For most individuals, ~1–3 g/d of exogenous creatine intake are required to maintain creatine stores depending on total muscle mass and physical activity levels (17, 18, 21). Endogenous *de novo* creatine synthesis occurs in the liver and kidney (15, 18) via a two-step process. First, arginine and glycine form ornithine and guanidinoacetic acid (GAA) by the enzyme arginine glycine amidinotransferase (AGAT). Second, creatine is formed by the transfer of the methyl group from S-adenosyl methionine to guanidinoacetate (22), as shown in **Figure 1**.

Creatine Supplementation During Resistance Training in Aging Adults

There is a growing body of literature examining the effects of creatine supplementation and resistance training in aging adults (**Table 1**). Individual studies involving aging males or aging males and females combined show mixed results. However, studies only involving aging females show more consistent results. This section will summarize findings across studies and discuss possible methodological reasons for the conflicting results. Furthermore, variables influencing the responsiveness to creatine supplementation are also proposed.

While it is difficult to compare results across studies in aging males, differences in training methodologies may be involved. In the Candow et al. (30) and Chrusch et al. (31) studies (both showing a positive effect from creatine), participants were directly supervised during each training session. However, in the Cooke et al. (32) study, participants were only supervised during weeks 1, 2, 6, 8, and 11. Supervised resistance training leads to greater muscle benefits compared to unsupervised training (44). Furthermore, the sample sizes were larger in the Candow et al. (30) and Chrusch et al. (31) studies which increased statistical power compared to the Cooke et al. (32) study. The study by Eijnde et al. (33) incorporated both resistance and aerobic exercise components into the training intervention which introduces the possibility of muscle interference [i.e., blunting of muscle growth and performance when performing both resistance-training and aerobic exercise in the same training program; (45)]. In addition, the resistance training protocol focused on developing muscular endurance (20–30 repetition range) rather than muscular strength, a primary dependent measure assessed.

Five studies have investigated the effects of creatine supplementation during resistance training in aging females, as shown in **Table 1**. In postmenopausal osteopenic or

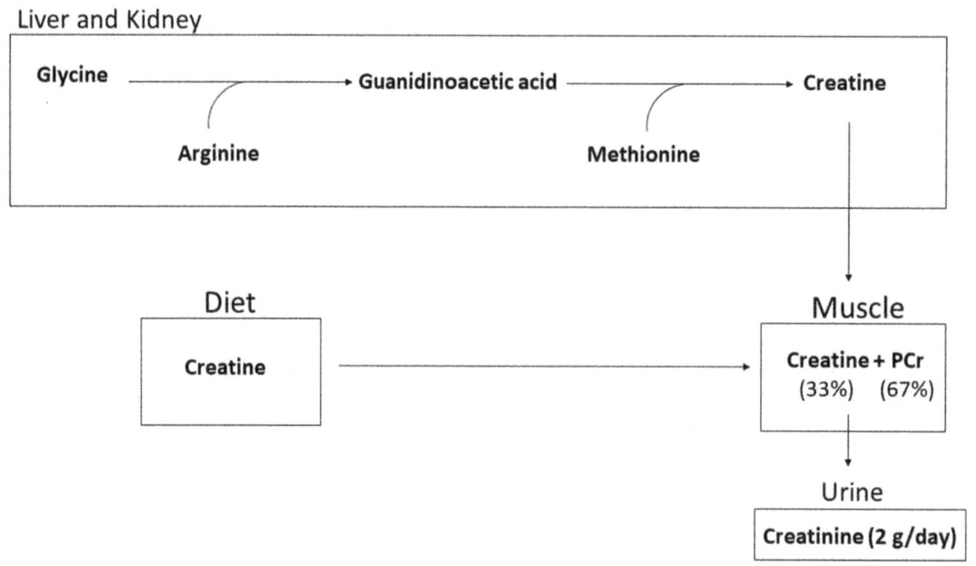

FIGURE 1 | Creatine is synthesized endogenously by a two step process from glycine, arginine, and methoione or through dietary intake. Ninety-five percent of creatine is taken up into the muscle and stored as free creatine (33%) or as phosphorylcreatine (67%). Approximately 2 g per day is broken down to creatinine and excreted.

osteoporotic females, Gualano et al. (26) showed that creatine supplementation during supervised resistance training produced greater gains (relative) in appendicular lean tissue mass (assessed by DXA) and upper-body (bench press) strength compared to placebo during resistance training. Previous work by Neves et al. (27) also found a beneficial effect from creatine on lower-limb lean tissue mass and indices of physical performance (timed-stand test) in postmenopausal women with knee osteoarthritis compared to placebo; however, there was no effect of creatine supplementation on total-body lean mass or muscle strength when compared to placebo. Additional work in postmenopausal women showed that creatine supplementation increased lean tissue mass, strength (bench press, knee extension, biceps curl), and tasks of physical performance (30-s chair stand, arm curl test, lying prone-to-stand test) compared to placebo (24). Chilibeck et al. (25) showed that postmenopausal females who ingested creatine daily during supervised whole-body resistance training experienced greater gains in relative upper-body maximal strength (bench press) compared to females on placebo. Finally, postmenopausal women who ingested creatine during a supervised strength training program had greater gains in lower-body (leg press) strength compared to females who ingested creatine or placebo but did not strength train. There were no differences between females who consumed creatine or placebo during training (23). Collectively, these results suggest that creatine supplementation during supervised resistance training is an effective lifestyle intervention for improving muscle mass and muscle/physical performance in aging postmenopausal women.

Research is limited regarding the effectiveness of creatine supplementation during resistance training in aging males and females combined, and therefore, there are only a few direct comparisons between males and females for responsiveness to creatine, as shown in **Table 1**. Brose et al. (36) showed that creatine supplementation increased lean tissue mass and isometric knee extension strength in aging adults compared to placebo. Males on creatine increased ankle-dorsiflexion isometric strength more than females on creatine. Candow et al. (37) and Pinto (42) found increases in strength and lean tissue mass with creatine and resistance training compared to placebo; however, no sex differences were found. Johannsmeyer et al. (41) showed that creatine supplementation increased whole-body lean tissue mass compared to placebo. Males on creatine increased upper-body strength (lat pull-down) and decreased urinary 3-methylhistidine excretion (indicator or whole-body protein catabolism) more than females on creatine. In contrast to these positive studies showing a beneficial effect from creatine, Bermon et al. (35) found no effect on strength or lean tissue mass. This study was limited by a small sample size ($n = 8$ per group) and a shorter training intervention (52 days) compared to the studies showing a positive effect from creatine (36, 37, 41, 42), and had participants perform a limited amount of work (3 exercises performed, 3 sets of 8 repetitions at 80% 1-RM). In two studies investigating disease populations, Deacon et al. (39) found no effect from creatine supplementation during 7 weeks of aerobic and resistance training on changes in muscle mass or performance in aging adults with chronic obstructive pulmonary disease (COPD) compared to those on placebo. In aging adults with type II diabetes, Gualano et al. (40) found no effect from creatine supplementation during 12 weeks of supervised aerobic and resistance combined training on muscle mass or strength compared to those on placebo. Both these disease state studies incorporated aerobic and resistance training into the exercise intervention which may have introduced the muscle interference

TABLE 1 | Resistance training and creatine studies in aging adults on performance and body composition changes.

References	Population	Supplement dose	Resistance training	Duration	Outcomes
WOMEN ONLY STUDIES					
Alves et al. (23)	*N* = 47; healthy women, Mean age = 66.8 years (range: 60–80 years)	CR (20 g/day for 5 days, followed by 5 g/day thereafter) or PLA with and without RT	RT = 2 days/week	24 weeks	↔ 1 RM strength compared to RT + PLA
Aguiar et al. (24)	*N* = 18; healthy women; Mean age = 65 years	CR (5 g/day) or PLA	RT = 3 days/week	12 weeks	CR ↑ gains in fat-free mass (+3.2%), muscle mass (+2.8%), 1 RM bench press, knee extension, and biceps curl compared to PLA
Chilibeck et al. (25)	*N* = 33; healthy women; Mean age = 57 years	CR (0.1 g/kg/day) or PLA	RT = 3 days/week	52 weeks	↔ lean tissue mass and muscle thickness gains between groups. ↑ relative bench press strength compared to PLA
Gualano et al. (26)	*N* = 30; "vulnerable" women; Mean age = 65.4 years	CR (20 g/day for 5 days; 5 g/day thereafter) or PLA with and without RT	RT = 2 days/week	24 weeks	CR + RT ↑ gains in 1 RM bench press and appendicular lean mass compared to PLA + RT
Neves et al. (27)	*N* = 24 (postmenopausal women with Knee osteoarthritis); Age = 55–65 years	CR (20 g/day for 1 week, followed by 5 g/day) or PLA	RT = 3 days/week	12 weeks	CR ↑ gains in limb lean mass. ↔ 1 RM leg press
MEN ONLY STUDIES					
Bemben et al. (28) and Eliot et al. (29)	*N* = 42; healthy men; age = 48–72 years	CR (5 g/day), protein (35 g/day), CR+ protein, or PLA	RT = 3 days/week	14 weeks	↔ lean tissue mass, 1 RM strength
Candow et al. (30)	*N* = 35; healthy men; age = 59–77 years	CR (0.1 g/kg/day) or CR + protein (0.3 g/kg/day) or PLA	RT = 3 days/week	10 weeks	CR and CR + protein conditions combined ↑muscle thickness compared to PLA. CR ↑1 RM bench press ↔ 1 RM leg press
Chrusch et al. (31)	*N* = 30; healthy men; age = 60–84 years	CR (0.3 g/kg/d for 5 days followed by 0.07 g/kg/day) or PLA	RT = 3 days/week	12 weeks	CR ↑ gains in lean tissue mass. CR ↑1 RM leg press, 1 RM knee extension, leg press endurance, and knee extension endurance. ↔ 1 RM bench press or bench press endurance.
Cooke et al. (32)	*N* = 20; healthy men; age = 55–70 years	CR (20 g/day for 7 days then 0.1 g/kg/day on training days)	RT = 3 days/week	12 weeks	↔ lean tissue mass, 1 RM bench press, 1 RM leg press
Eijnde et al. (33)	*N* = 46; healthy men; age = 55–75 years	CR (5 g/day) or PLA	Cardiorespiratory + RT = 2–3 days/week	26 weeks	↔ lean tissue mass or isometric maximal strength
Villanueva et al. (34)	*N* = 14; healthy men; age = 68.7 years	CR (0.3 g/kg/day for 5 days followed by 0.07 g/kg/day) + 35 g protein or PLA	RT = 3 days/week	12 weeks	↔ lean tissue mass or 1 RM bench press
MEN AND WOMEN STUDIES					
Bermon et al. (35)	*N* = 32 (16 men, 16 women); healthy; age = 67–80 years	CR (20 g/day for 5 days followed by 3 g/day) or PLA	RT = 3 days/week	7.4 weeks (52 days)	↔ lower limb muscular volume, 1-, 12-repetitions maxima, and the isometric intermittent endurance

(Continued)

TABLE 1 | Continued

References	Population	Supplement dose	Resistance training	Duration	Outcomes
Brose et al. (36)	*N* = 28 (15 men, 13 women); healthy; age: men = 68.7, women = 70.8 years	CR (5 g/day) or PLA	RT = 3 days/week	14 weeks	CR ↑ gains in lean tissue mass and isometric knee extension strength; ↔ type 1, 2a, 2x muscle fiber area
Candow et al. (37)	*N* = 39 (17 men, 22 women); healthy; age = 50–71 years	CR (0.1 g/kg) before RT, CR (0.1 g/kg) after RT, or PLA	RT = 3 days/week	32 weeks	CR after RT ↑ lean tissue mass, 1 RM leg press, 1 RM chest press compared to PLA
Collins et al. (38)	*N* = 16 (frail men and women); age = 70 years	CR (4 g/day) and protein (20 g/day) or protein	RT = 2 days/week	14 weeks	↔ lean tissue mass or muscle function
Deacon et al. (39)	*N* = 80 (50 men, 30 women); COPD; age = 68.2 years	CR (22 g/day for 5 day followed by 3.76 g/day) or PLA	RT = 3 days/week	7 weeks	↔ lean tissue mass or muscle strength
Gualano et al. (40)	*N* = 25 (9 men, 16 women); type 2 diabetes; age = 57 years	CR (5 g/day) or PLA	RT = 3 days/week	12 weeks	↔ lean tissue mass
Johannsmeyer et al. (41)	*N* = 31 (17 men, 14 women); healthy; age = 58 years	CR (0.1 g/kg/day) or PLA	RT = 3 days/week	12 weeks	CR ↑ gains in lean tissue mass and 1 RM strength in men only
Pinto et al. (42)	*N* = 27 (men and women); healthy; age = 60–80 years	CR (5 g/day) or PLA	RT = 3 days/week	12 weeks	CR ↑ gains in lean tissue mass. ↔ 10 RM bench press or leg press strength
Tarnopolsky et al. (43)	*N* = 39 (19 men, 20 women); healthy; age = 65–85 years	CR (5 g/day) + CLA (6 g/day) or PLA	RT = 2 days/week	26 weeks	CR + CLA ↑ gains in lean tissue mass, muscular endurance, isokinetic knee extension strength

CR, creatine; PLA, placebo; RT, resistance training; CLA, conjugated linoleic acid; RM, repetition maximum.

effect (45). It is important to note that no sex analyses were performed in the studies of Bermon et al. (35), Deacon et al. (39), and Gualano et al. (40).

Methodological Differences Between Studies

Collectively, inconsistent results across studies (independent of sex), may be related to differences in the exercise training intervention (i.e., supervision vs. non-supervision; duration and volume of training; combination of aerobic and resistance training), health status and sample size.

Furthermore, variables which influence an individual's responsiveness to creatine supplementation should also be considered (46–48).

Variables Influencing Individual Responses to Creatine

(A) Baseline Muscle Creatine Content

The magnitude of response to creatine supplementation is typically determined by initial muscle creatine concentration (47), which can be quite variable in aging individuals and across one's lifespan. Aging adults typically have significantly lower PCr and total creatine compared to young adults (49–52), however one study reported no differences between older and younger participants (53). In contrast, Rawson et al. (54) showed that aging adults ($n = 7$) had higher resting PCr stores compared to younger adult ($n = 8$) in the gastrocnemius muscle. Chilibeck et al. (14) performed a meta-analysis to assess PCr differences between young and aging adults. Results showed that when the quadriceps, gastrocnemius, and tibialis anterior muscle groups were combined, there were no differences in muscle PCr across age groups. However, when only studies that assessed the quadriceps were included, there was an age-related reduction in intramuscular PCr, suggesting that muscle groups may respond differently.

(B) Muscle Fiber Type Differences

The majority of intramuscular creatine is found in type II muscle fibers (46) which progressively decreases (quantity, size) with aging [for review see Larsson et al. (8)). Syrotuik and Bell (48) showed that individuals with the highest concentration and muscle cross-sectional area of type II fibers respond more favorably to creatine supplementation. Therefore, the age-related reduction in type II muscle fiber quantity and size may potentially attenuate the anabolic response to creatine.

(C) Impact of Habitual Dietary Intake of Creatine

Dietary intake of creatine may also influence the responsiveness to supplementation. Individuals with low dietary consumption of creatine-containing foods [i.e., meat, seafood, poultry; (15, 19)] typically have low intramuscular creatine concentrations and would therefore respond more favorably to creatine supplementation. For example, Burke et al. (55) showed that vegetarians experienced the greatest increase in intramuscular total creatine (PCr, free Cr) from 8 weeks of creatine supplementation (0.25 g/kg lean tissue mass/day for 7 days + 0.0625 g/kg lean tissue mass/day for 49 days) compared to

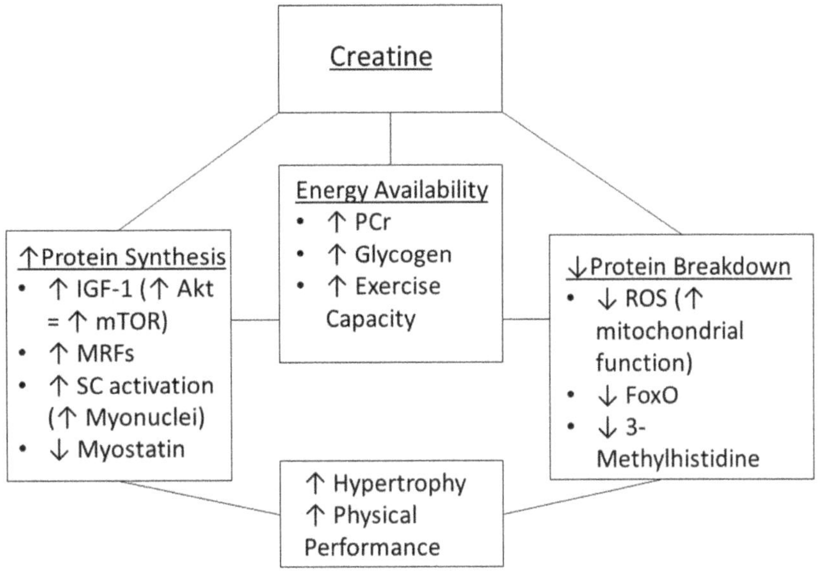

FIGURE 2 | Potential mechanisms of creatine supplementation to enhance muscle hypertrophy and physical performance. IGF-1, insulin-like growth factor 1; MRFs, myogenic regulatory factors; mTOR, mammalian target of rapamycin; PCr, phosphorylcreatine; ROS, reactive oxygen species; SC, satellite cells.

non-vegetarians who supplemented with creatine. Furthermore, in examining the effects of short-term creatine supplementation (0.3 g/day for 7 days) in omnivorous younger adults (n = 17, 29.18 ± 7.81 years) and aging individuals (n = 18, 71.78 ± 6.97 years), Solis et al. (52) showed that omnivores had higher dietary creatine intake pre-supplementation. Ingestion of creatine significantly increased PCr in aging individuals but not in the younger omnivore adults. There is evidence that meat consumption decreases with aging which may influence the response to creatine supplementation. We recommend that future research determine changes in intramuscular creatine concentration, type II muscle fiber quantity and size, and dietary intake of creatine so that a valid estimate regarding the effects of creatine supplementation in aging adults can be made.

Mechanisms by Which Creatine Supplementation Affects Muscle Mass in Aging Adults

Creatine supplementation may affect some of the mechanisms and pathways (those involving muscle protein synthesis and degradation) that contribute to sarcopenia (**Figure 2**). This section provides a review of mechanisms by which creatine may increase energy availability during resistance training, along with the effectiveness (or lack of effectiveness) of creatine supplementation for offsetting the effects of aging on muscle protein synthesis and degradation.

Increased Training Volume and Muscle Contraction With Creatine Supplementation Through Increased Energy Provision and Calcium Uptake Into the Sarcoplasmic Reticulum

Phosphocreatine (PCr) is important for buffering ATP levels during intense muscle contraction (i.e., resistance training). ATP, which is broken down to ADP and inorganic phosphate (Pi) during muscle contraction, can be quickly re-synthesized when PCr donates its phosphate to ADP (15). Low intramuscular PCr levels may not be able to sustain continued muscle contractions during resistance training. Aging adults have reduced intramuscular PCr levels in the upper-leg (vastus lateralis); whereas PCr levels are at normal levels in muscles of the lower-leg (gastrocnemius, tibialis anterior), those involved in low-intensity activities of daily living (i.e., walking) (14). Potentially, the reduction in PCr in the vastus lateralis may be associated with reduced participation in high-intensity physical activities (i.e., running, jumping) which involve recruitment of large muscle groups in the lower-limbs (56). There is strong evidence from studies measuring creatine and PCr levels either through muscle biopsies or ^{31}P-MRS that supplementation with creatine increases muscle creatine and/or PCr levels in muscle of aging adults (33, 36, 51, 52, 54). An animal model of senescence-accelerated mice indicated that creatine supplementation may lose its effectiveness over time due to down-regulation of the creatine transporter protein in muscle; however, this was not evident in aging humans (57).

Increased intramuscular PCr may provide greater capacity for ATP resynthesis during sustained intense muscular work or may enhance PCr recovery (i.e., and therefore greater recovery between sets of resistance training exercise) because an increase of creatine in the muscle would drive recovery of PCr through the reverse of the creatine kinase reaction (i.e., ATP + Cr → PCr + ADP) (51). Furthermore, creatine increases the rate of calcium uptake into the sarcoplasmic reticulum which may increase myofibrillar cross-bridge cycling leading to shortened muscle relaxation time and greater force development (58–60). Overall, this may lead to enhanced training volume during resistance training sessions in aging adults. In a study with full exercise supervision, where sets were performed with repetitions to failure, aging males (~70 years) were able to achieve a 31% greater training volume (defined as repetitions × kg) when supplemented with creatine compared to placebo during 12 weeks of resistance training (31). This has potential to stimulate greater training adaptations (i.e., greater increases in muscle mass and strength). This beneficial effect of creatine may not hold true however if resistance training is not performed to failure, which may be the case most of the time when older adults are performing resistance training non-supervised. Furthermore, in young participants, creatine supplementation was able to maintain resistance training volume and attenuate the interference effect of concurrent training (i.e., resistance and aerobic training) on strength adaptations (61). These results may have important implications in older adults, since both resistance and aerobic training are recommended and commonly practiced for optimal health.

Aside from PCr, glycogen is an important substrate that can drive re-phosphorylation of ATP during prolonged resistance training sessions, as evidenced by significant glycogen depletion during resistance training (62). Adults (> 50 years) with type II diabetes who supplemented with creatine (5 g/day) during 12 weeks exercise training (aerobic and resistance training, 3x/week) experienced a greater increase in membrane GLUT-4 content and membrane total GLUT-4 content ratio compared to adults on placebo (40). GLUT-4 is important for transport of glucose into muscle, and since glucose is a building block for glycogen, this has potential to enhance glycogen resynthesis following resistance training. Creatine supplementation in rats for 5 days before intermittent swimming spared gastrocnemius muscle glycogen when measured post-exercise (63). Blood lactate levels during exercise were also reduced with creatine supplementation suggesting that extra energy provided by phosphoryl creatine during the intermittent exercise resulted in a smaller requirement for anaerobic glycolysis, allowing sparing of glycogen. Potentially, the sparing of muscle glycogen would allow for greater exercise training capacity and volume to be performed leading to greater muscle mass and muscle/physical performance over time.

Aging and Pathways for Protein Synthesis—Effects of Creatine Supplementation

Resistance training increases the release of insulin-like growth factor-1 from muscle, which may stimulate activation of proteins called "myogenic regulatory factors" [MRFs; (64, 65)]. The MRFs are involved in activation, proliferation, and differentiation of satellite cells (66), which in turn are involved in muscle fiber repair/regeneration and thought to be important in the process of muscle hypertrophy (67). Satellite cells reside outside the muscle fiber between the sarcolemma and basal membrane and when activated they fuse with the muscle fiber membrane and cross the sarcolemma where they differentiate into myonuclei (67), which increases a muscle fiber's capacity for protein synthesis (68). Myostatin is a myokine (i.e., a hormone-like protein released from muscle) that has the opposite effect to MRFs and inhibits satellite cell activation (69). There is a reduction in satellite cell number with aging (70), and a reduced activation and proliferation of satellite cells in response to a session of resistance training (71). In young muscle, MRFs are increased and myostatin is reduced following a resistance training session, which leads to activation and proliferation of satellite cells (71). These responses are attenuated with aging (71). Although there is some evidence for creatine supplementation during resistance training to increase production of IGF-1, expression of MRFs, and activation of satellite cells in younger individuals (72–74), there is no evidence of this in aging adults. Males (55–70 years) had no increase (compared to placebo) in IGF-1 when supplemented with creatine (20 g/d for 5 days + 0.1 g/kg on training days thereafter) during 12 weeks of resistance training (32). In aging males (mean age 73 years) who supplemented with creatine (5 g/day) for 7 weeks, there was no greater increase in satellite cell's or expression of MRFs in response to resistance training compared to placebo (75). Furthermore, during surgical overload of the plantaris muscle in aging rats, creatine supplementation failed to affect myonuclear domain (i.e., the amount of myonuclei for a given muscle fiber area) and did not affect muscle fiber area compared to overload without creatine (76). This indicates unchanged satellite cell differentiation.

The pathway involving phosphatidylinositol 3-kinase [PI3K]-Akt/protein kinase B [PKB]-mammalian target of rapamycin [mTOR] is important for activation of translation within muscle and is therefore important for muscle protein synthesis in response to resistance training (77). Signaling through mTOR is reduced with aging (78) but there is no direct evidence that creatine supplementation influences mTOR in aging adults.

Aging and Pathways for Protein Degradation—Effects of Creatine Supplementation

In contrast to studies showing a lack of direct effect from creatine supplementation on mechanisms involved in protein synthesis, creatine supplementation may be effective for reducing muscle protein degradation. In younger males, but not females, acute supplementation with creatine (i.e., 20 g/day for 5 days followed by 5 g/day for 3–4 days) reduced leucine oxidation and the rate of appearance of leucine in blood after primed continuous intravenous infusion of radio-labeled leucine, indicating reduced protein degradation (79). This was accompanied by unchanged protein synthesis in both males and females (79). A global marker of muscle protein degradation, urinary 3-methylhistidine, is reduced in aging males (but not aging females) who supplemented with creatine during resistance training (30, 41). It is proposed that during the biological process of aging, there is damage to the mitochondria, causing defects in the respiratory chain, leading to production of reactive oxygen species (80). Reactive oxygen species can cause mutations in mitochondrial DNA (encoding for respiratory chain proteins) leading to further mitochondrial damage and a vicious cycle (80). Reactive oxygen species can damage cellular membranes, leading to inflammation, muscle damage, and muscle protein degradation. Supplementation with creatine may be effective in mitigating this mitochondrial damage, leading to reduced oxidative stress, inflammation, and cellular apoptosis (i.e., cell death). In cellular studies involving human umbilical vein endothelial cells (81) or skin cells (fibroblasts) (82), or mouse myoblasts (83) exposed to oxidative damage, incubation with creatine protected against mutations in mitochondrial DNA or mitochondrial damage. It was proposed that creatine is taken up by mitochondria, where it helps maintain energy status and function by transferring phosphate groups between sites of energy production (i.e., ATP) and sites of energy consumption (i.e., to re-phosphorylate ADP) (81). There is some support for creatine having a similar effect in aging adults. Compared to a placebo group, middle-aged males (mean age 48 years) who supplemented with 20 g/day of creatine for 7 days had reduced levels of proteolytic enzymes involved in apoptosis and DNA fragmentation, and upregulation of proteins involved in protection against mitochondrial damage after a muscle-damaging exercise session [i.e., 40 min of downhill running on a treadmill; ref. (84)]. In addition, aging males (mean age of 65 years) given a daily multi-ingredient nutritional supplement (containing 2.5 g of creatine) during 12 weeks of combined resistance and high-intensity interval training, had reduced levels of inflammation (as assessed by tumor necrosis factor- alpha and interleukin-6) compared to placebo (85). In this study, the nutritional supplement also contained calcium, vitamin D, and n-3 polyunsaturated fatty acids; therefore, the effects could not be attributed solely to the creatine. Finally, in an animal model of senescence-accelerated mice, a lifetime of creatine supplementation was effective at middle age (but not oldest age) for increasing muscle carnosine content (86). Carnosine has a number of protective mechanisms within muscle including prevention of glycosylation-induced protein damage, anti-oxidant effects, and pH buffering (86). Creatine supplementation was also effective at the middle-age mark for improving muscle function [i.e., attenuating fatigue in the slow-twitch soleus, and enhancing post-fatigue force recovery in fast-twitch extensor digitorum longus; (86)]. Future longer-term studies of creatine supplementation are needed to determine if there are similar benefits in older adults.

In summary, studies determining the mechanisms by which creatine supplementation may enhance muscle accretion in aging adults favor an effect from creatine on reducing muscle protein degradation, mainly through mitigation of mitochondrial damage.

Does the Timing of Creatine Ingestion Influence Aging Muscle?

It has been previously suggested that the strategic ingestion of creatine, in close proximity to resistance training, may help create a favorable environment for muscle growth (87). This section summarizes the limited body of research investigating the effects of the timing of creatine supplementation in response to resistance training.

In healthy aging adults who consumed creatine (0.1 g/kg) immediately before and cornstarch maltodextrin (0.1 g/kg) immediately after or cornstarch maltodextrin immediately before and creatine immediately after supervised whole-body resistance training sessions, significant improvements in upper-body (chest press) and lower-body (leg press) maximal strength were observed compared to placebo. There were no differences in strength gains between the creatine groups; however, only the group who consumed creatine post-exercise had statistically greater gains in lean tissue mass, compared to adults on placebo (37). Cribb and Hayes (88) found that a multi-ingredient supplement (including protein, carbohydrate, fat, and creatine monohydrate) in close proximity to training (i.e., immediately before and after) increased lean body mass and strength compared to ingesting the supplement in the morning and late evening (i.e., $>$ 5 h from training) in young resistance trained participants. However, caution is warranted with a multi-ingredient study, since the impact of any individual nutrient is unknown. A small meta-analysis involving 3 studies ($n = 80$, $>$ 18 years, ranging from 4 to 32 weeks) showed that post-exercise creatine supplementation led to greater gains in muscle mass compared to pre-exercise creatine [standardized mean difference 0.52, 95% CI 0.03–1.00, $p = 0.04$; (89)]. There were no differences between pre- and post-exercise creatine for effects on muscle strength. Loenneke et al. (90, 91) have recently provided evidence that exercise induced changes in muscle size do not contribute to exercise-induced changes in strength. Creatine has been shown to enhance training volume (24, 31), which is important for enhancing gains in muscle size, whereas training specificity seems to be more important for muscle strength (92). Although the mechanisms explaining the greater increase in muscle mass from post-exercise creatine remains to be determined, muscle contractions (during a resistance training session) stimulate creatine uptake into skeletal muscle, resulting in elevated intramuscular creatine stores (21). Greater intramuscular PCr is associated with greater muscle accretion in aging adults (36). Importantly, no study examining creatine timing has measured intramuscular creatine content, thus future research is warranted. Although the difference in muscle accumulation between pre- and post-exercise creatine is small, these results may be important for aging adults trying to maximize muscle accretion through the combination of creatine supplementation and resistance training.

Does the Combination of Creatine With Other Nutritional Supplements Augment Muscle Mass and Performance?

Research showing a beneficial effect from creatine, in combination with other nutritional supplements, is mixed. Aging males who supplemented with creatine ($n = 10$; 67.3 $\pm$ 3.1 years; 0.1 g/kg) and whey protein (0.3 g/kg) only on resistance-training days (3 days/week for 10 weeks) experienced greater gains in lean tissue mass (5.6 $\pm$ 0.9%), as measured by air-displacement plethysmography, and upper-body (bench press) strength compared to participants on creatine ($n = 13$, 65.5 $\pm$ 2.7 years; 2.2 $\pm$ 0.8%) or placebo ($n = 12$, 64.1 $\pm$ 3.1 years; 1.0 $\pm$ 1.0%) (30). However, in frail adults ($n = 18$, $\geq$65 years), the combination of creatine (5 g) and whey protein (20 g) during 12 weeks of resistance training failed to produce greater gains in lean tissue mass, handgrip strength, or indices of physical performance (time-up-and-go test, timed stand test) compared to whey protein alone (38). In aging males (48–72 years), the co-ingestion of creatine (5 g) and whey protein (35 g) during 14 weeks of resistance training increased whole-body lean tissue mass and measures of whole-body strength similarly to that of creatine or protein alone (28). Furthermore, Villanueva et al. (34) found no differences in muscle accretion, bench press strength, stair climbing power, or 400-m walk time from the combination of creatine (0.3 g/kg for 5 days + 0.07 g/kg for 68 days) and whey protein (35 g/day) during 12 weeks of resistance training compared to resistance training alone in aging males (68.1 ± 6.1 years). Results across individual studies suggest that the combination of creatine and protein does not provide additional muscle benefits compared to creatine or protein alone in aging adults.

The ingestion of a multi-ingredient supplement containing creatine (5 g), whey protein (60 g), vitamin D (1000 IU), EPA (2,800 mg), and DHA (1,780 mg) for 6 weeks significantly increased whole-body lean tissue mass (assessed by DXA), and upper-body strength in aging males ($n = 25$, 71 ± 1 years) compared to aging males on placebo ($n = 24$, 74 ± 1 years) (93). Interestingly, continued ingestion of the supplement during 12 weeks of supervised aerobic (1x/week) and resistance training (2x/week) did not lead to greater gains in lean tissue mass. Aging adults ($n = 21$, 65–85 years) who supplemented with creatine (5 g) and conjugated linoleic acid (CLA; 2 g) daily during 6 months of resistance training experienced greater gains in muscle accretion (2.1 kg) compared to those on placebo ($n = 18$; 0.9 kg increase) (43). The combination of creatine and CLA also increased lower-limb isokinetic strength and total-body muscle endurance (chest press, arm flexion, knee extension; females only). While it is difficult to determine whether creatine is responsible for the greater gains in muscle mass across individuals studies, a recent systematic review and meta-analysis performed by O'Bryan et al. (94) concluded that multi-ingredient supplements containing protein and creatine resulted in significantly greater gains in muscle mass compared to protein alone (1.01 kg; 95% CI [0.69, 1.33], $p < 0.00001$). Furthermore, Chilibeck et al. (14) showed that creatine supplementation during resistance training resulted in superior gains in muscle mass compared to placebo, even when studies involving protein and CLA were excluded from the meta-analysis.

Safety of Creatine Supplementation-Aging Adults and Clinical Populations

There is limited research regarding the safety profile of creatine supplementation. Self-reported adverse effects in aging adults from creatine include muscle cramping, muscle strains and gastrointestinal irritation. Using a retrospective questionnaire, Chrusch et al. (31) reported that 12 weeks of creatine supplementation (0.3 g/kg/day × 5 days + 0.07 g/kg/day thereafter) in aging males increased the incidence of muscle pulls and muscle strains compared to placebo. In aging adults ($n = 11$) who consumed creatine (0.3 g/kg) for 10 days, four adverse events were reports [pulled groin muscle, gastrointestinal irritation, constipation, bloating; (95)]. In aging postmenopausal women who ingested creatine (0.1 g/kg/day) during 52 weeks of resistance training, five participants reported symptoms of gastrointestinal irritation and two reported muscle cramping, which was higher ($p < 0.05$) than the adverse effects reported by females on placebo (25). However, several other studies indicate no adverse effects (self-reported) from creatine supplementation (23, 29, 37, 38).

There is no direct evidence that creatine supplementation causes cytotoxicity (urinary formaldehyde) in aging males (30) or has an adverse effect on kidney or liver function. Creatine supplementation (5 g/day) during 14 weeks of resistance training in frail adults resulted in no detrimental effect on kidney or liver function (38). In two studies involving aging post-menopausal females, creatine supplementation, with and without resistance training, had no effect on urinary albumin (96) or other markers of kidney (urea, microalbumin, urine protein, creatinine clearance) or liver function (bilirubin, aspartate aminotransferase, alanine aminotransferase, and alkaline phosphatase) (25). The co-ingestion of creatine and CLA during 6 months of resistance training had no effect on bilirubin or gamma glutamyltransferase protein in aging adults (43). From a clinical perspective, creatine supplementation did not alter kidney function (renal damage, hematuria, tubular damage, glomerular filtration rate, microalbumin) compared to placebo in aging patients with Parkinson Disease (97) or affect albuminuria, proteinuria, albumin: creatinine ratio, urea and creatinine and estimated creatinine clearance in aging adults with type II diabetes (40). In summary, self-reported adverse events from creatine supplementation include gastrointestinal issues and muscle pulls/strains. Direct assessment of kidney and liver function indicates no negative effect from creatine in aging adults.

CONCLUSIONS

Sarcopenia is an age-related muscle condition characterized by a reduction in muscle quantity, muscle performance (i.e., strength) and physical performance (i.e., tasks of functionality). Although multifactorial, sarcopenia may be caused by changes in muscle protein kinetics, neuromuscular function, inflammation, physical activity, and nutrition. Recent attention has focused on nutritional interventions as a potential therapeutic approach to counteract sarcopenia. When consumed during resistance training, creatine supplementation typically increases muscle mass and muscle/physical performance, possibly by influencing high-energy phosphate metabolism and calcium uptake, muscle protein kinetics, and inflammation. However, variability in the responsiveness to creatine supplementation is typically high in aging adults and factors such as initial intramuscular PCr concentration, type II muscle fiber content and size, and habitual dietary intake of creatine may possibly explain the inconsistent findings across individual studies. Furthermore, methodological issues such as sex, exercise training intervention, sample size, and participant health status may also influence study results.

AUTHOR CONTRIBUTIONS

DC, SF, PC, SC, JA, and RK contributed to the design, methodology, evaluation, writing, edits, and approval of the submission.

REFERENCES

1. Rosenberg IH. Sarcopenia: origins and clinical relevance. *J Nutr.* (1997) 127(5 Suppl.):991S. doi: 10.1093/jn/127.5.990S
2. Marty E, Liu Y, Samuel A, Or O, Lane J. A review of sarcopenia: enhancing awareness of an increasingly prevalent disease. *Bone.* (2017) 105:276–86. doi: 10.1016/j.bone.2017.09.008
3. Anker SD, Morley JE, von Haehling S. Welcome to the ICD-10 code for sarcopenia. *J Cachexia Sarcopenia Muscle.* (2016) 7:512–4. doi: 10.1002/jcsm.12147
4. Shafiee G, Keshtkar A, Soltani A, Ahadi Z, Larijani B, Heshmat R. Prevalence of sarcopenia in the world: a systematic review and meta-analysis of general population studies. *J Diabetes Metab Disord.* (2017) 16:21. doi: 10.1186/s40200-017-0302-x
5. Cruz-Jentoft AJ, Bahat G, Bauer J, Boirie Y, Bruyere O, Cederholm T, et al. Sarcopenia: revised European consensus on definition and diagnosis. *Age Ageing.* (2019) 48:16–31. doi: 10.1093/ageing/afy169
6. Ogawa S, Yakabe M, Akishita M. Age-related sarcopenia and its pathophysiological bases. *Inflamm Regen.* (2016) 36:5. doi: 10.1186/s41232-016-0022-5
7. Rizzoli R, Reginster JY, Arnal JF, Bautmans I, Beaudart C, Bischoff-Ferrari H, et al. Quality of life in sarcopenia and frailty. *Calcif Tissue Int.* (2013) 93:101–20. doi: 10.1007/s00223-013-9758-y
8. Larsson L, Degens H, Li M, Salviati L, Lee YI, Thompson W, et al. Sarcopenia: aging-related loss of muscle mass and function. *Physiol Rev.* (2019) 99:427–511. doi: 10.1152/physrev.00061.2017
9. Liguori I, Russo G, Aran L, Bulli G, Curcio F, Della-Morte D, et al. Sarcopenia: assessment of disease burden and strategies to improve outcomes. *Clin Interv Aging.* (2018) 13:913–27. doi: 10.2147/CIA.S149232
10. Robinson SM, Reginster JY, Rizzoli R, Shaw SC, Kanis JA, Bautmans I, et al. Does nutrition play a role in the prevention and management of sarcopenia? *Clin Nutr.* (2018) 37:1121–32. doi: 10.1016/j.clnu.2017.08.016
11. Dent E, Morley JE, Cruz-Jentoft AJ, Arai H, Kritchevsky SB, Guralnik J, et al. International clinical practice guidelines for sarcopenia (ICFSR): screening, diagnosis and management. *J Nutr Health Aging.* (2018) 22:1148–61. doi: 10.1007/s12603-018-1139-9
12. Candow DG, Chilibeck PD, Forbes SC. Creatine supplementation and aging musculoskeletal health. *Endocrine.* (2014) 45:354–61. doi: 10.1007/s12020-013-0070-4
13. Devries MC, Phillips SM. Creatine supplementation during resistance training in older adults-a meta-analysis. *Med Sci Sports Exerc.* (2014) 46:1194–203. doi: 10.1249/MSS.0000000000000220
14. Chilibeck PD, Kaviani M, Candow DG, Zello GA. Effect of creatine supplementation during resistance training on lean tissue mass and muscular strength in older adults: a meta-analysis. *Open Access J Sports Med.* (2017) 8:213–26. doi: 10.2147/OAJSM.S123529
15. Wyss M, Kaddurah-Daouk R. Creatine and creatinine metabolism. *Physiol Rev.* (2000) 80:1107–213. doi: 10.1152/physrev.2000.80.3.1107
16. Walker JB. Creatine: biosynthesis, regulation, and function. *Adv Enzymol Relat Areas Mol Biol.* (1979) 50:177–242. doi: 10.1002/9780470122952.ch4
17. Hultman E, Soderlund K, Timmons JA, Cederblad G, Greenhaff PL. Muscle creatine loading in men. *J Appl Physiol.* (1996) 81:232–37. doi: 10.1152/jappl.1996.81.1.232
18. Balsom PD, Soderlund K, Ekblom B. Creatine in humans with special reference to creatine supplementation. *Sports Med.* (1994) 18:268–80. doi: 10.2165/00007256-199418040-00005
19. Jung S, Bae YS, Kim HJ, Jayasena DD, Lee DD, Park HB, et al. Carnosine, anserine, creatine, and inosine 5'-monophosphate contents in breast and thigh meats from 5 lines of Korean native chicken. *Poultry Sci.* (2013) 92:3275–82. doi: 10.3382/ps.2013-03441
20. Kreider RB, Kalman DS, Antonio J, Ziegenfuss TN, Wildman R, Collins R, et al. International society of sports nutrition position stand: safety and efficacy of creatine supplementation in exercise, sport, and medicine. *J Int Soc Sports Nutr.* (2017) 14:18. doi: 10.1186/s12970-017-0173-z
21. Harris RC, Soderlund K, Hultman E. Elevation of creatine in resting and exercised muscle of normal subjects by creatine supplementation. *Clin Sci.* (1992) 83:367–74. doi: 10.1042/cs0830367
22. Paddon-Jones D, Borsheim E, Wolfe RR. Potential ergogenic effects of arginine and creatine supplementation. *J Nutr.* (2004) 134 (10 Suppl.):2894S; discussion 2895S. doi: 10.1093/jn/134.10.2888S
23. Alves CR, Merege Filho CA, Benatti FB, Brucki S, Pereira RM, de Sa Pinto AL, et al. Creatine supplementation associated or not with strength training upon emotional and cognitive measures in older women: a randomized double-blind study. *PLoS ONE.* (2013) 8:e76301. doi: 10.1371/journal.pone.0076301
24. Aguiar AF, Januario RS, Junior RP, Gerage AM, Pina FL, do Nascimento MA, et al. Long-term creatine supplementation improves muscular performance during resistance training in older women. *Eur J Appl Physiol.* (2013) 113:987–96. doi: 10.1007/s00421-012-2514-6
25. Chilibeck PD, Candow DG, Landeryou T, Kaviani M, Paus-Jenssen L. Effects of creatine and resistance training on bone health in postmenopausal women. *Med Sci Sports Exerc.* (2015) 47:1587–95. doi: 10.1249/MSS.0000000000000571
26. Gualano B, Macedo AR, Alves CR, Roschel H, Benatti FB, Takayama L, et al. Creatine supplementation and resistance training in vulnerable older women: a randomized double-blind placebo-controlled clinical trial. *Exp Gerontol.* (2014) 53:7–15. doi: 10.1016/j.exger.2014.02.003
27. Neves M, Gualano B, Roschel H, Fuller R, Benatti FB, Pinto AL, et al. Beneficial effect of creatine supplementation in knee osteoarthritis. *Med Sci Sports Exerc.* (2011) 43:1538–43. doi: 10.1249/MSS.0b013e3182118592
28. Bemben MG, Witten MS, Carter JM, Eliot KA, Knehans AW, Bemben DA. The effects of supplementation with creatine and protein on muscle strength following a traditional resistance training program in middle-aged and older men. *J Nutr Health Aging.* (2010) 14:155–9. doi: 10.1007/s12603-009-0124-8
29. Eliot KA, Knehans AW, Bemben DA, Witten MS, Carter J, Bemben MG. The effects of creatine and whey protein supplementation on body composition in men aged 48 to 72 years during resistance training. *J Nutr Health Aging.* (2008) 12:208–12. doi: 10.1007/BF02982622
30. Candow DG, Little JP, Chilibeck PD, Abeysekara S, Zello GA, Kazachkov M, et al. Low-dose creatine combined with protein during resistance training in older men. *Med Sci Sports Exerc.* (2008) 40:1645–52. doi: 10.1249/MSS.0b013e318176b310
31. Chrusch MJ, Chilibeck PD, Chad KE, Davison KS, Burke DG. Creatine supplementation combined with resistance training in older men. *Med Sci Sports Exerc.* (2001) 33:2111–7. doi: 10.1097/00005768-200112000-00021
32. Cooke MB, Brabham B, Buford TW, Shelmadine BD, McPheeters M, Hudson GM, et al. Creatine supplementation post-exercise does not enhance training-induced adaptations in middle to older aged males. *Eur J Appl Physiol.* (2014) 114:1321–32. doi: 10.1007/s00421-014-2866-1
33. Eijnde BO, Van Leemputte M, Goris M, Labarque V, Taes Y, Verbessem P, et al. Effects of creatine supplementation and exercise training on fitness in men 55-75 yr old. *J Appl Physiol.* (2003) 95:818–28. doi: 10.1152/japplphysiol.00891.2002
34. Villanueva MG, He J, Schroeder ET. Periodized resistance training with and without supplementation improve body composition and performance in older men. *Eur J Appl Physiol.* (2014) 114:891–905. doi: 10.1007/s00421-014-2821-1
35. Bermon S, Venembre P, Sachet C, Valour S, Dolisi C. Effects of creatine monohydrate ingestion in sedentary and weight-trained older adults. *Acta Physiol Scand.* (1998) 164:147–55. doi: 10.1046/j.1365-201X.1998.00427.x
36. Brose A, Parise G, Tarnopolsky MA. Creatine supplementation enhances isometric strength and body composition improvements following strength exercise training in older adults. *J Gerontol A Biol Sci Med Sci.* (2003) 58:11–9. doi: 10.1093/gerona/58.1.B11
37. Candow DG, Vogt E, Johannsmeyer S, Forbes SC, Farthing JP. Strategic creatine supplementation and resistance training in healthy older adults. *Appl Physiol Nutr Metab.* (2015) 40:689–94. doi: 10.1139/apnm-2014-0498
38. Collins J, Longhurst G, Roschel H, Gualano B. Resistance training and co-supplementation with creatine and protein in older subjects with frailty. *J Frailty Aging.* (2016) 5:126–34. doi: 10.14283/jfa.2016.85
39. Deacon SJ, Vincent EE, Greenhaff PL, Fox J, Steiner MC, Singh SJ, et al. Randomized controlled trial of dietary creatine as an adjunct therapy to physical training in chronic obstructive pulmonary disease. *Am J Respir Crit Care Med.* (2008) 178:233–9. doi: 10.1164/rccm.200710-1508OC

40. Gualano B, de Salles Painneli V, Roschel H, Artioli GG, Neves M, de Sa Pinto AL, et al. Creatine in type 2 diabetes: a randomized, double-blind, placebo-controlled trial. *Med Sci Sports Exerc.* (2011) 43:770–8. doi: 10.1249/MSS.0b013e3181fcee7d
41. Johannsmeyer S, Candow DG, Brahms CM, Michel D, Zello GA. Effect of creatine supplementation and drop-set resistance training in untrained aging adults. *Exp Gerontol.* (2016) 83:112–9. doi: 10.1016/j.exger.2016.08.005
42. Pinto CL, Botelho PB, Carneiro JA, Mota JF. Impact of creatine supplementation in combination with resistance training on lean mass in the elderly. *J Cachexia Sarcopenia Muscle.* (2016) 7:413–21. doi: 10.1002/jcsm.12094
43. Tarnopolsky M, Zimmer A, Paikin J, Safdar A, Aboud A, Pearce E, et al. Creatine monohydrate and conjugated linoleic acid improve strength and body composition following resistance exercise in older adults. *PLoS ONE.* (2007) 2:e991. doi: 10.1371/journal.pone.0000991
44. Mazzetti SA, Kraemer WJ, Volek JS, Duncan ND, Ratamess NA, Gomez AL, et al. The influence of direct supervision of resistance training on strength performance. *Med Sci Sports Exerc.* (2000) 32:1175–84. doi: 10.1097/00005768-200006000-00023
45. Fyfe JJ, Bishop DJ, Stepto NK. Interference between concurrent resistance and endurance exercise: molecular bases and the role of individual training variables. *Sports Med.* (2014) 44:743–62. doi: 10.1007/s40279-014-0162-1
46. Gualano B, Rawson ES, Candow DG, Chilibeck PD. Creatine supplementation in the aging population: effects on skeletal muscle, bone and brain. *Amino Acids.* (2016) 48:1793–805. doi: 10.1007/s00726-016-2239-7
47. Lemon PW. Dietary creatine supplementation and exercise performance: why inconsistent results? *Can J Appl Physiol.* (2002) 27:663–81. doi: 10.1139/h02-039
48. Syrotuik DG, Bell GJ. Acute creatine monohydrate supplementation: a descriptive physiological profile of responders vs. nonresponders. *J Strength Cond Res.* (2004) 18:610–7. doi: 10.1519/00124278-200408000-00039
49. Moller P, Bergstrom J, Furst P, Hellstrom K. Effect of aging on energy-rich phosphagens in human skeletal muscles. *Clin Sci.* (1980) 58:553–5. doi: 10.1042/cs0580553
50. Forsberg AM, Nilsson E, Werneman J, Bergstrom J, Hultman E. Muscle composition in relation to age and sex. *Clin Sci.* (1991) 81:249–56. doi: 10.1042/cs0810249
51. Smith SA, Montain SJ, Matott RP, Zientara GP, Jolesz FA, Fielding RA. Creatine supplementation and age influence muscle metabolism during exercise. *J Appl Physiol.* (1998) 85:1349–56. doi: 10.1152/jappl.1998.85.4.1349
52. Solis MY, Artioli GG, Otaduy MCG, Leite CDC, Arruda W, Veiga RR, et al. Effect of age, diet, and tissue type on PCr response to creatine supplementation. *J Appl Physiol.* (2017) 123:407–14. doi: 10.1152/japplphysiol.00248.2017
53. Kent-Braun JA, Ng AV. Skeletal muscle oxidative capacity in young and older women and men. *J Appl Physiol.* (2000) 89:1072–8. doi: 10.1152/jappl.2000.89.3.1072
54. Rawson ES, Clarkson PM, Price TB, Miles MP. Differential response of muscle phosphocreatine to creatine supplementation in young and old subjects. *Acta Physiol Scand.* (2002) 174:57–65. doi: 10.1046/j.1365-201x.2002.00924.x
55. Burke DG, Chilibeck PD, Parise G, Candow DG, Mahoney D, Tarnopolsky M. Effect of creatine and weight training on muscle creatine and performance in vegetarians. *Med Sci Sports Exerc.* (2003) 35:1946–55. doi: 10.1249/01.MSS.0000093614.17517.79
56. Candow DG, Chilibeck PD. Differences in size, strength, and power of upper and lower body muscle groups in young and older men. *J Gerontol A Biol Sci Med Sci.* (2005) 60:148–56. doi: 10.1093/gerona/60.2.148
57. Tarnopolsky M, Parise G, Fu MH, Brose A, Parshad A, Speer O, et al. Acute and moderate-term creatine monohydrate supplementation does not affect creatine transporter mRNA or protein content in either young or elderly humans. *Mol Cell Biochem.* (2003) 244:159–66. doi: 10.1007/978-1-4615-0247-0_24
58. Cooper R, Naclerio F, Allgrove J, Jimenez A. Creatine supplementation with specific view to exercise/sports performance: an update. *J Int Soc Sports Nutr.* (2012) 9:33. doi: 10.1186/1550-2783-9-33
59. Hespel P, Op't Eijnde B, Van Leemputte M. Opposite actions of caffeine and creatine on muscle relaxation time in humans. *J Appl Physiol.* (2002) 92:513–8. doi: 10.1152/japplphysiol.00255.2001
60. van Leemputte M, Vandenberghe K, Hespel P. Shortening of muscle relaxation time after creatine loading. *J Appl Physiol.* (1999) 86:840–4. doi: 10.1152/jappl.1999.86.3.840
61. de Salles Painelli V, Alves VT, Ugrinowitsch C, Benatti FB, Artioli GG, Lancha AH, et al. Creatine supplementation prevents acute strength loss induced by concurrent exercise. *Eur J Appl Physiol.* (2014) 114:1749–55. doi: 10.1007/s00421-014-2903-0
62. Haff GG, Koch AJ, Potteiger JA, Kuphal KE, Magee LM, Green SB, et al. Carbohydrate supplementation attenuates muscle glycogen loss during acute bouts of resistance exercise. *Int J Sport Nutr Exerc Metab.* (2000) 10:326–39. doi: 10.1123/ijsnem.10.3.326
63. Roschel H, Gualano B, Marquezi M, Costa A, Lancha AH. Creatine supplementation spares muscle glycogen during high intensity intermittent exercise in rats. *J Int Soc Sports Nutr.* (2010) 7:6. doi: 10.1186/1550-2783-7-6
64. Xu Q, Wu Z. The insulin-like growth factor-phosphatidylinositol 3-kinase-Akt signaling pathway regulates myogenin expression in normal myogenic cells but not in rhabdomyosarcoma-derived RD cells. *J Biol Chem.* (2000) 275:36750–7. doi: 10.1074/jbc.M005030200
65. Aguiar AF, Vechetti-Junior IJ, Alves de Souza RW, Castan EP, Milanezi-Aguiar RC, Padovani CR, et al. Myogenin, MyoD and IGF-I regulate muscle mass but not fiber-type conversion during resistance training in rats. *Int J Sports Med.* (2013) 34:293–301. doi: 10.1055/s-0032-1321895
66. Cornelison DD, Wold BJ. Single-cell analysis of regulatory gene expression in quiescent and activated mouse skeletal muscle satellite cells. *Dev Biol.* (1997) 191:270–83. doi: 10.1006/dbio.1997.8721
67. Petrella JK, Kim JS, Mayhew DL, Cross JM, Bamman MM. Potent myofiber hypertrophy during resistance training in humans is associated with satellite cell-mediated myonuclear addition: a cluster analysis. *J Appl Physiol.* (2008) 104:1736–42. doi: 10.1152/japplphysiol.01215.2007
68. Kao M, Columbus DA, Suryawan A, Steinhoff-Wagner J, Hernandez-Garcia A, Nguyen HV, et al. Enteral beta-hydroxy-beta-methylbutyrate supplementation increases protein synthesis in skeletal muscle of neonatal pigs. *Am J Physiol Endocrinol Metab.* (2016) 310:E1072–84. doi: 10.1152/ajpendo.00520.2015
69. Snijders T, Nederveen JP, McKay BR, Joanisse S, Verdijk LB, van Loon LJ, et al. Satellite cells in human skeletal muscle plasticity. *Front Physiol.* (2015) 6:283. doi: 10.3389/fphys.2015.00283
70. Kadi F, Charifi N, Denis C, Lexell J. Satellite cells and myonuclei in young and elderly women and men. *Muscle Nerve.* (2004) 29:120–7. doi: 10.1002/mus.10510
71. Snijders T, Verdijk LB, Smeets JS, McKay BR, Senden JM, Hartgens F, et al. The skeletal muscle satellite cell response to a single bout of resistance-type exercise is delayed with aging in men. *Age.* (2014) 36:9699. doi: 10.1007/s11357-014-9699-z
72. Burke DG, Candow DG, Chilibeck PD, MacNeil LG, Roy BD, Tarnopolsky MA, et al. Effect of creatine supplementation and resistance-exercise training on muscle insulin-like growth factor in young adults. *Int J Sport Nutr Exerc Metab.* (2008) 18:389–98. doi: 10.1123/ijsnem.18.4.389
73. Olsen S, Aagaard P, Kadi F, Tufekovic G, Verney J, Olesen JL, et al. Creatine supplementation augments the increase in satellite cell and myonuclei number in human skeletal muscle induced by strength training. *J Physiol.* (2006) 573(Pt. 2):525–34. doi: 10.1113/jphysiol.2006.107359
74. Willoughby DS, Rosene JM. Effects of oral creatine and resistance training on myogenic regulatory factor expression. *Med Sci Sports Exerc.* (2003) 35:923–9. doi: 10.1249/01.MSS.0000069746.05241.F0
75. Snijders T, Bell KE, Nederveen JP, Saddler NI, Mazara N, Kumbhare DA, et al. Ingestion of a multi-ingredient supplement does not alter exercise-induced satellite cell responses in older men. *J Nutr.* (2018) 148:891–9. doi: 10.1093/jn/nxy063
76. Schuenke MD, Brooks NE, Hikida RS. Interactions of aging, overload, and creatine supplementation in rat plantaris muscle. *J Aging Res.* (2011) 2011:393416. doi: 10.4061/2011/393416

77. Zanou N, Gailly P. Skeletal muscle hypertrophy and regeneration: interplay between the myogenic regulatory factors (MRFs) and insulin-like growth factors (IGFs) pathways. *Cell Mol Life Sci.* (2013) 70:4117–30. doi: 10.1007/s00018-013-1330-4
78. Li M, Verdijk LB, Sakamoto K, Ely B, van Loon LJ, Musi N. Reduced AMPK-ACC and mTOR signaling in muscle from older men, and effect of resistance exercise. *Mech Ageing Dev.* (2012) 133:655–64. doi: 10.1016/j.mad.2012.09.001
79. Parise G, Mihic S, MacLennan D, Yarasheski KE, Tarnopolsky MA. Effects of acute creatine monohydrate supplementation on leucine kinetics and mixed-muscle protein synthesis. *J Appl Physiol.* (2001) 91:1041–7. doi: 10.1152/jappl.2001.91.3.1041
80. Johnston AP, De Lisio M, Parise G. Resistance training, sarcopenia, and the mitochondrial theory of aging. *Appl Physiol Nutr Metab.* (2008) 33:191–9. doi: 10.1139/H07-141
81. Guidi C, Potenza L, Sestili P, Martinelli C, Guescini M, Stocchi L, et al. Differential effect of creatine on oxidatively-injured mitochondrial and nuclear DNA. *Biochim Biophys Acta.* (2008) 1780:16–26. doi: 10.1016/j.bbagen.2007.09.018
82. Berneburg M, Gremmel T, Kurten V, Schroeder P, Hertel I, von Mikecz A, et al. Creatine supplementation normalizes mutagenesis of mitochondrial DNA as well as functional consequences. *J Invest Dermatol.* (2005) 125:213–20. doi: 10.1111/j.0022-202X.2005.23806.x
83. Barbieri E, Guescini M, Calcabrini C, Vallorani L, Diaz AR, Fimognari C, et al. Creatine prevents the structural and functional damage to mitochondria in myogenic, oxidatively stressed C2C12 cells and restores their differentiation capacity. *Oxid Med Cell Longev.* (2016) 2016:5152029. doi: 10.1155/2016/5152029
84. Sheikholeslami-Vatani D, Faraji H. Influence of creatine supplementation on apoptosis markers after downhill running in middle-aged men: a crossover randomized, double-blind, and placebo-controlled study. *Am J Phys Med Rehabil.* (2018) 97:825–31. doi: 10.1097/PHM.0000000000000977
85. Bell KE, Snijders T, Zulyniak MA, Kumbhare D, Parise G, Chabowski A, et al. A multi-ingredient nutritional supplement enhances exercise training-related reductions in markers of systemic inflammation in healthy older men. *Appl Physiol Nutr Metab.* (2018) 43:299–302. doi: 10.1139/apnm-2017-0533
86. Derave W, Jones G, Hespel P, Harris RC. Creatine supplementation augments skeletal muscle carnosine content in senescence-accelerated mice (SAMP8). *Rejuvenation Res.* (2008) 11:641–7. doi: 10.1089/rej.2008.0699
87. Candow DG, Chilibeck PD. Timing of creatine or protein supplementation and resistance training in the elderly. *Appl Physiol Nutr Metab.* (2008) 33:184–90. doi: 10.1139/H07-139
88. Cribb PJ, Hayes A. Effects of supplement timing and resistance exercise on skeletal muscle hypertrophy. *Med Sci Sports Exerc.* (2006) 38:1918–25. doi: 10.1249/01.mss.0000233790.08788.3e
89. Forbes SC, Candow DG. Timing of creatine supplementation and resistance training: a brief review. *J Exerc Nutr.* (2018) 1:1.
90. Loenneke JP, Dankel SJ, Bell ZW, Buckner SL, Mattocks KT, Jessee MB, et al. Is muscle growth a mechanism for increasing strength? *Med Hypotheses.* (2019) 125:51–6. doi: 10.1016/j.mehy.2019.02.030
91. Loenneke JP, Buckner SL, Dankel SJ, Abe T. Exercise-induced changes in muscle size do not contribute to exercise-induced changes in muscle strength. *Sports Med.* (2019) 49:987–91. doi: 10.1007/s40279-019-01106-9
92. Schoenfeld BJ, Contreras B, Krieger J, Grgic J, Delcastillo K, Belliard R, et al. Resistance training volume enhances muscle hypertrophy but not strength in trained men. *Med Sci Sports Exerc.* (2019) 51:94–103. doi: 10.1249/MSS.0000000000001764
93. Bell KE, Snijders T, Zulyniak M, Kumbhare D, Parise G, Chabowski A, et al. A whey protein-based multi-ingredient nutritional supplement stimulates gains in lean body mass and strength in healthy older men: a randomized controlled trial. *PLoS ONE.* (2017) 12:e0181387. doi: 10.1371/journal.pone.0181387
94. O'Bryan KR, Doering TM, Morton RW, Coffey VG, Phillips SM, Cox GR. Do multi-ingredient protein supplements augment resistance training-induced gains in skeletal muscle mass and strength? A systematic review and meta-analysis of 35 trials. *Br J Sports Med.* (2019). doi: 10.1136/bjsports-2018-099889. [Epub ahead of print].
95. Chami J, Candow DG. Effect of creatine supplementation dosing strategies on aging muscle performance. *J Nutr Health Aging.* (2019) 23:281–5. doi: 10.1007/s12603-018-1148-8
96. Lobo DM, Tritto AC, da Silva LR, de Oliveira PB, Benatti FB, Roschel H, et al. Effects of long-term low-dose dietary creatine supplementation in older women. *Exp Gerontol.* (2015) 70:97–104. doi: 10.1016/j.exger.2015.07.012
97. Bender A, Samtleben W, Elstner M, Klopstock T. Long-term creatine supplementation is safe in aged patients with Parkinson disease. *Nutr Res.* (2008) 28:172–8. doi: 10.1016/j.nutres.2008.01.001

4

Obesity Alters the Muscle Protein Synthetic Response to Nutrition and Exercise

Joseph W. Beals [1], Nicholas A. Burd [2], Daniel R. Moore [3] and Stephan van Vliet [4]*

[1] Center for Human Nutrition, Washington University School of Medicine, St. Louis, MO, United States, [2] Department of Kinesiology and Community Health, University of Illinois at Urbana-Champaign, Urbana, IL, United States, [3] Faculty of Kinesiology and Physical Education, University of Toronto, Toronto, ON, Canada, [4] Duke Molecular Physiology Institute, Duke University Medical Center, Durham, NC, United States

***Correspondence:**
Joseph W. Beals
bealsjw@wustl.edu

Improving the health of skeletal muscle is an important component of obesity treatment. Apart from allowing for physical activity, skeletal muscle tissue is fundamental for the regulation of postprandial macronutrient metabolism, a time period that represents when metabolic derangements are most often observed in adults with obesity. In order for skeletal muscle to retain its capacity for physical activity and macronutrient metabolism, its protein quantity and composition must be maintained through the efficient degradation and resynthesis for proper tissue homeostasis. Life-style behaviors such as increasing physical activity and higher protein diets are front-line treatment strategies to enhance muscle protein remodeling by primarily stimulating protein synthesis rates. However, the muscle of individuals with obesity appears to be resistant to the anabolic action of targeted exercise regimes and protein ingestion when compared to normal-weight adults. This indicates impaired muscle protein remodeling in response to the main anabolic stimuli to human skeletal muscle tissue is contributing to poor muscle health with obesity. Deranged anabolic signaling related to insulin resistance, lipid accumulation, and/or systemic/muscle inflammation are likely at the root of the anabolic resistance of muscle protein synthesis rates with obesity. The purpose of this review is to discuss the impact of protein ingestion and exercise on muscle protein remodeling in people with obesity, and the potential mechanisms underlining anabolic resistance of their muscle.

Keywords: exercise, fat mass, muscle mass, mTORC1, p70S6K, inflammation, TLR4, anabolic resistance

INTRODUCTION

At present, 39% of adult Americans are obese (1), which is defined as having a body mass index (BMI) of 30 or higher. Obesity represents a growing societal problem as incidence has increased rapidly since the early 2000s when 30% of American were obese (2). If current trends continue, it is projected that nearly half of all US adults may be obese by 2030 (3). Obesity is associated with several chronic conditions including cancer, type 2 diabetes, cardiovascular disease, arthritis, liver and kidney disease, sleep apnea, mental illness (4, 5), and increased risk of all-cause mortality (6). The annual obesity-related healthcare costs in 2005 were estimated at $190.2 billion or nearly 21% of total medical spending in the US (7). Therefore, effective treatment strategies to prevent, halt, and reverse obesity are imperative to improve public health and reduce the societal (e.g., healthcare and economic) cost of obesity.

The frontline treatment of obesity is typically multifactorial and is predominantly centered around behavior strategies such as changes in nutrition and/or physical activity to elicit weight loss (8). Weight loss, however, commonly occurs with concomitant reductions in skeletal muscle mass (9), the prevention of which is a focus for several research groups (10, 11). These efforts are due to the recognized important contribution of skeletal muscle health to total body health (12).

Besides the obvious role in generating force for movement, skeletal muscle also contributes to health through the use and storage of macronutrients (13). Skeletal muscle is the primary determinant of meal-derived glucose (14) and lipid (15) uptake and utilizes a major portion of meal-derived amino acids (AA) released into systemic circulation to build new functional proteins (16, 17). Moreover, changes in the skeletal muscle's contribution to basal and/or postprandial macronutrient metabolism can have profound effects on disease risk (18). For example, impaired insulin sensitivity is a fundamental characteristic of Type 2 diabetes (19). Emerging data have revealed that obesity may also negatively alter muscle protein turnover, or the breaking down and rebuilding of functional proteins, with the myofibrillar proteins being particularly susceptible to anabolic resistance. The purpose of this review is to discuss the mechanisms by which obesity may hamper normal turnover of muscle proteins and ultimately impact muscle health (**Figure 1**). In addition, we discuss lifestyle strategies to improve the muscle protein synthetic response with obesity.

SKELETAL MUSCLE PROTEIN TURNOVER FOR HEALTHY MUSCLE

Tissue proteins are maintained through the coordination of rates of synthesis (from free AAs) and breakdown (replenishment of the free amino acid pool) under basal conditions. In skeletal muscle, protein synthesis appears to be more highly responsive to changes in plasma amino acid (AA) availability as compared to protein breakdown (MPB) (20–22). Proteins in skeletal muscle are degraded for a variety of reasons including to remodel the muscle in response to changes in metabolic demands (e.g., larger and stronger vs. more fatigue resistant muscles) (23, 24) or as they become old, damaged and subsequently need replacement (25–27). Moreover, as the body's largest pool of AAs, the muscle provides gluconeogenic precursors to other tissues during an overnight (28, 29) or prolonged fast (30). Therefore, the stimulation of muscle protein synthesis rates represents an important physiological process for maintaining the health and function of this tissue.

Regulation of muscle protein synthesis rates is coordinated by several extra- and intracellular signals, many of which are increased in response to nutrition (e.g., insulin and AAs; **Figure 2A**) and physical activity (e.g., muscle contraction; **Figure 2A**). Changes in protein phosphorylation and activity is fundamentally catalyzed by protein-protein interactions, the study of which has led to a greater understanding of and appreciation for the dynamic nature of mRNA translation regulation in human muscle (31). For example, mixed meal ingestion with protein and carbohydrate induces a rise in plasma aminoacidemia and insulinemia that directs the dissociation of Ras homolog-enriched in brain (Rheb) from its negative regulator tuberous sclerosis complex 2 (TSC2) in order to facilitate Rheb association with the mechanistic target of rapamycin (mTOR) to form the mTOR complex 1 (mTORC1) (32, 33). This complex subsequently moves to the lysosome and translocates toward the sarcolemma, which is more proximal to capillaries, AA transporters (e.g., the large neutral amino acid transporter, LAT1 or SLC7A5), and the ribosomal machinery (33–35). This intracellular positioning would presumably be ideally suited to detect and utilize exogenous nutrients for the postprandial muscle protein synthetic response at the level of mRNA translation. In addition, the kinase activity of mTORC1 is essential for the phosphorylation and activation of several proteins involved in ribosomal assembly (e.g., ribosomal protein S6, rpS6; eukaryotic translation initiation factor 4E-binding protein 1, 4EBP1; eukaryotic initiation factor 2, eIF2) either directly, or through downstream kinases (e.g., ribosomal protein S6 kinase 1, p70S6K1) (36, 37). Indeed, phosphorylation of mTOR and these downstream proteins are commonly used readouts of pathway activation (38–42), though it should be appreciated that changes in protein phosphorylation of these candidate markers do not always reflect their kinase activity (43) nor direct proportional changes in muscle protein synthesis (38) in human muscle. Importantly, these processes are also stimulated by muscle contraction (i.e., resistance exercise) with the peripheral targeting of mTORC1 persisting beyond the acute postprandial period (i.e., >3 h) (34), which likely contributes to the sustained p70S6K1 phosphorylation and myofibrillar (i.e., contractile proteins) protein synthetic response with exercise (44, 45). There is also *in vitro* evidence suggesting that, similar to glucose transport, an inducible pool of amino acid transporters (e.g., SNAT2) may also be recruited to the sarcolemma in response to anabolic stimuli, such as insulin, and contribute to the acute regulation of muscle protein synthesis (46). Thus, given the dynamic nature of anabolic signaling events and nutrient transport, any physical or biochemical changes within the skeletal muscle of people with obesity that interferes with these intracellular processes could ultimately contribute to the dysregulation of muscle protein synthesis.

Protein ingestion and exercise have been shown to be two primary anabolic stimuli to human skeletal muscle; protein ingestion being particularly important as it also provides the necessary substrate (i.e., essential AAs) for synthesizing new proteins. The factors involved in the regulation of muscle protein synthesis rates has been studied under a variety of conditions and different populations. From a protein nutrition perspective, a range of 20–40 g of high quality protein is required to ingest in a single meal to maximize the muscle protein synthetic response during the postprandial period in adult men (21, 47–50). Protein type (isolated vs. whole food), exercise pattern (resistance vs. endurance), BMI, and/or age of an individual may all be important factors that modulate the recommended amount of protein to consume in a meal to augment postprandial muscle protein synthesis rates as discussed elsewhere (51, 52).

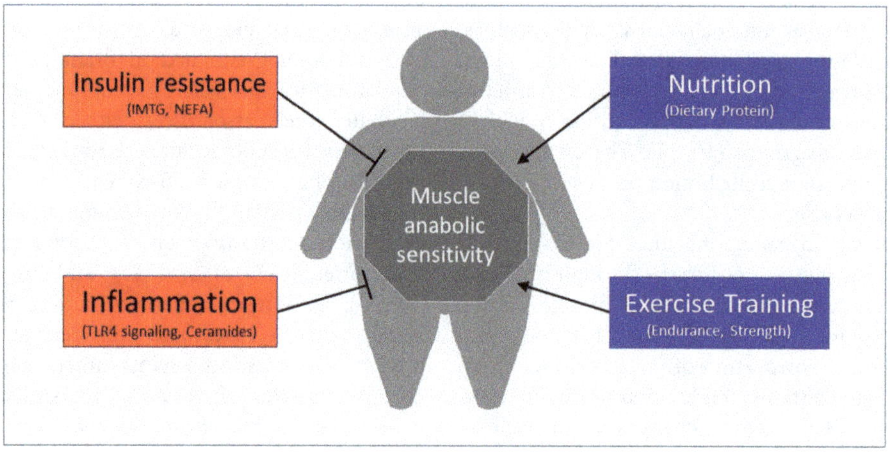

FIGURE 1 | Potential regulators of the postprandial muscle protein synthetic response with obesity.

Muscle protein synthesis, however, is a relatively generic term given the myriad of various structural and regulatory proteins within this tissue. Many studies, however, assess the synthesis of mixed muscle protein, or the entire muscle proteome. In healthy adults, the rates of protein synthesis are not equivalent across sub-fractions of the skeletal muscle (44, 53) and mixed muscle protein synthesis represents a weighted average of the rates of these sub-fractions. However, this approach may obscure important phenotypic differences in rates of protein synthesis occurring in specific protein sub-fractions in response to nutrition or exercise. For example, it has been shown that the stimulation of myofibrillar protein synthesis rates is more sensitive to feeding and exercise during early (i.e., ~5 h) and later (i.e., ~24 h) recovery when compared to the sarcoplasmic protein fraction in healthy adults (44, 54). More importantly, muscle sub-fractional protein synthesis rates are differentially responsive to common stimuli [e.g., insulin, exercise (38–40, 44, 55, 56)] and may be differentially impacted based on the population studied (39, 40, 57). Therefore, to obtain a more complete picture of the potential dysregulation of muscle protein metabolism in clinical populations such as the obese it is advantageous to investigate the response in specific sub-fractions.

THE IMPACT OF OBESITY ON MUSCLE PROTEIN TURNOVER

Basal muscle protein synthesis rates have been assessed in obese individuals in mixed muscle (41, 58) and within the myofibrillar (40, 42, 59–61), sarcoplasmic (40, 42, 61), and mitochondrial (41, 58, 62) protein sub-fractions and generally show no impairment when compared to healthy-weight counterparts. Though, lower basal mixed muscle (41) and mitochondrial (58) protein synthesis rates in individuals with obesity as compared to non-obese individuals have also been reported. The reasons for these discrepant findings are not clear, and may reflect the heterogeneity observed with obesity, which is discussed later on. However, obesity is characterized by several well-known impairments in macronutrient metabolism in skeletal muscle that results in altered regulation of blood glucose and lipids (63). Accumulating evidence also suggests that stimulation of muscle protein synthesis rates during the postprandial period is altered in obese individuals as compared to normal-weight controls (defined as a body mass index; BMI < 25 kg/m^2) (40–42, 58–60), although this finding is not universal (61, 62). Moreover, the specific alterations to muscle sub-fractions (e.g., mitochondrial, myofibrillar, and/or sarcoplasmic) are also not consistent among studies. These discrepancies between studies may relate to a lack of standardized participant grouping (e.g., healthy-weight (BMI < 25 kg/m^2) vs. non-obese individuals (BMI < 30 kg/m^2) as controls) and/or postprandial conditions (i.e., meal ingestion vs. AA infusions) among study designs. A summary of the above studies is presented in **Table 1** and their main findings will be discussed in the next sections.

Much of the earlier work studying the effects of obesity on the regulation of postprandial muscle protein synthesis rates centered on the intravenous delivery of AAs during a clamp procedure. Under hyperinsulinemic-hyperaminoacidemic clamp conditions, it has been reported that obese men exhibit lower rates of mixed muscle (58), myofibrillar (59), mitochondrial (58) protein synthesis when compared to controls, although evidence is also available that do not support these differences (41, 61). While a hyperinsulinemic-euglycemic clamp may represent the gold-standard for assessing insulin-sensitive glucose disposal, sustained hyperaminoacidemia (with or without hyperinsulinemia) is an atypical stimulus that may be associated with a refractory stimulation of muscle protein synthesis (64). Thus, the physiological relevance of clamp conditions for assessing the impact of protein nutrition on postprandial regulation of muscle protein synthesis is arguably limited.

Relatively few experiments have compared the stimulation of postprandial muscle protein synthesis rates in individuals with obesity vs. healthy-weight individuals under the typical applied setting of ingesting protein-dense foods (42, 60, 62). These experiments, which have incorporated the ingestion of a bolus of high-quality protein [i.e., milk (60) or lean pork (42, 62)],

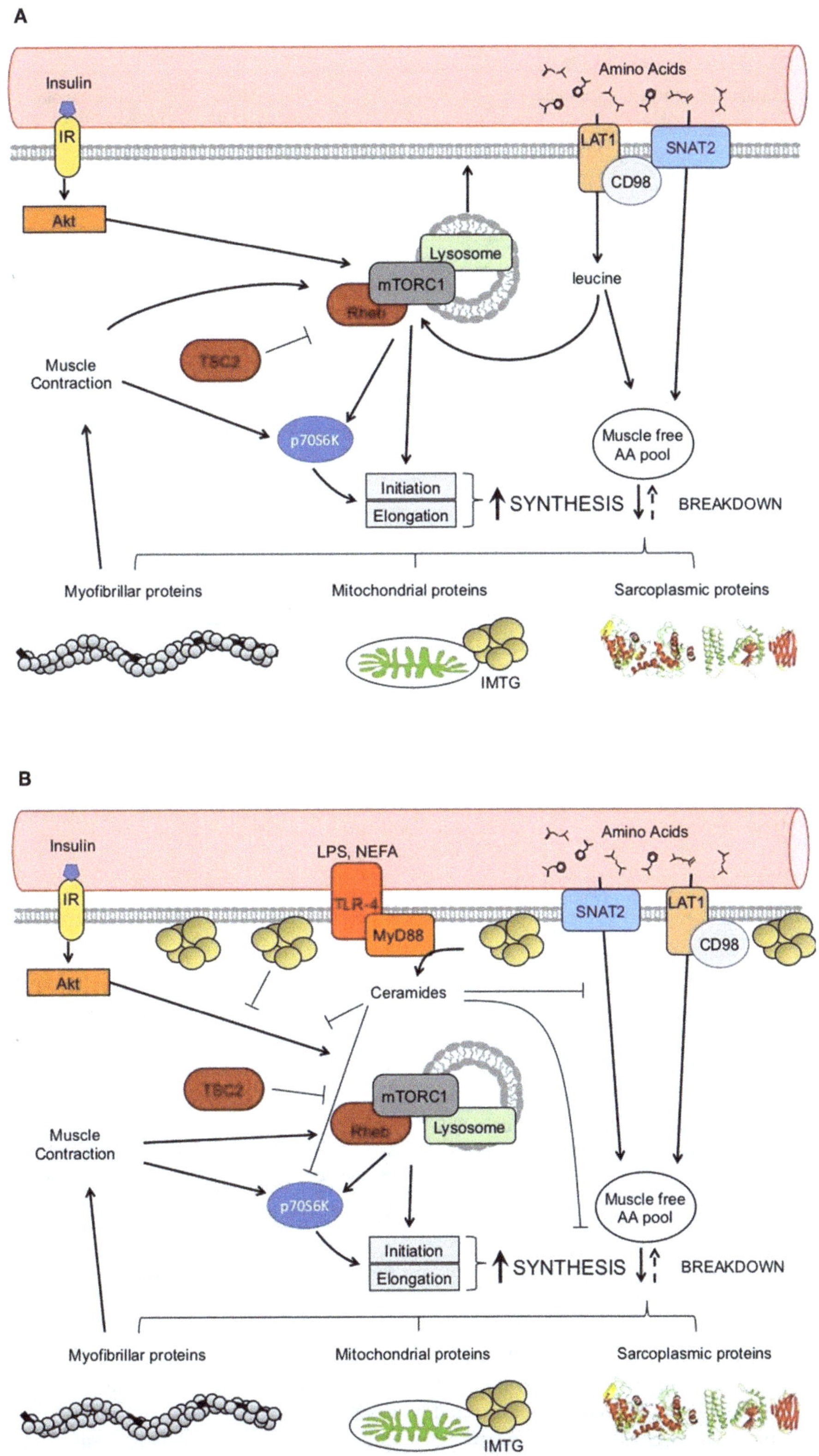

FIGURE 2 | Healthy anabolic signaling in the skeletal muscle **(A)**. Potential dysregulation to anabolic signaling with obesity **(B)**. → indicates a stimulation. ⊥ indicates an inhibition.

TABLE 1 | Effect of obesity on human muscle protein synthesis.

AMINO ACID INFUSION STUDIES						
Experiment	**Populations studied**	**Conditions**		**Basal MPS OB vs. CON**	**OB Postprandial MPS vs. basal**	**Postprandial MPS OB vs. CON**
Guillet et al. (58)	Young men	Hyper-AA		↓ Mixed	↑ Mixed	↓ Mixed
	OB vs. Non-OB (CON)	hyperinsulinemia		↓ Mito	↔ Mito	↓ Mito
Murton et. al. (59)	Older men	Hyper-AA		↔ Myo	↔ Myo	↓ Myo
	OB vs. HW (CON)	hyperinsulinemia				
Chevalier et al. (61)	Young men	Hyper-AA		↔ Myo	↑ Myo	↔ Myo
	OB vs. HW (CON)	hyperinsulinemia		↔ Sarc	↑ Sarc	↔ Sarc
Tran et al. (41)	Young men	Hyper-AA		↓ Mixed	↑ Mixed	↔ Mixed
	OB vs. HW (CON)			↓ Mito	↑ Mito	↔ Mito
PROTEIN INGESTION STUDIES						
Experiment	**Populations studied**	**Protein source**		**Basal MPS OB vs. CON**	**OB Postprandial MPS vs. basal**	**Postprandial MPS OB vs. CON**
Beals et al. (42)	Young adults	Lean pork (36 g)		↔ Myo	↔ Myo	↓ Myo
	OB vs. HW (CON)					
Beals et al. (62)	Young adults	Lean pork (36 g)		↔ Mito	↑ Mito	↔ Mito
	OB vs. HW (CON)					
Smeuninx et al. (60)	Older adults	Milk protein isolate (15 g)		↔ Myo	↔ Myo	↓ Myo
	OB vs. HW (CON)					
EXERCISE STUDIES						
Experiment	**Populations studied**	**Protein source**	**Exercise bout**	**Basal MPS OB vs. CON**	**OB Postexercise MPS vs. rest***	**Postexercise MPS OB vs. CON**
Hulston et al. (72)	Young adults	N/A	Unilateral knee	N/A	↑ Mixed	↔ Mixed
	OB vs. HW (CON)		extension 4 sets at 70% 1RM			
Beals et al. (40)	Young adults	Lean pork (36 g)	Unilateral knee	↔ Myo	↔ Myo	↓ Myo
	OB vs. HW (CON)		extension 4 sets at 65-70% 1RM	↔ Sarc	↔ Sarc	↔ Sarc

*OB, Obese; CON, control group; HW, healthy-weight; OW, overweight; AA, amino acids; MPS, muscle protein synthesis; Sarc, sarcoplasmic; Mito, mitochondrial; Myo, myofibrillar; Mixed, mixed muscle; ↔, no change/difference; ↑, increased/greater; ↓, decreased/lower. *these studies used a unilateral model—rest leg was used for this comparison.*

have revealed that myofibrillar (42, 60), but not mitochondrial protein synthesis rates (62), are reduced in people with obesity compared with healthy-weight individuals after the consumption of protein-dense foods. Indeed, protein-dense food ingestion results in a differential pattern of plasma amino acid availability when compared to directly infusing free AAs intravenously. For example, the ingestion of meat, milk and eggs, important sources of protein in many diet patterns, results in peak plasma amino acid availability occurring ~2 h after the meal, which wanes over the latter portion of a postprandial period (65, 66). The same pattern is also witnessed when observing plasma insulin concentrations after protein ingestion in healthy adults (67). By contrast, clamp conditions are on the other end of the continuum and attempt to alter concentrations of AA and/or insulin in a square wave fashion to maintain concentrations at postprandial or supraphysiological levels over an extended period of time, which may have unintended consequences on muscle protein synthesis rates (64). Clamp conditions also bypass the digestive tract, which plays several important roles in stimulating uptake of nutrients from a meal into peripheral tissues (68–70). Collectively, it is clear that the prime anabolic signals (dietary AAs) to muscle behave very differently when provided as a bolus vs. delivered intravenously, and underlines the value of using more practical approaches when characterizing the impact of nutrition on the regulation of muscle protein synthesis rates in a fraction specific manner with health and disease.

OBESITY-RELATED ANABOLIC RESISTANCE OF MUSCLE PROTEIN SYNTHESIS

Potential factors underpinning anabolic resistance of muscle protein synthesis with obesity are shown in **Figure 2B**. Somewhat contradictory to the above data regarding muscle protein synthesis rates, basal phosphorylation of anabolic signaling proteins such as mTOR^{S2448} (40–42), and its downstream target ribosomal protein S6 kinase (p70S6K^{T389}) (40, 71), are often quite elevated in people with obesity when compared to normal-weight individuals. These findings are suggestive of greater basal anabolic signaling in the muscle. However, an elevated phosphorylated-state of basal anabolic signaling mechanisms in people with obesity are not universal findings (59, 72), which again serves to reflect the heterogeneity in this condition. Total muscle mTOR protein content is also not always reported (41, 72), and presenting only ratios of phosphorylated: total protein can mask the true levels of phosphorylated mTOR as several studies have reported greater muscle mTOR protein content in individuals with obesity (40, 42). It is currently not fully understood how basal anabolic signals are maintained at these greater levels with obesity. Nevertheless, greater basal mTOR phosphorylation may prevent the characteristic postprandial increase in mTOR phosphorylation in those with obesity (41, 42), perhaps suggesting an upper limit for activation of anabolic signaling through this protein complex. For example, one study showing apparently normal basal mTOR phosphorylation in those with obesity, did show increased phosphorylation of mTOR during the postprandial period (59). Phosphorylation of other target proteins downstream of mTORC1 and/or p70S6K signaling [ribosomal protein S6, rpS6$^{S240/244}$ (58, 90); eukaryotic translation initiation factor 4E-binding protein 1, 4EBP1$^{T37/46}$ (58); eukaryotic initiation factor 2, eIF2^{S251} (44)] are unaltered by obesity indicating that proximal aspects of the anabolic signaling pathway are more disrupted compared to healthy-weight individuals.

INSULIN RESISTANCE AND MUSCLE ANABOLISM

Resistance to insulin was historically uncommon in the literature, initially only represented by case studies (73). However, by the 1950s it was recognized that a subset of people with type 2 diabetes were less responsive to insulin and this was accompanied with being overweight or obese (74). Given insulin's role in mTORC1 signaling, diminished responsiveness could be an important aspect of muscle protein metabolism during the postprandial period.

Obesity is often associated with elevated basal plasma circulating branched chain AAs (BCAA) levels (75, 76), which may relate to metabolic changes observed in the skeletal muscle of people with obesity (77). Greater plasma BCAAs concentrations are potentially linked to dysregulation of metabolism with obesity, mostly as it relates to insulin resistance (75, 78–81) and chronic activation of the mTORC1 signaling pathway (82, 83). These findings could be relevant to observations of elevated basal mTORC1 signaling in people with obesity (40–42). However, only one study that reported the effects of obesity on the mTORC1 signaling pathway and muscle protein synthesis has shown mild elevations (~20%) in plasma BCAAs in obese vs. lean individuals (61) with the majority reporting no differences (40–42, 58, 60, 84). Collectively this seems to suggest that elevated basal circulating BCAAs may not be significant nor consistent contributors to the dysregulated muscle protein anabolic response in obesity.

Obesity is also associated with elevated plasma non-esterified fatty acids (NEFA) (85). In fact, infusions of lipid with heparin, which increases plasma NEFAs, can blunt insulin sensitivity even in healthy, insulin-sensitive subjects (86). Lipid infusions also impair myofibrillar protein synthesis in healthy participants under hyperinsulinemic-hyperaminoacidemic conditions (87), which suggests a possible role for insulin resistance in the regulation of myofibrillar protein synthesis. A series of experiments examined the relationship between plasma NEFA concentrations and muscle protein synthesis rates in response to protein ingestion in obese participants and healthy-weight controls (42, 62). The participants with obesity in these studies had only subtle differences in postprandial plasma NEFAs, which did not appear to be related to either myofibrillar (42) or mitochondrial protein synthesis (62). In contrast, other have shown that greater intramyocellular lipids are associated with diminished postprandial myofibrillar protein synthesis in obese older adults (60). High intramyocellular lipid is classically associated with insulin resistance in sedentary populations (88), although the causality and mechanistic link for this relationship is not clear. It is worthwhile noting that intramyocellular lipid accumulation in obese human muscle (60) tends to be sub-sarcolemmal as compared to intermyofibrillar in athletic populations (89), which could impair mTORC1 translocation and subsequent downstream activity of this pathway. Alternatively, dysregulated insulin signaling is also attributed to changes in intracellular lipid metabolites (90–92) and in particular the sphingolipid ceramide (92, 93). An *in vitro* study showed that ceramide treatment reduced small neutral amino acid transporter (SNAT2)-mediated sarcolemmal translocation and amino acid transport in L6 myotubes, which translated in an attenuated phosphorylation of p70S6K^{T389} and amino acid induced stimulation of muscle protein synthesis (94). Thus, the relationship between intramyocellular lipid accumulation and/or ceramide production and the intracellular anabolic signaling (e.g., mTORC1) represents a fruitful area for further study.

Efficient delivery of AAs to peripheral tissues is important for the postprandial stimulation of muscle protein synthesis and may be mediated by an insulin-induced vasodilation of the capillary bed (95, 96). Muscle capillarity has been suggested to independently influence peripheral insulin sensitivity and postprandial myofibrillar protein synthesis rates in older adults (97–99), which could implicate a diminished muscle capillary network (100) and/or insulin-induced recruitment (101) in obese individuals as a contributing factor to the anabolic resistance of this population.

Thus, far the impact of obesity *per se* compared to its associated insulin resistance on the dysregulation of postprandial anabolic response is unknown. For instance, overweight young adults with apparently normal insulinemia and homeostatic model assessment of insulin resistance (HOMA-IR) have also been reported to have a blunted myofibrillar protein synthesis response to protein ingestion and greater basal mTOR phosphorylation (42). This could suggest that increased basal mTOR phosphorylation may occur early with weight gain prior to the development of discernible insulin resistance but concomitant with a blunted postprandial anabolic response. Indeed, substantial evidence has mounted that some individuals with obesity remain nearly as insulin sensitive as lean counterparts while other individuals with a similar degree of obesity become insulin resistant (102). Whether differences in insulin sensitivity are predictive of muscle anabolic sensitivity in obese individuals is currently not known.

INFLAMMATION AND MUSCLE PROTEIN SYNTHESIS

Obesity is associated with chronic low-grade inflammation (103), which has been linked to impaired glucose tolerance (104) and dyslipidemia (105). This includes elevated basal levels of plasma inflammatory biomarkers [i.e., CRP (42, 59, 60, 62, 72), IL-6 (42, 59, 62), TNFα (59)] in obese participants. Because of shared metabolic signaling pathways, skeletal muscle inflammation may also contribute to impaired protein anabolism in obese individuals [**Figure 2B** (106)]. Indeed, protein metabolism is dramatically altered by high levels of inflammation with trauma or severe illness [e.g., thermal injury (107) or end stage renal disease (108)], which may be related to direct effects of some inflammatory markers (e.g., CRP and TNFα) on suppressing muscle protein synthesis as demonstrated *in vitro* (109, 110).

A few studies have attempted to describe the muscle protein synthetic response to protein ingestion in humans with low-grade inflammation independent of obesity (111, 112). In healthy older men stratified by plasma C-reactive protein (CRP) concentrations, postprandial mixed muscle protein synthetic rates were not different between groups (111). Another group tested the effect of 1 week of ibuprofen or placebo administration on basal and postprandial myofibrillar protein responses to whey protein ingestion in older men with elevated CRP and compared these responses to those of healthy non-inflamed older men (112). In this study, basal and postprandial myofibrillar protein synthesis were not different between ibuprofen and placebo groups. Moreover, both intervention groups (ibuprofen and placebo) had similar basal and postprandial rates of myofibrillar protein synthesis compared with the non-inflamed control group (112). Despite the implication of CRP in attenuating muscle protein anabolism *in vitro* (109), results in humans, and especially obese individuals, are less clear. Nevertheless, elevated basal levels of plasma inflammatory biomarkers in individuals with obesity [i.e., CRP (42, 59, 60, 62, 72), IL-6 (42, 59, 62), TNFα (59)] are associated with basal muscle protein synthesis rates that are indistinguishable from healthy-weight non-inflamed controls, but blunted postprandial myofibrillar protein synthesis rates (42, 59, 60, 62), suggesting the impact of low-grade inflammation (e.g., elevated inflammatory cytokines) may depend on the nutrient environment. Moreover, as discussed above, the muscles of overweight individuals are also anabolic resistant (42), but this group does not show indications of systemic or muscle inflammation (62).

Data concerning the effect of muscle inflammation on postprandial muscle protein synthesis in people with obesity is largely limited to the toll-like receptor 4 (TLR4) signaling pathway. This receptor is involved in innate immunity and is primarily known for responding to endotoxin (113), but is also responsive to NEFA (114) and CRP (115) in circulation. TLR4 signaling involves docking with several intracellular proteins, among these is myeloid differentiation factor 88 (MyD88), which appears to potentiate the intracellular signaling of TLR4-induced insulin resistance (114, 116). Muscle TLR4 protein content correlates with body fat percentage in older adults (117) and is related to NEFA-induced insulin resistance (114). Although, one group found that muscle content of both TLR4 and MyD88 proteins are greater in obese, anabolic resistant adults compared with healthy-weight controls (62), discerning the impact of obesity or low-grade inflammation on differences in the postprandial muscle protein synthetic response is not possible from the experiment described above.

EXERCISE TO IMPROVE ANABOLIC SENSITIVITY WITH OBESITY

Leisure time physical activity is a potent treatment for health and its regular performance reduces mortality (118). Physical inactivity has been linked to numerous adverse health outcomes and is predictive of metabolic health with obesity (119). Physical inactivity has also been linked to anabolic resistance in obese older adults (60) and may contribute to the development of sarcopenic obesity (120). For interventions, exercise represents a structured manner to increase daily physical activity. Exercise training takes many forms, but most can be categorized as either endurance (aerobic) or resistance (strength) exercise, though those lines can be somewhat blurred (e.g., high intensity interval training). Each of these training modalities has differing effects on the muscle phenotype, but the effects on muscle tissue health (e.g., insulin sensitivity, endothelial function) appear to be more universal (121–124). Moreover, as physical activity is an essential component of strategies to improve body composition (125, 126), it is important to consider how the muscle adaptive response is affected by obesity.

Endurance training is commonly recommended to improve health and body composition in individuals with obesity. There is limited data studying the impact of endurance exercise on the muscle protein synthesis rates in individuals with obesity. However, in healthy, but untrained young men, an acute bout of endurance exercise appears to favor the stimulation of mitochondrial, over myofibrillar, muscle protein synthesis rates during the postprandial period, an effect which was not modified by a 10-wk training period (39). The same work also reported that resistance exercise tends to increase myofibrillar muscle protein synthesis, in particular after a period of training (39). These findings may be important for determining exercise prescription in those with obesity, given that myofibrillar protein synthesis seems to more affected by obesity (40, 42, 59–61) than muscle mitochondrial protein synthesis (41, 58, 62).

A single bout of resistance exercise can induce substantial alterations of macronutrient metabolism such as improvements in glucose tolerance (121) and postprandial lipemia (127) in healthy young men. Resistance exercise also potentiates muscle protein synthesis rates compared with feeding alone in healthy-weight young and older men (128), an effect that may persist for up to 2 days (54, 129). It appears that resistance exercise is particularly effective at enhancing the myofibrillar (more so than the sarcoplasmic or mitochondrial) sub-fractional protein synthetic response to protein ingestion in healthy adults (40, 44, 56). Therefore, resistance exercise would ostensibly be an ideal intervention for improving the obesity-related impairment in postprandial myofibrillar protein synthesis rates.

Two studies have assessed the impact of acute resistance exercise on muscle protein synthesis and related anabolic signaling mechanism in people with obesity, the findings of which are summarized in **Tables 1, 2** (40, 72). One investigation observed acute resistance exercise increased mixed muscle protein synthesis in the fasted state with no differences in protein synthetic rates nor anabolic signaling molecule phosphorylation (e.g., mTORC1) between obese and healthy-weight adults (72). However, mixed muscle protein synthetic responses represent an average of all muscle proteins, which can have markedly different rates of turnover and contraction and nutrient sensitivities (44, 130, 131). When sub-fractional protein synthetic responses to resistance exercise after protein ingestion are compared, the postprandial myofibrillar protein synthetic response was not further stimulated by resistance exercise in obese vs. healthy-weight groups whereas sarcoplasmic muscle protein synthesis rates were largely unaffected by obesity or exercise (40). We also reported that resistance exercise prior to protein ingestion did not augment phosphorylation of targets downstream of mTORC1 (p70S6K^{T389}, 4EBP1$^{T37/46}$) in those with obesity, which contrasted starkly with their healthy-weight counterparts. As highlighted previously, lysosomal targeting of mTORC1, which appears to be mediated by the production of phosphatidic acid (PA) (132–134), is integral to maximize post-exercise myofibrillar synthetic rates in the fed state (135). Interestingly, ceramide has also been reported to blunt PA production in L6 myoblasts (136), which may have contributed to the attenuated myofibrillar protein synthetic response to resistance exercise in obese individuals (40). Nevertheless, these studies collectively underscore the importance of assessing the

TABLE 2 | Effect of obesity on muscle anabolic signaling.

AMINO ACID INFUSION STUDIES						
Experiment	**Populations studied**	**Conditions**		**Basal OB vs. CON**	**OB Postprandial vs. basal**	**Postprandial OB vs. CON**
Murton et al. (59)	Older men	Hyper-AA		↔ mTOR^{S2448}	↑ mTOR^{S2448}	↔ mTOR^{S2448}
	OB vs. HW(CON)	hyperinsulinemia				
Chevalier et al. (61)	Young men	Hyper-AA		↔ p70S6K^{T389}	↑ p70S6K^{T389}	↓ p70S6K^{T389}
	OB vs. HW (CON)	hyperinsulinemia		↔ rpS6$^{S240/244}$	↑ rpS6$^{S240/244}$	↔ rpS6$^{S240/244}$
				↔ 4EBP1^{S65}	↑ 4EBP1^{S65}	↔ 4EBP1^{S65}
Tran et al. (41)	Young men	Hyper-AA		↑ mTOR^{S2448}	↔ mTOR^{S2448}	↑ mTOR^{S2448}
	OB vs. HW (CON)			↔ p70S6K^{T389}	↑ p70S6K^{T389}	↑ p70S6K^{T389}
				↔ eIF2^{S51}	↔ eIF2^{S51}	↔ eIF2^{S51}
Williamson et al. (71)	OB,T2D vs. HW (CON)	Hyperinsulinemia		↔ REDD1	↔ REDD1	↑ REDD1
				↑ p70S6K^{T389}	↓ p70S6K^{T389}	↔ p70S6K^{T389}
				↓ 4EBP1$^{T37/46}$	↔ 4EBP1$^{T37/46}$	↓ 4EBP1$^{T37/46}$
PROTEIN INGESTION STUDIES						
Experiment	**Populations studied**	**Protein source**		**Basal OB vs. CON**	**OB Postprandial vs. basal**	**Postprandial OB vs. CON**
Beals et al. (42)	Young adults	Lean pork (36 g)		↑ mTOR^{S2448}	↔ mTOR^{S2448}	↔ mTOR^{S2448}
	OB, OW vs. HW (CON)			↔ p70S6K^{T389}	↑ p70S6K^{T389}	↑ p70S6K^{T389}
Gran et al. (84)	Middle-aged men	Dairy protein (31 g)		N/A	↑ mTOR^{S2448}	↔ mTOR^{S2448}
	OB w/MetS vs. Non-OB (CON)				↔ p70S6K^{T389}	↓ p70S6K^{T389}
					↑ rpS6$^{S240/244}$	↔ rpS6$^{S240/244}$
		Soy protein (31 g)		N/A	↔ mTOR^{S2448}	↔ mTOR^{S2448}
					↔ p70S6K^{T389}	↓ p70S6K^{T389}
					↔ rpS6$^{S240/244}$	↔ rpS6$^{S240/244}$
EXERCISE STUDIES						
Experiment	**Populations studied**	**Protein source**	**Exercise bout**	**Basal OB vs. CON**	**OB Postexercise vs. rest***	**Postexercise OB vs. CON**
Hulston et al. (72)	Young adults	N/A	Unilateral knee	↔ mTOR^{S2448}	↑ mTOR^{S2448}	↔ mTOR^{S2448}
	OB vs. HW (CON)		extension 4	↔ p70S6K^{T389}	↑ p70S6K^{T389}	↔ p70S6K^{T389}
			sets at 70% 1RM	↔ 4EBP1$^{T37/46}$	↑ 4EBP1$^{T37/46}$	↔ 4EBP1$^{T37/46}$
Beals et al. (40)	Young adults	Lean pork (36 g)	Unilateral knee	↑ mTOR^{S2448}	↔ mTOR^{S2448}	↔ mTOR^{S2448}
	OB vs. HW (CON)		extension 4 sets	↑ p70S6K^{T389}	↔ p70S6K^{T389}	↓ p70S6K^{T389}
			at 65–70% 1RM	↔ 4EBP1$^{T37/46}$	↔ 4EBP1$^{T37/46}$	↓ 4EBP1$^{T37/46}$

*OB, obese; CON, control group; HW, healthy-weight; OW, overweight; AA, amino acids; mTORC1, mechanistic target of rapamycin; p70S6K, ribosomal protein S6 kinase; rpS6, ribosomal protein S6; 4EBP1, eukaryotic translation initiation factor 4E-binding protein 1; eIF2, eukaryotic initiation factor 2; REDD1, regulated in development and DNA damage 1; MetS, metabolic syndrome; ↔, No change/difference; ↑, increased/greater; ↓, decreased/lower; 1RM, one-repetition maximum strength. * Resting measurement was performed in contralateral non-exercised leg.*

sub-fractional protein synthetic responses to the independent and combined anabolic effect of resistance exercise and protein ingestion.

Combined endurance and resistance (i.e., concurrent) exercise training has been demonstrated to have beneficial effects on body composition in adults with overweight or obesity (137). An acute bout of concurrent exercise has been demonstrated to alleviate the suppressive effect of elevated NEFAs on postprandial mixed muscle protein synthesis rates in middle-aged men with overweight or obesity (138). There are relatively few studies that employed a longitudinal design incorporating a combined endurance and resistance exercise approach in obese older adults (139–141). These studies reported rates of mixed muscle protein synthesis before, during, and after exercise with somewhat equivocal results. Two reports showed that increased multi-modality physical activity (endurance + resistance) over a 3 month period increases basal mixed muscle protein synthesis rates, but the magnitude of postprandial stimulation of muscle protein synthesis rates was not affected (140). In contrast, the same group also reported, in a similar population, that weight loss over 12 months of caloric restriction with multi-modality physical activity does not change either basal or postprandial mixed muscle protein synthesis rates (141). That study did show that during active weight loss, measured at 3 months of the intervention, the postprandial mixed muscle protein synthesis rates were substantially elevated. The latter finding indicates that prolonged energy restriction with relatively low protein intake (1.0 g/kg/day) may hamper the muscle anabolic response to multi-modality exercise (141).

Several studies have shown that greater dietary protein (>1.2 g/kg/day) helps to preserve muscle protein synthesis rates during caloric restriction-induced weight loss (~40% energy restriction) in healthy-weight (142) and individuals with overweight or obesity (10, 143). In overweight and obese men, the amount of dietary protein required to sustain muscle protein synthesis rates during caloric restriction could be even greater when a high volume of exercise (resistance training and high-intensity intervals) is also performed (143). These studies (10, 141, 143) serve to underscore the importance of considering both nutrition and physical activity when designing interventions to treat obesity and/or its co-morbidities.

CONCLUSIONS

Protein ingestion is an important component of a healthy diet and has been touted for its potential to facilitate weight loss for those with obesity (144). When studies are considered together, obesity primarily affects the postprandial myofibrillar protein synthetic response to nutrition and exercise (**Table 1**), which is likely related to altered intramyocellular signaling cascades (**Table 2**). Identification of mechanisms responsible for greater basal anabolic signaling molecule phosphorylation could potentially yield novel therapeutic targets.

Obesity is an inherently variable condition, which likely explains the observations discussed throughout this review. For example, insulin resistance can manifest itself as impaired fasting glucose, glucose intolerance, or both (145). In fact, the variability in glucose metabolic outcomes with obesity has been extensively discussed (102, 145). With this in mind, differences in insulin sensitivity or inflammation may impact muscle protein synthetic responses and explain some of the variability observed in the various studies discussed in this review.

The studies of acute resistance exercise discussed above employed robust exercise protocols in excess of most recommendations for untrained weightlifters (146–148). It is remarkable that this exercise prescription was insufficient to augment myofibrillar protein synthesis rates after protein ingestion. There is potential that increasing the exercise volume could have a positive impact on postprandial myofibrillar protein synthesis rates; similar to improvements seen in older anabolic resistant adults (149). Future studies should focus on long-term interventions that include combined diet and exercise strategies to reduce obesity and examine the impact of weight loss and/or exercise training status on postprandial muscle protein synthesis and anabolic signaling. These long-term studies could also benefit from the use of deuterium oxide (heavy water) to determine free-living rates of muscle protein synthesis during an intervention period. However, differences between nutritional interventions (e.g., protein type, leucine dose) on acute rates of myofibrillar protein synthesis in response to a single meal ingestion with traditional primed constant infusions may be less pronounced when assessed by D2O in a free-living environment (150, 151), highlighting the need for additional research utilizing a variety of stable isotope methodologies to study the presence and consequence of obesity-related anabolic resistance. Dietary interventions should focus on ensuring adequate protein nutrition (~1.2 g/kg/day). Ideally, future studies would incorporate more comprehensive metabolic profiling (e.g., measures of insulin sensitivity) that would allow better insight as to how the phenomena of metabolic (ab)normality with obesity (102) affects muscle protein synthesis responses to dietary protein and exercise.

AUTHOR CONTRIBUTIONS

JB wrote the first draft of the manuscript. NB, DM, and SV critically revised the text and made substantial contributions to the manuscript. All authors approved the final version of the manuscript.

REFERENCES

1. Flegal KM, Kruszon-Moran D, Carroll MD, Fryar CD. Ogden CL Trends in obesity among adults in the united states, 2005 to 2014. *JAMA.* (2016) 315:2284–91. doi: 10.1001/jama.2016.6458
2. Hales CM, Carroll MD, Fryar CD, Ogden CL. Prevalence of obesity among adults and youth: United States, 2015-2016. *NCHS Data Brief.* (2017) 1–8.
3. Wang YC, McPherson K, Marsh T, Gortmaker SL, Brown M. Health and economic burden of the projected obesity trends in the USA and the UK. *Lancet Lond. Engl.* (2011) 378:815–25. doi: 10.1016/S0140-6736(11)60814-3

4. Gallagher EJ, LeRoith D. Obesity and diabetes: the increased risk of cancer and cancer-related mortality. *Physiol. Rev.* (2015) 95:727–48. doi: 10.1152/physrev.00030.2014
5. Pi-Sunyer X. The medical risks of obesity. *Postgrad. Med.* (2009) 121:21–33. doi: 10.3810/pgm.2009.11.2074
6. Aune D, Sen A, Prasad M, Norat T, Janszky I, Tonstad S, et al. BMI and all cause mortality: systematic review and non-linear dose-response meta-analysis of 230 cohort studies with 3.74 million deaths among 30.3 million participants. *BMJ.* (2016) 353:i2156. doi: 10.1136/bmj.i2156
7. Cawley J, Meyerhoefer C. The medical care costs of obesity: an instrumental variables approach. *J. Health Econ.* (2012) 31:219–30. doi: 10.1016/j.jhealeco.2011.10.003
8. Kushner RF. Weight loss strategies for treatment of obesity. *Prog. Cardiovasc. Dis.* (2014) 56:465–72. doi: 10.1016/j.pcad.2013.09.005
9. Gallagher D, Kelley DE, Thornton J, Boxt L, Pi-Sunyer X, Lipkin E, et al. Changes in skeletal muscle and organ size after a weight-loss intervention in overweight and obese type 2 diabetic patients. *Am J Clin Nutr.* (2017) 105:78–84. doi: 10.3945/ajcn.116.139188
10. Hector AJ, Marcotte GR, Churchward-Venne TA, Murphy CH, Breen L, Allmen M. et al. Whey protein supplementation preserves postprandial myofibrillar protein synthesis during short-term energy restriction in overweight and obese adults. *J Nutr.* (2015) 145:246–52. doi: 10.3945/jn.114.200832
11. Clamp LD, Hume DJ, Lambert EV, Kroff J. Successful and unsuccessful weight-loss maintainers: strategies to counteract metabolic compensation following weight loss. *J Nutr Sci.* (2018) 7:e20. doi: 10.1017/jns.2018.11
12. Wolfe RR. The underappreciated role of muscle in health and disease. *Am J Clin Nutr.* (2006) 84:475–82. doi: 10.1093/ajcn/84.3.475
13. Astrup A. Macronutrient balances and obesity: the role of diet and physical activity. *Public Health Nutr.* (1999) 2:341–7. doi: 10.1017/S1368980099000464
14. Baron AD, Brechtel G, Wallace P, Edelman SV. Rates and tissue sites of non-insulin- and insulin-mediated glucose uptake in humans. *Am J Physiol.* (1988) 255:E769–74. doi: 10.1152/ajpendo.1988.255.6.E769
15. Bickerton AST, Roberts R, Fielding BA, Hodson L, Blaak EE, Wagenmakers AJM, et al. Preferential uptake of dietary fatty acids in adipose tissue and muscle in the postprandial period. *Diabetes.* (2007) 56:168–76. doi: 10.2337/db06-0822
16. Groen BBL, Horstman AM, Hamer HM, de Haan M, van Kranenburg J, Bierau J, et al. Post-prandial protein handling: you are what you just ate. *PLoS ONE.* (2015) 10:141582. doi: 10.1371/journal.pone.0141582
17. Fouillet H, Gaudichon C, Mariotti F, Bos C, Huneau JF, Tomé D. Energy nutrients modulate the splanchnic sequestration of dietary nitrogen in humans: a compartmental analysis. *Am J Physiol Endocrinol Metab.* (2001) 281, E248–60. doi: 10.1152/ajpendo.2001.281.2.E248
18. Jacome-Sosa M, Parks EJ, Bruno RS, Tasali E, Lewis GF, Schneeman BO, et al. Postprandial metabolism of macronutrients and cardiometabolic risk: recent developments, emerging concepts, and future directions. *Adv Nutr Bethesda Md.* (2016) 7:364–74. doi: 10.3945/an.115.010397
19. DeFronzo RA, Tripathy, D. Skeletal muscle insulin resistance is the primary defect in type 2 diabetes. *Diabetes Care.* (2009) 32 (Suppl. 2):S157–63. doi: 10.2337/dc09-S302
20. Millward DJ, Garlick PJ, Nnanyelugo DO, Waterlow JC. The relative importance of muscle protein synthesis and breakdown in the regulation of muscle mass. *Biochem J.* (1976) 156:185–8. doi: 10.1042/bj1560185
21. Pennings B, Groen B, Gijsen AP, Zorenc AH, Senden JMG, Loon LJC, et al. van Amino acid absorption and subsequent muscle protein accretion following graded intakes of whey protein in elderly men. *Am J Physiol Endocrinol Metab.* (2012) 302:E992–9. doi: 10.1152/ajpendo.00517.2011
22. Biolo G, Tipton KD, Klein S, Wolfe RR. An abundant supply of amino acids enhances the metabolic effect of exercise on muscle protein. *Am J Physiol.* (1997) 273:E122–9. doi: 10.1152/ajpendo.1997.273.1.E122
23. Jones GM, Mayer RJ. Degradation of glucose-metabolizing enzymes in the rat small intestine during starvation. *Biochem J.* (1973) 132:657–61. doi: 10.1042/bj1320657a
24. Fritz PJ, Vesell ES, White EL, Pruitt KM. The roles of synthesis and degradation in determining tissue concentrations of lactate dehydrogenase-5*. *Proc Natl Acad Sci USA.* (1969) 62:558–65. doi: 10.1073/pnas.62.2.558
25. Jaleel A, Henderson GC, Madden BJ, Klaus KA, Morse DM, Gopala S, et al. Identification of *de novo* synthesized and relatively older proteins. *Diabetes.* (2010) 59:2366–74. doi: 10.2337/db10-0371
26. Ramamurthy B, Höök P, Jones AD, Larsson L. Changes in myosin structure and function in response to glycation. *FASEB J Off Publ Fed Am Soc Exp Biol.* (2001) 15:2415–22. doi: 10.1096/fj.01-0183com
27. Watanabe H, Ogasawara M, Suzuki N, Nishizawa N, Ambo K. Glycation of myofibrillar protein in aged rats and mice. *Biosci Biotechnol Biochem.* (1992) 56:1109–12. doi: 10.1271/bbb.56.1109
28. Odessey R, Khairallah EA, Goldberg AL. Origin and possible significance of alanine production by skeletal muscle. *J Biol Chem.* (1974) 249:7623–9.
29. Felig P, Marliss E, Pozefsky T, Cahill GF. Amino acid metabolism in the regulation of gluconeogenesis in man. *Am J Clin Nutr.* (1970) 23:986–92. doi: 10.1093/ajcn/23.7.986
30. Bak AM, Møller AB, Vendelbo MH, Nielsen TS, Viggers R, Rungby J, et al. Differential regulation of lipid and protein metabolism in obese vs. lean subjects before and after a 72-h fast. *Am J Physiol Endocrinol Metab.* (2016) 311:E224–35. doi: 10.1152/ajpendo.00464.2015
31. Hodson N, Philp A. The importance of mTOR trafficking for human skeletal muscle translational control. *Exerc Sport Sci Rev.* (2019) 47:46–53. doi: 10.1249/JES.0000000000000173
32. Hodson N, McGlory C, Oikawa SY, Jeromson S, Song Z, Ruegg MA, et al. Differential localisation and anabolic responsiveness of mTOR complexes in human skeletal muscle in response to feeding and exercise. *Am J Physiol Cell Physiol.* (2017) 313:C604–11. doi: 10.1152/ajpcell.00176.2017
33. Abou Sawan S, van Vliet S, Parel JT, Beals JW, Mazzulla M, West DWD, et al. Translocation and protein complex co-localization of mTOR is associated with postprandial myofibrillar protein synthesis at rest and after endurance exercise. *Physiol Rep.* (2018) 6:13628. doi: 10.14814/phy2.13628
34. Song Z, Moore DR, Hodson N, Ward C, Dent JR, O'Leary MF, et al. Resistance exercise initiates mechanistic target of rapamycin (mTOR) translocation and protein complex co-localisation in human skeletal muscle. *Sci Rep.* (2017) 7:5028. doi: 10.1038/s41598-017-05483-x
35. Hodson N, Brown T, Joanisse S, Aguirre N, West DWD, Moore DR, et al. Characterisation of L-Type amino acid transporter 1 (LAT1) expression in human skeletal muscle by immunofluorescent microscopy. *Nutrients.* (2017) 10:23. doi: 10.3390/nu10010023
36. Moro T, Ebert SM, Adams CM, Rasmussen BB. Amino acid sensing in skeletal muscle. *Trends Endocrinol Metab.* (2016) 27:796–806. doi: 10.1016/j.tem.2016.06.010
37. Kimball SR. Integration of signals generated by nutrients, hormones, and exercise in skeletal muscle. *Am J Clin Nutr.* (2014) 99:237S–42S. doi: 10.3945/ajcn.113.068387
38. Greenhaff PL, Karagounis LG, Peirce N, Simpson EJ, Hazell M, Layfield R, et al. Disassociation between the effects of amino acids and insulin on signaling, ubiquitin ligases, and protein turnover in human muscle. *Am J Physiol Endocrinol Metab.* (2008) *295*:E595–604. doi: 10.1152/ajpendo.90411.2008
39. Wilkinson SB, Phillips SM, Atherton PJ, Patel R, Yarasheski KE, Tarnopolsky MA, et al. Differential effects of resistance and endurance exercise in the fed state on signalling molecule phosphorylation and protein synthesis in human muscle. *J Physiol.* (2008) 586:3701–17. doi: 10.1113/jphysiol.2008.153916
40. Beals JW, Skinner SK, McKenna CF, Poozhikunnel EG, Farooqi SA, van Vliet S, et al. Altered anabolic signalling and reduced stimulation of myofibrillar protein synthesis after feeding and resistance exercise in people with obesity. *J Physiol.* (2018) 596:5119–33. doi: 10.1113/JP276210
41. Tran L, Kras KA, Hoffman N, Ravichandran J, Dickinson JM, D'Lugos A, et al. Lower fasted-state but greater increase in muscle protein synthesis in response to elevated plasma amino acids in obesity. *Obesity.* (2018) 26:1179–87. doi: 10.1002/oby.22213

42. Beals JW, Sukiennik RA, Nallabelli J, Emmons RS, van Vliet S, Young JR, et al. Anabolic sensitivity of postprandial muscle protein synthesis to the ingestion of a protein-dense food is reduced in overweight and obese young adults. *Am J Clin Nutr.* (2016) 104:1014–22. doi: 10.3945/ajcn.116.130385
43. McGlory C, White A, Treins C, Drust B, Close GL, Maclaren DPM, et al. Application of the [γ-32P] ATP kinase assay to study anabolic signaling in human skeletal muscle. *J Appl Physiol Bethesda Md.* (2014) 116:504–13. doi: 10.1152/japplphysiol.01072.2013
44. Moore DR, Tang JE, Burd NA, Rerecich T, Tarnopolsky MA, Phillips SM. Differential stimulation of myofibrillar and sarcoplasmic protein synthesis with protein ingestion at rest and after resistance exercise. *J Physiol.* (2009) 587:897–904. doi: 10.1113/jphysiol.2008.164087
45. Moore DR, Atherton PJ, Rennie MJ, Tarnopolsky MA, Phillips SM. Resistance exercise enhances mTOR and MAPK signalling in human muscle over that seen at rest after bolus protein ingestion. *Acta Physiol.* (2011) 201:365–72. doi: 10.1111/j.1748-1716.2010.02187.x
46. Hyde R, Peyrollier K, Hundal HS. Insulin promotes the cell surface recruitment of the SAT2/ATA2 system A amino acid transporter from an endosomal compartment in skeletal muscle cells. *J Biol Chem.* (2002) 277:13628–34. doi: 10.1074/jbc.M108609200
47. Yang Y, Breen L, Burd NA, Hector AJ, Churchward-Venne TA, Josse AR, et al. Resistance exercise enhances myofibrillar protein synthesis with graded intakes of whey protein in older men. *Br J Nutr.* (2012) 108:1780–8. doi: 10.1017/S0007114511007422
48. Moore DR, Churchward-Venne TA, Witard O, Breen L, Burd NA, Tipton KD, et al. Protein ingestion to stimulate myofibrillar protein synthesis requires greater relative protein intakes in healthy older versus younger men. *J Gerontol A Biol Sci Med Sci.* (2014) 70:57–62. doi: 10.1093/gerona/glu103
49. Moore DR, Robinson MJ, Fry JL, Tang JE, Glover EI, Wilkinson SB, et al. Ingested protein dose response of muscle and albumin protein synthesis after resistance exercise in young men. *Am J Clin Nutr.* (2009) 89:161–8. doi: 10.3945/ajcn.2008.26401
50. Robinson MJ, Burd NA, Breen L, Rerecich T, Yang Y, Hector AJ, et al. Dose-dependent responses of myofibrillar protein synthesis with beef ingestion are enhanced with resistance exercise in middle-aged men. *Appl Physiol Nutr Metab.* (2012) 38:120–5. doi: 10.1139/apnm-2012-0092
51. Burd NA, Beals JW, Martinez IG, Salvador AF, Skinner SK. Food-first approach to enhance the regulation of post-exercise skeletal muscle protein synthesis and remodeling. *Sports Med Auckl NZ.* (2019) 49:59–68. doi: 10.1007/s40279-018-1009-y
52. Phillips SM, Chevalier S, Leidy HJ. Protein "requirements" beyond the RDA: implications for optimizing health. *Appl Physiol Nutr Metab Physiol Appliquée Nutr Métabo.* (2016) 41:565–72. doi: 10.1139/apnm-2015-0550
53. Rooyackers OE, Balagopal P, Nair KS. Measurement of synthesis rates of specific muscle proteins using needle biopsy samples. *Muscle Nerve Suppl.* (1997) 5:S93–96.
54. Burd NA, West DWD, Moore DR, Atherton PJ, Staples AW, Prior T, et al. Enhanced amino acid sensitivity of myofibrillar protein synthesis persists for up to 24 h after resistance exercise in young men. *J Nutr.* (2011) 141:568–73. doi: 10.3945/jn.110.135038
55. Robinson MM, Soop M, Sohn TS, Morse DM, Schimke JM, Klaus KA, et al. High insulin combined with essential amino acids stimulates skeletal muscle mitochondrial protein synthesis while decreasing insulin sensitivity in healthy humans. *J Clin Endocrinol Metab.* (2014) 99:E2574–83. doi: 10.1210/jc.2014-2736
56. Donges CE, Burd NA, Duffield R, Smith GC, West DWD, Short MJ, et al. Concurrent resistance and aerobic exercise stimulates both myofibrillar and mitochondrial protein synthesis in sedentary middle-aged men. *J Appl Physiol.* (2012) 112:1992–2001. doi: 10.1152/japplphysiol.00166.2012
57. Rooyackers OE, Adey DB, Ades PA, Nair KS. Effect of age on *in vivo* rates of mitochondrial protein synthesis in human skeletal muscle. *Proc Natl Acad Sci USA.* (1996) 93:15364–69. doi: 10.1073/pnas.93.26.15364
58. Guillet C, Delcourt I, Rance M, Giraudet C, Walrand S, Bedu M, et al. Changes in basal and insulin and amino acid response of whole body and skeletal muscle proteins in obese men. *J Clin Endocrinol Metab.* (2009) 94:3044–50. doi: 10.1210/jc.2008-2216
59. Murton AJ, Marimuthu K, Mallinson JE, Selby AL, Smith K, Rennie MJ, et al. Obesity appears to be associated with altered muscle protein synthetic and breakdown responses to increased nutrient delivery in older men, but not reduced muscle mass or contractile function. *Diabetes.* (2015) 64:3160–71. doi: 10.2337/db15-0021
60. Smeuninx B, Mckendry J, Wilson D, Martin U, Breen L. Age-related anabolic resistance of myofibrillar protein synthesis is exacerbated in obese inactive individuals. *J Clin Endocrinol Metab.* (2017) 102:3535–45. doi: 10.1210/jc.2017-00869
61. Chevalier S, Burgos SA, Morais JA, Gougeon R, Bassil M, Lamarche M, et al. Protein and glucose metabolic responses to hyperinsulinemia, hyperglycemia, and hyperaminoacidemia in obese men. *Obesity.* (2015) 23:351–8. doi: 10.1002/oby.20943
62. Beals JW, Mackenzie RWA, van Vliet S, Skinner SK, Pagni BA, Niemiro GM, et al. Protein-rich food ingestion stimulates mitochondrial protein synthesis in sedentary young adults of different BMIs. *J Clin Endocrinol Metab.* (2017) 102:3415–24. doi: 10.1210/jc.2017-00360
63. Griffin ME, Marcucci MJ, Cline GW, Bell K, Barucci N, Lee D, et al. Free fatty acid-induced insulin resistance is associated with activation of protein kinase C theta and alterations in the insulin signaling cascade. *Diabetes.* (1999) 48:1270–4. doi: 10.2337/diabetes.48.6.1270
64. Bohé J, Low JFA, Wolfe RR, Rennie MJ. Latency and duration of stimulation of human muscle protein synthesis during continuous infusion of amino acids. *J Physiol.* (2001) 532:575–9. doi: 10.1111/j.1469-7793.2001.0575f.x
65. van Vliet S, Shy EL, Sawan SA, Beals JW, West DW, Skinner SK, et al. Consumption of whole eggs promotes greater stimulation of postexercise muscle protein synthesis than consumption of isonitrogenous amounts of egg whites in young men. *Am J Clin Nutr.* (2017) 106:1401–12. doi: 10.3945/ajcn.117.159855
66. Burd NA, Gorissen SH, van Vliet S, Snijders T, Loon LJ. van Differences in postprandial protein handling after beef compared with milk ingestion during postexercise recovery: a randomized controlled trial. *Am J Clin Nutr.* (2015) 102:828–36. doi: 10.3945/ajcn.114.103184
67. Sukkar MY, Hunter WM, Passmore R. Changes in plasma levels of insulin and growth-hormone levels after a protein meal. *Lancet.* (1967) 290:1020–2. doi: 10.1016/S0140-6736(67)90291-7
68. Mithieux G. Metabolic effects of portal vein sensing. *Diabetes Obes Metab.* (2014) 16:56–60. doi: 10.1111/dom.12338
69. de Lartigue G, Diepenbroek C. Novel developments in vagal afferent nutrient sensing and its role in energy homeostasis. *Curr Opin Pharmacol.* (2016) 31:38–43. doi: 10.1016/j.coph.2016.08.007
70. Lindgren O, Pacini G, Tura A, Holst JJ, Deacon CF, Ahrén B. Incretin effect after oral amino acid ingestion in humans. *J Clin Endocrinol Metab.* (2015) 100:1172–6. doi: 10.1210/jc.2014-3865
71. Williamson DL, Dungan CM, Mahmoud AM, Mey JT, Blackburn BK, Haus JM. Aberrant REDD1-mTORC1 responses to insulin in skeletal muscle from Type 2 diabetics. *Am J Physiol Regul Integr Comp Physiol.* (2015) 309:R855–63. doi: 10.1152/ajpregu.00285.2015
72. Hulston CJ, Woods RM, Dewhurst-Trigg R, Parry SA, Gagnon S, Baker L, et al. Resistance exercise stimulates mixed muscle protein synthesis in lean and obese young adults. *Physiol Rep.* (2018) 6:13799. doi: 10.14814/phy2.13799
73. Root HF, Carpenter TM. Studies of carbohydrate metabolism in cases of insulin resistance. *Trans Am Clin Climatol Assoc.* (1940) 56:1–11.
74. Lister J, Nash J, Ledingham U. Constitution and insulin sensitivity in diabetes mellitus. *Br Med J.* (1951) 1:376–9. doi: 10.1136/bmj.1.4703.376
75. Newgard CB, An J, Bain JR, Muehlbauer MJ, Stevens RD, Lien LF, et al. A branched-chain amino acid-related metabolic signature that differentiates obese and lean humans and contributes to insulin resistance. *Cell Metab.* (2009) 9:311–26. doi: 10.1016/j.cmet.2009.02.002
76. Felig P, Marliss E, Cahill GF. Plasma amino acid levels and insulin secretion in obesity. *N Engl J Med.* (1969) 281:811–6. doi: 10.1056/NEJM196910092811503
77. Lerin C, Goldfine AB, Boes T, Liu M, Kasif S, Dreyfuss JM, et al. Defects in muscle branched-chain amino acid oxidation contribute to impaired lipid metabolism. *Mol Metab.* (2016) 5:926–36. doi: 10.1016/j.molmet.2016.08.001
78. Tai ES, Tan MLS, Stevens RD, Low YL, Muehlbauer MJ, Goh DLM, et al. Insulin resistance is associated with a metabolic profile of altered protein metabolism in Chinese and Asian-Indian men. *Diabetologia.* (2010) 53:757–67. doi: 10.1007/s00125-009-1637-8

79. Boulet MM, Chevrier G, Grenier-Larouche T, Pelletier M, Nadeau M, Scarpa J, et al. Alterations of plasma metabolite profiles related to adipose tissue distribution and cardiometabolic risk. *Am J Physiol Endocrinol Metab.* (2015) 309:E736–46. doi: 10.1152/ajpendo.00231.2015
80. Würtz P, Mäkinen V-P, Soininen P, Kangas AJ, Tukiainen T, Kettunen J, et al. Metabolic signatures of insulin resistance in 7,098 young adults. *Diabetes.* (2012) 61:1372–80. doi: 10.2337/db11-1355
81. Wang TJ, Larson MG, Vasan RS, Cheng S, Rhee EP, McCabe E, et al. Metabolite profiles and the risk of developing diabetes. *Nat Med.* (2011) 17:448–53. doi: 10.1038/nm.2307
82. Gannon NP, Schnuck JK, Vaughan RA. BCAA metabolism and insulin sensitivity - dysregulated by metabolic status? *Mol Nutr Food Res.* (2018) 62:e1700756. doi: 10.1002/mnfr.201700756
83. Lynch CJ, Adams SH. Branched-chain amino acids in metabolic signalling and insulin resistance. *Nat Rev Endocrinol.* (2014) 10:723–36. doi: 10.1038/nrendo.2014.171
84. Gran P, Larsen AE, Bonham M, Dordevic AL, Rupasinghe T, Silva C, et al. Muscle p70S6K phosphorylation in response to soy and dairy rich meals in middle aged men with metabolic syndrome: a randomised crossover trial. *Nutr Metab.* (2014) 11:46. doi: 10.1186/1743-7075-11-46
85. Golay A, Swislocki AM, Chen YDI, Jaspan JB, Reaven GM. Effect of obesity on ambient plasma glucose, free fatty acid, insulin, growth hormone, and glucagon concentrations. *J Clin Endocrinol Metab.* (1986) 63:481–4. doi: 10.1210/jcem-63-2-481
86. Boden G, Jadali F, White J, Liang Y, Mozzoli M, Chen X, Coleman E, Smith, C. Effects of fat on insulin-stimulated carbohydrate metabolism in normal men. *J. Clin. Invest.* (1991) 88:960–6. doi: 10.1172/JCI115399
87. Stephens FB, Chee C, Wall BT, Murton AJ, Shannon CE, van Loon LJC, et al. Lipid induced insulin resistance is associated with an impaired skeletal muscle protein synthetic response to amino acid ingestion in healthy young men. *Diabetes.* (2014) 64:1615–20. doi: 10.2337/db14-0961
88. Goodpaster BH, He J, Watkins S, Kelley DE. Skeletal muscle lipid content and insulin resistance: evidence for a paradox in endurance-trained athletes. *J Clin Endocrinol Metab.* (2001) 86:5755–61. doi: 10.1210/jc.86.12.5755
89. Daemen S, Gemmink A, Brouwers B, Meex RCR, Huntjens PR, Schaart G, et al. Distinct lipid droplet characteristics and distribution unmask the apparent contradiction of the athlete's paradox. *Mol Metab.* (2018) 17:71–81. doi: 10.1016/j.molmet.2018.08.004
90. Lee JS, Pinnamaneni SK, Eo SJ, Cho IH, Pyo JH, Kim CK, et al. Saturated, but not n-6 polyunsaturated, fatty acids induce insulin resistance: role of intramuscular accumulation of lipid metabolites. *J Appl Physiol.* (2006) 100:1467–74. doi: 10.1152/japplphysiol.01438.2005
91. Perreault L, Newsom SA, Strauss A, Kerege A, Kahn DE, Harrison KA, et al. Intracellular localization of diacylglycerols and sphingolipids influences insulin sensitivity and mitochondrial function in human skeletal muscle. *JCI Insight.* (2018) 3:96805. doi: 10.1172/jci.insight.96805
92. Hla T, Kolesnick R. C16:0-ceramide signals insulin resistance. *Cell Metab.* (2014) 20:703–5. doi: 10.1016/j.cmet.2014.10.017
93. Bergman BC, Brozinick JT, Strauss A, Bacon S, Kerege A, Bui HH, et al. Muscle sphingolipids during rest and exercise: a C18:0 signature for insulin resistance in humans. *Diabetologia.* (2016) 59:785–98. doi: 10.1007/s00125-015-3850-y
94. Hyde R, Hajduch E, Powell DJ, Taylor PM, Hundal HS. Ceramide down-regulates System a amino acid transport and protein synthesis in rat skeletal muscle cells. *FASEB J.* (2004) 19:461–3. doi: 10.1096/fj.04-2284fje
95. Timmerman KL, Lee JL, Dreyer HC, Dhanani S, Glynn EL, Fry CS, et al. Insulin stimulates human skeletal muscle protein synthesis via an indirect mechanism involving endothelial-dependent vasodilation and mammalian target of rapamycin complex 1 signaling. *J Clin Endocrinol Metab.* (2010) 95:3848–57. doi: 10.1210/jc.2009-2696
96. Timmerman KL, Dhanani S, Glynn EL, Fry CS, Drummond MJ, Jennings K, et al. A moderate acute increase in physical activity enhances nutritive flow and the muscle protein anabolic response to mixed nutrient intake in older adults. *Am J Clin Nutr.* (2012) 95:1403–12. doi: 10.3945/ajcn.111.020800
97. Moore DR, Kelly RP, Devries MC, Churchward-Venne TA, Phillips SM, Parise G, et al. Low-load resistance exercise during inactivity is associated with greater fibre area and satellite cell expression in older skeletal muscle. *J Cachexia Sarcopenia Muscle.* (2018) 9:747–54. doi: 10.1002/jcsm.12306
98. Devries MC, Breen L, Von Allmen M, MacDonald MJ, Moore DR, Offord EA, et al. Low-load resistance training during step-reduction attenuates declines in muscle mass and strength and enhances anabolic sensitivity in older men. *Physiol Rep.* (2015) 3:12493. doi: 10.14814/phy2.12493
99. Snijders T, Nederveen JP, Verdijk LB, Houben AJHM, Goossens GH, Parise G, et al. Muscle fiber capillarization as determining factor on indices of insulin sensitivity in humans. *Physiol Rep.* (2017) 5:13278. doi: 10.14814/phy2.13278
100. Gavin TP, Stallings HW, Zwetsloot KA, Westerkamp LM, Ryan NA, Moore RA, et al. Lower capillary density but no difference in VEGF expression in obese vs. lean young skeletal muscle in humans. *J Appl Physiol Bethesda Md 1985.* (2005) 98:315–21. doi: 10.1152/japplphysiol.00353.2004
101. Clerk LH, Vincent MA, Jahn LA, Liu Z, Lindner JR, Barrett EJ. Obesity blunts insulin-mediated microvascular recruitment in human forearm muscle. *Diabetes.* (2006) 55:1436–42. doi: 10.2337/db05-1373
102. Samocha-Bonet D, Dixit VD, Kahn CR, Leibel RL, Lin X, Nieuwdorp M, et al. Metabolically healthy and unhealthy obese – the 2013 Stock Conference report. *Obes Rev Off J Int Assoc Study Obes.* (2014) 15:697–708. doi: 10.1111/obr.12199
103. Kitahara CM, Trabert B, Katki HA, Chaturvedi AK, Kemp TJ, Pinto LA, et al. Body mass index, physical activity, and serum markers of inflammation, immunity, and insulin resistance. *Cancer Epidemiol Biomarkers Prev.* (2014) 23:2840–9. doi: 10.1158/1055-9965.EPI-14-0699-T
104. Dali-Youcef N, Mecili M, Ricci R, Andrès E. Metabolic inflammation: connecting obesity and insulin resistance. *Ann Med.* (2013) 45:242–53. doi: 10.3109/07853890.2012.705015
105. Volpe CMO, Nogueira-Machado JA. The dual role of free fatty acid signaling in inflammation and therapeutics. *Recent Pat Endocr Metab Immune Drug Discov.* (2013) 7:189–97. doi: 10.2174/187153031131399 90041
106. Guillet C, Masgrau A, Walrand S, Boirie Y. Impaired protein metabolism: interlinks between obesity, insulin resistance and inflammation. *Obes Rev.* (2012) 13:51–7. doi: 10.1111/j.1467-789X.2012.01037.x
107. Porter C, Hurren NM, Herndon DN, Børsheim E. Whole body and skeletal muscle protein turnover in recovery from burns. *Int J Burns Trauma.* (2013) 3:9–17.
108. van Vliet S, Skinner SK, Beals JW, Pagni BA, Fang H-Y, Ulanov AV, et al. Dysregulated handling of dietary protein and muscle protein synthesis after mixed-meal ingestion in maintenance hemodialysis patients. *Kidney Int Rep.* (2018) 3:1403–15. doi: 10.1016/j.ekir.2018.08.001
109. Wåhlin-Larsson B, Wilkinson DJ, Strandberg E, Hosford-Donovan A, Atherton PJ, Kadi F. Mechanistic links underlying the impact of c-reactive protein on muscle mass in elderly. *Cell Physiol Biochem Int J Exp Cell Physiol Biochem Pharmacol.* (2017) 44:267–78. doi: 10.1159/000484679
110. Lang CH, Frost RA, Nairn AC, MacLean DA, Vary TC. TNF-alpha impairs heart and skeletal muscle protein synthesis by altering translation initiation. *Am J Physiol Endocrinol Metab.* (2002) 282:E336–47. doi: 10.1152/ajpendo.00366.2001
111. Buffière C, Mariotti F, Savary-Auzeloux I, Migné C, Meunier N, Hercberg S, et al. Slight chronic elevation of C-reactive protein is associated with lower aerobic fitness but does not impair meal-induced stimulation of muscle protein metabolism in healthy old men. *J Physiol.* (2015) 593:1259–72. doi: 10.1113/jphysiol.2014.286054
112. Dideriksen K, Reitelseder S, Malmgaard-Clausen NM, Bechshoeft R, Petersen RK, Mikkelsen UR, et al. No effect of anti-inflammatory medication on postprandial and postexercise muscle protein synthesis in elderly men with slightly elevated systemic inflammation. *Exp Gerontol.* (2016) 83:120–9. doi: 10.1016/j.exger.2016.07.016
113. Chow JC, Young DW, Golenbock DT, Christ WJ, Gusovsky F. Toll-like receptor-4 mediates lipopolysaccharide-induced signal transduction. *J Biol Chem.* (1999) 274:10689–92. doi: 10.1074/jbc.274.16.10689
114. Shi H, Kokoeva MV, Inouye K, Tzameli I, Yin H, Flier JS. TLR4 links innate immunity and fatty acid–induced insulin resistance. *J Clin Invest.* (2006) 116:3015–25. doi: 10.1172/JCI28898
115. Liu N, Liu J-T, Ji Y-Y, Lu P-P. C-reactive protein triggers inflammatory responses partly via TLR4/IRF3/NF-κB signaling pathway in rat vascular smooth muscle cells. *Life Sci.* (2010) 87:367–74. doi: 10.1016/j.lfs.2010.0 7.012

116. Kwon OS, Tanner RE, Barrows KM, Runtsch M, Symons JD, Jalili T, et al. MyD88 regulates physical inactivity-induced skeletal muscle inflammation, ceramide biosynthesis signaling, and glucose intolerance. *Am J Physiol Endocrinol Metab.* (2015) 309:E11–21. doi: 10.1152/ajpendo.00124.2015
117. Timmerman KL, Connors ID, Deal MA, Mott RE. Skeletal muscle TLR4 and TACE are associated with body fat percentage in older adults. *Appl Physiol Nutr Metab.* (2016) 41:446–51. doi: 10.1139/apnm-2015-0567
118. Ekelund U, Steene-Johannessen J, Brown WJ, Fagerland MW, Owen N, Powell KE, Bauman A, et al. Does physical activity attenuate, or even eliminate, the detrimental association of sitting time with mortality? A harmonised meta-analysis of data from more than 1 million men and women. *Lancet.* (2016) 388:1302–10. doi: 10.1016/S0140-6736(16)30370-1
119. Kanagasabai T, Thakkar NA, Kuk JL, Churilla JR, Ardern CI. Differences in physical activity domains, guideline adherence, and weight history between metabolically healthy and metabolically abnormal obese adults: a cross-sectional study. *Int J Behav Nutr Phys Act.* (2015) 12:227. doi: 10.1186/s12966-015-0227-z
120. Stenholm S, Harris TB, Rantanen T, Visser M, Kritchevsky SB, Ferrucci, L. Sarcopenic obesity - definition, etiology and consequences. *Curr Opin Clin Nutr Metab Care.* (2008) 11:693–700. doi: 10.1097/MCO.0b013e328312c37d
121. Koopman R, Manders RJF, Zorenc AHG, Hul GBJ, Kuipers H, Keizer HA, et al. A single session of resistance exercise enhances insulin sensitivity for at least 24 h in healthy men. *Eur J Appl Physiol.* (2005) 94:180–7. doi: 10.1007/s00421-004-1307-y
122. Whyte LJ, Ferguson C, Wilson J, Scott RA, Gill JMR. Effects of single bout of very high-intensity exercise on metabolic health biomarkers in overweight/obese sedentary men. *Metabolism.* (2013) 62:212–9. doi: 10.1016/j.metabol.2012.07.019
123. Short KR, Vittone JL, Bigelow ML, Proctor DN, Rizza RA, Coenen-Schimke JM, et al. Impact of aerobic exercise training on age-related changes in insulin sensitivity and muscle oxidative capacity. *Diabetes.* (2003) 52:1888–96. doi: 10.2337/diabetes.52.8.1888
124. Ashor AW, Lara J, Siervo M, Celis-Morales C, Oggioni C, Jakovljevic DG, et al. Exercise modalities and endothelial function: a systematic review and dose-response meta-analysis of randomized controlled trials. *Sports Med Auckl NZ.* (2015) 45:279–96. doi: 10.1007/s40279-014-0272-9
125. Paris HL, Foright RM, Werth KA, Larson LC, Beals JW, Cox-York K, et al. Increasing energy flux to decrease the biological drive toward weight regain after weight loss – A proof-of-concept pilot study. *Clin Nutr ESPEN.* (2015) 11:e12–20. doi: 10.1016/j.clnesp.2015.11.005
126. Manore MM, Larson-Meyer DE, Lindsay AR, Hongu N, Houtkooper L. Dynamic energy balance: an integrated framework for discussing diet and physical activity in obesity prevention—is it more than eating less and exercising more? *Nutrients.* (2017) 9:9080905. doi: 10.3390/nu9080905
127. Wilburn JR, Bourquin J, Wysong A, Melby CL. Resistance exercise attenuates high-fructose, high-fat-induced postprandial lipemia. *Nutr Metab Insights.* (2015) 8:29–35. doi: 10.4137/NMI.S32106
128. Pennings B, Koopman R, Beelen M, Senden JM, Saris WH, van Loon LJ. Exercising before protein intake allows for greater use of dietary protein-derived amino acids for *de novo* muscle protein synthesis in both young and elderly men. *Am J Clin Nutr.* (2011) 93:322–31. doi: 10.3945/ajcn.2010.29649
129. Phillips SM, Tipton KD, Ferrando AA, Wolfe RR. Resistance training reduces the acute exercise-induced increase in muscle protein turnover. *Am J Physiol Endocrinol Metab.* (1999) 276:E118–24. doi: 10.1152/ajpendo.1999.276.1.E118
130. Jaleel A, Short KR, Asmann YW, Klaus KA, Morse DM, Ford GC, Nair KS. *In vivo* measurement of synthesis rate of individual skeletal muscle mitochondrial proteins. *Am J Physiol Endocrinol Metab.* (2008) 295:E1255–68. doi: 10.1152/ajpendo.90586.2008
131. Mittendorfer B, Andersen J, Plomgaard P, Saltin B, Babraj J, Smith K, et al. Protein synthesis rates in human muscles: neither anatomical location nor fibre-type composition are major determinants. *J Physiol.* (2005) 563:203–11. doi: 10.1113/jphysiol.2004.077180
132. You J-S, Lincoln HC, Kim C-R, Frey JW, Goodman CA, Zhong X-P, et al. The role of diacylglycerol kinase ζ and phosphatidic acid in the mechanical activation of mammalian target of rapamycin (mTOR) signaling and skeletal muscle hypertrophy. *J Biol Chem.* (2014) 289:1551–63. doi: 10.1074/jbc.M113.531392
133. Hornberger TA, Chu WK, Mak YW, Hsiung JW, Huang SA, Chien S. The role of phospholipase D and phosphatidic acid in the mechanical activation of mTOR signaling in skeletal muscle. *Proc Natl Acad Sci U S A.* (2006) 103:4741–6. doi: 10.1073/pnas.0600678103
134. Jacobs BL, You J-S, Frey JW, Goodman CA, Gundermann DM, Hornberger TA. Eccentric contractions increase the phosphorylation of tuberous sclerosis complex-2 (TSC2) and alter the targeting of TSC2 and the mechanistic target of rapamycin to the lysosome. *J Physiol.* (2013) 591:4611–20. doi: 10.1113/jphysiol.2013.256339
135. Abou Sawan S, van Vliet S, West DWD, Beals JW, Paluska SA, Burd NA, et al. Whole egg, but not egg white, ingestion induces mTOR colocalization with the lysosome after resistance exercise. *Am J Physiol Cell Physiol.* (2018) 315:C537–43. doi: 10.1152/ajpcell.00225.2018
136. Mebarek S, Komati H, Naro F, Zeiller C, Alvisi M, Lagarde M, et al. Inhibition of *de novo* ceramide synthesis upregulates phospholipase D and enhances myogenic differentiation. *J Cell Sci.* (2007) 120:407–16. doi: 10.1242/jcs.03331
137. Sanal E, Ardic F, Kirac S. Effects of aerobic or combined aerobic resistance exercise on body composition in overweight and obese adults: gender differences. a randomized intervention study. *Eur J Phys Rehabil Med.* (2013) 49:1–11.
138. Smiles WJ, Churchward-Venne TA, van Loon LJC, Hawley JA, Camera DM. A single bout of strenuous exercise overcomes lipid-induced anabolic resistance to protein ingestion in overweight, middle-aged men. *FASEB J Off Publ Fed Am Soc Exp Biol.* (2019). doi: 10.1096/fj.201801917R. [Epub ahead of print].
139. Smith GI, Villareal DT, Sinacore DR, Shah K, Mittendorfer B. Muscle protein synthesis response to exercise training in obese, older men and women. *Med Sci Sports Exerc.* (2012) 44:1259–66. doi: 10.1249/MSS.0b013e3182496a41
140. Villareal DT, Smith GI, Sinacore DR, Shah K, Mittendorfer B. Regular multicomponent exercise increases physical fitness and muscle protein anabolism in frail, obese, older adults. *Obesity.* (2011) 19:312–8. doi: 10.1038/oby.2010.110
141. Villareal DT, Smith GI, Shah K, Mittendorfer B. Effect of weight loss on the rate of muscle protein synthesis during fasted and fed conditions in obese older adults. *Obes Silver Spring Md.* (2012) 20:1780–6. doi: 10.1038/oby.2011.280
142. Pasiakos SM, Cao JJ, Margolis LM, Sauter ER, Whigham LD, McClung JP, et al. Effects of high-protein diets on fat-free mass and muscle protein synthesis following weight loss: a randomized controlled trial. *FASEB J Off Publ Fed Am Soc Exp Biol.* (2013) 27:3837–47. doi: 10.1096/fj.13-230227
143. Hector AJ, McGlory C, Damas F, Mazara N, Baker SK, Phillips SM. Pronounced energy restriction with elevated protein intake results in no change in proteolysis and reductions in skeletal muscle protein synthesis that are mitigated by resistance exercise. *FASEB J Off Publ Fed Am SocExp Biol.* (2018) 32:265–75. doi: 10.1096/fj.201700158RR
144. Leidy HJ, Clifton PM, Astrup A, Wycherley TP, Westerterp-Plantenga MS, Luscombe-Marsh ND, et al. The role of protein in weight loss and maintenance. *Am J Clin Nutr.* (2015) 101:1320S—9S. doi: 10.3945/ajcn.114.084038
145. Perreault L, Bergman BC, Playdon MC, Dalla Man C, Cobelli C, Eckel RH. Impaired fasting glucose with or without impaired glucose tolerance: progressive or parallel states of prediabetes? *Am J Physiol Endocrinol Metab.* (2008) 295:E428–35. doi: 10.1152/ajpendo.90354.2008
146. American College of Sports Medicine. American college of sports medicine position stand. progression models in resistance training for healthy adults. *Med Sci Sports Exerc.* (2009) 41:687–708. doi: 10.1249/MSS.0b013e3181915670
147. CSEP. *Canadian Society for Exercise Physiology – Home.* Available online at: http://csep.ca/home (accessed March 14, 2018).
148. Donnelly JE, Blair SN, Jakicic JM, Manore MM, Rankin JW, Smith BK, American college of sports medicine american college of sports medicine position stand. appropriate physical activity intervention strategies for weight loss and prevention of weight regain for adults. *Med Sci Sports Exerc.* (2009) 41:459–71. doi: 10.1249/MSS.0b013e3181949333
149. Kumar V, Atherton PJ, Selby A, Rankin D, Williams J, Smith K, et al. Muscle protein synthetic responses to exercise: effects of age, volume, and intensity. *J Gerontol Ser A.* (2012) 67:1170–7. doi: 10.1093/gerona/gls141

150. Devries MC, McGlory C, Bolster DR, Kamil A, Rahn M, Harkness L, et al. Leucine, not total protein, content of a supplement is the primary determinant of muscle protein anabolic responses in healthy older women. *J Nutr.* (2018) 148:1088–95. doi: 10.1093/jn/nxy091

151. Devries MC, McGlory C, Bolster DR, Kamil A, Rahn M, Harkness L, et al. Protein leucine content is a determinant of shorter- and longer-term muscle protein synthetic responses at rest and following resistance exercise in healthy older women: a randomized, controlled trial. *Am J Clin Nutr.* (2018) 107:217–26. doi: 10.1093/ajcn/nqx028

5

Maximizing Post-Exercise Anabolism: The Case for Relative Protein Intakes

Daniel R. Moore*

Faculty of Kinesiology and Physical Education, University of Toronto, Toronto, ON, Canada

***Correspondence:**
Daniel R. Moore
dr.moore@utoronto.ca

Maximizing the post-exercise increase in muscle protein synthesis, especially of the contractile myofibrillar protein fraction, is essential to facilitate effective muscle remodeling, and enhance hypertrophic gains with resistance training. MPS is the primary regulated variable influencing muscle net balance with dietary amino acid ingestion representing the single most important nutritional variable enhancing post-exercise rates of muscle protein synthesis. Dose-response studies in average (i.e., ~80 kg) males have reported an absolute 20 g dose of high quality, rapidly digested protein maximizes mixed, and myofibrillar protein synthetic rates. However, it is unclear if these absolute protein intakes can be viewed in a "one size fits all" solution. Re-analysis of published literature in young adults suggests a relative single meal intake of ~0.31 g/kg of rapidly digested, high quality protein (i.e., whey) should be considered as a nutritional guideline for individuals of average body composition aiming to maximize post-exercise myofibrillar protein synthesis while minimizing irreversible amino acid oxidative catabolism that occurs with excessive intakes of this macronutrient. This muscle-specific bolus intake is lower than that reported to maximize whole body anabolism (i.e., ≥0.5 g/kg). Review of the available literature suggests that potential confounders such as the co-ingestion of carbohydrate, sex, and amount of active muscle mass do not represent significant barriers to the translation of this objectively determined relative protein intake. Additional research is warranted to elucidate the effective dose for proteins with suboptimal amino acid compositions (e.g., plant-based), and/or slower digestion rates as well as whether recommendations are appreciably affected by other physiological conditions such endurance exercise, high habitual daily protein ingestion, aging, obesity, and/or periods of chronic negative energy balance.

Keywords: muscle protein synthesis, muscle hypertrophy, resistance training, essential amino acids, dietary protein, lean body mass, recovery

INTRODUCTION

Lean body tissues, including skeletal muscle, are constantly being remodeled through the continuous and simultaneous processes of protein synthesis, and protein breakdown (collectively referred to as "turnover"). This constant turnover functions to breakdown old and/or damaged proteins and synthesize new proteins to help maintain protein mass and quality. Importantly, the algebraic difference between synthesis and breakdown determines net protein balance of a given tissue (e.g., muscle) and, ultimately, whether it is gaining or losing mass. To this end, resistance exercise increases muscle protein turnover for up to 48 h in the fasted state (1). Due to the greater stimulation of muscle protein synthesis compared to breakdown, muscle net balance is improved but, in the absence of exogenous amino acids, remains in a net negative balance (1, 2). It is only until a source of exogenous amino acids that net balance becomes positive due primarily the enhancement of muscle protein synthesis (3). Ultimately, the synergistic effects of resistance exercise and amino acid ingestion provides the requisite anabolic environment to support net tissue growth (i.e., muscle hypertrophy) characteristic of resistance training.

Notwithstanding the technical and logistical challenges associated with measuring rates of muscle protein breakdown in humans (especially in the postprandial state) (4), muscle protein synthesis is generally regarded as the prime-regulated variable in healthy humans in response to exercise and/or nutrition (5, 6). For example, the characteristic increase in muscle protein breakdown that occurs after resistance exercise in the fasted state is negated by the provision of exogenous amino acids, which subsequently supports greater rates of muscle protein synthesis, and an increased (and positive) net protein balance (3). The post-exercise increase in muscle protein synthesis that occurs with the ingestion of different dietary proteins (e.g., milk vs. soy) has also been shown to qualitatively predict training-induced increases in muscle hypertrophy and lean mass gains in young individuals (7–9). Importantly, measurement of the contractile myofibrillar protein subfraction, which is preferentially enhanced by resistance exercise and protein/amino acid ingestion (10–12), enhances the predictive ability of long-term (i.e., 24–48 h) rates of synthesis for muscle hypertrophy (13). Thus, identifying nutritional factors that may augment the exercise-induced increase in myofibrillar protein synthesis during this prolonged (i.e., >24 h) recovery period would ostensibly be an effective strategy to promote muscle hypertrophy. Therefore, the present review will focus on how dietary protein ingestion enhances post-exercise rates of muscle protein synthesis with a focus on the contractile myofibrillar protein fraction as a means to enhance recovery from, and adaptation to resistance exercise. The overall aim of this review will be to objectively determine the "optimal" relative bolus protein ingestion during the post-exercise recovery period as defined by one that maximizes myofibrillar protein synthesis while concomitantly minimizing estimated rates of amino acid oxidation. Potential biological (e.g., sex, age, body composition, active muscle mass), and nutritional (e.g., macronutrient co-ingestion, habitual protein intake, food matrix) confounders will be discussed to explore potential translational issues with recommending a per meal relative protein intake based on a preponderance of studies in young adults utilizing an isolated protein source (i.e., whey).

REGULATION OF MUSCLE PROTEIN SYNTHESIS AFTER EXERCISE BY DIETARY AMINO ACIDS

Since the first observations that skeletal muscle protein turnover is elevated in response to resistance exercise and that exogenous amino acids augment the increase in net protein balance of this tissue (2, 3), studies have investigated the nutritional factors that contribute to the optimal enhancement of post-exercise anabolism. This line of research has revealed that the most critical factor to enhance post-exercise muscle protein synthesis is the provision of dietary amino acids with the essential amino acids (EAA) primarily driving the response (14–17). A series of seminal studies from the Wolfe laboratory were the first to suggest a potential amino acid dose-response existed during recovery from resistance exercise in humans (15, 17, 18). These parallel studies demonstrated that lower EAA intakes (6–12 g) were associated with an apparent graded increase in muscle net balance (17, 18). When amino acid intakes were greater (i.e., 15 vs. 40 g EAA) there was a similar increase in post-exercise anabolism (15), suggestive of a potential ceiling effect. These seminal studies performed with crystalline amino acids provided the framework for future research into the nutritional regulation of post-exercise muscle protein synthesis. Importantly, as dietary amino acids are generally consumed as complete proteins, the next wave of muscle protein metabolism research investigated the ability of dietary protein to enhance post-exercise muscle remodeling.

ABSOLUTE PROTEIN INTAKE TO MAXIMIZE POST-EXERCISE MPS

The first study to address the post-exercise ingested protein dose-response required healthy young resistance trained subjects with an average body mass of ~86 kg to perform a bout of heavy bilateral leg-based resistance exercise (i.e., leg press, knee extension, leg curl) before ingesting a variable amount of egg protein to enhance mixed muscle protein synthesis (19). Consistent with earlier results using crystalline amino acids (17, 18, 20), it was observed that even small amounts of protein (i.e., 5 and 10 g) were sufficient to enhance post-exercise mixed muscle protein synthesis (19). Importantly, mixed muscle protein synthesis was further enhanced by 20 g of protein but revealed an apparent plateau as a doubling of ingested protein to 40 g had no additive effect on the post-exercise protein synthetic response. These data ultimately conformed to a one-phase exponential decay relationship (**Figure 1**) that is characteristic of many allosterically regulated enzymes of the body, such as those within the mTOR pathway that control mRNA translation and muscle protein synthesis (21, 22), and is consistent with a ingested protein dose-response curve. It was subsequently demonstrated that the myofibrillar protein fraction displays a similar ingested protein dose-response relationship with 20 g of whey protein eliciting a maximal synthetic response (23). A unique feature of the study by Witard et al. (23) was that the post-exercise whey protein dose-response occurred ~4 h after participants consumed a high protein (~30% energy) breakfast, highlighting that the pre-exercise nutritional state (i.e., fasted vs. fed) does not appear to have a substantial impact on the post-exercise protein requirement to maximize muscle protein synthesis. This may be particular relevant for many athletes who have reported to consume ~5 daily meals and would therefore be in a postprandial state for the majority of their waking hours (24). Therefore, similar to rested skeletal muscle (23), 20 g of high quality dietary protein appears to be sufficient to support maximal post-exercise

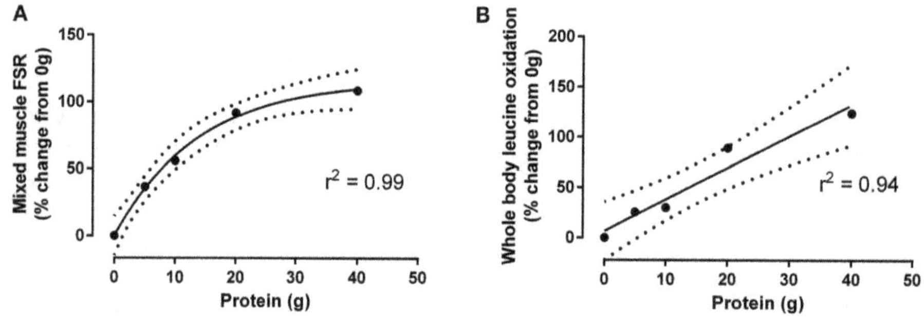

FIGURE 1 | Percent-change from fasted (i.e., 0 g protein ingestion) of mixed muscle protein synthesis **(A)** and whole body leucine oxidation **(B)** after resistance exercise in response to graded intakes of egg white protein, as adapted from Moore et al. (19). Data conform to one phase-exponential decay and linear correlation, respectively (Graphpad Prism V.6). Hashed line represents 95% CI.

rates of muscle protein synthesis in average weight (i.e., 80–85 kg) young adult males.

In contrast to the plateau observed with muscle protein synthesis, whole body leucine oxidation (a surrogate measure of protein oxidation) increases in a linear fashion with graded protein intakes (**Figure 1**) (19). This linear relationship may be related to the combination of a relatively low K_m for the rate-controlling enzyme for leucine oxidation (i.e., branched-chain ketoacid dehydrogenase) (25), and a greater overall substrate supply (i.e., leucine, valine, and isoleucine) with higher protein intakes. Importantly, this increase in leucine oxidation in conjunction with a concomitant increase in urea synthesis (23) highlights that dietary amino acids provided at levels that are in excess of their ability to be incorporated into new (muscle) proteins results in their deamination and, in the case of the branched chain amino acids, irreversible oxidation (**Figure 1**). This pattern of dietary amino acid oxidation is arguably an inefficient use of ingested protein if the specific goal is to maximize post-exercise muscle protein synthesis and anabolism. In fact, the marked increase in whole body leucine oxidation concomitant with a sustained elevation in blood amino acid concentration (19) is consistent with a metabolic pattern that has been suggested to be characteristic of an upper limit of intake for this macronutrient (26). Therefore, given the ability to induce a plateau in muscle protein synthesis yet minimize amino acid oxidation and urea synthesis (19, 23), 20 g of high quality protein (e.g., egg or whey protein) arguably represents an "optimal" or absolute protein intake to efficiently enhance muscle remodeling after resistance exercise in young adults.

RELATIVE PROTEIN INTAKE TO MAXIMIZE MYOFIBRILLAR PROTEIN SYNTHESIS

Based on previous studies that provided absolute protein intakes, the ingestion of 20 g of protein that was shown to maximize both mixed muscle and myofibrillar protein synthesis yet minimize whole body leucine oxidation, and ureagenesis in ~85 kg males translates into a relative protein intake of ~0.24 g protein/kg body weight. However, the ability to extrapolate these relative intakes into an "optimal" one-size-fits-all recommendation is arguably limited by the small sample size (i.e. $n = 54$) of "average" body mass individuals. In addition, the qualitative (albeit not statistically significant) ~10% increase in muscle protein synthetic rates between 20 and 40 g of protein could be interpreted as reflecting the "true" maximal intake as being within these two doses. Therefore, logical questions such as "would intakes greater than 20 g of protein further enhance muscle protein synthesis?" and "would 20 g of protein be the target intake for both 55 and 120 kg athletes?" naturally flow from these acute, absolute protein intake studies. In addition, recommendation of absolute meal protein intakes is at odds with daily recommendations for this macronutrient, which are almost universally prescribed relative to body mass.

To address these types of generalizability concerns, an unsystematic review was performed in Pubmed from its inception to July 1, 2019 consisting of keywords related to this review topic such as "whey," "myofibrillar protein synthesis," and "exercise." As maximizing post-exercise myofibrillar protein synthesis would be essential for those interested in enhancing muscle growth and potentially strength with training, studies investigating the synthesis of this muscle fraction were selected to increase homogeneity as well as reflect the greater contractile and nutrient sensitivity of this protein fraction (12). Moreover, studies that utilized a bolus protein feeding of whey protein after exercise and measured the synthesis of the myofibrillar protein fraction by traditional primed-constant stable isotope infusion during the subsequent 3–5 h postprandial period were included. Given that the preponderance of studies fitting these criteria have been performed in young adults, only this age group (i.e., <35 y) was included in the final dose-response analysis to minimize any confounding effects of age (see below for additional discussion). Finally, given the variability in fractional synthetic rates across different stable isotopes and precursor pools (27), post-exercise myofibrillar protein synthetic rates were expressed as a change from reported (when available) or estimated basal rates to better compare across studies. Details of the studies utilized for the subsequent analysis are presented in **Table 1**. Only articles in English were assessed with reference lists cross-checked for any additional relevant articles.

By utilizing a step-wise modeling comparison similar to our previous study at rest (39), it was observed that the increase in post-exercise myofibrillar protein synthesis in young adults

TABLE 1 | Overview of studies investigating the post-exercise stimulation of myofibrillar protein synthesis with bolus whey protein ingestion.

	Participants	Body mass (kg)	Absolute protein intake (g)	Relative protein intake (g/kg)	Exercise modality	Active muscle (kg)[a]	Post-exercise MPS[b]	MPS increase[c] (%)
Areta et al. (28)	$n = 8$ M	81 ± 11	20	~0.25	Bilateral KE	~7.2	1–4 h	~147
Areta et al. (28)	$n = 8$ M	84 ± 11	40	~0.48	Bilateral KE	~7.4	1–4 h	~134
Burd et al. (29)	$n = 8$ M	84 ± 9	20	~0.24	Unilateral KE	~3.8	0–5 h	~166
*Churchward-Venne et al. (30)	$n = 8$ M	77 ± 11	25	~0.32	Unilateral KE	~3.4	0–5 h	~171
†MacNaughton et al. (31)	$n = 15$ M	77 ± 5	20	~0.26	Bilateral CP, LPD, LP, KE, LC	~28.1	0–5 h	~47
†MacNaughton et al. (31)	$n = 15$ M	77 ± 5	40	~0.52	Bilateral CP, LPD, LP, KE, LC	~28.1	0–5 h	~84
†MacNaughton et al. (31)	$n = 15$ M	98 ± 8	20	~0.20	Bilateral CP, LPD, LP, KE, LC	~37.4	0–5 h	~58
†MacNaughton et al. (31)	$n = 15$ M	98 ± 8	40	~0.41	Bilateral CP, LPD, LP, KE, LC	~37.4	0–5 h	~83
McGlory et al. (32)	$n = 10$, M	80 ± 8	30	~0.37	Unilateral LP, KE	~10.8	0–3 h	~221
McKendry et al. (33)	$n = 8$, M	83 ± 11	25	~0.30	Bilateral LP, KE	~22.3	0–4 h	~139
Moore et al. (12)	$n = 7$ M	85 ± 12	25	~0.29	Unilateral KE, LP	~11.4	0–5 h	~180
Reidy et al. (34)	$n = 8$, M	76	17.3	~0.23	Bilateral KE	~6.7	3–5 h	~166
‡Reitelseder et al. (35)	$n = 9$ M	79 ± 9	17.5	~0.22	Unilateral KE	~3.5	1–6 h	~103
‡Reitelseder et al. (35)	$n = 8$ M	74 ± 6	0	0	Unilateral KE	~3.3	1–6 h	~81
*West et al. (36)	$n = 8$ M	84 ± 12	25	~0.30	Unilateral BC	~2.0	0–3 h	~150
*West et al. (36)	$n = 8$ M	84 ± 12	25	~0.30	Unilateral BC, Bilateral LP, KE, LC	~24.7	0–3 h	~129
West et al. (37)	$n = 8$ M	80 ± 10	25	~0.31	Bilateral KE	~7.1	1–5 h	~150
West et al. (38)	$n = 8$ M	77 ± 11	25	~0.32	Bilateral LP, KE, LC	~20.8	1–5 h	~160
West et al. (38)	$n = 8$ F	67 ± 6	25	~0.37	Bilateral LP, KE, LC	~19.5	1–5 h	~124
Witard et al. (23)	$n = 12$ M	83 ± 15	0	0	Unilateral KE	~3.7	0–4 h	~59
Witard et al. (23)	$n = 12$ M	84 ± 6	10	~0.12	Unilateral KE	~3.7	0–4 h	~84
Witard et al. (23)	$n = 12$ M	83 ± 7	20	~0.24	Unilateral KE	~3.7	0–4 h	~119
Witard et al. (23)	$n = 12$ M	79 ± 10	40	~0.51	Unilateral KE	~3.5	0–4 h	~141

MPS, myofibrillar protein synthesis; M, males; F, females; KE, knee extension; LP, leg press; BC, biceps curl; LC, leg curl; LPB, latissimus pull down; VL, vastus lateralis; BB, biceps brachii.
**Control MPS estimated from Moore et al. (39), which utilized identical ring-[$^{13}C_6$]phenylalanine tracer methodology.*
†Control MPS rested 0 g from Witard et al. (23).
‡Control MPS estimated as median value from Smith et al. (27) for L-[^{13}C]leucine infusion with [^{13}C]ketoisocaproate acid enrichment as the precursor.
[a]Active muscle mass estimated by first assuming total leg skeletal muscle mass represents ~29 and ~27% of total body mass for females and males, respectively, and total arm skeletal muscle mass represents ~9.5% of total body mass for males (40). These values were then divided in half to obtain the estimated single arm and single leg muscle mass and multiplied by 0.5 for BC exercise (i.e., ~50% of total arm muscle activated during arm flexion), 0.33 for KE exercise (i.e., ~33% of total leg muscle mass activated during knee extension), and 1.0 for LP exercise (i.e., ~100% of total leg muscle mass activated during leg press). Total active muscle mass was the sum of the estimated active muscle mass for each arm and/or leg.
[b]Represents duration over which MPS was measured after exercise.
[c]MPS increase above control MPS.

with protein ingestion displayed a bi-phase linear response that is consistent with the previous observation of a dose-response relationship (**Figure 2**). Breakpoint analysis revealed that the bi-phase linear response plateaued at ~0.31 g protein/kg body weight (i.e., estimated average requirement), which when accounting for a typical ~25% individual response variance in young adults (39) that would not be reflected in mean study responses could result in a safe intake of ~0.39 g/kg as an upper limit. This protein intake of ~0.31 g/kg is slightly higher than the relative intake calculated from the estimated plateau in protein synthesis and average group body weight previously determined in the mixed [~0.23 g/kg; (19)], and myofibrillar [~0.24 g/kg; (23)] protein fractions after the ingestion of 20 g of protein. This could explain in part the ~10% non-significant increases in protein synthesis from the 20 to 40 g doses (19, 23), which could suggest that the 20 g dose was not sufficient to maximize protein synthesis in all subjects whereas 40 g was clearly surfeit. In fact, the apparent lack of a true plateau in previous dose-response studies had led some to suggest that the protein intake to maximize muscle protein synthesis were within this range (i.e., >20 g) and that the upper level (i.e., 40 g) was necessary to obtain a maximal anabolic response (41).

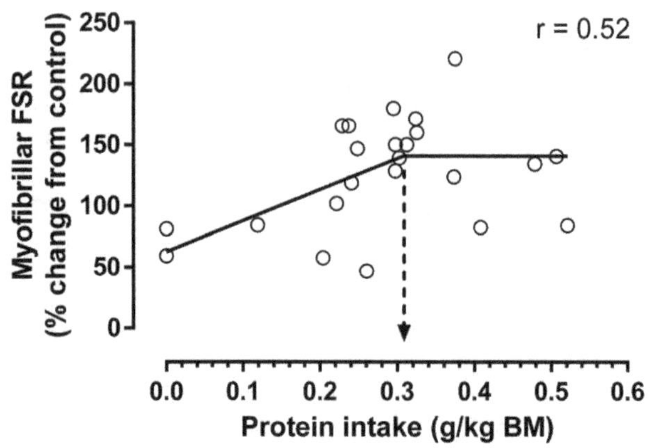

FIGURE 2 | Increase in post-exercise myofibrillar protein synthesis above control relative to ingested protein normalized to total body weight (for study details, see **Table 1**). Bi-phase linear regression was performed with the slope of the second line segment constrained to zero and the average protein intake to maximize myofibrillar protein synthesis determined by breakpoint analysis (indicated by hashed arrow; 0.31 ± 0.08 g protein/kg body weight; mean ± SE; $N = 23$ protein intakes; analysis performed by Graphpad Prism 6.0). Applying a typical ~25% variance when analyzing individual myofibrillar protein synthetic rates (39) as compared to a collapsed mean study response, a safe intake could represent ~0.38 g/kg. There was a strong trend for a bi-phasic linear regression model to explain a greater proportion of variance vs. a simple linear regression model ($r^2 = 0.27$ vs. 0.129, respectively; $P = 0.056$), suggesting the data conformed to a saturable dose-response relationship. First line segment described by: $y = 254x + 63$. Estimated maximal increase in myofibrillar protein synthesis above control is ~142% (as determined from equation above at 0.31 g protein/kg).

However, in contrast to the suggestion that 0.4–0.5 g protein/kg lean body mass (~0.34–0.43 g protein/kg body mass, assuming an average 15% body fat) should be ingested both before and after exercise (41), the data presented herein would suggest that only a moderately higher level of protein [i.e., ~0.31 vs. ~0.24 g/kg; (23)] should be ingested to reach a plateau in post-exercise myofibrillar protein synthesis.

WOULD SEX AFFECT THE RELATIVE PROTEIN REQUIREMENT?

Currently, research that evaluates the nutritional factors that enhance muscle protein synthesis after resistance exercise is primarily performed in young males with that of female athletes being unfortunately under-represented. For example, the only studies to evaluate the ingested protein dose-response, either at rest or after resistance exercise, have performed these investigations in males only (19, 23, 39, 42). The reason(s) for the unfortunate disparity in sex-based research is unclear but may include, in part, the potential influence of menstrual phase on protein kinetics, which has been reported to alter the basic requirements for some EAA (e.g., lysine) at rest (43) as well as influence whole body protein metabolism during endurance exercise (44). However, the stimulation of myofibrillar protein synthesis after resistance exercise is uninfluenced by the menstrual phase (45). Moreover, both the rested (46, 47), and the exercise-induced stimulation (48) of muscle protein synthesis are similar between young men and women in the fasted state, suggesting sex *per se* has little influence on the regulation of muscle protein remodeling in the absence of any nutritional manipulation.

With respect to the nutrient sensitivity of muscle protein synthesis, seminal work that investigated the nutritional factors that enhance post-exercise muscle anabolism reported no differences between males and females in their mixed study populations (15–18); this could suggest there are no overt differences in post-exercise nutrient sensitivity of muscle protein metabolism between sexes. It has also been demonstrated that the stimulation of myofibrillar protein synthesis with resistance exercise and a 25-g bolus of dietary protein ingestion is similar between young men and women (38). This study (38) provided an absolute amount of protein (25 g) to all participants that would likely translate into a saturating dose for both the men (~0.32 g/kg) and, especially, women (~37 g/kg), which makes it difficult to determine if potential sex differences exist at lower protein intakes. Nevertheless, the ability of whey protein to enhance post-exercise rates of myofibrillar protein synthesis during energy restriction is essentially identical between females and males when normalized to fat free mass (FFM) over a range of intakes (i.e., 0–0.8 g/kg FFM) (49). Therefore, despite a relative dearth of research studying the nutritional requirements of females after resistance exercise, it is difficult to envision, based on the current literature, a scenario in which acute protein requirements would be markedly disparate between the sexes.

CARBOHYDRATE CO-INGESTION

Carbohydrate ingestion during the recovery from resistance exercise is important for glycogen resynthesis (50, 51) and can contribute to the daily positive energy balance that is a general requisite to support muscle mass growth with training. Aside from providing additional energy during post-exercise recovery, it was first demonstrated that the co-ingestion of carbohydrate with crystalline amino acids improved post-exercise muscle net balance to a greater degree than amino acids alone (18). Subsequent studies revealed that this greater net anabolism was due primarily to an insulin-induced suppression of muscle protein breakdown rather than an augmentation of muscle protein synthesis (52, 53). In fact, as little as ~30 g of carbohydrate (and the associated insulin response) is sufficient to suppress post-exercise muscle protein catabolism (52). Provided dietary protein is provided at a level that would optimize muscle protein synthesis (i.e., ≥20 g), carbohydrate co-ingestion from 30–270 g has no additive effect on post-exercise muscle protein synthetic rates (52, 54, 55). Therefore, although it is unclear if carbohydrate co-ingestion may improve the synthetic effect of smaller (i.e., <20 g or <0.31 g/kg) amounts of dietary protein, it is clear that optimal protein ingestion is of paramount importance to maximize muscle protein synthesis after resistance exercise with mixed protein-carbohydrate beverages.

DOES THE AMOUNT OF ACTIVE MUSCLE MASS INFLUENCE POST-EXERCISE PROTEIN REQUIREMENTS?

It is customary for individuals engaged in resistance training for the goal of gaining muscle mass to perform whole body resistance exercise, which is in contrast to many acute studies aimed at understanding the local (i.e., muscle-specific) nutrient requirements to maximize muscle protein synthesis. This led MacNaughton et al. (31) to design an elegant study whereby groups of participants with markedly different body compositions were provided with moderate (20 g) and higher (40 g) doses of protein after a strenuous bout of whole body resistance exercise. The authors hypothesized that total lean body mass (LBM), and thus active lean (i.e., muscle) mass, would modify the acute requirement for dietary protein to maximize muscle protein synthesis during recovery. In contrast to their hypothesis and arguably the most compelling case against any impact of active muscle mass on acute protein requirements was the observation that participants with ~20 kg difference in LBM (i.e., ~59 vs. 79 kg LBM) had identical rates of myofibrillar protein synthesis after consumption of a moderate 20 g dose of whey protein. This finding is not without precedence as it has been shown previously that performing an intense bout of lower body resistance exercise (i.e., leg press, knee extension, leg curl), which would increase total body active muscle mass, does not impact blood flow during recovery to the arm nor post-exercise rates of myofibrillar protein synthesis with a moderate 25 g protein dose in the small biceps brachii (36, 56). Macnaughton et al. argued that the lower rates of myofibrillar protein synthesis in their whole body exercise protocol relative to a previous study utilizing unilateral leg resistance exercise (23) concomitant with statistically greater rates of synthesis with the larger (i.e., 40 g) dose were nevertheless indicative of greater post-exercise protein requirement with a greater active muscle mass (23). However, the study and cohort differences in myofibrillar synthesis rates are within the general inter-study variability (i.e., ±25%) for tracer-derived rates of human muscle protein synthesis (27). Arguably the most plausible reason for the greater myofibrillar synthetic rates with 40 as compare to 20 g of protein would be a greater statistical power to detect the relatively small ~20% difference between conditions, which the authors allude to in their discussion (31). For example, *post hoc* power analysis of previous absolute protein dose-response studies (19, 23) suggest that ~35 participants would be required to achieve statistical significance for the ~10% greater muscle protein synthetic rates with 40 g as compared to 20 g protein ingestion. This is markedly similar to the results in MacNaughton et al. (31) given that statistical significance between 20 and 40 g of protein was only achieved when the low and high LBM cohorts were collapsed (i.e., $n = 30$ total).

In order to more objectively estimate the impact of the amount of active muscle mass on post-exercise protein requirements, the increase in myofibrillar protein synthesis was compared to the amount of dietary protein ingested relative to the estimated active muscle mass (**Table 1**; **Figure 3**). If one were to expect the amount of active muscle mass influenced the ability of dietary protein to stimulate post-exercise muscle remodeling, then it would be likely that a greater protein intake per active muscle mass would also result in a greater increase in myofibrillar protein synthesis. Despite a greater than ~10-fold difference in relative protein intakes there was no observable relationship with the stimulation of myofibrillar protein synthesis, which suggests active muscle mass has little bearing on post-exercise protein requirement. The observation that the stimulation of muscle protein synthesis is apparently unrelated to the amount of protein ingested per unit of active muscle is not surprising given that resistance exercise is inherently anabolic and has been shown to improve intracellular amino acid recycling (1, 2). This enhanced intracellular amino acid reutilization would ultimately lessen the requirement for exogenous amino acids to support the exercise-induced stimulation of muscle protein synthesis, although protein/amino acid ingestion is still required to induce a net positive muscle protein balance. Therefore, presently available data suggest that the amount of active muscle mass has little bearing on the ability of or requirement for post-exercise protein ingestion to enhance muscle protein remodeling.

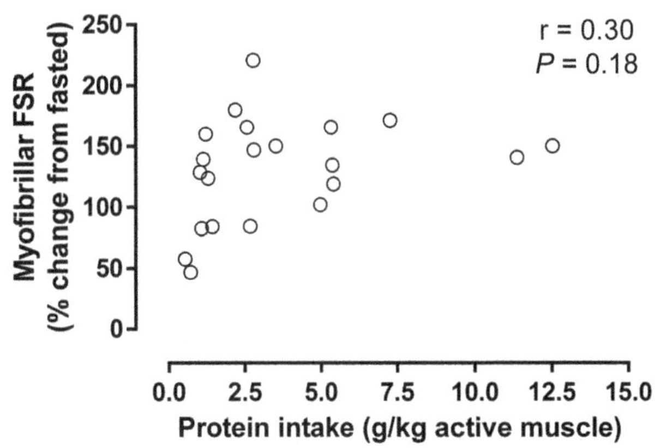

FIGURE 3 | Increase in myofibrillar protein synthesis above control after resistance exercise compared to ingested protein normalized to the estimated active muscle mass (for details, see **Table 1**). Data were analyzed using a linear correlation (Graphpad Prism V6). Non-significant slope defined by: $y = 3.91x + 116$ ($r = 0.30$; $P = 0.18$; $N = 21$ as only conditions with protein ingestion were included).

WHAT ABOUT MAXIMIZING WHOLE BODY ANABOLISM?

During the post-exercise recovery period muscle protein synthesis is maximized with the ingestion ~0.31 g/kg of protein whereas muscle protein breakdown has been demonstrated to be maximally suppressed with a moderate insulin response (e.g., from ~30 g of carbohydrate) (52). Collectively, this provides compelling evidence that muscle protein net balance is saturable and primarily dictated by the nutritional enhancement of rates of muscle protein synthesis, as highlighted previously (6). In contrast, it has recently been suggested that there is no practical maximal anabolic response to dietary protein at the whole body level given the hypothesized role of an inexhaustible ability to suppress protein breakdown at high protein intakes (57, 58). For example, ingesting 70 g (~0.82 g/kg) as compared to 40 g (~0.48 g/kg) of dietary protein has been shown to enhance whole body net protein balance, in the absence of any further increase in rested or post-exercise rates of mixed muscle protein synthesis, through a proportional reduction in estimates of whole body protein breakdown (59). Based on these findings as well as those from older adults (60), the authors recently collapsed their data across ages and reanalyzed using a linear model to support their suggestion of there being no practical limit (58). This appeared to confirm their previous hypothesis on this topic (57) and potentially influenced previous suggestions of a target meal protein intake for resistance-trained athletes of ~0.4–0.55 g/kg (61). However, we recently demonstrated that whole body net balance plateaus with dietary protein ingestion after resistance exercise in females (62) and variable intensity stop-and-go exercise in both sexes (63) despite a linear increase in estimates of amino acid deamination (i.e., increased urinary urea:creatinine ratio), and presumably oxidation. The apparent discrepancy may be related in part to the choice of statistical model in our research (62, 63) as compared to others (58) (i.e., biphase vs. linear regression, respectively). In potential support, extraction and reanalysis of whole body net protein balance data from just their young adults relative to body weight-normalized protein ingestion from Kim et al. (58) revealed that the data is better fit by a segmental bi-phase linear regression as compared to standard linear model (i.e., $r^2 = 0.62$ vs. 0.53, respectively; $P < 0.05$; Graphpad Prism V6). This analysis revealed a breakpoint in whole body net balance at ~0.71 g/kg, which is slightly greater than our recent estimates of ~0.5–0.6 g/kg (62, 63), and suggests that the capacity to assimilate dietary protein at the whole body level is substantially greater than at the muscle. While it has been suggested that these amino acids sequestered at the whole body level (e.g., within splanchnic tissues and/or circulating proteins) may be made available for muscle protein synthesis during the post-absorptive period (58), this possibility has yet to be empirically demonstrated. Some may also view these relatively higher per meal protein estimates as being unrealistic, although many Western populations with a skewed daily protein distribution routinely consume on average ~0.55 g/kg in their evening meal (64). Therefore, in contrast to prior suggested meal protein intakes of up to ~0.5 g/kg that are based on the supposition of no maximal whole body anabolism (61), it is argued that a more prudent "muscle-centric" target that maximizes muscle protein synthesis yet minimizes excess amino acid oxidative losses would place a more efficient intake at no more than ~0.39 g/kg.

POTENTIAL CAVEATS TO ACUTE RELATIVE PROTEIN REQUIREMENTS

The reanalysis of the relative protein intake to maximize post-exercise myofibrillar protein synthesis performed herein incorporates studies performed in healthy young individuals consuming a single, high-quality protein source (i.e., whey). While this approach increases homogeneity and allows for greater ease of comparison between studies, the results could be viewed as representing relative protein requirements under "ideal" conditions, notwithstanding the increased appreciation for the anabolic potential of whole foods (discussed in more detail below) (65–67). The following sections will briefly discuss conditions under which relative protein intakes may not be transferable and/or require further study.

Exercise Modality

Dietary protein is important for the remodeling of skeletal muscle after not only resistance exercise but also after high-intensity sprint exercise (68), steady-state endurance exercise (69), and combinations thereof (i.e., concurrent training) (70, 71). Unlike resistance exercise, which provides a predominantly muscle-specific stimulus (72), endurance exercise can increase whole body oxidative disposal of amino acids that must ultimately be replaced via dietary sources (73). This may contribute to the increased protein requirements of endurance athletes (74, 75). Studies from the same laboratory utilizing identical tracer methodology have demonstrated that the ingestion of 0 g (~0.057 vs. ~0.051%/h, respectively), and 20 g (~0.087 vs. ~0.070%/h, respectively) of whey protein elicit broadly similar rates of myofibrillar protein synthesis after 90 min of endurance exercise (~77% maximal aerobic capacity), and traditional resistance exercise (23, 69), which could be interpreted as reflecting a similar post-exercise protein requirement after these dichotomous exercise stimuli. However, it has recently been demonstrated in a group design that post-exercise rates of myofibrillar protein synthesis were ~16% greater after the ingestion of 20 g (~0.27 g/kg) of milk protein (whey, casein, and milk protein concentrate) compared to a protein-free control after an acute bout of concurrent exercise (71), which is slightly lower than the reported ~32% difference in myofibrillar protein synthetic rates between 25 g of whey (~0.32 g/kg) protein and a protein-free placebo after concurrent exercise in a crossover study (70). Although the relative differences in myofibrillar protein synthetic rates between 0 g protein and a moderate relative intake (i.e., ~0.26–0.32 g/kg) in these concurrent exercise studies seem muted compared to the present post-resistance exercise analysis (i.e., ~16–32 vs. ~79%), the estimated increase from basal may be moderately more comparable (i.e., ~78–147 vs. ~152%; **Figure 3**). Therefore, while the consumption of ~ 0.31 g/kg of protein would enhance myofibrillar remodeling after all forms of exercise, additional research may be warranted to confirm that this represents a saturable dose and/or is sufficient to fully replace any endurance exercise-induced oxidative amino acid losses. This is notwithstanding the other potential benefits of increased protein ingestion in endurance athletes during periods of intensified training that may be dissociated from myofibrillar remodeling, such as enhanced immune function and/or exercise performance (76, 77).

Population Age

Both young and old adults are capable of mounting an enhanced muscle protein synthetic response after resistance exercise in the fasted state (78, 79), which is consistent with the ability to increase muscle mass with this type of training across the lifespan (80). However, it has been observed that the combined effects of resistance exercise and amino acid ingestion on the enhancement of muscle protein synthesis may be delayed (81), and/or blunted in older adults (82, 83), suggesting nutrient sensitivities may be compromised with advancing age. In potential support, it has been shown that the ingestion of 40 g (~0.49 g/kg) of whey protein enhanced rates of post-exercise myofibrillar protein synthesis over and above that observed with 20 g (~0.25 g/kg) in older (~70 y) adults (82). However, the relative dose may not be substantially greater than younger adults as 30 g (~0.37 g/kg) of milk protein concentrate was recently demonstrated to enhance post-exercise myofibrillar protein synthetic rates in healthy older adults with no further benefit at 45 g (~0.56 g/kg) (84). Given that the anabolic potential of exercise and/or nutrition may be intimately tied to the "biological" age of a muscle as dictated by its habitual activity (85, 86), additional research is needed to confirm whether greater relative intakes are required to maximize post-exercise anabolism in older age and, if so, what lifestyle and/or biological factors may need to be considered (e.g., daily step count, presence/absence of sub-clinical chronic inflammation, excess body fat, etc.).

Protein Type

The studies examining the post-exercise ingested protein dose-response utilized high quality (i.e., enriched in EAA), rapidly digested protein sources (i.e., egg and whey) (19, 23). Moreover, the estimates for the relative protein requirements derived herein were obtained with studies utilizing whey protein, which due to its rapid digestion (37), and/or greater leucine content (87, 88) elicits an early (i.e., within 3 h) and robust post-exercise stimulation of muscle protein synthesis. In contrast, proteins that contain lower quantities of the branched-chain amino acids (e.g., plant-based, caseinate), and/or are slowly digested (e.g., micellar casein) generally result in a suboptimal muscle protein synthetic response compared to an equal amount of whey protein (88), although recent research with dairy proteins may not support this "rapid rate of leucinemia" requirement for post-exercise myofibrillar remodeling (89). Nevertheless, studies have suggested that proteins with suboptimal essential amino acid and/or leucine content may ultimately be compensated for by ingesting a greater absolute protein amount. For example, it has been reported that the post-exercise stimulation of mixed muscle protein synthesis over 5 h (90), and myofibrillar protein synthesis over 3–5 h (34) of recovery is similar with the ingestion of ~20 g of a mixed protein (i.e., whey, casein, soy blend) and ~17 g of whey. Therefore, the optimal intake of proteins that may be relatively deficient in EAA and/or leucine and/or slowly digested may need to be addressed in future studies. Alternatively, individuals who prefer to ingest lower quality proteins (insofar as the stimulation of muscle protein synthesis is concerned) may consider consuming intakes at the upper "safe" intake of ~0.39 g/kg.

Food Matrix

Early studies investigating the nutritional regulation of muscle protein synthesis have primarily provided dietary protein in beverage form. However, recent focus has been placed on the importance of studying whole foods (e.g., egg, beef) given these are typically nutrient-dense and arguably more representative of "normal" habitual dietary patterns (66, 67). Inasmuch as the peak and/or the rate of change in blood amino acid concentration regulates post-exercise muscle protein synthesis (37), the typically delayed digestion and absorption of solid foods may result in an attenuated muscle protein synthetic response (91). In this event, it is unclear if consuming a greater protein intake to account for any attenuated hyperaminoacidemia from solid food ingestion may be required to maximize post-exercise muscle protein synthesis. However, digestion rate may not be the only (or even primary) variable that influences the anabolic potential of whole food as minced beef has been demonstrated to induce a more rapid postprandial aminoacademia than skim milk but a lower early (i.e., <2 h), and potentially cumulative (i.e., 0–5 h) post-exercise myofibrillar protein synthetic response (92). Other studies have also demonstrated whole milk as more anabolic than skim milk (93) and skim milk more anabolic than soy juice (8) during post-exercise recovery. Finally, we recently demonstrated that whole egg supports a greater post-exercise myofibrillar protein synthetic response than an isonitrogenous quantity of egg white protein, which was supported by a greater lysosomal targeting of the mechanistic target of rapamycin (mTOR) as the potential underlying physiological mechanism (94, 95). This could suggest there may be circumstances whereby whole, nutrient-dense foods may require a lower relative intake to maximize post-exercise anabolism than other isolated protein sources. Although additional research is warranted to define the anabolic potential of whole food and its associated dose-response relationship to post-exercise anabolism, a target of ~0.31 g/kg protein could arguably represent a reasonable starting point for individuals aiming to enhance myofibrillar protein synthetic rates in the interim.

Habitual Protein Intake

Although it is generally accepted that daily protein requirements are elevated in strength athletes (96), habitual intakes of populations engaged in chronic resistance training generally far exceed most recommendations (i.e., >2 g/kg/d) (97). Habitually high protein diets increase the capacity for protein catabolism and amino acid oxidation as a means to manage this excess macronutrient load (98). From an acute feeding standpoint, rodent models have demonstrated that adaptation to a high protein intake is accompanied by a greater splanchnic extraction of dietary nitrogen, which results in an attenuated post-prandial delivery to and deposition of dietary nitrogen in peripheral tissues (99). In this way, the gut may act as a buffer to ensure amino acid delivery to peripheral tissues (including muscle) is relatively constant regardless of habitual dietary protein intake. This has some support in humans as there is reduced dietary amino acid availability after consumption of 25 g of milk protein when adapted to a moderate (1.5 g/kg/d) as compared to low (0.7 g/kg/d) protein diet (100), suggesting a potentially greater splanchnic amino acid sequestration. Although rested postprandial rates of myofibrillar protein synthesis were non-statistically attenuated by ~50% in the moderate compared to the low protein group in the study by Gorissen et al. (100), Pasiakos et al. (101) demonstrated that the postprandial stimulation of mixed muscle protein synthesis by 20 g of protein was attenuated when consuming 1.6 vs. 0.8 g/kg/d and was not enhanced with a 2.4 g/kg/d controlled diet. Collectively these data could suggest that individuals habituated to lower protein diet approximating the recommended dietary allowance (RDA; 0.83 g/kg/d) may be able to support maximal rates of muscle protein synthesis after exercise with intakes lower than ~0.31 g/kg. In contrast, those adapted to higher habitual intakes, as is common in many strength athletes, may require a greater relative intake to account for an attenuated peripheral dietary amino acid appearance and/or enhanced amino acid oxidative capacity. However, the threshold at which this greater acute requirement may manifest could be relatively high (e.g., ~3x the RDA) given that previous post-exercise dose-response studies recruited participants with relatively high self-reported habitual intakes (i.e., 1.4–2.3 g/kg/d) yet still demonstrated approximate plateaus in muscle protein synthetic rates with 20 g (~0.24 g/kg) protein ingestion (19, 23).

Negative Energy Balance

Muscle protein synthesis is an energetically expensive process and is down-regulated during periods of cellular energy stress, such as during a diet-induced negative energy balance (49, 102). The post-exercise stimulation of myofibrillar protein synthesis with dietary protein ingestion is not affected by low levels of muscle glycogen (103), highlighting that acute energy restriction does not constrain post-exercise muscle remodeling with exogenous amino acid ingestion. In contrast, more chronic periods of negative energy balance (i.e., 5–10 d) suppress resting mixed and myofibrillar protein synthesis (49, 102, 104). In addition, after a 5-day moderate protein (i.e., 1.4 g/kg/d) low energy (30 kcal/kg fat-free mass/d) diet, post-exercise myofibrillar protein synthesis is increased in a linear dose-dependent fashion with 15 and 30 g of dietary protein (49). Although the maximal absolute protein intake was lower than previous dose-response studies during energy balance (i.e., 30 vs. 40 g) (19, 23), there was no apparent plateau in post-exercise myofibrillar protein synthesis within the range of relative protein intakes studied (i.e., up to ~0.5 g/kg body weight) (49). Additionally, the estimated maximal myofibrillar protein synthesis with 30 g protein ingestion (determined by the group mean response) was ~82% above the rested fasted rate during energy deficit (49), which is less than the estimated plateau of ~142% during energy balance in the present review and could suggest a saturable protein intake was not provided during this negative energy balance. While it is possible that maximal rates of myofibrillar protein synthesis may generally be constrained during chronic diet-induced negative energy balance, the lack of a plateau and the relatively modest increase in myofibrillar protein synthesis with 30 g of protein could also suggest that the protein intake required to maximize post-exercise myofibrillar protein synthesis is slightly greater during a period of energy restriction. This would generally be in line with the observations that high daily dietary protein intakes (i.e., at least ~2 times the RDA) are required to maintain lean body mass and muscle protein synthesis during a negative energy diet with (104, 105) or without resistance exercise (101). Additional benefits for higher protein intakes during negative energy balance could be increased satiety and post-prandial thermogenesis (106), both of which would help support weight loss goals. Therefore, although it has been suggested that 0.25–0.3 g protein/kg body weight should be targeted after exercise in athletes aiming to maintain lean body mass during weight loss (107), the ~0.31 g protein/kg body mass determined herein could be viewed as a minimum intake with a safe intake closer to ~0.4 g/kg for individuals consuming a sub-optimal energy intake.

Obesity

Beyond traditional derangements in glucose metabolism, it is becoming appreciated that excess body fat may also be an independent factor contributing to the dysregulation of muscle protein synthesis in obese populations (108). For example, obesity has been associated with a blunted myofibrillar protein synthetic response to dietary protein ingestion (i.e., 36 g or ~0.35 g/kg) (109), and resistance exercise (110). In addition, this anabolic resistance, which is not reported in relatively active obese individuals (i.e., ~7,400 steps/day) (111), may be exacerbated by inactivity (112), which suggests this anabolic resistance of obesity, similar to older adults (85, 86), has a strong lifestyle component to its manifestation and severity. Thus, inasmuch as this anabolic resistance extends to the post-exercise sensitivity to dietary amino acids, it could be argued that obese individuals may require a greater relative protein intake than their lean counterparts when normalized to the metabolically active lean body mass. However, studies used in the present analysis that yielded a relative protein intake of ~0.31 g/kg included participants of average body fat (~15%). Therefore, providing recommendations relative to total body mass would result in a greater dose per kg lean body mass in obese individuals (i.e., ~0.34 vs. ~0.41 g/kg lean body mass, respectively, assuming 30% body fat), which subsequently may be sufficient to overcome any obesity-related anabolic resistance.

PRACTICAL APPLICATION OF ACUTE RELATIVE PROTEIN INTAKES

A single bout of resistance exercise can increase muscle protein synthesis for up to 24–48 h with the duration for which it is elevated influenced by training history of the athlete (13, 113) and the specific exercise stimulus (11), which ultimately factor into the general inability of single acute (i.e., <6 h) "snapshots" of myofibrillar protein synthesis to predict training-induced muscle hypertrophy (114). However, individuals who are able to support greater rates of myofibrillar protein synthesis over this 24–48 h post-exercise recovery period have been shown to experience greater training-induced gains in muscle hypertrophy (13). Given that individuals who engage in resistance training for the goal of enhancing muscle mass and/or muscle strength typically train 3–5 times per week (115), athletes are generally in some state of post-exercise recovery. Dietary protein consumed at any point during this prolonged 24–48 h recovery period would ultimately contribute to the remodeling of skeletal muscle. Outside of the response after a single meal, the pattern and distribution of dietary protein ingestion has been shown to influence muscle protein synthesis over 12–24 h both at rest (116) and after resistance exercise (28, 117, 118). For example, the repeated ingestion of 20 g of whey protein (~0.25 g/kg) at 3 h intervals has been shown to support the greatest rates of myofibrillar protein synthesis and whole body net protein balance over the 12 h after an acute bout of resistance exercise (28, 117). This has led to the suggesting that 4–5 meal occasions, which is the typical feeding frequency already adopted by many elite athletes (24), would be the most favorable and metabolically efficient means to consume one's daily protein intake if the goal is to maximize skeletal muscle remodeling while simultaneously minimizing irreversible amino acid oxidative catabolism (28, 117). Therefore, if one were to take a "muscle-centric" view for the daily protein requirement then the optimal amount and pattern of protein intake would translate into ~1.24–1.55 g/kg/d for a resistance-trained individual aiming to maximize skeletal muscle remodeling and/or net protein accretion. Even if one were to apply a conservative ~20% correction-factor (i.e., ~0.37 g/kg) to account for less anabolic proteins [e.g., plant-based; (88)], then this pattern of protein intake would provide ~1.48–1.85 g/kg/d. Both of these estimates are within the range of intakes suggested to maximize lean mass growth with training (119) and are in line with current sports science consensus recommendations for daily protein intake (96).

CONCLUSION

The present review puts forth the argument that protein recommendations should be normalized to the body weight of an individual for a greater ease of translation of the dose that maximizes muscle protein synthesis and minimizes amino acid oxidation during the recovery from resistance exercise. Based on re-analysis of previously published literature, an intake of ~0.31 g/kg of high quality protein represents a suitable target to maximize myofibrillar protein synthesis during recovery from resistance exercise, regardless of sex, and quantity of active muscle mass. Though additional research is warranted to confirm whether acute protein requirements to maximize post-exercise rates of muscle protein synthesis are influenced by age, chronic energy status, and/or food matrix, a moderate intake of ~0.31 g/kg of high quality protein represents a good approximation for individuals of all body sizes aiming to efficiently enhance the repair, remodeling, and net synthesis of skeletal muscle tissue after resistance exercise.

AUTHOR CONTRIBUTIONS

DM wrote and approved the final version the manuscript.

REFERENCES

1. Phillips SM, Tipton KD, Aarsland A, Wolf SE, Wolfe RR. Mixed muscle protein synthesis and breakdown after resistance exercise in humans. *Am J Physiol.* (1997) 273(1 Pt 1):E99–107. doi: 10.1152/ajpendo.1997.273.1.E99
2. Biolo G, Maggi SP, Williams BD, Tipton KD, Wolfe RR. Increased rates of muscle protein turnover and amino acid transport after resistance exercise in humans. *Am J Physiol.* (1995) 268(3 Pt 1):E514–20. doi: 10.1152/ajpendo.1995.268.3.E514
3. Biolo G, Tipton KD, Klein S, Wolfe RR. An abundant supply of amino acids enhances the metabolic effect of exercise on muscle protein. *Am J Physiol.* (1997) 273(1 Pt 1):E122–9. doi: 10.1152/ajpendo.1997.273.1.E122
4. Kumar V, Atherton P, Smith K, Rennie MJ. Human muscle protein synthesis and breakdown during and after exercise. *J Appl Physiol.* (2009) 106:2026–39. doi: 10.1152/japplphysiol.91481.2008
5. Rennie MJ, Wackerhage H, Spangenburg EE, Booth FW. Control of the size of the human muscle mass. *Annu Rev Physiol.* (2004) 66:799–828. doi: 10.1146/annurev.physiol.66.052102.134444
6. Rasmussen BB, Phillips SM. Contractile and nutritional regulation of human muscle growth. *Exerc Sport Sci Rev.* (2003) 31:127–31 doi: 10.1097/00003677-200307000-00005
7. Hartman JW, Tang JE, Wilkinson SB, Tarnopolsky MA, Lawrence RL, Fullerton AV, et al. Consumption of fat-free fluid milk after resistance exercise promotes greater lean mass accretion than does consumption of soy or carbohydrate in young, novice, male weightlifters. *Am J Clin Nutr.* (2007) 86:373–81. doi: 10.1093/ajcn/86.2.373
8. Wilkinson SB, Tarnopolsky MA, Macdonald MJ, Macdonald JR, Armstrong D, Phillips SM. Consumption of fluid skim milk promotes greater muscle protein accretion after resistance exercise than does consumption of an isonitrogenous and isoenergetic soy-protein beverage. *Am J Clin Nutr.* (2007) 85:1031–40. doi: 10.1093/ajcn/85.4.1031
9. Josse AR, Tang JE, Tarnopolsky MA, Phillips SM. Body composition and strength changes in women with milk and resistance exercise. *Med Sci Sports Exerc.* (2010) 42:1122–30. doi: 10.1249/MSS.0b013e3181c854f6
10. Burd NA, West DW, Moore DR, Atherton PJ, Staples AW, Prior T, et al. Enhanced amino acid sensitivity of myofibrillar protein synthesis persists for up to 24 h after resistance exercise in young men. *J Nutr.* (2011) 141:568–73. doi: 10.3945/jn.110.135038
11. Burd NA, West DW, Staples AW, Atherton PJ, Baker JM, Moore DR, et al. Low-load high volume resistance exercise stimulates muscle protein synthesis more than high-load low volume resistance exercise in young men. *PLoS ONE.* (2010) 5:e12033. doi: 10.1371/journal.pone.0012033
12. Moore DR, Tang JE, Burd NA, Rerecich T, Tarnopolsky MA, Phillips SM. Differential stimulation of myofibrillar and sarcoplasmic protein synthesis with protein ingestion at rest and after resistance exercise. *J Physiol.* (2009) 587(Pt 4):897–904. doi: 10.1113/jphysiol.2008.164087
13. Damas F, Phillips SM, Libardi CA, Vechin FC, Lixandrao ME, Jannig PR, et al. Resistance training-induced changes in integrated myofibrillar protein synthesis are related to hypertrophy only after attenuation of muscle damage. *J Physiol.* (2016) 594:5209–22. doi: 10.1113/JP272472
14. Rasmussen BB, Tipton KD, Miller SL, Wolf SE, Wolfe RR. An oral essential amino acid-carbohydrate supplement enhances muscle protein anabolism after resistance exercise. *J Appl Physiol.* (2000) 88:386–92 doi: 10.1152/jappl.2000.88.2.386
15. Tipton KD, Ferrando AA, Phillips SM, Doyle Jr D, Wolfe RR. Postexercise net protein synthesis in human muscle from orally administered amino acids. *Am J Physiol.* (1999) 276(4 Pt 1):E628–34. doi: 10.1152/ajpendo.1999.276.4.E628
16. Tipton KD, Borsheim E, Wolf SE, Sanford AP, Wolfe RR. Acute response of net muscle protein balance reflects 24-h balance after exercise and amino acid ingestion. *Am J Physiol Endocrinol Metab.* (2003) 284:E76–89. doi: 10.1152/ajpendo.00234.2002
17. Borsheim E, Tipton KD, Wolf SE, Wolfe RR. Essential amino acids and muscle protein recovery from resistance exercise. *Am J Physiol Endocrinol Metab.* (2002) 283:E648–57. doi: 10.1152/ajpendo.00466.2001
18. Miller SL, Tipton KD, Chinkes DL, Wolf SE, Wolfe RR. Independent and combined effects of amino acids and glucose after resistance exercise. *Med Sci Sports Exerc.* (2003) 35:449–55. doi: 10.1249/01.MSS.0000053910.63105.45

19. Moore DR, Robinson MJ, Fry JL, Tang JE, Glover EI, Wilkinson SB, et al. Ingested protein dose response of muscle and albumin protein synthesis after resistance exercise in young men. *Am J Clin Nutr.* (2009) 89:161–8. doi: 10.3945/ajcn.2008.26401
20. Tang JE, Manolakos JJ, Kujbida GW, Lysecki PJ, Moore DR, Phillips SM. Minimal whey protein with carbohydrate stimulates muscle protein synthesis following resistance exercise in trained young men. *Appl Physiol Nutr Metab.* (2007) 32:1132–8. doi: 10.1139/H07-076
21. Drummond MJ, Dreyer HC, Fry CS, Glynn EL, Rasmussen BB. Nutritional and contractile regulation of human skeletal muscle protein synthesis and mTORC1 signaling. *J Appl Physiol.* (2009) 106:1374–84. doi: 10.1152/japplphysiol.91397.2008
22. Deldicque L, Sanchez Canedo C, Horman S, De Potter I, Bertrand L, Hue L, et al. Antagonistic effects of leucine and glutamine on the mTOR pathway in myogenic C2C12 cells. *Amino Acids.* (2008) 35:147–55. doi: 10.1007/s00726-007-0607-z
23. Witard OC, Jackman SR, Breen L, Smith K, Selby A, Tipton KD. Myofibrillar muscle protein synthesis rates subsequent to a meal in response to increasing doses of whey protein at rest and after resistance exercise. *Am J Clin Nutr.* (2014) 99:86–95. doi: 10.3945/ajcn.112.055517
24. Burke LM, Slater G, Broad EM, Haukka J, Modulon S, Hopkins WG. Eating patterns and meal frequency of elite Australian athletes. *Int J Sport Nutr Exerc Metab.* (2003) 13:521–38. doi: 10.1123/ijsnem.13.4.521
25. Phillips SM. A brief review of critical processes in exercise-induced muscular hypertrophy. *Sports Med.* (2014) 44(Suppl 1):S71–7. doi: 10.1007/s40279-014-0152-3
26. Pencharz PB, Elango R, Ball RO. An approach to defining the upper safe limits of amino acid intake. *J Nutr.* (2008) 138:1996s–2002s. doi: 10.1093/jn/138.10.1996S
27. Smith GI, Patterson BW, Mittendorfer B. Human muscle protein turnover–why is it so variable? *J Appl Physiol.* (2011) 110:480–91. doi: 10.1152/japplphysiol.00125.2010
28. Areta JL, Burke LM, Ross ML, Camera DM, West DW, Broad EM, et al. Timing and distribution of protein ingestion during prolonged recovery from resistance exercise alters myofibrillar protein synthesis. *J Physiol.* (2013) 591:2319–31. doi: 10.1113/jphysiol.2012.244897
29. Burd NA, Holwerda AM, Selby KC, West DW, Staples AW, Cain NE, et al. Resistance exercise volume affects myofibrillar protein synthesis and anabolic signalling molecule phosphorylation in young men. *J Physiol.* (2010) 588(Pt 16):3119–30. doi: 10.1113/jphysiol.2010.192856
30. Churchward-Venne TA, Burd NA, Mitchell CJ, West DW, Philp A, Marcotte GR, et al. Supplementation of a suboptimal protein dose with leucine or essential amino acids: effects on myofibrillar protein synthesis at rest and following resistance exercise in men. *J Physiol.* (2012) 590:2751–65. doi: 10.1113/jphysiol.2012.228833
31. Macnaughton LS, Wardle SL, Witard OC, McGlory C, Hamilton DL, Jeromson S, et al. The response of muscle protein synthesis following whole-body resistance exercise is greater following 40 g than 20 g of ingested whey protein. *Physiol Rep.* (2016) 4:e12893. doi: 10.14814/phy2.12893
32. McGlory C, Wardle SL, Macnaughton LS, Witard OC, Scott F, Dick J, et al. Fish oil supplementation suppresses resistance exercise and feeding-induced increases in anabolic signaling without affecting myofibrillar protein synthesis in young men. *Physiol Rep.* (2016) 4:e12715. doi: 10.14814/phy2.12715
33. McKendry J, Perez-Lopez A, McLeod M, Luo D, Dent JR, Smeuninx B, et al. Short inter-set rest blunts resistance exercise-induced increases in myofibrillar protein synthesis and intracellular signalling in young males. *Exp Physiol.* (2016) 101:866–82. doi: 10.1113/EP085647
34. Reidy PT, Walker DK, Dickinson JM, Gundermann DM, Drummond MJ, Timmerman KL, et al. Soy-dairy protein blend and whey protein ingestion after resistance exercise increases amino acid transport and transporter expression in human skeletal muscle. *J Appl Physiol.* (2014) 116:1353–64. doi: 10.1152/japplphysiol.01093.2013
35. Reitelseder S, Agergaard J, Doessing S, Helmark IC, Lund P, Kristensen NB, et al. Whey and casein labeled with L-[1-13C]leucine and muscle protein synthesis: effect of resistance exercise and protein ingestion. *Am J Physiol Endocrinol Metab.* (2011) 300:E231–42. doi: 10.1152/ajpendo.0051 3.2010
36. West DW, Kujbida GW, Moore DR, Atherton P, Burd NA, Padzik JP, et al. Resistance exercise-induced increases in putative anabolic hormones do not enhance muscle protein synthesis or intracellular signalling in young men. *J Physiol.* (2009) 587(Pt 21):5239–47. doi: 10.1113/jphysiol.2009.177220
37. West DW, Burd NA, Coffey VG, Baker SK, Burke LM, Hawley JA, et al. Rapid aminoacidemia enhances myofibrillar protein synthesis and anabolic intramuscular signaling responses after resistance exercise. *Am J Clin Nutr.* (2011) 94:795–803. doi: 10.3945/ajcn.111.013722
38. West DW, Burd NA, Churchward-Venne TA, Camera DM, Mitchell CJ, Baker SK, et al. Sex-based comparisons of myofibrillar protein synthesis after resistance exercise in the fed state. *J Appl Physiol.* (2012) 112:1805–13. doi: 10.1152/japplphysiol.00170.2012
39. Moore DR, Churchward-Venne TA, Witard O, Breen L, Burd NA, Tipton KD, et al. Protein ingestion to stimulate myofibrillar protein synthesis requires greater relative protein intakes in healthy older versus younger men. *J Gerontol A Biol Sci Med Sci.* (2015) 70:57–62. doi: 10.1093/gerona/glu103
40. Gallagher D, Visser M, De Meersman RE, Sepulveda D, Baumgartner RN, Pierson RN, et al. Appendicular skeletal muscle mass: effects of age, gender, and ethnicity. *J Appl Physiol.* (1997) 83:229–39. doi: 10.1152/jappl.1997.83.1.229
41. Aragon AA, Schoenfeld BJ. Nutrient timing revisited: is there a post-exercise anabolic window? *J Int Soc Sports Nutr.* (2013) 10:5. doi: 10.1186/1550-2783-10-5
42. Cuthbertson D, Smith K, Babraj J, Leese G, Waddell T, Atherton P, et al. Anabolic signaling deficits underlie amino acid resistance of wasting, aging muscle. *Faseb J.* (2005) 19:422–4. doi: 10.1096/fj.04-2640fje
43. Kriengsinyos W, Wykes LJ, Goonewardene LA, Ball RO, Pencharz PB. Phase of menstrual cycle affects lysine requirement in healthy women. *Am J Physiol Endocrinol Metab.* (2004) 287:E489–96. doi: 10.1152/ajpendo.00262.2003
44. Phillips SM, Atkinson SA, Tarnopolsky MA, MacDougall JD. Gender differences in leucine kinetics and nitrogen balance in endurance athletes. *J Appl Physiol.* (1993) 75:2134–41. doi: 10.1152/jappl.1993.75.5.2134
45. Miller BF, Hansen M, Olesen JL, Flyvbjerg A, Schwarz P, Babraj JA, et al. No effect of menstrual cycle on myofibrillar and connective tissue protein synthesis in contracting skeletal muscle. *Am J Physiol Endocrinol Metab.* (2006) 290:E163–8. doi: 10.1152/ajpendo.00300.2005
46. Fujita S, Rasmussen BB, Bell JA, Cadenas JG, Volpi E. Basal muscle intracellular amino acid kinetics in women and men. *Am J Physiol Endocrinol Metab.* (2007) 292:E77–83. doi: 10.1152/ajpendo.0017 3.2006
47. Jahn LA, Barrett EJ, Genco ML, Wei L, Spraggins TA, Fryburg DA. Tissue composition affects measures of postabsorptive human skeletal muscle metabolism: comparison across genders. *J Clin Endocrinol Metab.* (1999) 84:1007–10. doi: 10.1210/jc.84.3.1007
48. Dreyer HC, Fujita S, Glynn EL, Drummond MJ, Volpi E, Rasmussen BB. Resistance exercise increases leg muscle protein synthesis and mTOR signalling independent of sex. *Acta Physiol.* (2010) 199:71–81. doi: 10.1111/j.1748-1716.2010.02074.x
49. Areta JL, Burke LM, Camera DM, West DW, Crawshay S, Moore DR, et al. Reduced resting skeletal muscle protein synthesis is rescued by resistance exercise and protein ingestion following short-term energy deficit. *Am J Physiol Endocrinol Metab.* (2014) 306:E989–97. doi: 10.1152/ajpendo.00590.2013
50. Alghannam AF, Gonzalez JT, Betts JA. Restoration of muscle glycogen and functional capacity: role of post-exercise carbohydrate and protein co-ingestion. *Nutrients.* (2018) 10:E253. doi: 10.3390/nu10020253
51. Burke LM, Hawley JA, Wong SH, Jeukendrup AE. Carbohydrates for training and competition. *J Sports Sci.* (2011) 29(Suppl 1):S17–27. doi: 10.1080/02640414.2011.585473
52. Glynn EL, Fry CS, Drummond MJ, Dreyer HC, Dhanani S, Volpi E, et al. Muscle protein breakdown has a minor role in the protein anabolic response to essential amino acid and carbohydrate intake following resistance exercise. *Am J Physiol Regul Integr Comp Physiol.* (2010) 299:R533–40. doi: 10.1152/ajpregu.00077.2010
53. Borsheim E, Cree MG, Tipton KD, Elliott TA, Aarsland A, Wolfe RR. Effect of carbohydrate intake on net muscle protein synthesis during recovery from resistance exercise. *J Appl Physiol.* (2004) 96:674–8. doi: 10.1152/japplphysiol.00333.2003

54. Staples AW, Burd NA, West DW, Currie KD, Atherton PJ, Moore DR, et al. Carbohydrate does not augment exercise-induced protein accretion versus protein alone. *Med Sci Sports Exerc.* (2011) 43:1154–61. doi: 10.1249/MSS.0b013e31820751cb
55. Koopman R, Beelen M, Stellingwerff T, Pennings B, Saris WH, Kies AK, et al. Coingestion of carbohydrate with protein does not further augment postexercise muscle protein synthesis. *Am J Physiol Endocrinol Metab.* (2007) 293:E833–42. doi: 10.1152/ajpendo.00135.2007
56. West DW, Cotie LM, Mitchell CJ, Churchward-Venne TA, MacDonald MJ, Phillips SM. Resistance exercise order does not determine postexercise delivery of testosterone, growth hormone, and IGF-1 to skeletal muscle. *Appl Physiol Nutr Metab.* (2013) 38:220–6. doi: 10.1139/apnm-2012-0397
57. Deutz NE, Wolfe RR. Is there a maximal anabolic response to protein intake with a meal? *Clin Nutr.* (2013) 32:309–13. doi: 10.1016/j.clnu.2012.11.018
58. Kim IY, Deutz NEP, Wolfe RR. Update on maximal anabolic response to dietary protein. *Clin Nutr.* (2018) 37:411–8. doi: 10.1016/j.clnu.2017.05.029
59. Kim IY, Schutzler S, Schrader A, Spencer HJ, Azhar G, Ferrando AA, et al. The anabolic response to a meal containing different amounts of protein is not limited by the maximal stimulation of protein synthesis in healthy young adults. *Am J Physiol Endocrinol Metab.* (2016) 310:E73–80. doi: 10.1152/ajpendo.00365.2015
60. Kim IY, Schutzler S, Schrader A, Spencer H, Kortebein P, Deutz NE, et al. Quantity of dietary protein intake, but not pattern of intake, affects net protein balance primarily through differences in protein synthesis in older adults. *Am J Physiol Endocrinol Metab.* (2015) 308:E21–8. doi: 10.1152/ajpendo.00382.2014
61. Schoenfeld BJ, Aragon AA. How much protein can the body use in a single meal for muscle-building? Implications for daily protein distribution. *J Int Soc Sports Nutr.* (2018) 15:10. doi: 10.1186/s12970-018-0215-1
62. Malowany JM, West DWD, Williamson E, Volterman KA, Abou Sawan S, Mazzulla M, et al. Protein to maximize whole-body anabolism in resistance-trained females after exercise. *Med Sci Sports Exerc.* (2019) 51:798–804. doi: 10.1249/MSS.0000000000001832
63. Mazzulla M, Volterman KA, Packer JE, Wooding DJ, Brooks JC, Kato H, et al. Whole-body net protein balance plateaus in response to increasing protein intakes during post-exercise recovery in adults and adolescents. *Nutr Metab.* (2018) 15:62. doi: 10.1186/s12986-018-0301-z
64. Almoosawi S, Winter J, Prynne CJ, Hardy R, Stephen AM. Daily profiles of energy and nutrient intakes: are eating profiles changing over time? *Eur J Clin Nutr.* (2012) 66:678–86. doi: 10.1038/ejcn.2011.210
65. Gorissen SH, Remond D, van Loon LJ. The muscle protein synthetic response to food ingestion. *Meat Sci.* (2015) 109:96–100. doi: 10.1016/j.meatsci.2015.05.009
66. Burd NA, Beals JW, Martinez IG, Salvador AF, Skinner SK. Food-first approach to enhance the regulation of post-exercise skeletal muscle protein synthesis and remodeling. *Sports Med.* (2019) 49(Suppl 1):59–68. doi: 10.1007/s40279-018-1009-y
67. Burd NA, McKenna CF, Salvador AF, Paulussen KJM, Moore DR. Dietary protein quantity, quality, and exercise are key to healthy living: a muscle-centric perspective across the lifespan. *Front Nutr.* (2019) 6:83. doi: 10.3389/fnut.2019.00083
68. Coffey VG, Moore DR, Burd NA, Rerecich T, Stellingwerff T, Garnham AP, et al. Nutrient provision increases signalling and protein synthesis in human skeletal muscle after repeated sprints. *Eur J Appl Physiol.* (2011) 111:1473–83. doi: 10.1007/s00421-010-1768-0
69. Breen L, Philp A, Witard OC, Jackman SR, Selby A, Smith K, et al. The influence of carbohydrate-protein co-ingestion following endurance exercise on myofibrillar and mitochondrial protein synthesis. *J Physiol.* (2011) 589(Pt 16):4011–25. doi: 10.1113/jphysiol.2011.211888
70. Camera DM, West DW, Phillips SM, Rerecich T, Stellingwerff T, Hawley JA, et al. Protein ingestion increases myofibrillar protein synthesis after concurrent exercise. *Med Sci Sports Exerc.* (2015) 47:82–91. doi: 10.1249/MSS.0000000000000390
71. Churchward-Venne TA, Pinckaers PJM, Smeets JSJ, Peeters WM, Zorenc AH, Schierbeek H, et al. Myofibrillar and mitochondrial protein synthesis rates do not differ in young men following the ingestion of carbohydrate with milk protein, whey, or micellar casein after concurrent resistance- and endurance-type exercise. *J Nutr.* (2019) 149:198–209. doi: 10.1093/jn/nxy244
72. Roy BD, Fowles JR, Hill R, Tarnopolsky MA. Macronutrient intake and whole body protein metabolism following resistance exercise. *Med Sci Sports Exerc.* (2000) 32:1412–8. doi: 10.1097/00005768-200008000-00009
73. Mazzulla M, Parel JT, Beals JW, Van VS, Abou Sawan S, West DWD, et al. Endurance exercise attenuates postprandial whole-body leucine balance in trained men. *Med Sci Sports Exerc.* (2017) 49:2585–92. doi: 10.1249/MSS.0000000000001394
74. Kato H, Suzuki K, Bannai M, Moore DR. Branched-chain amino acids are the primary limiting amino acids in the diets of endurance-trained men after a bout of prolonged exercise. *J Nutr.* (2018) 148:925–31. doi: 10.1093/jn/nxy048
75. Kato H, Suzuki K, Bannai M, Moore DR. Protein requirements are elevated in endurance athletes after exercise as determined by the indicator amino acid oxidation method. *PLoS ONE.* (2016) 11:e0157406. doi: 10.1371/journal.pone.0157406
76. Witard OC, Turner JE, Jackman SR, Kies AK, Jeukendrup AE, Bosch JA, et al. High dietary protein restores overreaching induced impairments in leukocyte trafficking and reduces the incidence of upper respiratory tract infection in elite cyclists. *Brain Behav Immun.* (2014) 39:211–9. doi: 10.1016/j.bbi.2013.10.002
77. Williamson E, Kato H, Volterman KA, Suzuki K, Moore DR. The effect of dietary protein on protein metabolism and performance in endurance-trained males. *Med Sci Sports Exerc.* (2019) 51:352–60. doi: 10.1249/MSS.0000000000001791
78. Kumar V, Selby A, Rankin D, Patel R, Atherton P, Hildebrandt W, et al. Age-related differences in the dose-response relationship of muscle protein synthesis to resistance exercise in young and old men. *J Physiol.* (2009) 587:211–7. doi: 10.1113/jphysiol.2008.164483
79. Balagopal P, Schimke JC, Ades P, Adey D, Nair KS. Age effect on transcript levels and synthesis rate of muscle MHC and response to resistance exercise. *Am J Physiol Endocrinol Metab.* (2001) 280:E203–8. doi: 10.1152/ajpendo.2001.280.2.E203
80. Roth SM, Ivey FM, Martel GF, Lemmer JT, Hurlbut DE, Siegel EL, et al. Muscle size responses to strength training in young and older men and women. *J Am Geriatr Soc.* (2001) 49:1428–33. doi: 10.1046/j.1532-5415.2001.4911233.x
81. Drummond MJ, Dreyer HC, Pennings B, Fry CS, Dhanani S, Dillon EL, et al. Skeletal muscle protein anabolic response to resistance exercise and essential amino acids is delayed with aging. *J Appl Physiol.* (2008) 104:1452–61. doi: 10.1152/japplphysiol.00021.2008
82. Yang Y, Breen L, Burd NA, Hector AJ, Churchward-Venne TA, Josse AR, et al. Resistance exercise enhances myofibrillar protein synthesis with graded intakes of whey protein in older men. *Br J Nutr.* (2012) 108:1780–8. doi: 10.1017/S0007114511007422
83. Churchward-Venne TA, Holwerda AM, Phillips SM, and van Loon LJ. What is the optimal amount of protein to support post-exercise skeletal muscle reconditioning in the older adult? *Sports Med.* (2016) 46:1205–12. doi: 10.1007/s40279-016-0504-2
84. Holwerda AM, Paulussen KJM, Overkamp M, Goessens JPB, Kramer IF, Wodzig W, et al. Dose-dependent increases in whole-body net protein balance and dietary protein-derived amino acid incorporation into myofibrillar protein during recovery from resistance exercise in older men. *J Nutr.* (2019) 149:221–30. doi: 10.1093/jn/nxy263
85. Burd NA, Wall BT, van Loon LJ. The curious case of anabolic resistance: old wives' tales or new fables? *J Appl Physiol.* (2012) 112:1233–5. doi: 10.1152/japplphysiol.01343.2011
86. Moore, DR. Keeping older muscle "young" through dietary protein and physical activity. *Adv Nutr.* (2014) 5:599s—607s. doi: 10.3945/an.113.005405
87. Churchward-Venne TA, Breen L, Di Donato DM, Hector AJ, Mitchell CJ, Moore DR, et al. Leucine supplementation of a low-protein mixed macronutrient beverage enhances myofibrillar protein synthesis in young men: a double-blind, randomized trial. *Am J Clin Nutr.* (2014) 99:276–86. doi: 10.3945/ajcn.113.068775
88. Tang JE, Moore DR, Kujbida GW, Tarnopolsky MA, Phillips SM. Ingestion of whey hydrolysate, casein, or soy protein isolate: effects on mixed muscle protein synthesis at rest and following resistance exercise in young men. *J Appl Physiol.* (2009) 107:987–92. doi: 10.1152/japplphysiol.000 76.2009

89. Chan AH, D'Souza RF, Beals JW, Zeng N, Prodhan U, Fanning AC, et al. The degree of aminoacidemia after dairy protein ingestion does not modulate the postexercise anabolic response in young men: a randomized controlled trial. *J Nutr.* (2019). doi: 10.1093/jn/nxz099. [Epub ahead of print].
90. Reidy PT, Walker DK, Dickinson JM, Gundermann DM, Drummond MJ, Timmerman KL, et al. Protein blend ingestion following resistance exercise promotes human muscle protein synthesis. *J Nutr.* (2013) 143:410–6. doi: 10.3945/jn.112.168021
91. Burke LM, Winter JA, Cameron-Smith D, Enslen M, Farnfield M, Decombaz J. Effect of intake of different dietary protein sources on plasma amino acid profiles at rest and after exercise. *Int J Sport Nutr Exerc Metab.* (2012) 22:452–62. doi: 10.1123/ijsnem.22.6.452
92. Burd NA, Gorissen SH, van Vliet S, Snijders T, van Loon LJ. Differences in postprandial protein handling after beef compared with milk ingestion during postexercise recovery: a randomized controlled trial. *Am J Clin Nutr.* (2015) 102:828–36. doi: 10.3945/ajcn.114.103184
93. Elliot TA, Cree MG, Sanford AP, Wolfe RR, Tipton KD. Milk ingestion stimulates net muscle protein synthesis following resistance exercise. *Med Sci Sports Exerc.* (2006) 38:667–74. doi: 10.1249/01.mss.0000210190.64458.25
94. Abou Sawan S, van Vliet S, Parel JT, Beals JW, Mazzulla M, West DWD, et al. Translocation and protein complex co-localization of mTOR is associated with postprandial myofibrillar protein synthesis at rest and after endurance exercise. *Physiol Rep.* (2018) 6. doi: 10.14814/phy2.13628
95. van Vliet S, Shy EL, Abou Sawan S, Beals JW, West DW, Skinner SK, et al. Consumption of whole eggs promotes greater stimulation of postexercise muscle protein synthesis than consumption of isonitrogenous amounts of egg whites in young men. *Am J Clin Nutr.* (2017) 106:1401–12. doi: 10.3945/ajcn.117.159855
96. Thomas DT, Erdman KA, Burke LM. American college of sports medicine joint position statement. nutrition and athletic performance. *Med Sci Sports Exerc.* (2016) 48:543–68. doi: 10.1249/MSS.0000000000000852
97. Phillips SM. Protein requirements and supplementation in strength sports. *Nutrition.* (2004) 20:689–95. doi: 10.1016/j.nut.2004.04.009
98. Millward DJ. Metabolic demands for amino acids and the human dietary requirement: millward and rRvers (1988) revisited. *J Nutr.* (1998) 128(12 Suppl):2563s–76s. doi: 10.1093/jn/128.12.2563S
99. Morens C, Gaudichon C, Fromentin G, Marsset-Baglieri A, Bensaid A, Larue-Achagiotis C, et al. Daily delivery of dietary nitrogen to the periphery is stable in rats adapted to increased protein intake. *Am J Physiol Endocrinol Metab.* (2001) 281:E826–36. doi: 10.1152/ajpendo.2001.281.4.E826
100. Gorissen SH, Horstman AM, Franssen R, Kouw IW, Wall BT, Burd NA, et al. Habituation to low or high protein intake does not modulate basal or postprandial muscle protein synthesis rates: a randomized trial. *Am J Clin Nutr.* (2017) 105:332–42. doi: 10.3945/ajcn.115.129924
101. Pasiakos SM, Cao JJ, Margolis LM, Sauter ER, Whigham LD, McClung JP, et al. Effects of high-protein diets on fat-free mass and muscle protein synthesis following weight loss: a randomized controlled trial. *Faseb J.* (2013) 27:3837–47. doi: 10.1096/fj.13-230227
102. Pasiakos SM, Vislocky LM, Carbone JW, Altieri N, Konopelski K, Freake HC, et al. Acute energy deprivation affects skeletal muscle protein synthesis and associated intracellular signaling proteins in physically active adults. *J Nutr.* (2010) 140:745–51. doi: 10.3945/jn.109.118372
103. Camera DM, West DW, Burd NA, Phillips SM, Garnham AP, Hawley JA, et al. Low muscle glycogen concentration does not suppress the anabolic response to resistance exercise. *J Appl Physiol.* (2012) 113:206–14. doi: 10.1152/japplphysiol.00395.2012
104. Hector AJ, McGlory C, Damas F, Mazara N, Baker SK, Phillips SM. Pronounced energy restriction with elevated protein intake results in no change in proteolysis and reductions in skeletal muscle protein synthesis that are mitigated by resistance exercise. *Faseb J.* (2018) 32:265–75. doi: 10.1096/fj.201700158RR
105. Longland TM, Oikawa SY, Mitchell CJ, Devries MC, Phillips SM. Higher compared with lower dietary protein during an energy deficit combined with intense exercise promotes greater lean mass gain and fat mass loss: a randomized trial. *Am J Clin Nutr.* (2016) 103:738–46. doi: 10.3945/ajcn.115.119339
106. Paddon-Jones D, Westman E, Mattes RD, Wolfe RR, Astrup A, Westerterp-Plantenga W. Protein, weight management, and satiety. *Am J Clin Nutr.* (2008) 87:1558s–61s. doi: 10.1093/ajcn/87.5.1558S
107. Murphy CH, Hector AJ, Phillips SM. Considerations for protein intake in managing weight loss in athletes. *Eur J Sport Sci.* (2015) 15:21–8. doi: 10.1080/17461391.2014.936325
108. Beals JW, Burd NA, Moore DR, van Vliet S. Obesity alters the muscle protein synthetic response to nutrition and exercise. *Front Nutr.* (2019) 6:87. doi: 10.3389/fnut.2019.00087
109. Beals JW, Sukiennik RA, Nallabelli J, Emmons RS, van Vliet S, Young JR, et al. Anabolic sensitivity of postprandial muscle protein synthesis to the ingestion of a protein-dense food is reduced in overweight and obese young adults. *Am J Clin Nutr.* (2016) 104:1014–22. doi: 10.3945/ajcn.116.130385
110. Beals JW, Skinner SK, McKenna CF, Poozhikunnel EG, Farooqi SA, van Vliet S, et al. Altered anabolic signalling and reduced stimulation of myofibrillar protein synthesis after feeding and resistance exercise in people with obesity. *J Physiol.* (2018) 596:5119–33. doi: 10.1113/JP276210
111. Kouw IWK, van Dijk JW, Horstman AMH, Kramer IF, Goessens JPB, van Dielen FMH, et al. Basal and postprandial myofibrillar protein synthesis rates do not differ between lean and obese middle-aged men. *J Nutr.* (2019). doi: 10.1093/jn/nxz104. [Epub ahead of print].
112. Smeuninx B, McKendry J, Wilson D, Martin U, Breen L. Age-related anabolic resistance of myofibrillar protein synthesis is exacerbated in obese inactive individuals. *J Clin Endocrinol Metab.* (2017) 102:3535–45. doi: 10.1210/jc.2017-00869
113. Tang JE, Perco JG, Moore DR, Wilkinson SB, Phillips SM. Resistance training alters the response of fed state mixed muscle protein synthesis in young men. *Am J Physiol Regul Integr Comp Physiol.* (2008) 294:R172–8. doi: 10.1152/ajpregu.00636.2007
114. Mitchell CJ, Churchward-Venne TA, Parise G, Bellamy L, Baker SK, Smith K, et al. Acute post-exercise myofibrillar protein synthesis is not correlated with resistance training-induced muscle hypertrophy in young men. *PLoS ONE.* (2014) 9:e89431. doi: 10.1371/journal.pone.0089431
115. Wernbom M, Augustsson J, Thomee R. The influence of frequency, intensity, volume and mode of strength training on whole muscle cross-sectional area in humans. *Sports Med.* (2007) 37:225–64. doi: 10.2165/00007256-200737030-00004
116. Mamerow MM, Mettler JA, English KL, Casperson SL, Arentson-Lantz E, Sheffield-Moore M, et al. Dietary protein distribution positively influences 24-h muscle protein synthesis in healthy adults. *J Nutr.* (2014) 144:876–80. doi: 10.3945/jn.113.185280
117. Moore DR, Areta J, Coffey VG, Stellingwerff T, Phillips SM, Burke LM, et al. Daytime pattern of post-exercise protein intake affects whole-body protein turnover in resistance-trained males. *Nutr Metab.* (2012) 9:91. doi: 10.1186/1743-7075-9-91
118. Res PT, Groen B, Pennings B, Beelen M, Wallis GA, Gijsen AP, et al. Protein ingestion before sleep improves postexercise overnight recovery. *Med Sci Sports Exerc.* (2012) 44:1560–9. doi: 10.1249/MSS.0b013e31824cc363
119. Morton RW, Murphy KT, McKellar SR, Schoenfeld BJ, Henselmans M, Helms E, et al. A systematic review, meta-analysis and meta-regression of the effect of protein supplementation on resistance training-induced gains in muscle mass and strength in healthy adults. *Br J Sports Med.* (2018) 52:376–84. doi: 10.1136/bjsports-2017-097608

6

Influence of Fish Oil-Derived n-3 Fatty Acid Supplementation on Changes in Body Composition and Muscle Strength During Short-Term Weight Loss in Resistance-Trained Men

*Jordan D. Philpott[1], Niels J. Bootsma[1], Nidia Rodriguez-Sanchez[1], David Lee Hamilton[1,2], Elizabeth MacKinlay[3], James Dick[3], Samuel Mettler[4], Stuart D. R. Galloway[1], Kevin D. Tipton[5] and Oliver C. Witard[1,6]**

[1] Physiology, Exercise and Nutrition Research Group, Faculty of Health Sciences and Sport, University of Stirling, Stirling, United Kingdom, [2] Institute for Physical Activity and Nutrition (IPAN), School of Exercise and Nutrition Sciences, Deakin University, Geelong, VIC, Australia, [3] Institute of Aquaculture, University of Stirling, Stirling, United Kingdom, [4] Department of Health Sciences and Technology, ETH Zurich, Zurich, Switzerland, [5] Department of Sport and Exercise Sciences, Faculty of Social Sciences and Health, Durham University, Durham, United Kingdom, [6] Centre for Human and Applied Physiological Sciences, School of Basic and Medical Biosciences, Faculty of Life Sciences and Medicine, King's College London, London, United Kingdom

***Correspondence:**
Oliver C. Witard
oliver.witard@kcl.ac.uk

Background: A detrimental consequence of diet-induced weight loss, common in athletes who participate in weight cutting sports, is muscle loss. Dietary omega-3 polyunsaturated fatty acids (n-3PUFA) exhibit a protective effect on the loss of muscle tissue during catabolic situations such as injury-simulated leg immobilization. This study aimed to investigate the influence of dietary n-3PUFA supplementation on changes in body composition and muscle strength following short-term diet-induced weight loss in resistance-trained men.

Methods: Twenty resistance-trained young (23 ± 1 years) men were randomly assigned to a fish oil group that supplemented their diet with 4 g n-3PUFA, 18 g carbohydrate, and 5 g protein (FO) or placebo group containing an equivalent carbohydrate and protein content (CON) over a 6 week period. During weeks 1–3, participants continued their habitual diet. During week 4, participants received all food items to control energy balance and a macronutrient composition of 50% carbohydrate, 35% fat, and 15% protein. During weeks 5 and 6, participants were fed an energy-restricted diet equivalent to 60% habitual energy intake. Body composition and strength were measured during weeks 1, 4, and 6.

Results: The decline in total body mass (FO = −3.0 ± 0.3 kg, CON = −2.6 ± 0.3 kg), fat free mass (FO = −1.4 ± 0.3 kg, CON = −1.2 ± 0.3 kg) and fat mass (FO = −1.4 ± 0.2 kg, CON = −1.3 ± 0.3 kg) following energy restriction was similar between groups (all $p > 0.05$; d: 0.16–0.39). Non-dominant leg extension 1 RM increased (6.1 ± 3.4%) following energy restriction in FO ($p < 0.05$, $d = 0.29$), with no changes observed in CON ($p > 0.05$, $d = 0.05$). Dominant leg extension 1 RM tended to increase following energy restriction in FO ($p = 0.09$, $d = 0.29$), with no changes in CON ($p > 0.05$, $d = 0.06$).

Changes in leg press 1 RM, maximum voluntary contraction and muscular endurance following energy restriction were similar between groups ($p > 0.05$, $d = 0.05$).

Conclusion: Any possible improvements in muscle strength during short-term weight loss with n-3PUFA supplementation are not related to the modulation of FFM in resistance-trained men.

Keywords: omega-3 polyunsaturated fatty acids, energy restriction, fat-free mass, fat mass, performance, athletes

INTRODUCTION

The application of diet-induced weight loss extends beyond clinical (overweight and obese) populations. Athletic populations competing in weight-category sports (e.g., boxing), or sports where a high power-to-body mass ratio (sprinting) or aesthetics (gymnastics) are pre-requisites for success also routinely periodize their training programme to include short-term periods of energy restriction (1). However, a counterproductive feature of diet-induced weight loss in athletes that accompanies the reduction in fat mass includes the decline in fat-free mass (FFM), specifically of skeletal muscle tissue (2, 3).

Changes in body composition during diet-induced weight loss can be manipulated with nutrition (4). Most notably, experimental studies demonstrate that increasing dietary protein intake confers an effective nutritional strategy to promote high-quality weight loss during energy restriction, i.e., loss of fat mass while maintaining muscle mass during short-term weight loss (2, 5). However, the preservation of muscle mass during energy restriction with a higher protein intake did not translate into the better maintenance of exercise performance in resistance-trained young men (2). The importance of other nutrients for maintaining FFM during diet-induced weight loss has been proposed (2, 5), but few experimental studies have addressed the effectiveness of these nutrients on changes in body composition during weight loss.

Another potentially effective nutritional intervention to promote high-quality weight loss during energy restriction in athletic populations is the ingestion of omega-3 polyunsaturated fatty acid (n-3PUFA). Both *in vitro* cell line experiments (6, 7) and *in vivo* human studies (8–10) support the notion that n-3PUFA exhibit anabolic properties, in particular the omega-3 species eicosapentaenoic acid (EPA). Previous proof-of-principle studies have demonstrated that fish oil-derived n-3PUFA supplementation potentiated the response of muscle protein synthesis (MPS) to the infusion of amino acids and insulin (9, 10), and enhanced muscle mass (11) and strength (12, 13) in older adults. The mechanism most commonly proposed to underpin the anabolic action of n-3PUFA relates to modifying the lipid profile of the muscle phospholipid membrane. This structural change in integrity of the muscle membrane is understood to activate intracellular signaling proteins (e.g., mTORC1-p70S6k1) (9, 14) that upregulate muscle protein synthesis (MPS), thus modulating muscle mass.

Based on current evidence from experimental studies, the metabolic role of n-3PUFA in regulating muscle mass is most evident under catabolic conditions. Consistent with this notion, fish oil-derived n-3PUFA supplementation was shown to exhibit protective roles in preserving muscle mass in a clinical population of cancer cachexia patients (15) and following a short-term period of leg immobilization in healthy recreationally-active young women (8). Another catabolic situation is diet-induced weight loss, whereby the intracellular activation of AMPK signals an energy deficit within the muscle cell (16). Given that MPS is an energetically expensive process, requiring ~4 moles of ATP to bind each amino acid during the elongation process of translation (17), this activation of AMPK acts to conserve energy during weight loss by down-regulating basal rates of MPS (16, 18, 19). To our knowledge, all studies to date that have investigated the impact of fish oil supplementation on body composition during weight loss have been conducted in a clinical setting with overweight and/or obese patients (20, 21). Given the link between dietary n-3PUFA intake, MPS and muscle mass during injury-simulated leg immobilization in trained young women (8), there is strong rationale to support a protective role of n-3PUFA in maintaining muscle mass and strength during energy-restricted weight loss in athletes.

The primary aim of this study was to investigate the influence of fish oil-derived n-3PUFA supplementation during short-term diet-induced weight loss on changes in body composition and muscle strength in resistance-trained young men. We hypothesized that n-3PUFA supplementation would attenuate the loss of lean body mass and better maintain lower limb muscle strength following a 2 week period of an energy-restricted diet compared to placebo.

METHODS

Study Design

Using a parallel research design adapted from Mettler et al. (2) (**Figure 1**), participants were randomly assigned to one of two groups: a fish oil supplement group (FO) or an energy and macronutrient matched control group (CON). Participants consumed their assigned supplement twice daily for the entire 6-week study period. Participants consumed their habitual diet for the first 3 weeks of the study, with week 1 used to assess energy intake and energy expenditure. During week 4, all food items and fluids were supplied by researchers, providing 100% of habitual energy intake. During weeks 5 and 6, the energy content of the diet was reduced to 60% of habitual intake. At the end of weeks 1, 4, and 6, measurements of body mass, body composition, and muscle performance were obtained under controlled laboratory conditions using dual energy x-ray absorptiometry (DXA), leg extension and leg press fixed

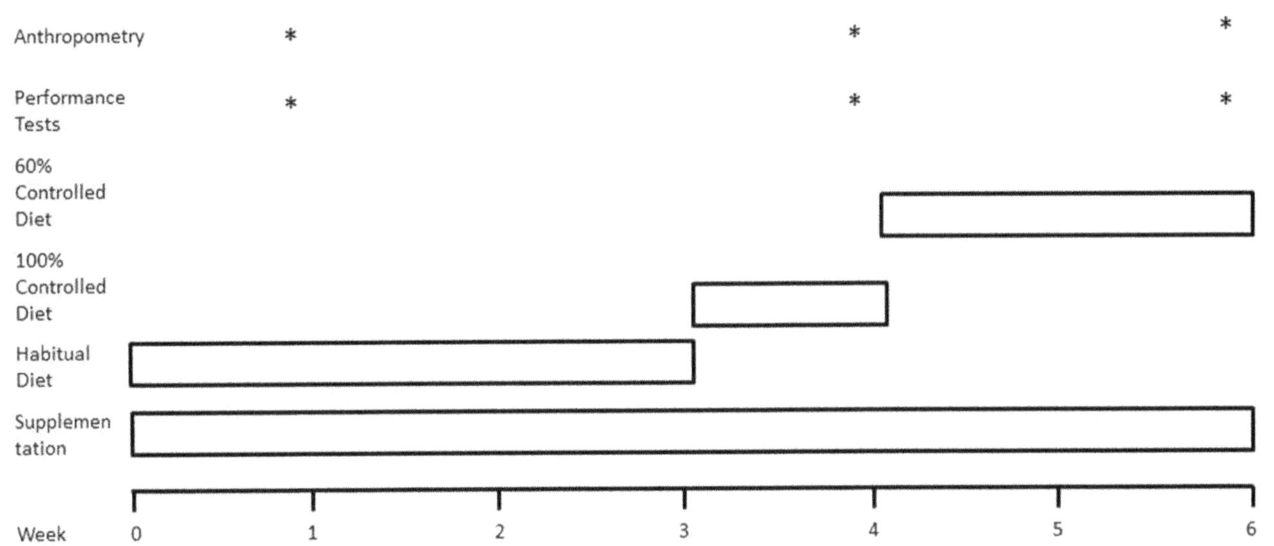

FIGURE 1 | Schematic overview of study design. Weeks 0–3, participants consumed their habitual diet under free-living conditions. Week 4, all food items were supplied by researchers to ensure participants consumed a diet constituting 100% of habitual energy intake and a macronutrient composition of 50% carbohydrate, 35% fat, and 15% protein. Weeks 5 and 6, all food items provided to ensure energy-restricted diet was equivalent to 60% of habitual energy intake. *Represents when the category occurs displayed in the figure.

resistance machines (Cybex International, Illinois, USA) and isokinetic dynamometry technology.

Participant Recruitment and Ethical Approval

Twenty healthy (no known metabolic disorders as determined by health questionnaire) young resistance-trained males were recruited from local sports clubs. All participants had undertaken resistance training for at least the previous 6 months, were currently training $\geq$2 times per week, and were not consuming supplements containing n-3PUFA at the time of study enrolment. Participants were asked to continue their habitual training throughout the 6-week study period. The West of Scotland Research Ethics Service approved the study procedures.

Dietary Control and Supplementation

In a single blinded fashion, participants were divided equally between supplement conditions, consuming 2 × 200 mL volume juice-based drinks (1 × morning and 1 × evening) daily over the 6 week supplementation period (Smartfish Sports Nutrition, Ltd). Drinks were provided to match energy and macronutrient composition of the two diets. However, the FO beverage contained an additional 2 g of n-3PUFA per drink. Supplements were taste-matched and equal in protein and carbohydrate content. The experimental supplement condition contained 2 g of fish oil (~1 g of EPA and ~1 g of DHA) whereas the placebo condition did not contain fish oil. The additional energy provided by the fish oil supplement in the experimental condition was accounted for by modifying the energy content of the background diet.

Trial Days and Measurements

Testing sessions commenced at ~07:00 on weeks 1 (day 7), 4 (day 27), and 6 (day 41) following an overnight fast and having consumed 500 ml of water 1–2 h prior to arriving at the laboratory. Participants were instructed to empty their bladder before body weight was measured using standard laboratory scales (Seca Quadra 808, Birmingham, UK) with participants wearing underwear only. Body composition was measured using a narrowed fan-beamed dual-energy x-ray absorptiometry (iDXA GE Healthcare) with analysis performed using GE Encore 13.40.038 Software (GE Healthcare). All DXA scans followed procedures previously described by Rodriguez-Sanchez and Galloway (22) and were performed by the same trained technician.

Muscle Strength and Endurance

The first test of muscle strength was a single leg isokinetic/eccentric maximum voluntary contraction (MVC) of the knee flexors using an isokinetic dynamometer (Biodex Corporation, New York). Participants were seated on the dynamometer with their upper body, hips, and thigh securely strapped into the seat and the hip at a 90° angle to the legs. The lower leg was attached to the arm of the dynamometer 1 cm above the lateral malleolus ankle joint with the axis of rotation of the dynamometer arm aligned with the lateral femoral condyle. The dynamometer arm was set to start and stop at angles 90° and 0°, respectively, at the knee joint. Participants were asked to use maximum effort resist the dynamometer arm from moving the knee joint from a 90° to a 0° angle. Each participant performed 3 × 3 sets/reps of this MVC protocol with a 60 s rest between sets. Each participant's greatest peak torque from the three sets was recorded.

Following 5 min rest, unilateral 1 RM for leg extension was assessed using a previously validated protocol (23) on a fixed resistance machine (Cybex International Inc, Cybex International, MA). Seat and knee position was recorded during testing session and was replicated during weeks 4 and 6. On the same day, following a 10 min rest period, unilateral muscular endurance was measured. Participants completed as many repetitions as possible on leg extension and leg press, with resistance set at 60% of individual baseline 1 RM. Participants completed repetitions at their own pace but were instructed to cease exercising as soon as a rest between repetitions was required. In total, testing sessions were completed within 180 min.

Diet

During weeks 1–3, all participants consumed their habitual diet but were asked to refrain from eating oily fish to ensure that supplementation accounted for changes in blood lipid profiles. During week 1, energy intake and energy expenditure were measured. Energy intake was measured using a 3-d food report. On the same days as the food report, energy expenditure was measured using the physical activity questionnaire (24) and from Actiheart data (CamNtech Ltd, Papworth Everard, England). All measures of energy intake and expenditure were averaged to give a 100% energy value. During week 4, participants were instructed to consume only the food provided by researchers that contained 100% of their habitual diet with a macronutrient composition of 50% carbohydrate, 35% fat, and 15% protein. The energy content of the supplement was taken into account when calculating the habitual energy intake of each participant. The only exceptions were water and diet soft drinks that could be consumed *ad libitum*. Participants were asked to provide feedback on the volume of food consumed. If a participant reported feeling hungry, the energy content of the diet was increased. Conversely, if the volunteer was unable to eat all food provided, the energy content of the diet was reduced. Participants also were asked to monitor their body weight throughout week 4 to ensure body weight stability. During weeks 5 and 6, dietary energy intake was reduced to 60% of habitual intake, however macronutrient composition remained constant. Throughout weeks 4–6, foods rich in omega-3 fatty acids such as oily fish (tuna, salmon, mackerel), walnuts and margarine were omitted from the diet. The diets were individually tailored to compensate for individual eating patterns and preferences and therefore maximize diet compliance. During weeks 4–6, participants were asked to return any food that was not consumed to researchers for weighing. Returned food was then weighed and an energy content was calculated. The energy content not consumed by the participant was added on to the following day's diet. Every attempt was made to provide participants with the confidence to honestly report any non-compliance without any consequences.

Blood Analysis

Approximately 1 mL of venous blood was dispensed onto specialized Whatman 903 blood collection cards (GE Healthcare Ltd, Forest Farm Industrial Estate, Cardiff, CF 14 7YT, UK). Cards were dried for 3 h after which the dried whole blood sample was detached from the collection device using forceps and placed into a screw-cap vial containing 1 mL of methylating solution (1.25 M methanol/HCl). Vials were then placed in a hot block at 70°C for 1 h. The vials were allowed to cool to room temperature before adding 2 mL of distilled water and 2 mL of saturated KCl solution. Fatty acid methyl esters (FAME) were then extracted using 1 × 2 mL of isohexane + BHT followed by a second extraction using 2 mL of isohexane alone. This extraction method has been previously validated as a reliable measure of whole blood fatty acid composition in our own laboratories (25). FAME were then separated and quantified by gas liquid chromatography (ThermoFisher Trace, Hemel Hempstead, England) using a 60 m × 0.32 mm × 0.25 μm film thickness capillary column (ZB Wax, Phenomenex, Macclesfield, UK). Hydrogen was used as carrier gas at a flow rate of 4.0 mL·min−1 and the temperature program was from 50 to 150°C at 40°C·min−1 then to 195°C at 2°C·min−1 and finally to 215°C at 0.5°C·min−1. Individual FAME were identified compared to well-characterized in house standards as well as commercial FAME mixtures (Supelco™ 37 FAME mix, Sigma- Aldrich Ltd., Gillingham, England).

Data Presentation and Statistical Analysis

Data were analyzed using Statistical Package for Social Sciences 21 (IBM SPSS, Chicago, IL). All data were found to be normally distributed based on the Shapiro-Wilk test. Differences across time for body composition, muscle strength and muscular endurance were analyzed by a mixed-design, two-way (time and supplement group) ANOVA. Two between-subject variables (FO and PLA) and either three within-subject (weeks 1 (habitual diet), 4 (100% diet), and 6 (60% diet) time-points) or 2 within-subjects (week 4 and week 6) variables were modeled within the two-way ANOVA. Where a significant time × supplement group interaction was detected, a Bonferroni *post hoc* test was performed to locate the timepoint(s) whereby differences existed between supplement groups. Statistical significance was set at the level of ≤0.05. Cohen's effect sizes (d) were calculated to compare differences between conditions. Effect sizes of 0.2 were considered small, 0.5 considered medium, and >0.8 were considered large (26). All data were expressed as means ± SD, unless otherwise stated.

RESULTS

Supplement Control

All participants consumed all of the supplements provided to them. No adverse events occurred due to the fish oil or placebo supplementation.

Dietary Intake During Energy Restriction

No differences in energy or macronutrient intakes were observed between FO and CON during the habitual diet, 100% diet, and 60% diet periods ($p > 0.05$, **Figure 2**). Energy intake was lower during the 60% diet period compared to the 100% diet period in both conditions ($p < 0.001$).

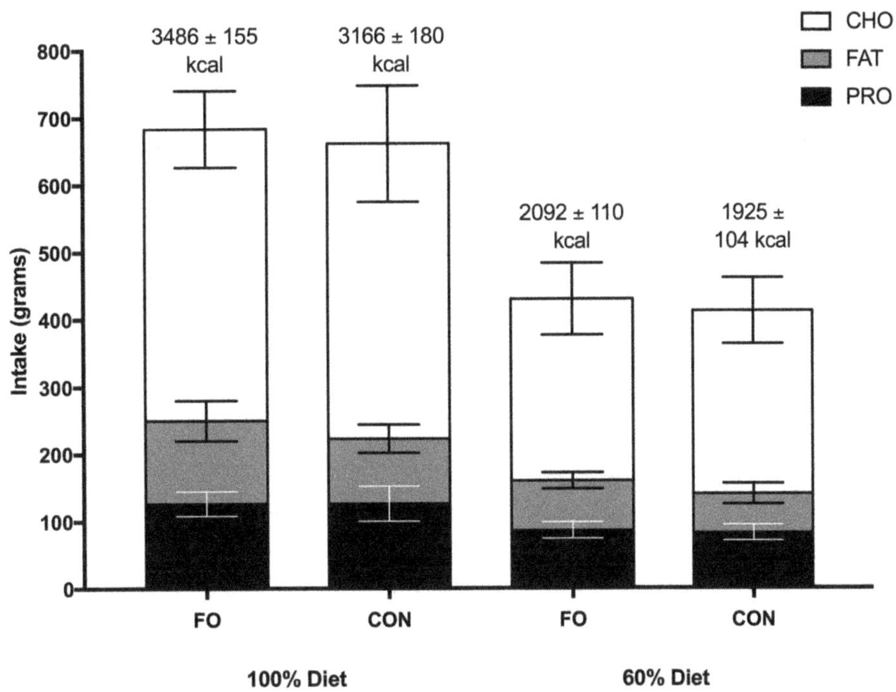

FIGURE 2 | Energy intake (kcal) and macronutrient composition (grams) during the 100% diet period and the 60% diet period in fish oil (FO) and control (CON) supplement groups. Values are means ± SD. CHO, carbohydrate; PRO, protein.

Blood n-3PUFA Composition

Baseline (pre) blood % n-3PUFA/totalPUFA composition was similar between groups ($p < 0.01$, **Figure 3**). Blood n-3PUFA composition increased by ~60% following 6 weeks of supplementation in FO, whereas no change was observed in CON. At the individual level, blood % n-3PUFA/totalPUFA composition increased in all 10 participants after supplementation in FO.

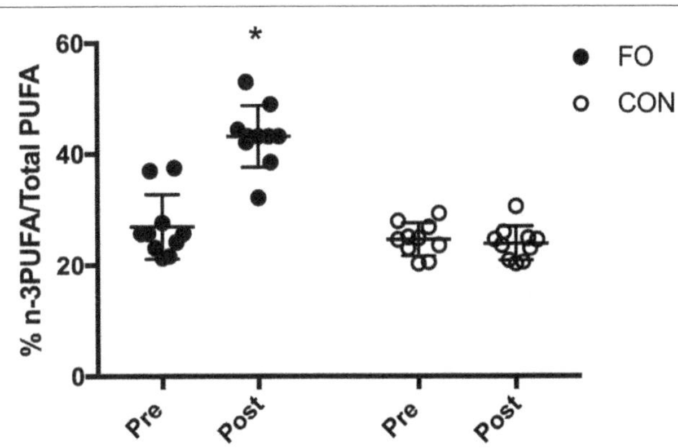

FIGURE 3 | Blood % n-3PUFA/total PUFA composition before (Pre) and after (Post) 6 week of supplementation. Data are expressed as means ± SD and also as individual values. *Significant difference vs. baseline (Pre) in corresponding supplement group.

Body Composition

Total body mass (pre: 83.6 ± 3.6 kg; post: 80.8 ± 3.5 kg, $p < 0.001$), lean body mass (pre: 64.4 ± 2.3 kg; post: 63.0 ± 2.3 kg, $p < 0.001$), and fat mass (pre: 15.8 ± 1.6 kg; post: 14.4 ± 1.6 kg, $p < 0.001$) for all participants, decreased from baseline (pre) following 2 weeks of energy restriction (**Figure 4A**), with no differences between conditions. Individual changes in body mass, lean body mass and fat mass are presented in **Figures 4B–D**. Regional changes in total body mass, lean body mass, and fat mass were similar between FO and CON (see **Supplementary Table**).

Muscle Strength

Leg press and leg extension 1RM remained constant between week 1 and week 4 for both dominant and non-dominant legs (all $p > 0.30$, **Figure 5**). Leg extension 1 RM for the non-dominant leg increased by 6.1 ± 3.4% following energy restriction (weeks 4–6) compared with energy balance (weeks 0–4) in FO ($p < 0.05$, $d = 0.29$), with no changes in CON across the 6 week period. Leg extension 1 RM for the dominant leg tended to increase following energy restriction in FO ($p = 0.092$, $d = 0.29$), whereas no changes were observed in CON. No differences in leg press 1 RM for either leg were observed between weeks 4 (pre 100% diet period) and 6 (post 60% diet period) in either supplement group.

There were no differences in MVC for the dominant leg across diet periods or between supplement groups (**Figure 6**). MVC for the non-dominant leg decreased by 5.7 ± 7.9% from week 1 to 4 ($p = 0.03$, $d = 0.31$) and by 7.4 ± 11.8% from week 1 to 6 ($p = 0.016$, $d = 0.42$), with no differences between supplement groups.

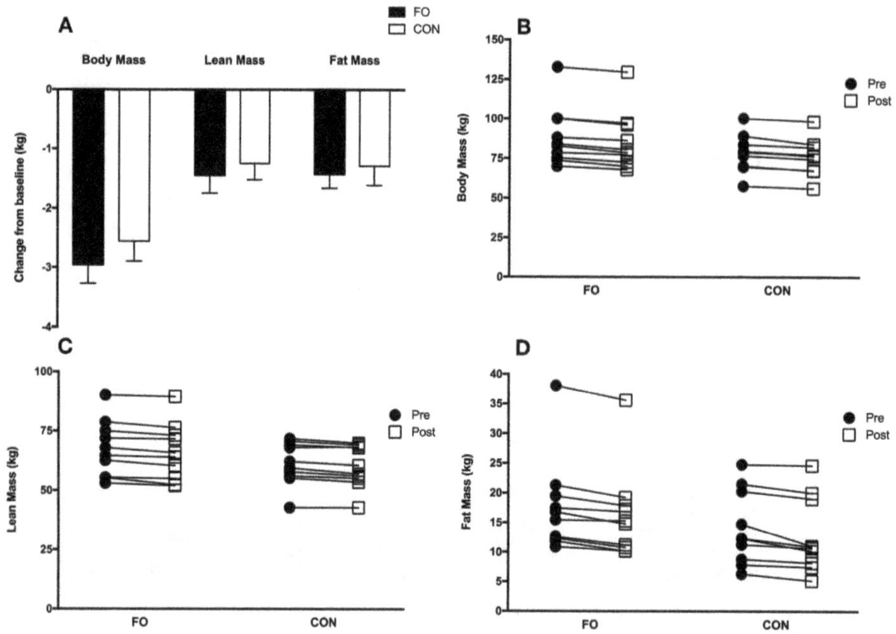

FIGURE 4 | Group **(A)** and individualized changes in total body mass **(B)**, lean body mass **(C)**, and fat mass **(D)** from baseline (average of the two measurements collected during week 1 (Habitual diet) and 4 (100% diet) prior to weight loss) following 2 weeks of 40% energy restriction in fish oil (FO) and control (CON) supplement groups. Values are means ± SEM.

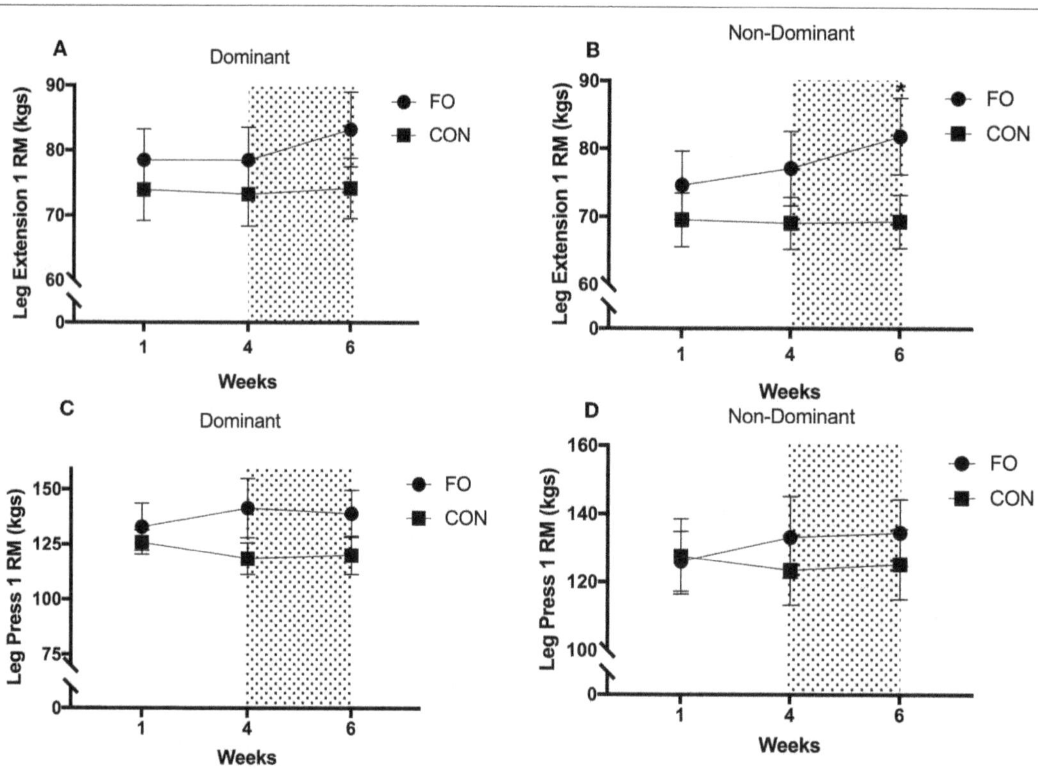

FIGURE 5 | One repetition maximum for **(A)** dominant leg extension, **(B)** non-dominant leg extension, **(C)** dominant leg press, and **(D)** non-dominant leg press during weeks 1 (habitual diet), 4 (100% diet), and 6 (60% diet) of study. Shaded area represents the 2 week period of energy restriction. Values are means ± SEM. *Significant difference compared to weeks 1 and 4 in corresponding supplement group ($p < 0.05$).

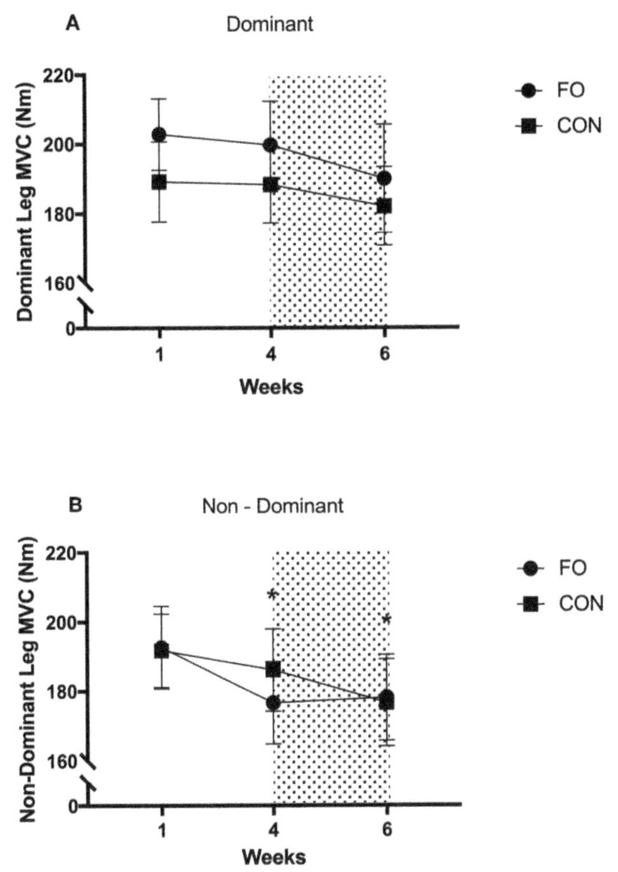

FIGURE 6 | Maximum Voluntary Contraction of dominant and non-dominant legs during week 1 (habitual diet), week 4 (100% diet), and week 6 (60% diet). Shaded area represents 2 week period of energy restriction. Values are mean ± SEM. **(A)** dominant leg. **(B)** non-dominant leg. *Significant difference compared to week 1.

Muscular Endurance

There were no differences in muscular endurance across diet periods or between supplement groups in either the dominant or non-dominant leg for leg extension or leg press exercises (all $p > 0.05$, **Figure 7**).

DISCUSSION

The primary aim of this study was to investigate the influence of dietary fish oil-derived n-3PUFA supplementation on changes in body composition and muscle strength during a short-term period of weight loss in resistance-trained young men. Our findings indicate that n-3PUFA supplementation resulted in a partial improvement in muscle strength following 2 weeks of 40% energy restriction, i.e., a small improvement in 1 RM leg extension in FO, but changes in MVC we similar between FO and CON groups. However, refuting our original hypothesis, n-3PUFA supplementation failed to modulate changes in body composition or attenuate the decline in muscle endurance induced by short-term weight loss. The practical implications of these preliminary data remain unclear, but suggest that dietary n-3PUFA supplementation may maintain, if not improve, some components of muscle strength during short-term weight loss in athletes competing in weight category sports and/or sports that depend on a high power-to-body mass ratio. However, the causal mechanism(s) that underpin this muscle adaptive response does not appear to be related to the modulation of lean body mass.

Changes in muscle strength induced by diet and exercise training are often associated with changes in muscle mass. Despite the improvement in 1 RM leg extension with n-3PUFA supplementation following the 2 week period of diet-induced weight loss, the decline in fat-free mass was comparable between supplement groups. Our laboratory previously demonstrated that 4 weeks of fish oil supplementation markedly increased n-3PUFA concentrations in the muscle cell (14). The uptake of n-3PUFA into the muscle cell membrane has been suggested to prime the muscle translational machinery inside the cell to respond to anabolic stimuli in both young (10) and older (9) adults. Moreover, a recent study demonstrated that fish oil supplementation attenuated the decline in muscle mass following 2 weeks of limb immobilization in trained young women, as mediated by a greater integrated response of MPS (8). Given that the primary locus of control for the regulation of muscle mass in resistance-trained young men is MPS (27), we hypothesized that any improvement in muscle strength during weight loss with n-3PUFA supplementation would be mediated by the preservation of lean body mass. However, in the present study, non-dominant leg extension 1 RM increased by >6% with n-3PUFA supplementation following 2 week of diet-induced weight loss, despite a 1.4 kg decrease in FFM. This apparent disconnect between muscle strength and FFM is not uncommon (28) and cannot be explained from this proof-of-principle study. Nonetheless, even if the incorporation of n-3PUFA into the phospholipid layer of the muscle cell membrane led to an upregulation of the muscle protein synthetic machinery, it did not appear to mediate the improvement in muscle strength observed following diet-induced weight loss in the n-3PUFA group.

A feasible alternative explanation for the improvement in 1 RM leg extension following energy restriction with n-3PUFA supplementation, in the absence of any changes in lean body mass, may relate to neuromuscular function. Consistent with this notion, a previous study demonstrated a reduction in electro-mechanical delay, defined as the time taken for a specific muscle to respond to a stimulus, with n-3PUFA supplementation, albeit in older adult women (12). From a mechanistic standpoint, DHA is an essential component of the phospholipid membrane of neurons localized in brain tissue (29). Moreover, previous animal and human studies have reported strong associations between increased DHA concentrations in brain tissue (30), improvements in brain function and increased muscle strength (31). In the present study, we report a marked increase in blood n-3PUFA concentrations following 4 weeks of n-3PUFA supplementation containing 2 g of DHA per day. On the basis of comparable findings using a rodent model (32), it is reasonable to assume that DHA concentrations also increased in the neural tissue of our resistance-trained men.

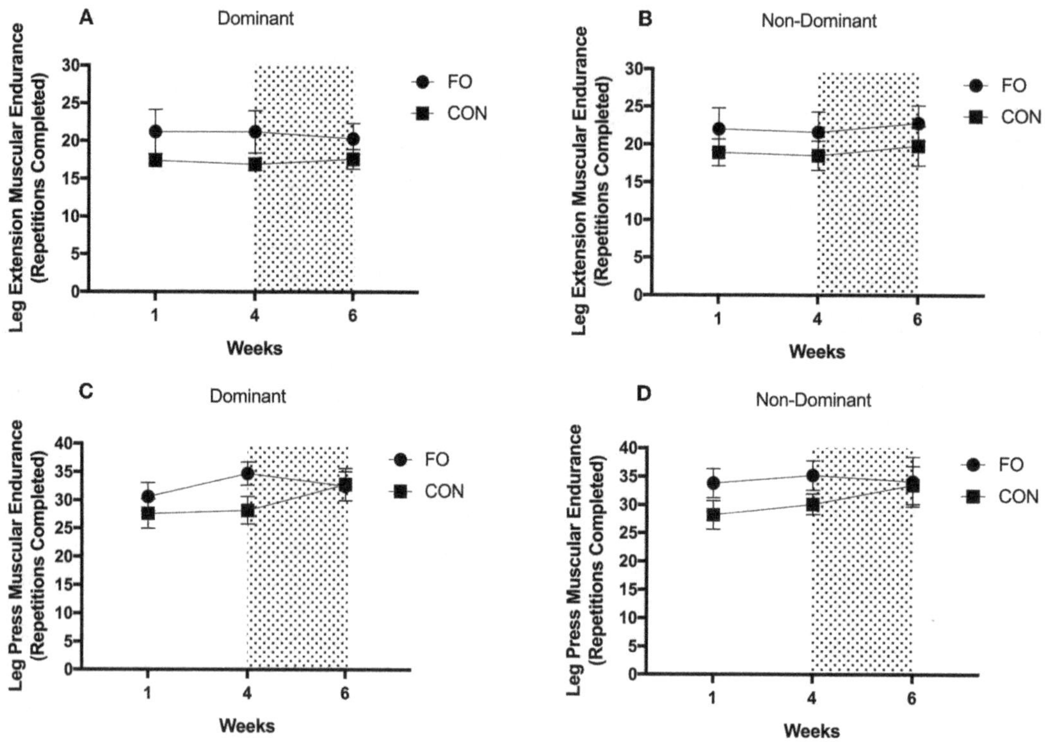

FIGURE 7 | Muscular endurance for **(A)** leg extension on dominant leg, **(B)** leg extension on non-dominant leg, **(C)** leg press on dominant leg, and **(D)** leg press on non-dominant leg during weeks 1 (habitual diet), 4 (100% diet), and 6 (60% diet) of study protocol. Shaded area represents a 2 week period of energy restriction. Values are means ± SEM.

Although speculative, these data provide preliminary support for the notion that neuromuscular mechanisms may underpin the current observation of a maintenance, if not increase, in muscle strength following an energy-restricted diet in the n-3PUFA group.

The divergent response of leg press strength and leg extension strength to weight loss between groups further supports the notion that n-3PUFA supplementation enhanced neural adaptations. Although we observed an improvement in leg extension 1 RM with n-3PUFA supplementation, no difference in strength was observed for leg press 1 RM between groups. A possible explanation for this differential finding relates to the recruitment and activation of different muscle groups between exercises. Based on electromyography data, only the quadricep muscle group is activated during leg extension (33), whereas multiple muscle groups, including gastrocnemius, quadriceps and gluteus maximus are activated during the leg press (34). We report a regional decline in FFM in both left and right legs following weight loss in both groups (**Supplementary Table**). Expressed relative to total muscle mass activated during the exercise test, the decline in FFM in muscles activated during the leg extension was less than leg press. Hence, we speculate that the incorporation of DHA into neural tissue altered the interaction between the central nervous system and muscle tissue, potentially improving firing rate and recruitment of motor neurons during the 1 RM leg extension. Further research is warranted to substantiate this notion and to examine the influence of n-3PUFA supplementation on neuromuscular activity during leg press and leg extension exercises both under conditions of weight maintenance and weight loss.

The effective modification of body composition during weight loss with nutrition, and more specifically with manipulation of dietary protein, has been demonstrated previously in both clinical (35, 36) and athletic (18, 37) populations. In this regard, the protein content of an energy-restricted diet has been shown to modulate the magnitude of muscle loss during weight loss (2, 5). Recent evidence suggests an interactive effect of protein and n-3PUFA in the regulation of muscle protein metabolism. For example, Smith et al. (10) demonstrated a potentiated response of MPS to the intravenous infusion of amino acids following 8 weeks of n-3PUFA supplementation in young adults. Based on this observation, it is possible that a higher dietary protein intake was required in the present study for n-3PUFA supplementation to elicit a protective effect on lean body mass during weight loss. By design, in the present study dietary protein intake was reduced during the 2 week weight loss period in proportion to the energy deficit imposed. The basis for this methodological decision was to examine a proof-of-concept, i.e., testing the impact of n-3PUFA supplementation on body composition and muscle strength during weight loss rather than saturate any beneficial response with a high protein intake. Accordingly, during the energy restriction period, protein intake was 5% lower in FO and 7% lower in PLA compared to the habitual diet, equating to a reduction of 310 and 340 kcals, respectively. We also cannot discount the possibility that the combination of an energy deficit and reduction in dietary protein intake may have potentiated the decline in lean body mass during weight loss in both groups, thus countering any potential enhancement of n-3PUFA on MPS. Consistent with this notion, a negative nitrogen balance was reported for at least 10 days during a period of reduced protein intake (38). This negative nitrogen balance is indicative of a net loss of protein at the whole-body level. Conversely, increasing the protein content of the diet is known to increase nitrogen balance during energy restriction (37). The measurement of nitrogen balance was beyond the scope of the present study. However, based on previous work (39), we speculate that participants in both supplement conditions were in negative nitrogen balance. Future research in athletes is warranted to examine the influence of n-3PUFA supplementation on changes in body composition and muscle performance during energy restriction within a more practical situation when combined with a protein intake that meets recently published guidelines (4).

Although there are many strengths to the present study, including dietary control and the measurement of blood omega-3 concentrations, there also are limitations. Firstly, DEXA was the only measure of body composition and we acknowledge that DEXA measurements alone are not sufficient for the accurate assessment of muscle mass (40). Therefore, although all attempts were made to standardize the DEXA protocol (i.e., body positioning, hydration status), we cannot discount the possibility that our study incurred a type II statistical error with regards to examining the influence of FO supplementation on changes in body composition during short-term weight loss. Combining DEXA with measurements of bioelectrical impedance and air displacement plethysmography for calculating the four-compartmental model of body composition may provide more accurate results. Secondly, the participants that took part in this study were not a homogenous group. Although participants were resistance trained for at least 6 months, there were individuals and with different resistance abilities with different experience as well as being different types of athletes, i.e., power athletes or team-sports athletes. Thirdly, although we were able to fully control diet, we could only reliably control diet during the energy restriction phase for 2 weeks. A longer period of energy restriction may have allowed for further differences between the groups to have been observed.

To conclude, dietary supplementation with 4 g/d of n-3PUFA may maintain, or even improve, leg extension 1 RM strength following 2 weeks of energy restriction. However, this strength adaptation was not mediated by the increased preservation of lean body mass during diet-induced weight loss. The practical application of these preliminary data remains unclear but implies a potential role for n-3PUFA supplementation in improving muscle performance during weight loss in athletic populations. However, follow-up mechanistic work is warranted to establish the influence of n-3PUFA supplementation on changes in body composition, muscle performance and neuromuscular function during more prolonged periods of energy restriction in athletic populations.

AUTHOR CONTRIBUTIONS

The study was designed by JP, NB, DH, SM, SG, KT, and OW. Data were collected by JP, NB, and NR-S. Analyzed by JP, NB, EM, and JD. Data interpretation and manuscript preparation were undertaken by JP, NB, NR-S, DH, SG, KT, and OW.

REFERENCES

1. Tipton KD. Efficacy and consequences of very-high-protein diets for athletes and exercisers. *Proc Nutri Soc.* (2011) 70:205–14. doi: 10.1017/S0029665111000024
2. Mettler S, Mitchell N, Tipton KD. Increased protein intake reduces lean body mass loss during weight loss in athletes. *Med Sci Sports Exerc.* (2010) 42:326–37. doi: 10.1249/MSS.0b013e3181b2ef8e
3. Racette SB, Rochon J, Uhrich ML, Villareal DT, Das SK, Fontana L, et al. Effects of two years of calorie restriction on aerobic capacity and muscle strength. *Med Sci Sports Exerc.* (2017) 49:2240–9. doi: 10.1249/MSS.0000000000001353
4. Witard OC, Garthe I, Phillips SM. Dietary protein for training adaptation and body composition manipulation in track and field athletes. *Int J Sport Nutri Exerc Metab.* (2019) 29:165–174. doi: 10.1123/ijsnem.2018-0267
5. Longland TM, Oikawa SY, Mitchell CJ, Devries MC, Phillips SM. Higher compared with lower dietary protein during an energy deficit combined with intense exercise promotes greater lean mass gain and fat mass loss: a randomized trial. *Am J Clin Nutr.* (2016) 103:738–46. doi: 10.3945/ajcn.115.119339
6. Kamolrat T, Gray SR. The effect of eicosapentaenoic and docosahexaenoic acid on protein synthesis and breakdown in murine C2C12 myotubes. *Biochem Biophys Res Commun.* (2013) 432:593–8. doi: 10.1016/j.bbrc.2013.02.041
7. Jeromson S, Mackenzie I, Doherty MK, Whitfield PD, Bell G, Dick J, et al. Lipid remodeling and an altered membrane-associated proteome may drive the differential effects of EPA and DHA treatment on skeletal muscle glucose uptake and protein accretion. *Am J Physiol Endocrinol Metab.* (2018) 314:E605–19. doi: 10.1152/ajpendo.00438.2015
8. McGlory C, Gorissen SHM, Kamal M, Bahniwal R, Hector AJ, Baker SK, et al. Omega-3 fatty acid supplementation attenuates skeletal muscle disuse atrophy during two weeks of unilateral leg immobilization in healthy young women. *FASEB J.* (2019) 33:4586–97. doi: 10.1096/fj.201801857RRR
9. Smith GI, Atherton P, Reeds DN, Mohammed BS, Rankin D, Rennie MJ, et al. Dietary omega-3 fatty acid supplementation increases the rate of muscle protein synthesis in older adults: a randomized controlled trial. *Am J Clin Nutri.* (2011) 93:402–12. doi: 10.3945/ajcn.110.005611
10. Smith GI, Atherton P, Reeds DN, Mohammed BS, Rankin D, Rennie MJ, et al. Omega-3 polyunsaturated fatty acids augment the muscle protein anabolic response to hyperinsulinaemia-hyperaminoacidaemia in healthy young and middle-aged men and women. *Clin Sci.* (2011) 121:267–78. doi: 10.1042/CS20100597
11. Smith GI, Julliand S, Reeds DN, Sinacore DR, Klein S, Mittendorfer B. Fish oil-derived n-3 PUFA therapy increases muscle mass and

function in healthy older adults. *Am J Clin Nutri.* (2015) 102:115–22. doi: 10.3945/ajcn.114.105833

12. Rodacki CLN, Rodacki ALF, Pereira G, Naliwaiko K, Coelho I, Pequito D, et al. Fish-oil supplementation enhances the effects of strength training in elderly women. *Am J Clin Nutri.* (2012) 95:428–36. doi: 10.3945/ajcn.111.0 21915
13. Da Boit M, Sibson R, Sivasubramaniam S, Meakin JR, Greig CA, Aspden RM, et al. Sex differences in the effect of fish-oil supplementation on the adaptive response to resistance exercise training in older people: a randomized controlled trial. *Am J Clin Nutri.* (2017) 105:151–8. doi: 10.3945/ajcn.116.140780
14. McGlory C, Galloway SDR, Hamilton DL, McClintock C, Breen L, Dick JR, et al. Temporal changes in human skeletal muscle and blood lipid composition with fish oil supplementation. *Prostaglandins Leukot Essent Fatty Acids.* (2014) 90:199–206. doi: 10.1016/j.plefa.2014.03.001
15. Murphy RA, Mourtzakis M, Chu QSC, Baracos VE, Reiman T, Mazurak VC. Nutritional intervention with fish oil provides a benefit over standard of care for weight and skeletal muscle mass in patients with nonsmall cell lung cancer receiving chemotherapy. *Cancer.* (2011) 117:1775–82. doi: 10.1002/cncr.25709
16. Pasiakos SM, Vislocky LM, Carbone JW, Altieri N, Konopelski K, Freake HC, et al. Acute energy deprivation affects skeletal muscle protein synthesis and associated intracellular signaling proteins in physically active adults. *J Nutri.* (2010) 140:745–51. doi: 10.3945/jn.109.1 18372
17. Browne GJ, Proud CG. A novel mTOR-regulated phosphorylation site in elongation factor 2 kinase modulates the activity of the kinase and its binding to calmodulin. *Mol Cell Biol.* (2004) 24:2986–97. doi: 10.1128/MCB.24.7.2986-2997.2004
18. Areta JL, Burke LM, Camera DM, West DWD, Crawshay S, Moore DR, et al. Reduced resting skeletal muscle protein synthesis is rescued by resistance exercise and protein ingestion following short-term energy deficit. *Am J Physiol Endocrinol Metab.* (2014) 306:E989–97. doi: 10.1152/ajpendo.00590.2013
19. Hector AJ, McGlory C, Damas F, Mazara N, Baker SK, Phillips SM. Pronounced energy restriction with elevated protein intake results in no change in proteolysis and reductions in skeletal muscle protein synthesis that are mitigated by resistance exercise. *FASEB J.* (2018) 32:265–75. doi: 10.1096/fj.201700158RR
20. Kunesová M, Braunerová R, Hlavatý P, Tvrzická E, Stanková B, Skrha J, et al. The influence of n-3 polyunsaturated fatty acids and very low calorie diet during a short-term weight reducing regimen on weight loss and serum fatty acid composition in severely obese women. *Physiol Res.* (2006) 55:63–72.
21. Munro IA, Garg ML. Weight loss and metabolic profiles in obese individuals using two different approaches. *Food Function.* (2011) 2:611–6. doi: 10.1039/c1fo10143a
22. Rodriguez-Sanchez N, Galloway SDR. Errors in dual energy x-ray absorptiometry estimation of body composition induced by hypohydration. *Int J Sport Nutri Exerc Metab.* (2015) 25:60–8. doi: 10.1123/ijsnem.201 4-0067
23. Baechle TR, Earle RW. *Essentials of Strength Training and Conditioning.* 3rd ed. Champaign, IL: Human Kinetics (2008).
24. Bouchard C, Tremblay A, Leblanc C, Lortie G, Savard R, Thériault G. A method to assess energy expenditure in children and adults. *Am J Clin Nutri.* (1983) 37:461–7. doi: 10.1093/ajcn/37.3.461
25. Bell GJ, MacKinlay E, Dick J, Younger I, Lands B, Gilhooly T. Using a fingertip whole blood sample for rapid fatty acid measurement: method validation and correlation with erythrocyte polar lipid compositions in UK subjects. *Br J Nutr.* (2011) 106:1408–15. doi: 10.1017/S00071145110 01978
26. Cohen J. *Statistical Power Analysis for the Behavioral Sciences.* Oxford: Routledge (2013). doi: 10.4324/9780203771587
27. Atherton PJ, Smith K. Muscle protein synthesis in response to nutrition and exercise. *J Physiol.* (2012) 590:1049–57. doi: 10.1113/jphysiol.2011.225003
28. Dankel SJ, Buckner SL, Jessee MB, Grant Mouser J, Mattocks KT, Abe T, et al. Correlations do not show cause and effect: not even for changes in muscle size and strength. *Sports Med.* (2018) 48:1–6. doi: 10.1007/s40279-017-0774-3
29. Lauritzen L, Hansen HS, Jørgensen MH, Michaelsen KF. The essentiality of long chain n-3 fatty acids in relation to development and function of the brain and retina. *Prog Lipid Res.* (2001) 40:1–94. doi: 10.1016/S0163-7827(00)00017-5
30. Brenna JT, Salem N, Sinclair AJ, Cunnane SC, International Society for the Study of Fatty Acids and Lipids, ISSFAL. alpha-Linolenic acid supplementation and conversion to n-3 long-chain polyunsaturated fatty acids in humans. *Prostaglandins Leuk Essent Fatty Acids.* (2009) 80:85–91. doi: 10.1016/j.plefa.2009.01.004
31. Pentikäinen H, Savonen K, Komulainen P, Kiviniemi V, Paajanen T, Kivipelto M, et al. Muscle strength and cognition in ageing men and women: the DR's EXTRA study. *Eur Geriatric Med.* (2017) 8:275–7. doi: 10.1016/j.eurger.2017.04.004
32. Valentini KJ, Pickens CA, Wiesinger JA, Fenton JI. The effect of fish oil supplementation on brain DHA and EPA content and fatty acid profile in mice. *Int J Food Sci Nutri.* (2018) 69:705–17. doi: 10.1080/09637486.2017.1413640
33. Jakobsen MD, Sundstrup E, Andersen CH, Bandholm T, Thorborg K, Zebis MK, et al. Muscle activity during knee-extension strengthening exercise performed with elastic tubing and isotonic resistance. *Int J Sports Phys Ther.* (2012) 7:606–16.
34. Da Silva EM, Brentano MA, Cadore EL, De Almeida APV, Kruel LFM. Analysis of muscle activation during different leg press exercises at submaximum effort levels. *J Strength Cond Res.* (2008) 22:1059–65. doi: 10.1519/JSC.0b013e3181739445
35. Mojtahedi MC, Thorpe MP, Karampinos DC, Johnson CL, Layman DK, Georgiadis JG, et al. The effects of a higher protein intake during energy restriction on changes in body composition and physical function in older women. *J Gerontol.* (2011) 66:1218–25. doi: 10.1093/gerona/g lr120
36. Kempen KP, Saris WH, Westerterp KR. Energy balance during an 8-wk energy-restricted diet with and without exercise in obese women. *Am J Clin Nutri.* (1995) 62:722–9. doi: 10.1093/ajcn/ 62.4.722
37. Walberg JL, Leidy MK, Sturgill DJ, Hinkle DE, Ritchey SJ, Sebolt DR. Macronutrient content of a hypoenergy diet affects nitrogen retention and muscle function in weight lifters. *Int J Sports Med.* (1988) 9:261–6. doi: 10.1055/s-2007-1025018
38. Quevedo MR, Price GM, Halliday D, Pacy PJ, Millward DJ. Nitrogen homoeostasis in man: diurnal changes in nitrogen excretion, leucine oxidation and whole body leucine kinetics during a reduction from a high to a moderate protein intake. *Clin Sci.* (1994) 86:185–93. doi: 10.1042/cs08 60185
39. Oi Y, Okuda T, Koishi H, Koh H, Waki M, Kurata M, et al. Relationship between protein intake and nitrogen balance in obese patients on low energy diet. *J Nutri Sci Vitaminol.* (1987) 33:219–26. doi: 10.3177/jnsv. 33.219
40. Wilson JP, Strauss BJ, Fan B, Duewer FW, Shepherd JA. Improved 4-compartment body-composition model for a clinically accessible measure of total body protein. *Am J Clin Nutri.* (2013) 97:497–504. doi: 10.3945/ajcn.112.0 48074

7

Impact of a High Protein Intake on the Plasma Metabolome in Elderly Males: 10 Week Randomized Dietary Intervention

*Brenan Durainayagam[1,2], Cameron J. Mitchell[1,3], Amber M. Milan[1,4], Nina Zeng[1], Pankaja Sharma[1], Sarah M. Mitchell[1], Farha Ramzan[1], Scott O. Knowles[4], Anders Sjödin[5], Karl-Heinz Wagner[6], Nicole C. Roy[7,8,9], Karl Fraser[7,8,9] and David Cameron-Smith[1,9,10]**

[1] Liggins Institute, University of Auckland, Auckland, New Zealand, [2] Division of Systems Medicine and Digestive Medicine, Department of Metabolism, Digestion and Reproduction, Imperial College London, London, United Kingdom, [3] School of Kinesiology, The University of British Columbia, Vancouver, BC, Canada, [4] Food Nutrition & Health Team, AgResearch, Palmerston North, New Zealand, [5] Department of Nutrition, Exercise and Sport, Copenhagen University, Copenhagen, Denmark, [6] Department of Nutritional Sciences and Research Platform Active Ageing, University of Vienna, Vienna, Austria, [7] The High-Value Nutrition National Science Challenge, Auckland, New Zealand, [8] Food & Bio-based Products Group, AgResearch, Palmerston North, New Zealand, [9] Riddet Institute, Massey University, Palmerston North, New Zealand, [10] Clinical Nutrition Research Centre, Singapore Institute for Clinical Sciences, Agency for Science, Technology, and Research, Singapore, Singapore

***Correspondence:**
David Cameron-Smith
d.cameron-smith@auckland.ac.nz

High protein diets may improve the maintenance of skeletal muscle mass in the elderly, although it remains less clear what broader impact such diets have on whole body metabolic regulation in the elderly. Non-targeted polar metabolomics analysis using HILIC HPLC-MS was used to profile the circulating plasma metabolome of elderly men ($n = 31$; 74.7 ± 4.0 years) who were randomized to consume for 10 weeks a diet designed to achieve either protein (RDA; $0.8 \cdot g^{-1} \cdot kg^{-1}$) or that doubled this recommend intake (2RDA; $1.6.g.kg^{-1}$). A limited number of plasma metabolites ($n = 24$) were significantly differentially regulated by the diet. These included markers of protein anabolism, which increased by the 2RDA diet, including; urea, creatine, and glutarylcarnitine. Whilst in response to the RDA diet; glutamine, glutamic acid, and proline were increased, relative to the 2RDA diet ($p < 0.05$). Metaboanalyst identified six major metabolic pathways to be influenced by the quantity of protein intake, most notably the arginine and proline pathways. Doubling of the recommended protein intake in older males over 10 weeks exerted only a limited impact on circulating metabolites, as determined by LC-MS. This metabolomic response was almost entirely due to increased circulating abundances of metabolites potentially indicative of altered protein anabolism, without evidence of impact on pathways for metabolic health.

Trial Registration: This trial was registered on 3rd March 2016 at the Australia New Zealand Clinical Trial Registry (www.anzctr.org.au) at ACTRN 12616000310460.

Keywords: dietary protein, plasma metabolomics, older adults, pathway mapping, nutritional interventions

BACKGROUND

An adequate intake of dietary protein is essential for the maintenance of health in the elderly. Yet considerable debate exists as to how much protein is required for maintaining optimal health in the aging population (1). Recent analysis has shown that dietary intakes only meeting the World Health Organization (WHO) recommended daily allowance (RDA) for dietary protein (0.8 $g{\cdot}kg^{-1}{\cdot}d^{-1}$) increase the risk of progressive skeletal muscle and muscular strength and/or function loss in the elderly (2–4). This loss of muscle mass and function, known as sarcopenia, is a major risk factor for the loss of independence, increasing the likelihood for institutionalized care and mortality risk (5). Recent meta-analysis of both intervention and cohort studies provides additional evidence that diets that have protein intakes greater than the RDA offer protection against muscle loss in the elderly (6, 7). Recent expert opinions and consensus statements have therefore suggested that older people should be aiming to consume diets that provide well in excess of the RDA, with recommendations ranging from 1.0 to 1.5 $g{\cdot}kg^{-1}{\cdot}d^{-1}$ (8–10).

Whilst there is emerging evidence of the potential benefits of higher intakes of protein for maintenance of muscle mass and function, the value and importance of dietary protein in the context of various changes in digestive and metabolic function, and the associated changes in liver and renal function, in the elderly, require careful consideration (11, 12). It must be considered whether elevated protein impacts on the already established heightened risk and a wide range of complex diseases, including many cancers, type 2 diabetes and cardiovascular disease, that is experienced in the elderly (13, 14). To date, analysis of the impact of dietary protein in the elderly on metabolic disease risk is limited, with studies demonstrating an adverse effect of diets rich in animal proteins, with the possible exception of dairy protein (15, 16).

In order to define evidence-based protein intake recommendations, it is therefore important to comprehensively understand the metabolic implications of an increase in dietary protein intake. These metabolic adaptations are undoubtedly complex, as altered protein intake impacts on digestive hormones, circulating amino acids and their metabolites, but also exerts an as yet poorly defined impact on the human gut microbiome (16, 17). A range of nutritional intervention studies have utilized either targeted or untargeted metabolomics approaches to profile the complex metabolic adaptations to diet (18–20). Profiling of either plasma or urinary metabolites has been able to identify major features of metabolic adaptation and possible mechanisms by which health status is altered (12, 21). These studies have also provided significant insight into a range of metabolites that form predictive biomarkers of dietary intake and habits that can be subsequently applied to the analysis of habitual diet or adherence to a dietary intervention (22, 23).

Abbreviations: WHO, World Health Organization; RDA, recommended daily allowance; HILIC-MS, hydrophilic interaction liquid chromatography-mass spectrometry; BMI, body mass index; ANOVA, analysis of variance; BCAAs branched chain amino acids; TMAO, trimethylamine *N*-Oxide; CVD, cardiovascular disease.

Recently, we have reported on the primary outcomes of a 10-week intervention altering protein intake in older men, in which it was demonstrated that a controlled whole food diet intervention that doubled the WHO recommendation resulted in reduced loss of skeletal muscle size and function, than a diet only meeting the WHO protein recommendation (7). Thus, in a secondary analysis, this study aimed to further examine the impacts of a high protein diet on metabolic function using a global/untargeted metabolomics analysis of polar metabolites via hydrophilic interaction liquid chromatography-mass spectrometry (HILIC-MS) (24). It is hypothesized that a 10 week diet that doubles the RDA for protein (2RDA: 1.6 $g{\cdot}kg^{-1}{\cdot}d^{-1}$) in comparison to a diet that meets the RDA (RDA: 0.8 $g{\cdot}kg^{-1}{\cdot}d^{-1}$) would result in a significant alteration of polar metabolites related primarily to amino acid oxidation and anabolism, with additional adaptation in pathways related to metabolic regulation of carbohydrate and lipid metabolic homeostasis.

METHODS

Ethics Statement

Written informed consent was obtained from all participants before participation in the trial. The study was reviewed and approved by the Southern Health and Disability Ethics Committee (New Zealand; 15/STH/236) and was conducted in accordance with the Declaration of Helsinki. The study was prospectively registered with the Australian and New Zealand Clinical Trial Registry (www.anzctr.org.au) as ACTRN12616000310460 on March 9, 2016.

Participants

Healthy elderly men, ≥70 years were recruited through advertisements to participate in the study. All participants were free-living individuals who had a body mass index (BMI; kg/m^2) ranging from 18 to 35. All were non-smokers who did not consume any dietary supplements 1 month before participating in the study. Exclusion criteria to those potential participants were those who consumed a restricted diet, including vegetarians or with self-reported food allergies (e.g., nuts, fish, dairy). Further exclusion was applied to those with a prior history of cancer, diabetes, thyroid disease or conditions affecting neuromuscular function.

Experimental Design

The design of this study has been previously described in Mitchell et al. (7). Participants were randomized into two groups (equal allocation ratio) where they either received a controlled diet of 0.8 protein $kg^{-1}{\cdot}d^{-1}$ (RDA) or 1.6 g protein $kg^{-1}{\cdot}d^{-1}$ (2RDA) for 10 weeks. All meals consumed by the participants during the 10-week study were provided. Energy from fat was standardized (28–31% of energy), with the difference being made up of carbohydrates. All diets adhered to Eating and Activity Guidelines for New Zealand (25). Adults met the recommendations for intake of fruit and vegetables. All participants completed dietary records to ensure all food provided was consumed, and food selection was adjusted to participants' preferences to maintain high compliance. Any non-study food consumed was also asked to be recorded. The energy content of the intervention diet was individually calculated to match participants estimated energy needs based on the Harris-Benedict equation (26) and adjusted for physical activity, which was assessed by wrist-worn accelerometers (Fitbit Charge HR). The estimated energy needs were calculated before the intervention and adjusted fortnightly based on participant weight maintenance and satiety to ensure participants consumed adequate protein relative to energy intake. Throughout the study protein and energy were distributed between breakfast, lunch and dinner as 30, 30, and 40%, respectively. During the intervention, participants were instructed to maintain their normal lifestyle, and prepared meals were delivered to their homes. All testing was conducted at the University of Auckland Nutrition and Mobility Clinic.

Metabolomics Analysis

Fasted plasma was collected pre-intervention and at the completion of 10 weeks of diet intervention. Extraction of metabolites was performed using a previously described bi-phasic method (27). Briefly, 100 μl of plasma was mixed with 800 μl of cold (−20°C) $CHCl_3$/MeOH (50:50, v/v), agitated for 30 s and stored at −20°C for 60 min to allow for protein precipitation. Subsequently, 400 μl water was added, the mixture was vortexed (2 × 15 s) and centrifuged for 10 min at 14,000 rpm and 4°C to separate the aqueous (upper) and organic (lower) phases.

The lower organic phase is the lipid portion of the extract and was not analyzed as the interest in this clinical trial was around the impact of prolonged increased protein intake on the metabolome. Thus, any changes are likely to occur in the polar metabolome rather than the lipidome.

The aqueous phase (200 μl) was collected, dried under a stream of nitrogen and reconstituted in 200 μl of acetonitrile: water (50:50, v/v) containing 10 μg/ml d_2-tyrosine as an internal standard. Samples were placed in the LC-auto-sampler at 4°C for HILIC-MS analysis. Blank procedure samples were prepared exactly as the samples, but plasma was replaced with Milli-Q water. To avoid any systematic analytical effects, samples were randomized before analysis. To verify and/or maintain data quality within each mode, a QC sample (comprising a pooled extract of all samples) was also injected once for every 10 samples. Retention time, signal/intensity, and mass error of internal standards were monitored constantly to check instrument response variability and retention time shifts.

Plasma extracts were analyzed by HILIC LC-MS (Thermo Fisher Scientific, Waltham, MA, USA) using both positive and negative ionization modes. HILIC-MS conditions have been previously described in Fraser et al. (24). Briefly, compounds were separated using a 5 μm ZIC-pHILIC column (100 × 2.1 mm, 5 μm; Merck Darmstadt, Germany) eluted with solvent A: acetonitrile with 0.1% formic acid, and solvent B: 16 mM ammonium formate in water, at a flow rate of 250 μl/min. Initial conditions of the solvent gradient were set at 97:3 (A:B), which was held for 1 min, where after that the gradient was changed linearly to give a ratio 10:90 (A:B) at 14.5 min and maintained till 17 min. At this time and up to 24 min, the column was allowed to return to initial conditions and re-equilibrate. The column effluent was connected to an electrospray source of a high-resolution mass spectrometer (Exactive Orbitrap, Thermo, San Jose, CA, USA). Mass spectral data were collected in profile data acquisition mode covering a mass range of $m/z = 55–1,100$ with a mass resolution setting of 25,000 and a maximum trap fill time of 250 ms using the Xcalibur software package (Thermo, San Jose, CA, USA).

Data processing consisted of a series of procedures aimed at converting raw mass spectrometry data to data matrices suitable for further statistical analyses. Peak detection, alignment, grouping, and noise elimination were performed using XCMS software (28). The resultant peak intensity table was subjected to run-order correction and batch normalization utilizing pooled QC samples and applying the lowess regression model (29). This was evaluated on the open-source online platform Workflow4metabolomics (https://workflow4metabolomics.org) (30). Finally, features with a CV of >30% within the pooled QC samples were removed.

Statistical Analysis

Principal component analysis (PCA) was used to validate the quality of the analytical system performance and observe possible outliers using the commercial package SIMCA-P+ version 14.1 software (Umetrics, Umea, Sweden). Two-way repeated measures ANOVA was used to determine differences in groups with time (pre vs. post) as a repeated factor and diet as a fixed factor using R (version 3.4.2). *Post-hoc* comparisons were conducted by Holm-Sidak corrections. False discovery rate adjustment of *P*-values (FDR) was applied using the Benjamini-Hochberg method.

Peak Identification

Peak identification was performed by verifying the accuracy of mass measurements, the retention time and the tandem mass spectrometry results against an in-house database, which contained over 600 authentic standard compounds. Where a feature did not match the library, the molecular and co-eluting ions were manually inspected. The source voltage applied created a small amount of source induced fragmentation which could be used to facilitate annotation of the unknown features. Thus, pseudo MS^2 spectral data was validated by inspecting each metabolite for perfectly co-eluting fragment and molecular ions. These were matched to the MS/MS data provided on public libraries such as METLIN (31) and the Human Metabolome Database (HMDB) (32). The use of pseudo MS^2 spectral data to validate the molecular ion has been previously described as an acceptable approach (33) and has been applied in large cohort trials such as the HUSWERMET project (34). Each metabolite was assigned a confidence level defined by the Metabolomics Standard Initiative (35). Therefore, the level 2 annotation is based on co-eluting accurate mass fragment ions observed with the accurate mass of the molecular ion.

Network Analysis and Metabolic Pathway Construction

MetaboAnalyst (version 4.0) was used for pathway enrichment analysis utilizing the Kyoto Encyclopedia of Genes and Genomes (KEGG) database, which can provide valuable information by integrating two pathway analysis approaches; pathway enrichment analysis and pathway topology analysis (32). The hypergeometric test was selected to evaluate whether a particular metabolite set was represented more than once (36). The relative-betweenness centrality algorithm was applied for pathway topology analysis measuring the numbers of shortest paths going through a node in the network. This takes into consideration the global network structure, not only the immediate neighbor of the current node (37). The acquired impact value represents the accumulative percentage of importance for the matched metabolite nodes involved in a pathway. Network construction was performed by Cytoscape (version 3.4.0) (38) utilizing the plugin Metscape and topological parameters were analyzed using the network analyser tool (39). To confirm the most important metabolites of the network, two well-established node centrality measures were used to estimate node importance; the degree of each node and betweenness.

RESULTS

Subject Characteristics and Dietary Intake

The participants were randomly assigned to either the RDA ($n = 16$) or 2RDA ($n = 15$) diet; of these one subject withdrew his consent before the start of the dietary intervention (RDA group) and one subject from the 2RDA group did not complete the 10-week intervention due to failed diet compliance (**Table 1**). Based on dietary records, compliance was 98.9% for both protein and energy intake in the RDA group and 97.5% and 98.4% for protein and energy intake, respectively in the 2RDA group, with no compliance difference between the two groups. As previously reported, both groups shared a small energy deficit of 209 ± 213 and 145 ± 214 kcal/d in the RDA and 2RDA groups, respectively, with no energy deficit difference between the two groups. Detailed changes in body composition and macronutrient information can be found in Mitchell et al. (7).

Metabolomics Analysis

The stability and reproducibility of the current data were evaluated by the QC samples measured during the whole experimental period. PCA score plot representation analysis on the whole data matrix, which included all features (*m/z* and retention time) showed no obvious run-order effects for metabolite profiles obtained in positive and negative ion modes (**Supplementary Figure 1**). This result demonstrated good stability and reproducibility in the current metabolomic dataset. After data processing, 170 and 275 features were detected in positive and negative ionization mode respectively, which were pooled together to visualize in a volcano plot (**Figure 1**). The total number of features (445) were separated by significance (post-intervention *t*-test) and fold change (>1.2).

TABLE 1 | Physical characteristics of participants.

	RDA ($n = 15$)	2RDA ($n = 14$)
Age (years)	74.9 ± 1.1	73.8 ± 0.9
Height (cm)	171.8 ± 2.0	172.1 ± 1.6
Weight (kg)	83.9 ± 5.4	83.0 ± 2.4
BMI (kg/m^2)	28.2 ± 1.4	28.0 ± 0.9

Values are means ± standard error of the mean. The RDA is 0.8 g protein·kg^{-1}·d^{-1}, 2RDA is 1.6 protein·kg^{-1}·d^{-1}. BMI, Body mass index, RDA, Recommended dietary allowance.

Two-way repeated measure ANOVA revealed 24 metabolites exhibiting changes between and within diet groups ($p < 0.05$). These differentially regulated metabolites are classified by using the four levels of certainty as defined by Sumner et al. (35) (**Supplementary Table 1**). After 10 weeks, nine metabolites demonstrated increases only within the 2RDA group. Glutrylcarnitine (**Figure 2A**), trigonelline (**Figure 2B**), trimethylamine *N*-Oxide (TMAO; **Figure 2C**), glycocyamine (**Figure 2D**), creatinine (**Figure 2E**), and urea (**Figure 2F**) all increased within the 2RDA group ($p < 0.05$ each, respectively), whereas there were no changes in the RDA group for these metabolites. Furtheremore, these metabolites were significantly elevated in the 2RDA group compared to the RDA group post-intervention ($p < 0.05$ each, respectively). Two pyrimidines, dihydrothymine (**Figure 2G**) and uridine (**Figure 2H**), along with an unknown metabolite (**Supplementary Figure 2A**) increased within the 2RDA group after 10 weeks but were not higher than the RDA group at the post-intervention stage ($p < 0.05$ each, respectively).

Ten metabolites demonstrated changes within the RDA group after the 10 week intervention. Tryptophan (**Figure 3A**), creatine (**Figure 3B**) and methylimidazoleacetic acid (**Figure 3C**) all reduced within the RDA group and post-intervention were lower in the RDA group compared to the 2RDA group ($p < 0.05$ each, respectively). Furthermore, the 2RDA diet increased the level of tryptophan ($p = 0.04$) and creatine ($p = 0.001$) after the 10 week intervention. Glutamine (**Figure 3D**), uric acid (**Figure 3E**) and unknown metabolite M160T639 (**Supplementary Figure 2B**) increased within the RDA group with not changes obeserved within the 2RDA group ($p < 0.05$ each, respectively). Post-intervention, the RDA group was higher than the 2RDA group for uric acid ($p = 0.02$) and glutamine ($p = 0.03$). Threonine (**Figure 3F**) and glutamic acid (**Figure 3G**) along with unknown metabolite M145T531 (**Supplementary Figure 2C**) increased only within the RDA group with no difference observed between groups post-intervention ($p < 0.05$ each, respectively). 2-aminoadipic acid (**Figure 3H**) did not show any changes within diet groups but was elevated in the 2RDA group compared RDA group post-intervention ($p = 0.04$).

At baseline, four metabolites were different among the 30 participants, which converged at the end of the 10-week period. Lenticin (**Figure 4A**) and proline (**Figure 4B**) increased within the RDA group ($p < 0.05$ each, respectively). Indoleacrylic acid increased within both the RDA (**Figure 4C**; $p = 0.03$) and 2RDA

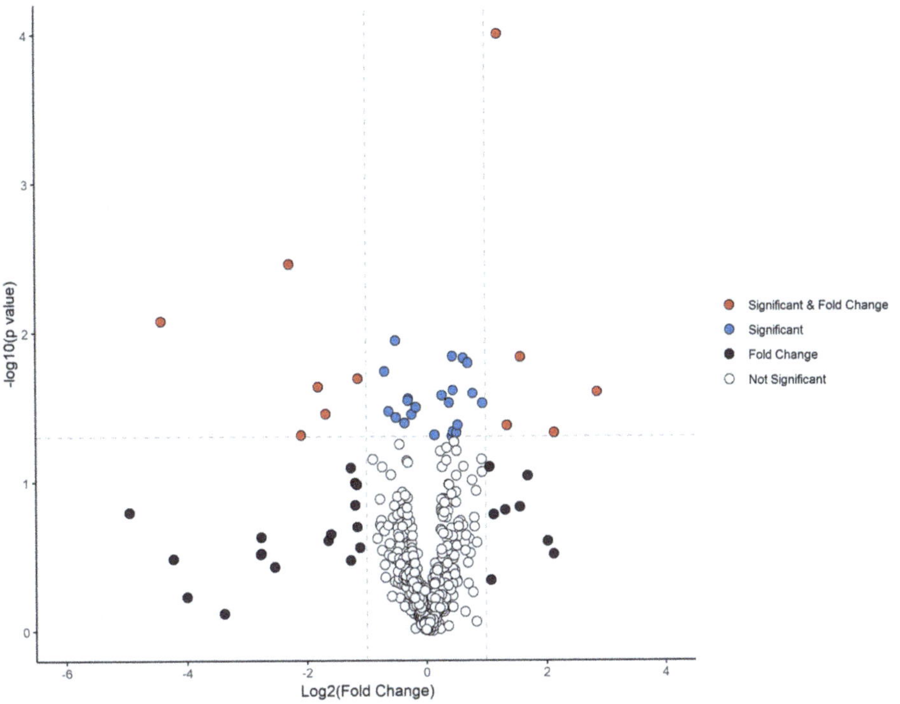

FIGURE 1 | Volcano plot analysis of metabolite changes after 10 weeks dietary intervention. Red dots denote significant ($p < 0.05$) and fold change (>1.2) features. Blue dots represent significant features ($p < 0.05$), black dots designate fold change (>1.2), and clear dots represent neither no significance ($p > 0.05$) or fold change of <1.2.

group ($p = 0.003$). Arginine (**Figure 4D**) was also different at baseline ($p = 0.02$) but demonstrated no changes within diet and at the post-intervention stage. Dimethylglycine (**Figure 4E**) decreased in both diet groups with no pre or post difference ($p < 0.05$ each, respectively).

Pathway Analysis

Six pathways were statistically significant as determined by MetaboAnalyst; five pathways relating to amino acid metabolism are ranked in descending order in **Table 2**. Arginine and proline metabolism was the most significant with eight identified metabolites. The pathways were composed of metabolites that increased within the RDA group such as; glutamine, glutamate, and proline. In addition, metabolites that increased within 2RDA group; urea, glycocyamine, creatinine, creatine, and tryptohan were also important components in the pathways identified.

Metabolic Network Analysis

Figure 5 displays a network visualization, where it demonstrates the centrality of glutamine, glutamic acid, arginine, and uridine and their connectivity to an array of metabolites and enzymes. These metabolites are considered hub metabolites based on measures of degree >10 and betweenness centrality (>0.1), where they are not only components of pathways but are also integral to pathway performance (**Table 3**).

DISCUSSION

Comprehensive polar metabolomics analysis via HILIC-LCMS was applied to the plasma samples from elderly males who consumed a diet that contained foods to achieve the RDA for protein or when the diet was manipulated to achieve twice the RDA (2RDA). The key finding was centered on amino acid metabolism, with very few significant changes in metabolites not directly related to amino acid metabolism. Eleven metabolites were different between the RDA and 2RDA groups at the end of the interevention. Adherence to a diet that met the minimum dietary recommendations (RDA) resulted in increased circulatory concentrations of a limited subset of non-essential amino acids, including; glutamine, glutamic acid, and proline. These amino acids, along with arginine, have been identified as integral hubs where metabolic pathways overlap and may be indicative of increased overall tissue catabolism. With an increased protein consumption (2RDA), there were alterations in the circulatory metabolome consistent with increased amino acid flux and nitrogenous oxidative metabolism. There was also a shift in circulating metabolites that may be indicative of induction of anabolic pathways (40, 41). This metabolomic analysis provides evidence of how changes in dietary protein may impact the regulation of muscle mass. In this study, these results provide support for our previously published findings of increased muscle mass and physical strength in the older men who consumed the higher protein diet (7).

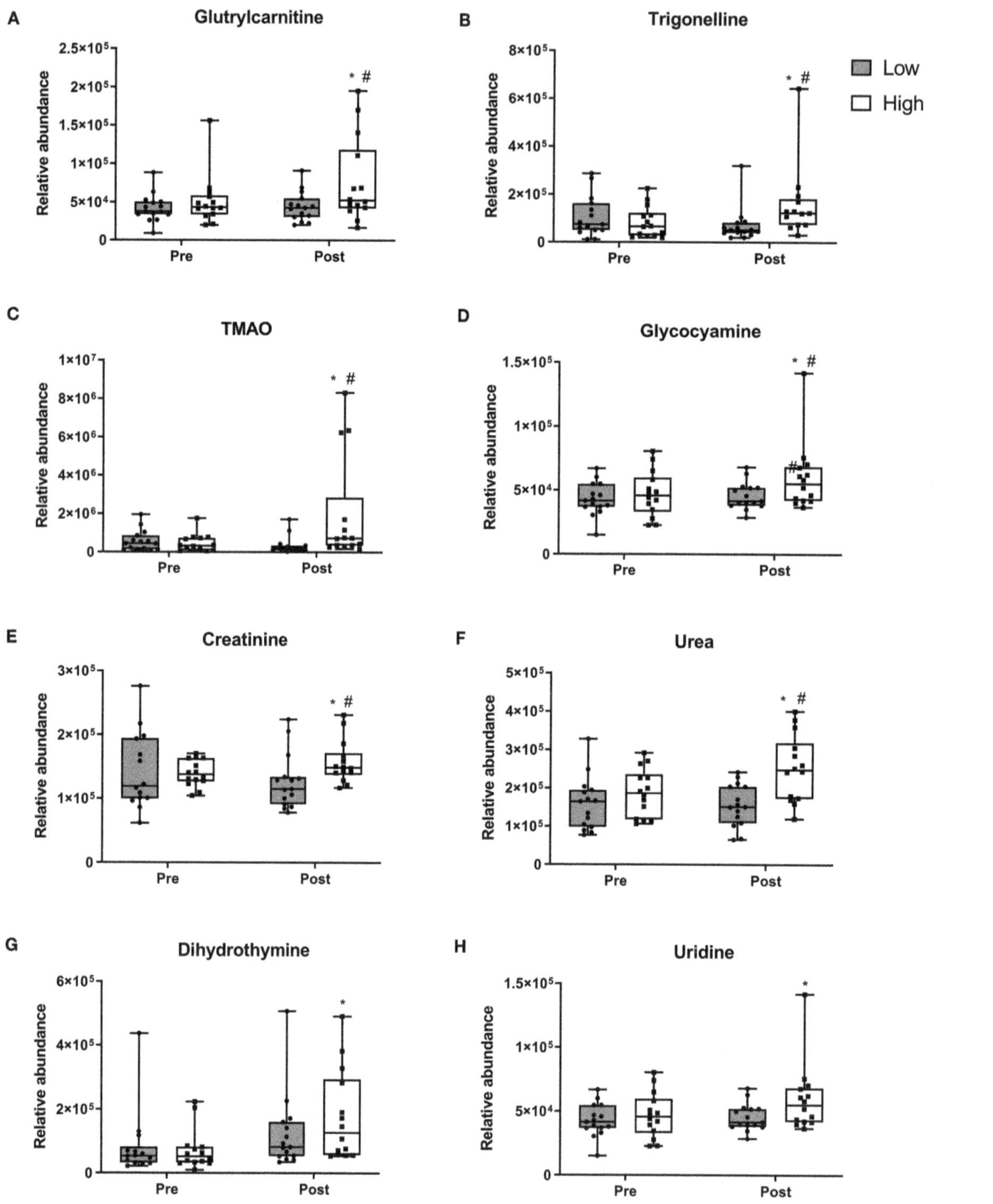

FIGURE 2 | Metabolites which increased in the 2RDA diet. Box and whisker plot showing median, first, and third quartiles, and maximum and minimum values. **(A)** glutrylcarnitine, **(B)** trigonelline, **(C)** TMAO, **(D)** glycocyamine, **(E)** creatinine, **(F)** urea, **(G)** dihydrothymine, and **(H)** uridine increased within the 2RDA group. # denotes the significant differences of metabolites between 2RDA and RDA. *Represents the significant differences of metabolites between pre and post intervention within each group.

Arginine and Proline Metabolism

Greatest statistical discrimination between the diets related to arginine and proline pathways, which comprised of eight metabolites with fold changes ranging between 1.2 and 2.7. The high centrality of arginine places it as a key metabolic hub, acting as a precursor for downstream targets. In this pathway, arginine

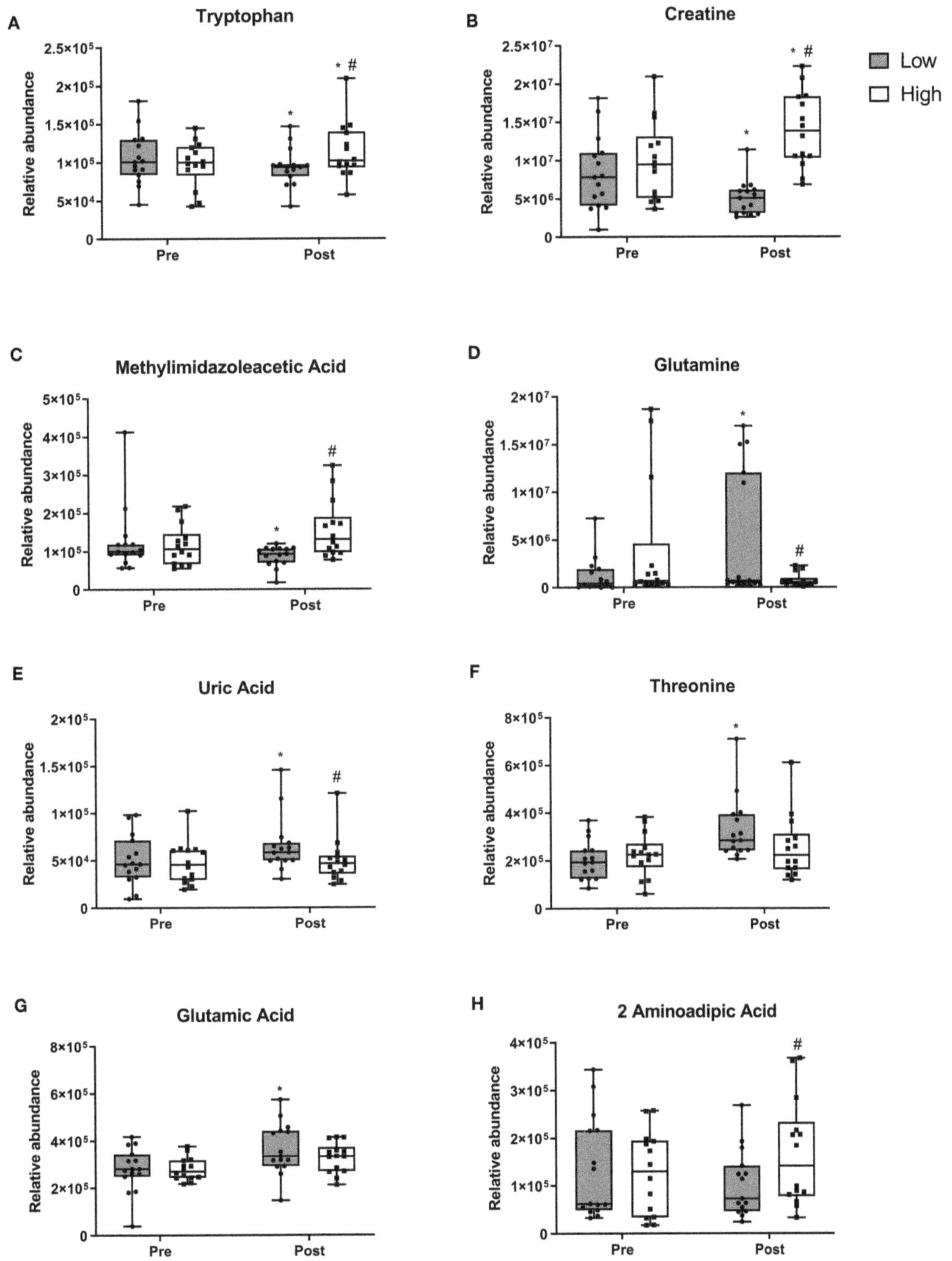

FIGURE 3 | Metabolite responses to 2RDA or RDA after 10 week intervention. Box and whisker plots showing median, first, and third quartiles, and maximum and minimum values. **(A)** tryptophan, **(B)** creatine, **(C)** methylimidazoleacetic acid increased in the 2RDA group. **(D)** glutamine **(E)** uric acid, **(F)** threonine, **(G)** glutamic acid all increased in the RDA group. **(H)** 2-aminoadipic acid was higher in the 2RDA group compared to the RDA group. #denotes the significant differences of metabolites between 2RDA and RDA. *Represents the significant differences of metabolites between pre and post intervention within each group.

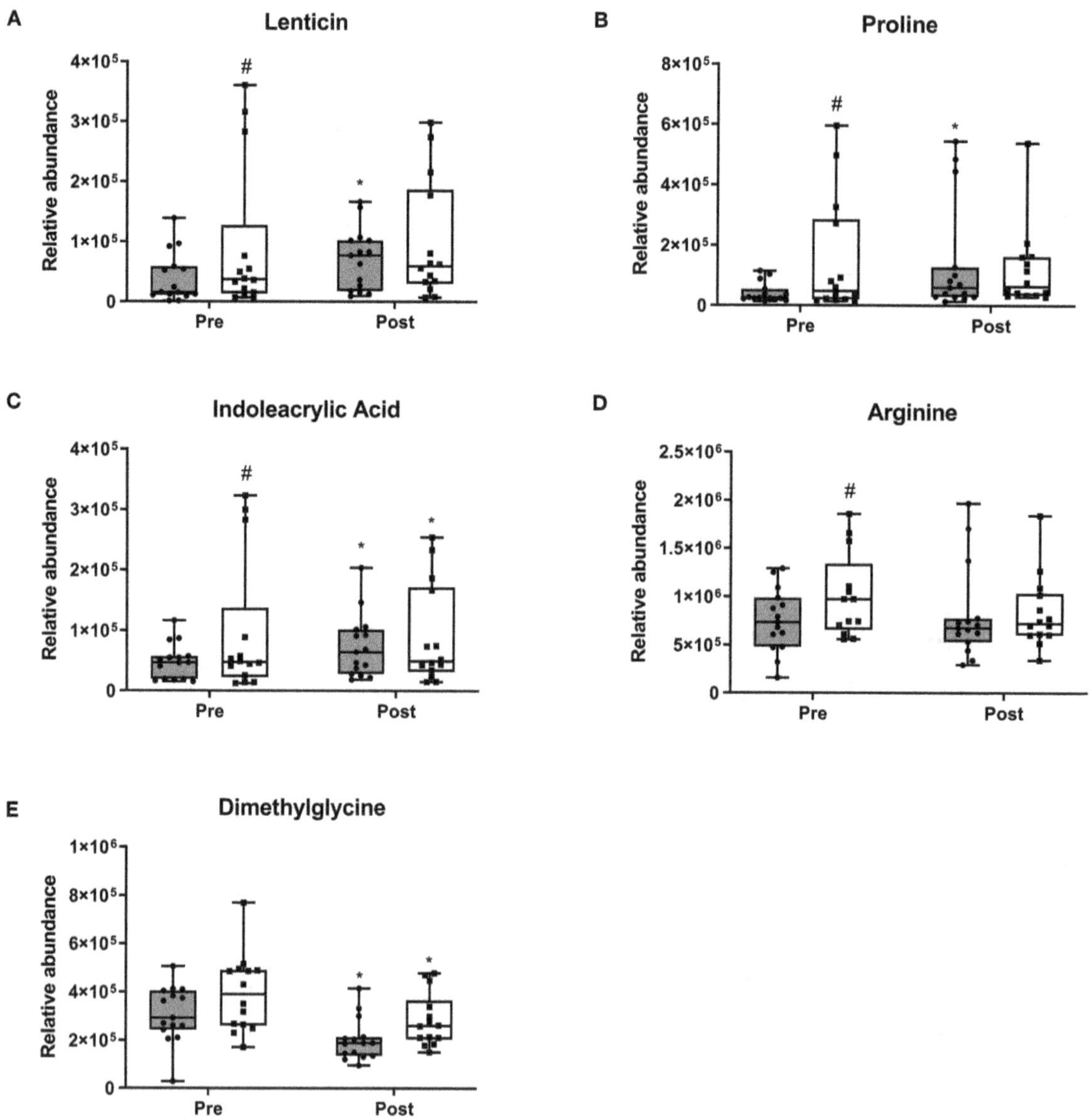

FIGURE 4 | Pre-intervention metabolite differences. Box and whisker plots show median, first, and third quartiles, and maximum and minimum values. There were four metabolites which exhibited pre-intervention differences **(A)** lenticin, **(B)** proline, **(C)** indoleacrylic acid, and **(D)** arginine. **(E)** dimethylglycine decreased in both diet groups. # denotes the significant differences of metabolites between 2RDA and RDA. *Represents the significant differences between pre and post-intervention within each group.

is converted by arginase-1 to urea and is also the precursor to creatine through the intermediate glycocyamine. Urea and creatine are widely used markers of protein intake (42). Arginine is also important in overall skeletal muscle protein balance as a key substrate for nitric oxide, an endogenous regulator of vascular homeostasis (43). Evidence suggests nitric oxide is integral to skeletal muscle contractile function, blood flow, and glucose homeostasis, further highlighting the importance of arginine (44). Also part of the arginine-proline pathway is glutamic acid, the precursor to proline, which increased 3-fold in the RDA group. High levels of proline have been previously implicated as a risk factor for sarcopenia and frailty (45). Therefore, in the current study, the post-intervention difference between diet groups by the observed approximate 30% elevations in urea, glycocyamine, and creatine in the 2RDA group together with the alterations in the arginine and proline pathways, is indicative of a metabolomic milleau potentially favorable to sustaining anabolism.

Glycine, Serine, and Threonine Metabolism

Five metabolites from the glycine, serine, and threonine metabolism pathway were regulated by protein intake, including; glycocyamine, creatine, and tryptophan all of which were higher in the 2RDA group compared to the RDA group. Of these, it

TABLE 2 | Description of the total number of compounds in the pathway.

Pathway name	Total compound[a]	Hits[b]	Raw p[c]	-Log (p)	Impact[d]
Arginine & proline metabolism	77	8	2.57E-08	2.06E-06	0.356
Aminoacyl-tRNA biosynthesis	75	6	1.03E-05	0.00041	0.0563
Glycine, serine & threonine metabolism	48	5	1.80E-05	0.00048	0.137
Pyridine metabolism	60	4	0.00821	0.0164	0.0355
Nitrogen metabolism	39	3	0.00271	0.0372	0.000
Glutamine & glutamate metabolism	11	2	0.00279	0.0372	0.139
Alanine, aspartate & glutamate metabolism	24	2	0.0132	0.151	0.384

[a] *Total compound is the number of compounds involved in the pathway.*
[b] *Hits is the matched number from the user uploaded data.*
[c] *The raw p is the original p-value calculated from the enrichment analysis.*
[d] *Impact value is calculated from pathway topology analysis for comparison among different pathways. It represents the cumulative percentage of importance for the matched metabolite nodes involved in a pathway. The importance of each metabolite node is calculated from centrality measures and represents the percentage with regard to the total pathway importance.*

has been shown that glycine, serine, and threonine metabolism are central to providing precursors for the synthesis of proteins, nucleic acids, and lipids (46). Threonine was increased by 60% in the RDA group and has been shown to follow the changes of branch chain amino acids (BCAAs) in situations of muscle catabolism (47, 48). Dimethylglycine which was identified to be part of the same cycle is produced from betaine and metabolized to glycine, decreased in both RDA and 2RDA groups. Dimenthylglycine is a degradation product for one-carbon metabolism, which supports multiple physiological processes such as; amino acid metabolism, and biosynthesis of purines (46). Tryptophan has multiple biological roles and whilst it has not been directly implicated in tissue anabolism, it is the precursor of serotonin and reflected in mood and cognition (49). Therefore, while its role is difficult to ascertain, tryptophan's fasting plasma levels may be of significant interest as an indicator of nutritional status beyond anabolism. Contrasting observations have been reported for relationships between tryptophan and skeletal muscle. Moaddel et al. (50) associated higher levels of tryptophan with low muscle quality, while in Toyoshima et al. (45) tryptophan was lower in sarcopenic participants. Our findings for tryptophan are in agreement with Toyoshima et al. (45) where the 2RDA group increased the plasma level of tryptophan by 16% and was higher than the RDA group at the end of the intervention.

Aminoacyl-tRNA Biosynthesis, Nitrogen Metabolism, and Pyrimidine Metabolism

Metabolism of the aminoacyl-tRNA biosynthesis and nitrogen metabolism pathway also discriminated between 2RDA and RDA with six and three identified metabolites, respectively. Glutamine and glutamic acid are components of both aminoacyl-tRNA and nitrogen metabolism, which along with threonine, proline, and arginine (which demonstrated a trend), increased in the RDA group. Aminoacyl-tRNA substrates are the essential first steps for protein synthesis. Dysregulation of these pathways has been linked with aging muscle (51). Based on our previous demonstration of reduced appendicular lean mass in the RDA group (7), these data suggest the circulatory alterations both aminoacyl-tRNAs and nitrogen metabolism are reflective of this loss of muscle mass.

Uridine, dihydrothymine, and urea, were metabolites identified to be components of pyrimidine metabolism where glucose and glutamine serve as precursors. These metabolites were each increased in the 2RDA group, by at least 60%. Pyrimidine metabolism, is integral to cell cycle regulation, and tightly linked to the ability of the cell to acquire nutrients, generate metabolic energy, and to drive anabolism, including nucleotide/nucleic acid biosynthesis (52). Glutamine is an important component of muscle protein, and helps repair and build muscle (53). Furthermore, glutamine deficiency stimulates cell apoptosis, which may thereby trigger a low-level inflammatory process and increase the rate of sarcopenic progression (54). In times of catabolic stress, glutamine derived by *de novo* synthesis from skeletal BCAAs are used to form glutamic acid. Glutamic acid displays remarkable metabolic versatility being highly abundant in liver, kidney, skeletal muscle, and the brain, illustrating its utility (55). In this study, glutamine increased 3-fold and glutamic acid was elevated by 30% in the RDA group. which is concomitant with physical changes of reduced lean muscle (7).

Markers of Specific Diet Consumption

The findings of the current study are complex in that there were observed baseline differences revealed by the 2-way repeated measures ANOVA, prior to the dietary interventions, in a small subset of metabolites. This was despite the cohort being relatively homogenous in terms of age, BMI, background diet and general metabolic and cardiovascular health. It is unclear whether these differences are then reflective of the complexity associated with inter-individual variability or indicative of a difference in habitual diet or associated lifestyle factor(s). Notable amongst the pre-intervention differences was lenticin, found in lentil extracts and is detected in blood after lentil consumption (56). These observed baseline differences were normalized with the 10 week intervention, as the participants adhered to the well-designed meals matched for micronutrients, macronutrients, and food structure, except protein.

In this study, uric acid, the end product of purine metabolism, was increased by 30% in the RDA diet. Increased concentrations of uric acid is a causative factor in gout (57), where previously, it has been postulated that higher consumption of dietary protein

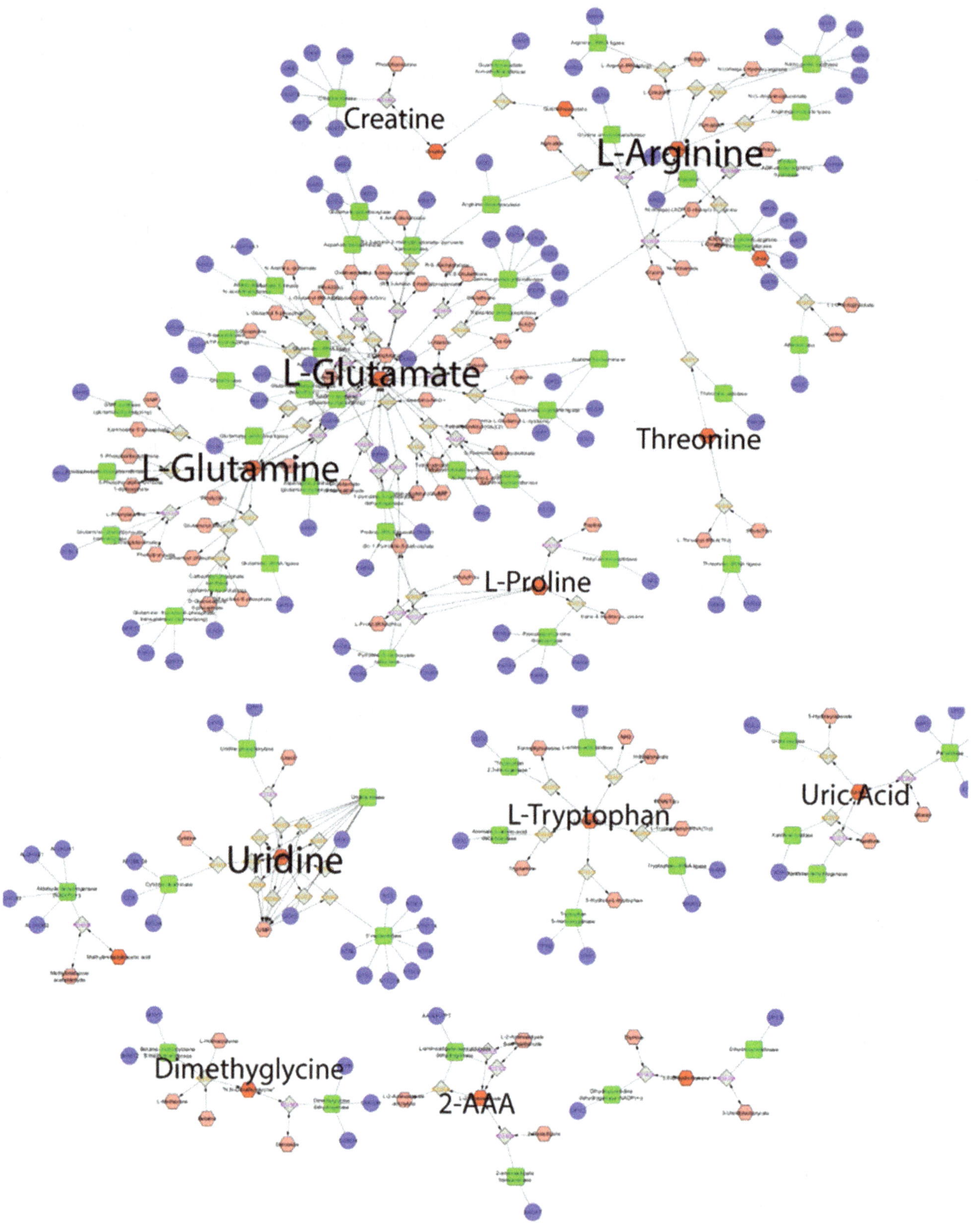

FIGURE 5 | Global metabolic network pathways. Nodes correspond to the identified plasma metabolite, and edges indicate a significant correlation between nodes. Red hexagons represent inputted metabolites; pink hexagons represent compounds, blue circles represent genes, green quadrangles represent enzymes, gray quadrangles represent reaction paths.

TABLE 3 | Topological parameters of key metabolites.

Metabolite	KeggID	Degree	Betweenness centrality	Pathways
Glutamic acid	C00025	39	0.670	Arginine & proline metabolism, Aminoacyl-tRNA biosynthesis, Nitrogen metabolism, Glutamine & glutamate metabolism, Alanine, aspartate & glutamate metabolism
Glutamine	C00064	19	0.645	Arginine & proline metabolism, Aminoacyl-tRNA biosynthesis, Nitrogen metabolism, Glutamine & glutamate metabolism, Alanine, aspartâte & glutamate metabolism, Pyrimidine metabolism
Arginine	C00062	16	0.444	Argine & proline metabolism, Aminoacyl-tRNA biosynthesis
Uridine	C00299	12	1.000	Pyrimidine metabolism

The degree of a node is the number of edges associated with it, and the betweenness centrality of a node is the number of shortest communication paths between different pairs of nodes.

increases uric acid excretion, thereby reducing circulatory uric acid (58, 59). TMAO is generated from choline, betaine, and carnitine by gut microbial metabolism, increased in the 2RDA group by 5-fold with no change in the RDA group. The specific increase of TMAO in the 2RDA is similar to previous observations of well-known protein sources; fish (60) and meat (61). Whilst, the role of TMAO remains speculative toward gut health and CVD risk (62), the present finding suggests it can be regarded as a marker of high protein intake.

Limitations

This trial applied an untargeted HILIC-MS approach to cover polar metabolites, yet the metabolome is vast in number and diverse in nature. There is opportunity for future studies to implement more comprehensive untargeted metabolomics analysis to cover greater diversity of the metabolome by utilizing reverse phase (RP)-MS and lipidomic analysis and to include other biological matricies such a urine and feces. These types of analysis could provide a more holistic understanding of the impact of nutritional interventions on metabolism and physiology. Lastly, while the findings of this discovery study can be explained and make sense biologically, it is recommended that discovery studies should be followed-up with a targeted approach to quantify findings and replicated in independent and larger cohorts.

CONCLUSIONS

In the current study, untargeted metabolomics analyses were carried out to discriminate the polar plasma metabolome changes associated with a prescribed protein intake at RDA ($0.8\ g{\cdot}kg^{-1}{\cdot}d^{-1}$) or 2RDA ($1.6\ g{\cdot}kg^{-1}{\cdot}d^{-1}$) for 10 weeks. Post-intervention, two-way repeated measures ANOVA revealed metabolites of increased amino acid flux such as urea and creatinine were higher in the 2RDA diet compared to the RDA diet. Further metabolites were different between the two diet groups such as tryptophan and creatine and glutamine, which are components of the arginine and proline metabolism and nitrogen metabolism. These metabolites and pathways are indicative of changes in key aspects of skeletal muscle metabolism, which showed a good association with reduced maintenance of mass and function (7). Conversely, in the 2RDA group biomarkers of increased amino acid flux were increased, such as urea and uridine. Along with pathways these are involved in (glycine, serine, and threonine metabolism and aminoacyl-tRNA metabolism) allow us to speculate these alterations in metabolites are indicative of induction of tissue anabolism. Overall, this study demonstrated shifts in the metabolome induced by a higher protein diet is very limited in its metabolomic impact. Of those few metabolites that were statistically altered, it can be suggested that these are indicative of a possible induction of pathways supporting tissue anabolism and maintenance of muscle mass. In contrast, reducing protein intake to current minimum requirements resulted in a more catabolic metabolomic profile, potentially congruent with changes in skeletal muscle phenotype previously reported in the same cohort.

AUTHOR CONTRIBUTIONS

CM, AM, SK, NR, AS, K-HW, and DC-S designed the research. CM, AM, SM, NZ, FR, and PS conducted the research. BD, CM, and KF conducted the statistical analysis. BD wrote the manuscript. DC-S had primary responsibility for the final content of manuscript. All authors provided content and feedback to the manuscript and read and approved the final manuscript.

FUNDING

This study was supported by New Zealand Ministry of Business, Innovation and Employment International Relationships and the European Union (IRSES-318962-BIOAGE) and AgResearch Limited Strategic Science Investment Fund (A21246: Food Nutrition; Nutritional strategies for an aging population). The funders had no role in the design, data collection, analysis, decision to publish or in preparation of the manuscript.

REFERENCES

1. Traylor DA, Gorissen SHM, Phillips SM. Perspective: protein requirements and optimal intakes in aging: are we ready to recommend more than the recommended daily allowance? *Adv Nutr.* (2018) 9:171–82. doi: 10.1093/advances/nmy003
2. Landi F, Calvani R, Tosato M, Martone AM, Ortolani E, Savera G, et al. Protein intake and muscle health in old age: from biological plausibility to clinical evidence. *Nutrients.* (2016) 8:E295. doi: 10.3390/nu8050295
3. Houston DK, Nicklas BJ, Ding J, Harris TB, Tylavsky FA, Newman AB, et al. Dietary protein intake is associated with lean mass change in older, community-dwelling adults: the Health, Aging, and Body Composition (Health ABC) Study. *Am J Clin Nutr.* (2008) 87:150–5. doi: 10.1093/ajcn/87.1.150
4. WHO/FAO/UNU Expert *Consultation. Protein and amino acid requirements in human nutrition. World Health Organ Tech Rep Ser.* (2007). p. 1–265.
5. Filippin LI, Teixeira VN, da Silva MPM, Miraglia F, da Silva FS. Sarcopenia: a predictor of mortality and the need for early diagnosis and intervention. *Aging Clin Exp Res.* (2015) 27:249–54. doi: 10.1007/s40520-014-0281-4
6. Isanejad M, Mursu J, Sirola J, Kröger H, Rikkonen T, Tuppurainen M, et al. Dietary protein intake is associated with better physical function and muscle strength among elderly women. *Br J Nutr.* (2016) 115:1281–91. doi: 10.1017/S000711451600012X
7. Mitchell CJ, Milan AM, Mitchell SM, Zeng N, Ramzan F, Sharma P, et al. The effects of dietary protein intake on appendicular lean mass and muscle function in elderly men: a 10-wk randomized controlled trial. *Am J Clin Nutr.* (2017) 106:1375–83. doi: 10.3945/ajcn.117.160325
8. Loenneke JP, Loprinzi PD, Murphy CH, Phillips SM. Per meal dose and frequency of protein consumption is associated with lean mass and muscle performance. *Clin Nutr.* (2016) 35:1506–11. doi: 10.1016/j.clnu.2016.04.002
9. Wolfe RR, Cifelli AM, Kostas G, Kim I-Y. Optimizing protein intake in adults: interpretation and application of the recommended dietary allowance compared with the acceptable macronutrient distribution range. *Adv Nutr An Int Rev J.* (2017) 8:266–75. doi: 10.3945/an.116.013821
10. Phillips SM, Chevalier S, Leidy HJ. Protein "requirements" beyond the RDA: implications for optimizing health. *Appl Physiol Nutr Metab.* (2016) 41:565–72. doi: 10.1139/apnm-2015-0550
11. Westerterp-Plantenga MS, Lemmens SG, Westerterp KR. Dietary protein - Its role in satiety, energetics, weight loss and health. *Br J Nutr.* (2012) 108(Suppl. 2):S105–12. doi: 10.1017/S0007114512002589
12. Playdon MC, Moore SC, Derkach A, Reedy J, Subar AF, Sampson JN, et al. Identifying biomarkers of dietary patterns by using metabolomics. *Am J Clin Nutr.* (2017) 105:450–65. doi: 10.3945/ajcn.116.144501
13. North BJ, Sinclair DA. The intersection between aging and cardiovascular disease. *Circ Res.* (2012) 110:1097–108. doi: 10.1161/CIRCRESAHA.111.246876
14. Protogerou AD, Safar ME, Iaria P, Safar H, Le Dudal K, Filipovsky J, et al. Diastolic blood pressure and mortality in the elderly with cardiovascular disease. *Hypertension.* (2007) 50:172–80. doi: 10.1161/HYPERTENSIONAHA.107.089797
15. Virtanen HEK, Voutilainen S, Koskinen TT, Mursu J, Tuomainen T-P, Virtanen JK. Intake of different dietary proteins and risk of heart failure in men. *Circ Hear Fail.* (2018) 11:e004531. doi: 10.1161/CIRCHEARTFAILURE.117.004531
16. Song M, Fung TT, Hu FB, Willett WC, Longo VD, Chan AT, et al. Association of animal and plant protein intake with all-cause and cause-specific mortality. *JAMA Intern Med.* (2016) 176:1453–63. doi: 10.1001/jamainternmed.2016.4182
17. Beaumont M, Portune KJ, Steuer N, Lan A, Cerrudo V, Audebert M, et al. Quantity and source of dietary protein influence metabolite production by gut microbiota and rectal mucosa gene expression: a randomized, parallel, double-blind trial in overweight humans. *Am J Clin Nutr.* (2017) 106:1005–19. doi: 10.3945/ajcn.117.158816
18. Esko T, Hirschhorn JN, Feldman HA, Hsu YHH, Deik AA, Clish CB, et al. Metabolomic profiles as reliable biomarkers of dietary composition. *Am J Clin Nutr.* (2017) 105:547–54. doi: 10.3945/ajcn.116.144428
19. Hernández-Alonso P, Giardina S, Cañueto D, Salas-Salvadó J, Cañellas N, Bulló M. Changes in plasma metabolite concentrations after a low-glycemic index diet intervention. *Mol Nutr Food Res.* (2018) 63:e1700975. doi: 10.1002/mnfr.201700975
20. Garcia-Perez I, Posma JM, Gibson R, Chambers ES, Hansen TH, Vestergaard H, et al. Objective assessment of dietary patterns by use of metabolic phenotyping: a randomised, controlled, crossover trial. *Lancet Diabetes Endocrinol.* (2017) 5:184–95. doi: 10.1016/S2213-8587(16)30419-3
21. Andersen MBS, Rinnan A, Manach C, Poulsen SK, Pujos-Guillot E, Larsen TM, et al. Untargeted metabolomics as a screening tool for estimating compliance to a dietary pattern. *J Proteome Res.* (2014) 13:1405–18. doi: 10.1021/pr400964s
22. Gibbons H, Carr E, McNulty BA, Nugent AP, Walton J, Flynn A, et al. Metabolomic-based identification of clusters that reflect dietary patterns. *Mol Nutr Food Res.* (2017) 61:1–11. doi: 10.1002/mnfr.201601050
23. Sullivan AO, Gibney MJ, Brennan L. Dietary intake patterns are reflected in metabolomic profiles : potential role in dietary assessment studies 1–3. *Am J Clin Nutr.* (2011) 93:314–21. doi: 10.3945/ajcn.110.000950
24. Fraser K, Harrison SJ, Lane GA, Otter DE, Hemar Y, Quek SY, et al. Non-targeted analysis of tea by hydrophilic interaction liquid chromatography and high resolution mass spectrometry. *Food Chem.* (2012) 134:1616–23. doi: 10.1016/j.foodchem.2012.03.045
25. Ministry of Healthy. *Easting and Activity Guidelines for New Zealand Adults.* Wellington: Ministry of Health (2015).
26. Farooqi N, Slinde F, Carlsson M, Håglin L, Sandström T. Predicting energy requirement with pedometer-determined physical-activity level in women with chronic obstructive pulmonary disease. *Int J Chron Obstruct Pulmon Dis.* (2015) 10:1129–37. doi: 10.2147/COPD.S80616
27. Armirotti A, Basit A, Realini N, Caltagirone C, Bossù P, Spalletta G, et al. Sample preparation and orthogonal chromatography for broad polarity range plasma metabolomics: application to human subjects with neurodegenerative dementia. *Anal Biochem.* (2014) 455:48–54. doi: 10.1016/j.ab.2014.03.019
28. Smith CA, Want EJ, O'Maille G, Abagyan R, Siuzdak G. XCMS: processing mass spectrometry data for metabolite profiling using nonlinear peak alignment, matching, and identification. *Anal Chem.* (2006) 78:779–87. doi: 10.1021/ac051437y
29. Van Der Kloet FM, Bobeldijk I, Verheij ER, Jellema RH. Analytical error reduction using single point calibration for accurate and precise metabolomic phenotyping. *J Proteome Res.* (2009) 8:5132–41. doi: 10.1021/pr900499r
30. Giacomoni F, Le Corguillé G, Monsoor M, Landi M, Pericard P, Pétéra M, et al. Workflow4Metabolomics: a collaborative research infrastructure for computational metabolomics. *Bioinformatics.* (2015) 31:1493–5. doi: 10.1093/bioinformatics/btu813
31. Guijas C, Montenegro-Burke JR, Domingo-Almenara X, Palermo A, Warth B, Hermann G, et al. METLIN: a technology platform for identifying knowns and unknowns. *Anal Chem.* (2018) 90:3156–64. doi: 10.1021/acs.analchem.7b04424
32. Wishart DS, Feunang YD, Marcu A, Guo AC, Liang K, Vázquez-Fresno R, et al. HMDB 4.0: the human metabolome database for 2018. *Nucleic Acids Res.* (2018) 46:D608–17. doi: 10.1093/nar/gkx1089
33. Lynn KS, Cheng ML, Chen YR, Hsu C, Chen A, Lih TM, et al. Metabolite identification for mass spectrometry-based metabolomics using multiple types of correlated ion information. *Anal Chem.* (2015) 87:2143–51. doi: 10.1021/ac503325c
34. Dunn WB, Lin W, Broadhurst D, Begley P, Brown M, Zelena E, et al. Molecular phenotyping of a UK population: defining the human serum metabolome. *Metabolomics.* (2014) 11:9–26. doi: 10.1007/s11306-014-0707-1
35. Sumner LW, Amberg A, Barrett D, Beale MH, Beger R, Daykin CA, et al. Proposed minimum reporting standards for chemical analysis. *Metabolomics.* (2007) 3:211–21. doi: 10.1007/s11306-007-0082-2
36. Brunelli L, Ristagno G, Bagnati R, Fumagalli F, Latini R, Fanelli R, et al. A combination of untargeted and targeted metabolomics approaches unveils changes in the kynurenine pathway following cardiopulmonary resuscitation. *Metabolomics.* (2013) 9:839–52. doi: 10.1007/s11306-013-0506-0
37. Wang L, Hou E, Wang L, Wang Y, Yang L, Zheng X, et al. Reconstruction and analysis of correlation networks based on GC-MS metabolomics

data for young hypertensive men. *Anal Chim Acta.* (2015) 854:95–105. doi: 10.1016/j.aca.2014.11.009

38. Shannon P, Markiel A, Ozier O, Baliga NS, Wang JT, Ramage D, et al. Cytoscape: a software environment for integrated models of biomolecular interaction networks. *Genome Res.* (2003) 13:2498–504. doi: 10.1101/gr.1239303
39. Karnovsky A, Weymouth T, Hull T, Glenn Tarcea V, Scardoni G, Laudanna C, et al. Metscape 2 bioinformatics tool for the analysis and visualization of metabolomics and gene expression data. *Bioinformatics.* (2012) 28:373–80. doi: 10.1093/bioinformatics/btr661
40. Mitchell WK, Phillips BE, Wilkinson DJ, Williams JP, Rankin D, Lund JN, et al. Supplementing essential amino acids with the nitric oxide precursor, L-arginine, enhances skeletal muscle perfusion without impacting anabolism in older men. *Clin Nutr.* (2017) 36:1573–9. doi: 10.1016/j.clnu.2016.09.031
41. Chow LS. Mechanism of insulin's anabolic effect on muscle: measurements of muscle protein synthesis and breakdown using aminoacyl-tRNA and other surrogate measures. *AJP Endocrinol Metab.* (2006) 291:E729–36. doi: 10.1152/ajpendo.00003.2006
42. Schwingshackl L, Hoffmann G. Comparison of high vs. normal/low protein diets on renal function in subjects without chronic kidney disease: a systematic review and meta-analysis. *PLoS ONE.* (2014) 9:e97656. doi: 10.1371/journal.pone.0097656
43. Newsholme P, Brennan L, Bender K. Amino acid metabolism, β-cell function, and diabetes. *Diabetes.* (2006) 55(Suppl. 2):S39–47. doi: 10.2337/db06-S006
44. da Boit M, Tommasi S, Elliot D, Zinellu A, Sotgia S, Sibson R, et al. Sex differences in the associations between L-arginine pathway metabolites, skeletal muscle mass and function, and their responses to resistance exercise, in old age. *J Nutr Health Aging.* (2017) 22:534–40. doi: 10.1007/s12603-017-0964-6
45. Toyoshima K, Nakamura M, Adachi Y, Imaizumi A, Hakamada T, Abe Y, et al. Increased plasma proline concentrations are associated with sarcopenia in the elderly. *PLoS ONE.* (2017) 12:e0185206. doi: 10.1371/journal.pone.0185206
46. Ducker GS, Rabinowitz JD. One-carbon metabolism in health and disease. *Cell Metab.* (2016) 25:27–42. doi: 10.1016/j.cmet.2016.08.009
47. Mirisola MG, Taormina G, Fabrizio P, Wei M, Hu J, Longo VD. Serine- and threonine/valine-dependent activation of PDK and Tor orthologs converge on Sch9 to promote aging. *PLoS Genet.* (2014) 10:e1004113. doi: 10.1371/journal.pgen.1004113
48. Volpi E, Kobayashi H, Sheffield-Moore M, Mittendorfer B, Wolfe RR. Essential amino acids are primarily responsible for the amino acid stimulation of muscle protein anabolism in healthy elderly adults. *Am J Clin Nutr.* (2003) 78:250–8. doi: 10.1093/ajcn/78.2.250
49. Palego L, Betti L, Rossi A, Giannaccini G. Tryptophan biochemistry: structural, nutritional, metabolic, and medical aspects in humans. *J Amino Acids.* (2016) 2016:8952520. doi: 10.1155/2016/8952520
50. Moaddel R, Fabbri E, Khadeer MA, Carlson OD, Gonzalez-Freire M, Zhang P, et al. Plasma biomarkers of poor muscle quality in older men and women from the Baltimore longitudinal study of aging. *J Gerontol Ser A Biol Sci Med Sci.* (2016) 71:1266–72. doi: 10.1093/gerona/glw046
51. Dillon EL. Nutritionally essential amino acids and metabolic signaling in aging. *Amino Acids.* (2013) 45:431–41. doi: 10.1007/s00726-012-1438-0
52. Lane AN, Fan TWM. Regulation of mammalian nucleotide metabolism and biosynthesis. *Nucleic Acids Res.* (2015) 43:2466–85. doi: 10.1093/nar/gkv047
53. Mittendorfer B, Volpi E, Wolfe RR. Whole body and skeletal muscle glutamine metabolism in healthy subjects. *Am J Physiol Endocrinol Metab.* (2001) 280:E323–33. doi: 10.1152/ajpendo.2001.280.2.E323
54. Meynial-Denis D. Glutamine metabolism in advanced age. *Nutr Rev.* (2016) 74:225–36. doi: 10.1093/nutrit/nuv052
55. Brosnan JT. Glutamate, at the interface between amino acid and carbohydrate metabolism. *J Nutr.* (2000) 130:988S–90S. doi: 10.1093/jn/130.4.988S
56. Bondia-Pons I, Martinez JA, de la Iglesia R, Lopez-Legarrea P, Poutanen K, Hanhineva K, et al. Effects of short- and long-term mediterranean-based dietary treatment on plasma LC-QTOF/MS metabolic profiling of subjects with metabolic syndrome features: The Metabolic Syndrome Reduction in Navarra (RESMENA) randomized controlled trial. *Mol Nutr Food Res.* (2015) 59:711–28. doi: 10.1002/mnfr.201400309
57. Zhang Y, Chen C, Choi H, Chaisson C, Hunter D, Niu J, et al. Purine-rich foods intake and recurrent gout attacks. *Ann Rheum Dis.* (2012) 71:1448–53. doi: 10.1136/annrheumdis-2011-201215
58. Villegas R, Xiang YB, Elasy T, Xu WH, Cai H, Cai Q, et al. Purine-rich foods, protein intake, and the prevalence of hyperuricemia: The Shanghai Men's Health Study. *Nutr Metab Cardiovasc Dis.* (2012) 22:409–16. doi: 10.1016/j.numecd.2010.07.012
59. Gibson T, Rodgers AV, Simmonds HA, Court-Brown F, Todd E, Meilton V. A controlled study of diet in patients with gout. *Ann Rheum Dis.* (1983) 42:123–7. doi: 10.1136/ard.42.2.123
60. Cheung W, Keski-Rahkonen P, Assi N, Ferrari P, Freisling H, Rinaldi S, et al. A metabolomic study of biomarkers of meat and fish intake. *Am J Clin Nutr.* (2017) 105:600–8. doi: 10.3945/ajcn.116.146639
61. Krüger R, Merz B, Rist MJ, Ferrario PG, Bub A, Kulling SE, et al. Associations of current diet with plasma and urine TMAO in the KarMeN study: direct and indirect contributions. *Mol Nutr Food Res.* (2017) 61:1700363. doi: 10.1002/mnfr.201700363
62. Velasquez MT, Ramezani A, Manal A, Raj DS. Trimethylamine N-oxide: the good, the bad and the unknown. *Toxins.* (2016) 8:E326. doi: 10.3390/toxins8110326

8

Nutritional Strategies to Combat Type 2 Diabetes in Aging Adults: The Importance of Protein

*Kayleigh M. Beaudry and Michaela C. Devries**

Department of Kinesiology, Faculty of Applied Health Sciences, University of Waterloo, Waterloo, ON, Canada

***Correspondence:**
Michaela C. Devries
m4devrie@uwaterloo.ca

The prevalence of pre-diabetes (PD) and type II diabetes (T2D) has risen dramatically in recent years affecting an estimated 422 million adults worldwide. The risk of T2D increases with age, with the sharpest rise in diagnosis occurring after age 40. With age, there is also a progressive decline in muscle mass starting after the age of 30. The decline in muscle mass and function due to aging is termed sarcopenia and immediately precedes the sharp rise in T2D. The purpose of the current review is to discuss the role of protein to attenuate declines in muscle mass and insulin sensitivity to prevent T2D and sarcopenia in aging adults. The current recommended dietary allowance for protein consumption is set at 0.8 g/kg/day and is based on dated studies on young healthy men and may not be sufficient for older adults. Protein consumption upwards of 1.0–1.5 g/kg/day in older adults is able to induce improvements in glycemic control and muscle mass. Obesity, particularly central or visceral obesity is a major risk factor in the development of PD and T2D. However, the tissue composition of weight loss in older adults includes both lean body mass and fat mass and therefore may have adverse metabolic consequences in older adults who are already at a high risk of lean body mass loss. High protein diets have the ability to increase weight loss while preserving lean body mass therefore inducing "high-quality weight loss," which provides favorable metabolic changes in older adults. High protein diets also induce beneficial outcomes on glycemic markers due to satiety, lowered post-prandial glucose response, increased thermogenesis, and the ability to decrease rates of muscle protein breakdown (MPB). The consumption of dairy specific protein consumption has also been shown to improve insulin sensitivity by improving body composition, enhancing insulin release, accelerating fat oxidation, and stimulating rates of muscle protein synthesis (MPS) in older adults. Exercise, specifically resistance training, also works synergistically to attenuate the progression of PD and T2D by further stimulating rates of MPS thereby increasing muscle mass and inducing favorable changes in glycemic control independent of lean body mass increases.

Keywords: protein, dairy, aging, type 2 diabetes, sarcopenia, resistance exercise

INTRODUCTION

The average lifespan has increased by 20 years, increasing the age of the population worldwide (1). At the same time, the rates of obesity have also increased radically (2). In 2015, 603.7 million adults were considered obese, which is nearly double that reported in 1980 (2). Obesity is associated with a multitude of co-morbidities such as cardiovascular disease, metabolic syndrome, and type 2

with metabolic alterations including T2D, including the thought that dietary protein would adversely raise blood glucose levels and have a detrimental effect on kidney function (44). The belief that dietary protein is converted into glucose upon consumption and adversely increases blood glucose concentrations is thought to have originated from a study by Janney conducted in 1915 where 3.5 g of glucose was produced from consuming 6.25 g of protein from meat (51). These findings have been discredited by several studies, the first of which was conducted in 1924 involving participants with and without diabetes who were fed 50 g of protein and showed no change in blood glucose concentrations (52). Furthermore, a study conducted in 1936 that found that consuming even large amounts of protein (1.3 pounds) in a single serving does not raise blood glucose concentrations (53). This remains true in individuals with diabetes and impaired glucose control, with dietary protein exhibiting insulinotropic effects and enhancing blood glucose clearance from the blood (54–56). The second reason why higher protein intakes were not encouraged for individuals with diabetes pertains to the theory that increased dietary protein intake would lead to kidney disease, a theory that has also been discredited. A recent meta-analysis conducted by Devries et al. (57) indicated that high protein diets (≤1.5 g/kg/ body weight or ≤20% energy intake or ≤100 g protein per day) did not adversely influence kidney function on glomerular filtration rate in adults without kidney disease. Furthermore, a sub-analysis revealed that increased protein consumption did not adversely affect kidney function in individuals with type 2 diabetes (57). More recent evidence now supports a positive effect of a protein-rich diet in diabetes (44) and sarcopenia (11). These positive outcomes are thought to be due to several mechanisms, including an increase in protein anabolism, weight loss, enhanced glycemic control, daily appetite control, and satiety (47, 58) (**Figure 2**).

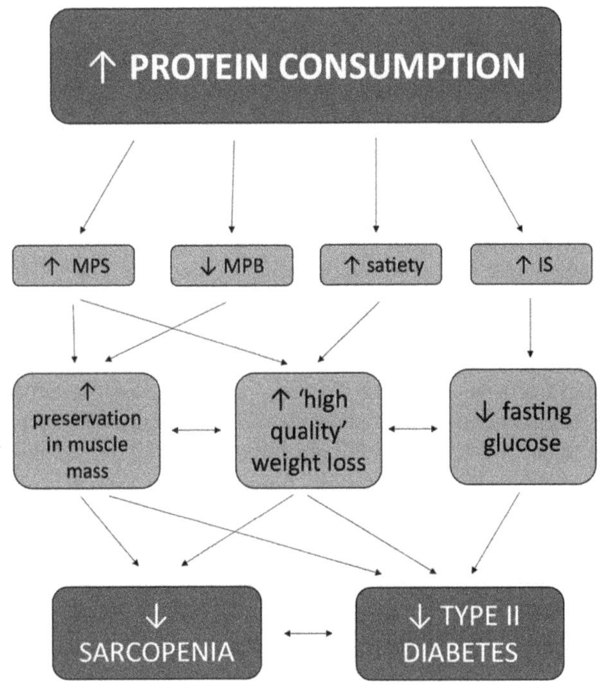

FIGURE 2 | Interrelated effects of increased protein consumption on factors related to both sarcopenia and type II diabetes in older adults.

Protein Intake and Its Effect on Insulin Sensitivity and Glycemic Control

Obesity, particularly central or visceral obesity, is a risk factor for the development of T2D and is common in PD and T2D (59). Weight loss remains a dominant determinant of reducing the risk of diabetes, with a weight loss of ~5 kg accounting for an ~55% reduction in the risk of T2D in overweight or obese individuals with impaired glucose control (60). Weight loss, even modest weight loss in overweight and obese subjects has been shown to improve markers of glycemic control in T2D (61–63). Energy-restricted high protein, low carbohydrate diets have been successful in improving weight loss and glucose control in T2D (49). However, it is not just the amount of weight loss that is important, but also the composition of weight loss. While traditional energy restriction leads to weight loss, this type of weight loss induces not only a loss of fat mass (~75% of mass lost), but also a loss of muscle mass (~25% of mass lost), which could have adverse metabolic consequences particularly in older adults who are already losing muscle mass (64–66). In fact, it has been shown that in older adults, total weight loss was represented by a higher proportion of lean mass loss compared to fat mass, whereas weight gain was largely represented by an increase in fat mass (67). This decrease in lean body mass can have adverse metabolic consequences and accelerate the development of T2D and sarcopenia in older adults.

Higher protein diets may be especially important to improve IS in older adults with PD or T2D as higher protein intakes during weight loss can help preserve muscle mass (66, 68), inducing what is known as "high-quality" weight loss. A study by Piatti et al. (69) found that while hypocaloric high protein and high carbohydrate diets had similar effects on the total amount of weight loss, the high protein diet was able to improve insulin sensitivity and spare lean body mass whereas the high carbohydrate diet did not. Furthermore, a study by Wycherley et al. (70) found that as compared with a standard protein diet, a high protein diet induced a greater reduction in fat mass (2.1 kg) in men and women with T2D. Glycemic control and insulin concentrations improved in all groups with no difference between groups; however, the change in insulin concentration was related to the extent of fat mass loss, suggesting that a higher protein diet may exert a more favorable effect on glycemic control than a standard protein diet (70). Promotion of "high quality" weight loss may be particularly important in older adults who are already losing muscle mass (16, 66). By inducing energy restriction while increasing or maintaining the consumption of protein at 1.6 g/kg/day or 30% of energy intake, the amount of lean mass that is lost is reduced (71, 72). The sparing of lean muscle mass is an important aspect to consider as skeletal muscle mass is an extremely metabolically active tissue and the loss of lean tissue mass may be in part responsible for the plateau in weight loss or weight regain following weight loss programs (73, 74).

In addition to inducing "high-quality" weight loss, energy restricted, higher protein diets have also been found to induce greater weight loss than traditional low-fat, standard energy restricted diets (75), likely at least in part, due to the effects of protein consumption on satiety. Satiety or the perceived feeling of fullness after a meal has been shown to be significantly higher following high protein meals (47). Post-prandially there are reductions in perceived hunger and increases in perceived fullness after consuming a high protein meal compared to a standard protein meal (47). When dietary protein intake is increased from 15 to 30% of energy intake and carbohydrate remains constant there is a decrease in *ad libitum* caloric intake due to increased leptin sensitivity (76). Mechanistically this is due to the effect of protein consumption on the gut hormone response. Specifically, after the consumption of a high protein meal there are reductions in the hunger stimulating hormone ghrelin as well as increases in the satiety-stimulating hormones PYY and GLP-1 (47, 77). The impact of protein consumption on satiety is significant as higher protein diets may help regulate appetite control, satiety and prevent increased caloric intake and overeating, which can help facilitate weight loss and/or weight maintenance.

Higher protein diets also assert beneficial effects on IS and glycemic control independent of weight loss. A study by Gannon and Nuttall (78) found that in diabetic men after 5 weeks on a high protein, low carbohydrate diet there was a decrease in fasting blood glucose levels and glycohemoglobin content with no significant changes in body weight. Another study from the same research group confirmed these findings by showing that a high protein, low carbohydrate diet lowered the postprandial glucose response and improved overall glucose control in diabetic men and women despite no changes in body weight compared to a more traditional high carbohydrate diet (79). Together these studies suggest that consuming a higher protein diet is beneficial to improve glycemic control in individuals with T2D during periods of weight maintenance. Considering that weight loss is not always recommended in older adults due to the effects of weight loss on lean body mass (67, 80), these findings are important as they suggest that a higher protein diet may be efficacious to improve glycemic control in older individuals with IR, PD, or T2D without weight loss; however, studies in IR older adults are required.

The Special Case for Dairy-Based Protein Consumption to Improve Muscle Mass and Insulin Sensitivity in Older Adults

The consumption of dairy products has also has been shown to improve IS (81). A study by Choi et al. (82) found that each additional serving per day of dairy was associated with a 9% lower risk of T2D in men. The protective effect of dairy intake was seen regardless of body mass index, physical activity levels, and family history (82). This relationship has been confirmed in women irrespective of age, BMI, physical activity level, and family history, with each additional dairy serving per day associated with a 4% lower risk for T2D (83). Furthermore, an inverse relationship between frequency of dairy intake and insulin resistance syndrome (IRS) in overweight adults was also observed in the CARDIA study (84). IRS was defined as the presence of 2 or more of abnormal glucose homeostasis, obesity, elevated blood pressure, and dyslipidemia, all which increase the risk of developing T2D. In this study the 10-year incidence of IRS was two thirds lower in overweight adults who consumed more than 5 servings/day of dairy products compared to those who consumed <1.5 servings/day (84).

Results from prospective trials examining whether increasing dairy consumption can enhance IS have been promising. A study by Rideout et al. (81) found that consumption of 4 servings/day of low-fat dairy milk and yogurt products reduced fasting plasma insulin by 9% and improved IR by 11% in overweight and obese adults over a 6-month time period. Yogurt may be especially effective at enhancing IS due to its probiotic content. Certain species of probiotics have been found to prevent weight gain, prevent obesity, improve energy metabolism, and enhance insulin sensitivity (85). Several studies have shown that the consumption of probiotic yogurt reduces fasting blood glucose concentration and glycosylated hemoglobin levels in patients with T2D (86) and induces positive changes in lipid profiles and insulin sensitivity (85). This suggests that the composition and/or diversity of the gut microbiota may contribute to the development of T2D and that supplementing with probiotics could be useful in preventing IR (87). A protective effect of probiotic cultures on gut permeability and gut barrier function is one potential mechanism that has been suggested to explain the positive effects of probiotic yogurt on IR (87). Decreases in gut barrier function may be linked to diet-induced changes that lead to the development of IR and T2D in animal models by increased endotoxemia which allows harmful macromolecules and microorganisms through the barrier (88). Taken together, the results from these studies suggest that increasing dairy consumption, particularly yogurt, may help in the prevention and management of T2D.

There are several potential mechanisms by which increased dairy intake can improve IS, thus preventing T2D. The milk proteins, casein and particularly whey, have insulinotropic properties, meaning they enhance the release of insulin, while maintaining a low glycemic response (83, 89). In a study by Pal et al. (90), 12 weeks of whey protein supplementation (54 g/day) decreased fasting plasma insulin levels by 11% and IR by 10% in overweight and obese older adults. Similarly, in T2D men and women, when whey protein was added to the breakfast and lunch meals there was a 31 and 57% increased insulin response after breakfast and lunch, respectively, which resulted in a lower blood glucose response to the lunch meal (91). Mechanistically this may be due to the effect of whey to increase incretin secretion. In particular, whey protein is a potent stimulus for the secretion of glucagon-like peptide (83) and glucose-dependent insulinotropic polypeptide (91), both of which stimulate insulin secretion and inhibits glucagon secretion, inhibiting hepatic glucose production and thereby lowering blood glucose concentrations (92).

Dairy products are also excellent sources of magnesium, calcium, lactose, and dairy protein, which have been shown to increase satiety, which may protect against weight gain and obesity (82–84) and promote greater weight loss during energy restriction (93). Vitamin D is also recognized for its insulin sensitizing effect through regulation of insulin receptor expression and stimulation of insulin release by the beta-cells of the pancreas (94, 95). Together, these data support a role for multiple components of dairy products to work synergistically to enhance IS through different mechanisms, decreasing the risk of developing T2D.

Of particular pertinence to older adults with IR, PD, or T2D, increased dairy consumption has also been found to induce favorable effects on body composition (8). Dairy products contain high levels of calcium, which has been shown to accelerate fat loss, while maintaining lean body mass, by increasing fecal fat excretion (96), decreasing fat absorption (97), increasing fat oxidation (98) and increasing the thermic effect of food (99). Furthermore, dairy products are an excellent source of whey protein and whey protein consumption leads to greater increases in MPS than other proteins due to its rich leucine content (90, 100), suggesting that it may induce favorable effects on lean body mass. Indeed, whey protein has been shown to enhance lean mass in numerous populations including young (101), older adults (102), and PD/T2D (103) as well as preserve muscle anabolism and lean body mass during weight loss (104, 105). These findings suggest that increased dairy consumption may promote "high quality" weight loss, which as detailed above, would be favorable for the prevention and management of T2D in older adults. Indeed, a study by Josse et al. (66) in overweight and obese, premenopausal women found significantly greater fat loss with a gain in lean body mass during a 16-week hypo-energetic diet with 30% of energy intake from dietary protein, with one half of the total protein intake from dairy sources. Higher intakes of dairy protein combined with an aerobic exercise intervention 7 day/week with an additional 2 day/week of resistance training, induced greater total and visceral fat losses and greater lean mass gains compared to those who consumed diets lower in protein lacking dairy foods (66). Furthermore, a recent meta-analysis of 27 randomized controlled trials found that consumption of 2–4 servings/day of dairy foods or 20–84 g/day of whey protein resulted in a greater loss of body weight and fat mass and a smaller loss of lean mass as compared with low dairy control diets (93). Increased dairy consumption may therefore be particularly beneficial for older adults with impaired glucose control like PD and T2D due to the combined effect of dairy on both IS and lean body mass.

EXERCISE, TYPE 2 DIABETES, AND SARCOPENIA

Exercise has long been known for its ability to decrease or attenuate the progression of PD and T2D (19, 106). Exercise induces positive effects on glucose handling in both healthy individuals and those with impaired glucose handling (19, 107–109), such that a single bout of exercise can markedly increase post-exercise glucose control up to 20-fold for up to 72 h, depending on exercise type, intensity and duration (19, 107, 109–112). Although the beneficial effects of exercise are well-known in relation to T2D and all-cause mortality, individuals with T2D are among the least likely population to exercise and the adherence rate of physical activity are exceptionally low (113). Some barriers to exercise in these individuals include poor health, lack of company, lack of interest and lack of time (113). While increasing physical activity and/or exercise is considered a fundamental treatment for the prevention and management of T2D and the benefits of aerobic exercise are well-known (109, 114), we are going to focus on the effects of resistance exercise on IS since it is the most efficacious exercise strategy to improve muscle mass and thus may be the most effective strategy to prevent sarcopenia and T2D.

Protein Enhances the Effects of Resistance Exercise on Muscle Mass and IS

Resistance exercise is the primary mode of exercise to elicit positive changes in muscle mass (115) by significantly increasing the rate of MPS (25), which over time leads to muscle hypertrophy. A recent meta-analysis found that resistance training increases lean body mass by ~1 kg in older adults (116). While this 1 kg increase may appear modest, this increase is in contrast to the ~0.18 kg/year decline in lean body mass that occurs beyond the age of 50 (116). Although the effect of resistance training alone may not be enough to promote a net positive protein balance, when protein is consumed after a bout of resistance exercise rates of MPS can be elevated for up to 24 h (117), which may attenuate the decline in lean body mass in older adults. Indeed, while 24 weeks of resistance training in frail older adults improved muscle strength and functional performance, only the group supplemented with protein also had a significant increase in skeletal muscle mass (118). Therefore, it may be the synergistic approach of repeated bouts of resistance exercise and protein consumption that results in the greatest skeletal muscle hypertrophy (119). Support for this theory comes from a recent meta-analysis that found that protein consumption during resistance training induced a 0.3 kg greater increase in lean body mass in young and older adults (120). Thus, the combination of resistance exercise and protein consumption may be especially beneficial for older adults with IR, PD, or T2D to attenuate declines in lean body mass.

Resistance exercise can also directly improve glycemic control through several mechanisms including, (1) increasing muscle mass, which in turn will increase glucose storage capacity, (2) upregulating insulin signaling proteins, and (3) inducing GLUT 4 translocation to the cell membrane to facilitate glucose clearance from circulation during and immediately after exercise (121). While high protein diets alone induce improvements in body composition and IS in older adults with impaired glucose control (69, 122), the addition of resistance exercise exerts an added benefit on IS and glucose handling. A study by Castaneda et al.

(123) involving 16 weeks of resistance training in older men and women with T2D, found increases in muscle glycogen stores, reduced plasma glycosylated hemoglobin levels and increases in fat free mass. This shows that resistance exercise is also a viable method for producing favorable changes in body composition but also improving the insulin signaling pathway, independent of increases in lean body mass. A subsequent study found that resistance training increases markers of IS and glycemic control that is independent of changes in muscle mass in T2D men and women (124). They found that resistance exercise of no more than 30 min in duration, three times per week increased GLUT4 protein content, insulin receptor content and glycogen synthase content (124). The combination of protein supplementation and resistance exercise also have a synergistic affect in diabetic populations. When a high protein diet and a resistance training program 3 times per week was combined in T2D men and women there was an approximate 2-fold reduction in insulin concentrations compared to control groups (70). However, the synergistic effects of a combined high protein and resistance training warrant future research in diabetic populations as it seems to be the most effective strategy to simultaneously increase lean body mass, decrease total body weight, and improve markers of glucose control independent of weight loss and thus may ultimately have the greatest effect in older adults at risk of developing or with PD/T2D.

CONCLUSIONS

With age there is a loss of muscle mass and the development of IR, increasing the risk of sarcopenia and T2D. When these two conditions coincide, they can create a vicious cycle whereby IR induces greater muscle mass loss, leading to a further reduction in IS and vice versa. Protein has emerged as a potential strategy to combat the decline in muscle mass and IS that occur with increasing age, potentially preventing the development of T2D and sarcopenia. However, protein intake recommendations in older adults are currently insufficient at 0.8 g/kg/day, despite many groups advocating for increased requirements of 1.0–1.2 g/kg/day in older adults and 1.2–1.5 g/kg/day in those who are at risk of malnutrition. While trials in older, IR/PD/T2D populations are lacking, the evidence to date does support a role for higher protein intakes to attenuate declines in muscle mass and IS, particularly when combined with resistance exercise. Further work examining the effectiveness of higher protein intakes, with and without resistance training, in older adults with IR to prevent the development of sarcopenia and T2D are warranted.

AUTHOR CONTRIBUTIONS

MD and KB conceived, wrote, and edited the manuscript.

REFERENCES

1. Centers for Disease Control and Prevention (CDC). Trends in aging–United States and worldwide. *MMWR Morb Mortal Wkly Rep.* (2003) 52:101–4; 106.
2. Afshin A, Forouzanfar MH, Reitsma MB, Sur P, Estep K, Lee A, et al. Health effects of overweight and obesity in 195 countries over 25 years. *N Engl J Med.* (2017) 377:13–27. doi: 10.1056/NEJMoa1614362
3. Leong KS, Wilding JP. Obesity and diabetes. *Best Pract Res Clin Endocrinol Metab.* (1999) 13:221–37. doi: 10.1053/beem.1999.0017
4. Roglic G. WHO global report on diabetes: a summary. *Int J Noncummun Dis.* (2016) 1:3–8. doi: 10.4103/2468-8827.184853
5. Mann S, Beedie C, Balducci S, Zanuso S, Allgrove J, Bertiato F, et al. Changes in insulin sensitivity in response to different modalities of exercise: a review of the evidence. *Diabetes Metab Res Rev.* (2014) 30:257–68. doi: 10.1002/dmrr.2488
6. Public Health Agency of Canada. *Daibetes in Canada: Facts and Figures From a Public Health Perspective.* (2011). Available online at: http://www.phac-aspc.gc.ca/cd-mc/publications/diabetes-diabete/facts-figures-faits-chiffres-2011/chap1-eng.php
7. Paddon-Jones A, Rasmussen B. Dietary protein recommendations and the prevention of sarcopenia. *Curr Opin Clin Nutr Metab Care.* (2009) 12: 86–90. doi: 10.1097/MCO.0b013e32831cef8b
8. Radavelli-Bagatini S, Zhu K, Lewis JR, Dhaliwal SS, Prince RL. Association of dairy intake with body composition and physical function in older community-dwelling women. *J Acad Nutr Diet.* (2013) 113:1669–74. doi: 10.1016/j.jand.2013.05.019
9. Guillet C, Boirie Y. Insulin resistance: a contributing factor to age-related muscle mass loss? *Diabetes Metab.* (2005) 31(Spec No. 2):5s20–6. doi: 10.1016/S1262-3636(05)73648-X
10. Santilli V, Bernetti A, Mangone M, Paoloni M. Clinical definition of sarcopenia. *Clin Cases Miner Bone Metab.* (2014) 11:177–80. doi: 10.11138/ccmbm/2014.11.3.177
11. Beasley JM, Shikany JM, Thomson CA. The role of dietary protein intake in the prevention of sarcopenia of aging. *Nutr Clin Pract.* (2013) 28:684–90. doi: 10.1177/0884533613507607
12. Landi F, Onder G, Bernabei R. Sarcopenia and diabetes: two sides of the same coin. *J Am Med Dir Assoc.* (2013) 14:540–1. doi: 10.1016/j.jamda.2013.05.004
13. Morley JE, Malmstrom TK, Rodriguez-Manas L, Sinclair AJ. Frailty, sarcopenia and diabetes. *J Am Med Dir Assoc.* (2014) 15:853–9. doi: 10.1016/j.jamda.2014.10.001
14. Umegaki H. Sarcopenia and diabetes: Hyperglycemia is a risk factor for age-associated muscle mass and functional reduction. *J Diabetes Investig.* (2015) 6:623–4. doi: 10.1111/jdi.12365
15. Wang T, Feng X, Zhou J, Gong H, Xia S, Wei Q, et al. Type 2 diabetes mellitus is associated with increased risks of sarcopenia and pre-sarcopenia in Chinese elderly. *Sci Rep.* (2016) 6:38937. doi: 10.1038/srep38937
16. Trierweiler H, Kisielewicz G, Hoffmann Jonasson T, Rasmussen Petterle R, Aguiar Moreira C, Zeghbi Cochenski Borba V. Sarcopenia: a chronic complication of type 2 diabetes mellitus. *Diabetol Metab Syndr.* (2018) 10:25. doi: 10.1186/s13098-018-0326-5
17. DeFronzo R, Jacot E, Jequier E, Maeder E, Wahren J, Felber J. The effect of insulin on the disposal of intravenous glucose. Results from indirect calorimetry and hepatic and femoral venous catherterization. *Diabetes.* (1981) 30:1000–7. doi: 10.2337/diab.30.12.1000
18. Scott D, de Courten B, Ebeling PR. Sarcopenia: a potential cause and consequence of type 2 diabetes in Australia's ageing population? *Med J Aust.* (2016) 205:329–33. doi: 10.5694/mja16.00446
19. Riddell MC, Sigal RJ. Physical activity, exercise and diabetes. *Can J Diabetes.* (2013) 37:359–60. doi: 10.1016/j.jcjd.2013.10.001
20. Kortebein P, Ferrando A, Lombeida J, Wolfe R, Evans WJ. Effect of 10 days of bed rest on skeletal muscle in healthy older adults. *JAMA.* (2007) 297:1769–74. doi: 10.1001/jama.297.16.1772-b
21. Paddon-Jones D, Sheffield-Moore M, Urban RJ, Sanford AP, Aarsland A, Wolfe RR, et al. Essential amino acid and carbohydrate supplementation ameliorates muscle protein loss in humans during 28 days bedrest. *J Clin Endocrinol Metab.* (2004) 89:4351–8. doi: 10.1210/jc.2003-032159

22. Paddon-Jones D. Interplay of stress and physical inactivity on muscle loss: nutritional countermeasures. *J Nutr.* (2006) 136:2123–6. doi: 10.1093/jn/136.8.2123
23. Paddon-Jones D, Short KR, Campbell WW, Volpi E, Wolfe RR. Role of dietary protein in the sarcopenia of aging. *Am J Clin Nutr.* (2008) 87:1562S–66S. doi: 10.1093/ajcn/87.5.1562S
24. Wolfe RR. The underappreciated role of muscle in health and disease. *Am J Clin Nutr.* (2006) 84:475–82. doi: 10.1093/ajcn/84.3.475
25. Morton RW, McGlory C, Phillips SM. Nutritional interventions to augment resistance training-induced skeletal muscle hypertrophy. *Front Physiol.* (2015) 6:245. doi: 10.3389/fphys.2015.00245
26. Biolo G, Maggi SP, Williams BD, Tipton KD, Wolfe RR. Increased rates of muscle protein turnover and amino acid transport after resistance exercise in humans. *Am J Physiol.* (1995) 268(3 Pt 1):E514–20. doi: 10.1152/ajpendo.1995.268.3.E514
27. Abdulla H, Smith K, Atherton PJ, Idris I. Role of insulin in the regulation of human skeletal muscle protein synthesis and breakdown: a systematic review and meta-analysis. *Diabetologia.* (2016) 59:44–55. doi: 10.1007/s00125-015-3751-0
28. Phillips SM. Protein requirements and supplementation in strength sports. *Nutrition.* (2004) 20:689–95. doi: 10.1016/j.nut.2004.04.009
29. Murphy CH, Oikawa SY, Phillips SM. Dietary protein to maintain muscle mass in aging: a case for per-meal protein recommendations. *J Frailty Aging.* (2016) 5:49–58. doi: 10.14283/jfa.2016.80
30. Welle S, Thornton C, Jozefowicz R, Statt M. Myofibrillar protein synthesis in young and old men. *Am J Physiol.* (1993) 264(5 Pt 1):E693–8. doi: 10.1152/ajpendo.1993.264.5.E693
31. Yarasheski KE, Zachwieja JJ, Bier DM. Acute effects of resistance exercise on muscle protein synthesis rate in young and elderly men and women. *Am J Physiol.* (1993) 265(2 Pt 1):E210–4. doi: 10.1152/ajpendo.1993.265.2.E210
32. Rooyackers OE, Adey DB, Ades PA, Nair KS. Effect of age on *in vivo* rates of mitochondrial protein synthesis in human skeletal muscle. *Proc Natl Acad Sci USA.* (1996) 93:15364–9. doi: 10.1073/pnas.93.26.15364
33. Trappe T, Williams R, Carrithers J, Raue U, Esmarck B, Kjaer M, et al. Influence of age and resistance exercise on human skeletal muscle proteolysis: a microdialysis approach. *J Physiol.* (2004) 554(Pt 3):803–13. doi: 10.1113/jphysiol.2003.051755
34. Volpi E, Mittendorfer B, Rasmussen BB, Wolfe RR. The response of muscle protein anabolism to combined hyperaminoacidemia and glucose-induced hyperinsulinemia is impaired in the elderly. *J Clin Endocrinol Metab.* (2000) 85:4481–90. doi: 10.1210/jc.85.12.4481
35. Guillet CM, Prod'homme M, Balage M, Gachon P, Giraudet C, Morin L, et al. Impaired anabolic response of muscle protein synthesis is associated with S6K1 dysregulation in elderly humans. *FASEB J.* (2004) 18:1586–7. doi: 10.1096/fj.03-1341fje
36. Cuthbertson D, Smith K, Babraj J, Leese G, Waddell T, Atherton P, et al. Anabolic signaling deficits underlie amino acid resistance of wasting, aging muscle. *FASEB J.* (2005) 19:422–4. doi: 10.1096/fj.04-2640fje
37. Katsanos CS, Kobayashi H, Sheffield-Moore M, Aarsland A, Wolfe RR. Aging is associated with diminished accretion of muscle proteins after the ingestion of a small bolus of essential amino acids. *Am J Clin Nutr.* (2005) 82:1065–73. doi: 10.1093/ajcn/82.5.1065
38. Smith GI, Reeds DN, Hall AM, Chambers K, Finck BN, Mittendorfer B. Sexually dimorphic effect of aging on skeletal muscle protein synthesis. *Biol Sex Differ.* (2012) 3:11. doi: 10.1186/2042-6410-3-11
39. Adeva MM, Calvino J, Souto G, Donapetry C. Insulin resistance and the metabolism of branched-chain amino acids in humans. *Amino Acids.* (2012) 43:171–81. doi: 10.1007/s00726-011-1088-7
40. Park SW, Goodpaster BH, Lee JS, Kuller L, Boudreau R, de Rekeneire N, et al. Excessive loss of skeletal muscle mass in older adults with type 2 diabetes. *Diabetes Care.* (2009) 32:1993–7. doi: 10.2337/dc09-0264
41. Walls HL, Magliano DJ, Stevenson CE, Backholer K, Mannan HR, Shaw JE, et al. Projected progression of the prevalence of obesity in Australia. *Obesity.* (2012) 20:872–8. doi: 10.1038/oby.2010.338
42. Srikanthan P, Karlamangla AS. Relative muscle mass is inversely associated with insulin resistance and prediabetes. Findings from the third National Health and Nutrition Examination Survey. *J Clin Endocrinol Metab.* (2011) 96:2898–903. doi: 10.1210/jc.2011-0435
43. Wolfe RR, Miller SL, Miller KB. Optimal protein intake in the elderly. *Clin Nutr.* (2008) 27:675–84. doi: 10.1016/j.clnu.2008.06.008
44. Campbell AP, Rains TM. Dietary protein is important in the practical management of prediabetes and type 2 diabetes. *J Nutr.* (2015) 145:164–9s. doi: 10.3945/jn.114.194878
45. Bauer J, Biolo G, Cederholm T, Cesari M, Cruz-Jentoft AJ, Morley JE, et al. Evidence-based recommendations for optimal dietary protein intake in older people: a position paper from the PROT-AGE Study Group. *J Am Med Dir Assoc.* (2013) 14:542–59. doi: 10.1016/j.jamda.2013.05.021
46. Deutz NE, Bauer JM, Barazzoni R, Biolo G, Boirie Y, Bosy-Westphal A, et al. Protein intake and exercise for optimal muscle function with aging: recommendations from the ESPEN Expert Group. *Clin Nutr.* (2014) 33:929–36. doi: 10.1016/j.clnu.2014.04.007
47. Paddon-Jones D, Leidy H. Dietary protein and muscle in older persons. *Curr Opin Clin Nutr Metab Care.* (2014) 17:5–11. doi: 10.1097/MCO.0000000000000011
48. Tieland M, Borgonjen-Van den Berg KJ, van Loon LJ, de Groot LC. Dietary protein intake in community-dwelling, frail, and institutionalized elderly people: scope for improvement. *Eur J Nutr.* (2012) 51:173–9. doi: 10.1007/s00394-011-0203-6
49. Evert AB, Boucher JL, Cypress M, Dunbar SA, Franz MJ, Mayer-Davis EJ, et al. Nutrition therapy recommendations for the management of adults with diabetes. *Diabetes Care.* (2013) 36:3821–42. doi: 10.2337/dc13-2042
50. Breen L, Phillips SM. Skeletal muscle protein metabolism in the elderly: Interventions to counteract the 'anabolic resistance' of ageing. *Nutr Metab.* (2011) 8:68. doi: 10.1186/1743-7075-8-68
51. Janney NW. The metabolic relationship of the proteins to glucose. *J Biol Chem.* (1915) 20:132–50.
52. MacLean H. *Modern Methods in the Diagnosis and Treatment of Glycosuria and Diabetes.* London: Constable & Co. Ltd. (1924).
53. Conn JW, Newburgh LH. The glycemic response to isoglucogenic quantities of protein and carbohydrate. *J Clin Invest.* (1936) 15:665–71. doi: 10.1172/JCI100818
54. Nuttall FQ, Mooradian AD, Gannon MC, Billington C, Krezowski P. Effect of protein ingestion on the glucose and insulin response to a standardized oral glucose load. *Diabetes Care.* (1984) 7:465–70. doi: 10.2337/diacare.7.5.465
55. Gannon MC, Nuttall FQ, Lane JT, Burmeister LA. Metabolic response to cottage cheese or egg white protein, with or without glucose, in type II diabetic subjects. *Metab Clin Exp.* (1992) 41:1137–45. doi: 10.1016/0026-0495(92)90300-Y
56. Gannon MC, Nuttall FQ, Grant CT, Ercan-Fang S, Ercan-Fang N. Stimulation of insulin secretion by fructose ingested with protein in people with untreated type 2 diabetes. *Diabetes Care.* (1998) 21:16–22. doi: 10.2337/diacare.21.1.16
57. Devries MC, Sithamparapillai A, Brimble KS, Banfield L, Morton RW, Phillips SM. Changes in kidney function do not differ between healthy adults consuming higher- compared with lower- or normal-protein diets: a systematic review and meta-analysis. *J Nutr.* (2018) 148:1760–75. doi: 10.1093/jn/nxy197
58. Layman DK, Baum JI. Dietary protein impact on glycemic control during weight loss. *J Nutr.* (2004) 134:968s–73s. doi: 10.1093/jn/134.4.968S
59. Tchernof A, Despres JP. Pathophysiology of human visceral obesity: an update. *Physiol Rev.* (2013) 93:359–404. doi: 10.1152/physrev.00033.2011
60. Hamman RF, Wing RR, Edelstein SL, Lachin JM, Bray GA, Delahanty L, et al. Effect of weight loss with lifestyle intervention on risk of diabetes. *Diabetes Care.* (2006) 29:2102–7. doi: 10.2337/dc06-0560
61. Norris SL, Zhang X, Avenell A, Gregg E, Bowman B, Schmid C, et al. Long-term effectiveness of weight-loss interventions in adults with pre-diabetes: a review. *Am J Prev Med.* (2005) 28:126–39. doi: 10.1016/j.amepre.2004.08.006
62. Wing RR, Lang W, Wadden TA, Safford M, Knowler W, Bertoni AG, et al. Benefits of modest weight loss in improving cardiovascular risk factors in overweight and obese individuals with type 2 diabetes. *Diabetes Care.* (2011) 34:1481–6. doi: 10.2337/dc10-2415
63. Franz MJ, Boucher JL, Rutten-Ramos S, VanWormer JJ. Lifestyle weight-loss intervention outcomes in overweight and obese adults with type 2 diabetes: a systematic review and meta-analysis of randomized clinical trials. *J Acad Nutr Diet.* (2015) 115:1447–63. doi: 10.1016/j.jand.2015.02.031

64. Hunter GR, Byrne NM, Sirikul B, Fernandez JR, Zuckerman PA, Darnell BE, et al. Resistance training conserves fat-free mass and resting energy expenditure following weight loss. *Obesity.* (2008) 16:1045–51. doi: 10.1038/oby.2008.38
65. Campbell RK. Type 2 diabetes: where we are today: an overview of disease burden, current treatments, and treatment strategies. *J Am Pharm Assoc.* (2003) 49(Suppl 1):S3–9. doi: 10.1331/JAPhA.2009.09077
66. Josse AR, Atkinson SA, Tarnopolsky MA, Phillips SM. Increased consumption of dairy foods and protein during diet- and exercise-induced weight loss promotes fat mass loss and lean mass gain in overweight and obese premenopausal women. *J Nutr.* (2011) 141:1626–34. doi: 10.3945/jn.111.141028
67. Newman AB, Lee JS, Visser M, Goodpaster BH, Kritchevsky SB, Tylavsky FA, et al. Weight change and the conservation of lean mass in old age: the health, aging and body composition study. *Am J Clin Nutr.* (2005) 82:872–8; quiz 915–6. doi: 10.1093/ajcn/82.4.872
68. Verreijen AM, Verlaan S, Engberink MF, Swinkels SJ, de Vogel-van den Bosch J, Weijs PJ. A high whey protein–, leucine-, and vitamin D–enriched supplement preserves muscle mass during intentional weight loss in obese older adults: a double-blind randomized controlled trial. *Am J Clin Nutr.* (2014) 101:279–86. doi: 10.3945/ajcn.114.090290
69. Piatti PM, Monti F, Fermo I, Baruffaldi L, Nasser R, Santambrogio G, et al. Hypocaloric high-protein diet improves glucose oxidation and spares lean body mass: comparison to hypocaloric high-carbohydrate diet. *Metab Clin Exp.* (1994) 43:1481–7. doi: 10.1016/0026-0495(94)90005-1
70. Wycherley TP, Noakes M, Clifton PM, Cleanthous X, Keogh J, Brinkworth GD. A high-protein diet with resistance exercise training improves weight loss and body composition in overweight and obese patients with type 2 diabetes. *Diabetes Care.* (2010) 33:969–76. doi: 10.2337/dc09-1974
71. Parker B, Noakes M, Luscombe N, Clifton P. Effect of a high-protein, high–monounsaturated fat weight loss diet on glycemic control and lipid levels in type 2 diabetes. *Diabetes Care.* (2002) 25:425–30. doi: 10.2337/diacare.25.3.425
72. Layman DK, Boileau RA, Erickson DJ, Painter J, Shiue H, Sather C, et al. A reduced ratio of dietary carbohydrate to protein improves body composition and blood lipid profiles during weight loss in adult women. *J Nutr.* (2003) 133:411–7. doi: 10.1093/jn/133.2.411
73. Strychar I, Lavoie ME, Messier L, Karelis AD, Doucet E, Prud'homme D, et al. Anthropometric, metabolic, psychosocial, and dietary characteristics of overweight/obese postmenopausal women with a history of weight cycling: a MONET (Montreal Ottawa New Emerging Team) study. *J Am Diet Assoc.* (2009) 109:718–24. doi: 10.1016/j.jada.2008.12.026
74. Hunter GR, Brock DW, Byrne NM, Chandler-Laney P, Del Corral P, Gower BA. Exercise training prevents regain of visceral fat for 1 year following weight loss. *Obesity.* (2010) 18:690–5. doi: 10.1038/oby.2009.316
75. Wycherley TP, Moran LJ, Clifton PM, Noakes M, Brinkworth GD. Effects of energy-restricted high-protein, low-fat compared with standard-protein, low-fat diets: a meta-analysis of randomized controlled trials. *Am J Clin Nutr.* (2012) 96:1281–98. doi: 10.3945/ajcn.112.044321
76. Weigle DS, Breen PA, Matthys CC, Callahan H, Meeuws KE, Burden VR, et al. A high-protein diet induces sustained reductions in appetite, *ad libitum* caloric intake, and body weight despite compensatory changes in diurnal plasma leptin and ghrelin concentrations. *Am J Clin Nutr.* (2005) 82:41–8. doi: 10.1093/ajcn/82.1.41
77. van der Klaauw AA, Keogh JM, Henning E, Trowse VM, Dhillo WS, Ghatei MA, et al. High protein intake stimulates postprandial GLP1 and PYY release. *Obesity.* (2013) 21:1602–7. doi: 10.1002/oby.20154
78. Gannon, MC, Nuttall FQ. "Effect of a high-protein, low-carbohydrate diet on blood glucose control in people with type 2 diabetes." *Diabetes.* (2004) 53:2375–82. doi: 10.2337/diabetes.53.9.2375
79. Gannon MC, Nuttall FQ, Saeed A, Jordan K, Hoover H. An increase in dietary protein improves the blood glucose response in persons with type 2 diabetes. *Am J Clin Nutr.* (2003) 78:734–41. doi: 10.1093/ajcn/78.4.734
80. Frimel TN, Sinacore DR, Villareal DT. Exercise attenuates the weight-loss-induced reduction in muscle mass in frail obese older adults. *Med Sci Sports Exerc.* (2008) 40:1213–9. doi: 10.1249/MSS.0b013e31816a85ce
81. Rideout TC, Marinangeli CPF, Martin H, Browne RW, Rempel CB. Consumption of low-fat dairy foods for 6 months improves insulin resistance without adversely affecting lipids or bodyweight in healthy adults: a randomized free-living cross-over study. *Nutr J.* (2013) 12:56. doi: 10.1186/1475-2891-12-56
82. Choi HK, Willett WC, Stampfer MJ, Rimm E, Hu B. Dairy consumption and risk of type 2 diabetes mellitus in men - a prospective study. *Arch Intern Med.* (2005) 165:997–1003. doi: 10.1001/archinte.165.9.997
83. Liu S, Choi HK, Ford E, Song Y, Klevak A, Buring JE, et al. A prospective study of dairy intake and the risk of type 2 diabetes in women. *Diabetes Care.* (2006) 29:1579–84. doi: 10.2337/dc06-0256
84. Pereira MA, Jacobs DR, Van Horn L, Slattery ML, Kartashov AI, Ludwig DS. Dairy consumption, obesity, and the insulin resistance syndrome in young adults - The CARDIA study. *J Am Med Assoc.* (2002) 287:2081–9. doi: 10.1001/jama.287.16.2081
85. Madjd A, Taylor MA, Mousavi N, Delavari A, Malekzadeh R, Macdonald IA, et al. Comparison of the effect of daily consumption of probiotic compared with low-fat conventional yogurt on weight loss in healthy obese women following an energy-restricted diet: a randomized controlled trial. *Am J Clin Nutr.* (2016) 103:323–9. doi: 10.3945/ajcn.115.120170
86. Ejtahed HS, Mohtadi-Nia J, Homayouni-Rad A, Niafar M, Asghari-Jafarabadi M, Mofid V. Probiotic yogurt improves antioxidant status in type 2 diabetic patients. *Nutrition.* (2012) 28:539–43. doi: 10.1016/j.nut.2011.08.013
87. Hulston CJ, Churnside AA, Venables MC. Probiotic supplementation prevents high-fat, overfeeding-induced insulin resistance in human subjects. *Br J Nutr.* (2015) 113:596–602. doi: 10.1017/S0007114514004097
88. Serino M, Luche E, Gres S, Baylac A, Berge M, Cenac C, et al. Metabolic adaptation to a high-fat diet is associated with a change in the gut microbiota. *Gut.* (2012) 61:543–53. doi: 10.1136/gutjnl-2011-301012
89. Liljeberg Elmstahl H, Bjorck I. Milk as a supplement to mixed meals may elevate postprandial insulinaemia. *Eur J Clin Nutr.* (2001) 55:994–9. doi: 10.1038/sj.ejcn.1601259
90. Pal S, Ellis V, Dhaliwal S. Effects of whey protein isolate on body composition, lipids, insulin and glucose in overweight and obese individuals. *Br J Nutr.* (2010) 104:716–23. doi: 10.1017/S0007114510000991
91. Frid AH, Nilsson M, Holst JJ, Bjorck IM. Effect of whey on blood glucose and insulin responses to composite breakfast and lunch meals in type 2 diabetic subjects. *Am J Clin Nutr.* (2005) 82:69–75. doi: 10.1093/ajcn/82.1.69
92. Cho YM, Fujita Y, Kieffer TJ. Glucagon-like peptide-1: glucose homeostasis and beyond. *Annu Rev Physiol.* (2014) 76: 535–59. doi: 10.1146/annurev-physiol-021113-170315
93. Stonehouse W, Wycherley T, Luscombe-Marsh N, Taylor P, Brinkworth G, Riley M. Dairy intake enhances body weight and composition changes during energy restriction in 18-50-year-old adults-a meta-analysis of randomized controlled trials. *Nutrients.* (2016) 8:E394. doi: 10.3390/nu8070394
94. Maestro B, Campion J, Davila N, Calle C. Stimulation by 1,25-dihydroxyvitamin D3 of insulin receptor expression and insulin responsiveness for glucose transport in U-937 human promonocytic cells. *Endocr J.* (2000) 47:383–91. doi: 10.1507/endocrj.47.383
95. Borissova AM, Tankova T, Kirilov G, Dakovska L, Kovacheva R. The effect of vitamin D3 on insulin secretion and peripheral insulin sensitivity in type 2 diabetic patients. *Int J Clin Pract.* (2003) 57:258–61.
96. Jacobsen R, Lorenzen JK, Toubro S, Krog-Mikkelsen I, Astrup A. Effect of short-term high dietary calcium intake on 24-h energy expenditure, fat oxidation, and fecal fat excretion. *Int J Obes.* (2005) 29:292–301. doi: 10.1038/sj.ijo.0802785
97. Lorenzen JK, Nielsen S, Holst JJ, Tetens I, Rehfeld J, Astrup A. Effect of dairy calcium or supplementary calcium intake on postprandial fat metabolism, appetite, and subsequent energy intake. *Am J Clin Nutr.* (2007) 85:678–87. doi: 10.1093/ajcn/85.3.678
98. Melanson EL, Donahoo WT, Dong F, Ida T, Zemel MB. Effect of low- and high-calcium dairy-based diets on macronutrient oxidation in humans. *Obes Res.* (2005) 13:2102–12. doi: 10.1038/oby.2005.261
99. Shi H, Dirienzo D, Zemel MB. Effects of dietary calcium on adipocyte lipid metabolism and body weight regulation in energy-restricted aP2-agouti transgenic mice. *FASEB J.* (2001) 15:291–3. doi: 10.1096/fj.00-0584fje

100. Layman DK, Walker DA. Potential importance of leucine in treatment of obesity and the metabolic syndrome. *J Nutr.* (2006) 136(1 Suppl):319s–23s. doi: 10.1093/jn/136.1.319S

101. Volek JS, Volk BM, Gomez AL, Kunces L, Kupchak BR, Freidenreich DJ, et al. Whey protein supplementation during resistance training augments lean body mass. *J Am Coll Nutr.* (2013) 32:122–35. doi: 10.1080/07315724.2013.793580

102. Bauer JM, Verlaan S, Bautmans I, Brandt K, Donini LM, Maggio M, et al. Effects of a vitamin D and leucine-enriched whey protein nutritional supplement on measures of sarcopenia in older adults, the PROVIDE study: a randomized, double-blind, placebo-controlled trial. *J Am Med Dir Assoc.* (2015) 16:740–7. doi: 10.1016/j.jamda.2015.05.021

103. Flaim C, Kob M, Di Pierro AM, Herrmann M, Lucchin L. Effects of a whey protein supplementation on oxidative stress, body composition and glucose metabolism among overweight people affected by diabetes mellitus or impaired fasting glucose: a pilot study. *J Nutr Biochem.* (2017) 50:95–102. doi: 10.1016/j.jnutbio.2017.05.003

104. Frestedt JL, Zenk JL, Kuskowski MA, Ward LS, Bastian ED. A whey-protein supplement increases fat loss and spares lean muscle in obese subjects: a randomized human clinical study. *Nutr Metab.* (2008) 5:8. doi: 10.1186/1743-7075-5-8

105. Hector AJ, Marcotte GR, Churchward-Venne TA, Murphy CH, Breen L, von Allmen M, et al. Whey protein supplementation preserves postprandial myofibrillar protein synthesis during short-term energy restriction in overweight and obese adults. *J Nutr.* (2015) 145:246–52. doi: 10.3945/jn.114.200832

106. Holloszy JO. Exercise-induced increase in muscle insulin sensitivity. *J Appl Physiol.* (1985) 99:338–43. doi: 10.1152/japplphysiol.00123.2005

107. American Diabetes Association. Physical activity/exercise and diabetes. *Diabetes Care.* (2004) 27:S58–62. doi: 10.2337/diacare.27.2007.S58

108. Sigal RJ, Kenny GP, Wasserman DH, Castaneda-Sceppa C. Physical activity/exercise and type 2 diabetes. *Diabetes Care.* (2004) 27:2518–39. doi: 10.2337/diacare.27.10.2518

109. Sigal RJ, Kenny GP, Boule NG, Wells G, Prud'homme D, Fortier M, et al. Effects of aerobic training, resistance training, or both on glycemic control in type 2 diabetes - a randomized trial. *Ann Intern Med.* (2007) 147:357–69. doi: 10.7326/0003-4819-147-6-200709180-00005

110. Holloszy JO, Schultz J, Kusnierkiewicz J, Hagberg JM, Ehsani, A. Effects of exercise on glucose-tolerance and insulin resistance - brief review and some preliminary-results. *Acta Med Scand.* (1986) 711:55–65. doi: 10.1111/j.0954-6820.1986.tb08932.x

111. Goodyear LJ, Kahn BB. Exercise, glucose transport, and insulin sensitivity. *Annu Rev Med.* (1998) 49:235–61. doi: 10.1146/annurev.med.49.1.235

112. Richter EA, Derave W, Wojtaszewski JF. Glucose, exercise and insulin: emerging concepts. *J Physiol.* (2001) 535(Pt 2):313–22. doi: 10.1111/j.1469-7793.2001.t01-2-00313.x

113. Qiu SH, Sun ZL, Cai X, Liu L, Yang B. Improving patients' adherence to physical activity in diabetes mellitus: a review. *Diabetes Metab J.* (2012) 36:1–5. doi: 10.4093/dmj.2012.36.1.1

114. Yang Z, Scott CA, Mao C, Tang J, Farmer A. Resistance exercise versus aerobic exercise for type 2 diabetes: a systematic review and meta-analysis. *Sports Med.* (2014) 44:487–99. doi: 10.1007/s40279-013-0128-8

115. Schoenfeld BJ, Peterson MD, Ogborn D, Contreras B, Sonmez G. Effects of low- vs. high-load resistance training on muscle strength and hypertrophy in well-trained men. *J Strength Cond Res.* (2015) 29:2954–63. doi: 10.1519/JSC.0000000000000958

116. Peterson MD, Sen A, Gordon PM. Influence of resistance exercise on lean body mass in aging adults: a meta-analysis. *Med Sci Sports Exerc.* (2011) 43:249–58. doi: 10.1249/MSS.0b013e3181eb6265

117. Burd NA, West DW, Moore DR, Atherton P, Staples AW, Prior T, et al. Enhanced amino acid sensitivity of myofibrillar protein synthesis persists for up to 24 h after resistance exercise in young men. *J Nutr.* (2011) 141:568–73. doi: 10.3945/jn.110.135038

118. Tieland M, Dirks ML, van der Zwaluw N, Verdijk LB, van de Rest O, de Groot LC, et al. Protein supplementation increases muscle mass gain during prolonged resistance-type exercise training in frail elderly people: a randomized, double-blind, placebo-controlled trial. *J Am Med Dir Assoc.* (2012) 13:713–9. doi: 10.1016/j.jamda.2012.05.020

119. Cermak NM, Res PT, de Groot LC, Saris W, van Loon LJ. Protein supplementation augments the adaptive response of skeletal muscle to resistance-type exercise training: a meta-analysis. *Am J Clin Nutr.* (2012) 96:1454–64. doi: 10.3945/ajcn.112.037556

120. Morton RW, Murphy KT, McKellar SR, Schoenfeld B, Henselmans M, Helms E, et al. A systematic review, meta-analysis and meta-regression of the effect of protein supplementation on resistance training-induced gains in muscle mass and strength in healthy adults. *Br J Sports Med.* (2018) 52:376–84. doi: 10.1136/bjsports-2017-097608

121. Cuff DJ, Meneilly GS, Martin A, Ignaszewski A, Tildesley H, Frohlich JJ. Effective exercise modality to reduce insulin resistance in women with type 2 diabetes. *Diabetes Care.* (2003) 26:2977–82. doi: 10.2337/diacare.26.11.2977

122. Gannon MC, Nuttall FQ. Effect of a high-protein, low-carbohydrate diet on blood glucose control in people with type 2 diabetes. *Diabetes.* (2004) 53:2375–82. doi: 10.2337/diabetes.53.9.2375

123. Castaneda C, Layne JE, Munoz-Orians L, Gordon PL, Walsmith J, Foldvari M, et al. A randomized controlled trial of resistance exercise training to improve glycemic control in older adults with type 2 diabetes. *Diabetes Care.* (2002) 25:2335–41. doi: 10.2337/diacare.25.12.2335

124. Holten MK, Zacho M, Gaster M, Juel C, Wojtaszewski JF, Dela F. Strength training increases insulin-mediated glucose uptake, GLUT4 content, and insulin signaling in skeletal muscle in patients with type 2 diabetes. *Diabetes.* (2004) 53:294–305. doi: 10.2337/diabetes.53.2.294

9

Voluntary Resistance Running as a Model to Induce mTOR Activation in Mouse Skeletal Muscle

Gommaar D'Hulst[1], Andrew S. Palmer[2], Evi Masschelein[1], Ori Bar-Nur[2] and Katrien De Bock[1]*

[1] Laboratory of Exercise and Health, Department of Health Sciences and Technology, Swiss Federal Institute of Technology (ETH) Zurich, Zurich, Switzerland, [2] Laboratory of Regenerative and Movement Biology, Department of Health Sciences and Technology, Swiss Federal Institute of Technology (ETH) Zurich, Zurich, Switzerland

***Correspondence:**
Katrien De Bock
katrien-debock@ethz.ch

Long-term voluntary resistance running has been shown to be a valid model to induce muscle growth in rodents. Moreover, the mammalian target of rapamycin complex 1 (mTORC1) is a key signaling complex regulating exercise/nutrient-induced alterations in muscle protein synthesis. How acute resistance running affects mTORC1 signaling in muscle and if resistance applied to the wheel can modulate mTORC1 activation has not yet been fully elucidated. Here, we show that both acute resistance running and acute free running activated mTORC1 signaling in the *m. gastrocnemius, m. soleus, and m. plantaris*, but not in *m. tibialis anterior* of mice when compared to sedentary controls. Furthermore, only the low threshold oxidative part in the m. gastrocnemius showed increased mTORC1 signaling upon running and acute heavy-load resistance running evoked higher downstream mTORC1 signaling in both m. soleus and m. plantaris than free running without resistance, pointing toward mechanical load as an important independent regulator of mTORC1. Collectively, in this study, we show that voluntary resistance running is an easy-to-use, time-efficient and low stress model to study acute alterations in mTORC1 signaling upon high-load muscular contractions in mice.

Keywords: mTORC1, signaling, resistance running, load, acute

INTRODUCTION

Maintaining skeletal muscle mass throughout life is critical as loss of muscle mass is associated with increased mortality (Szulc et al., 2010), higher disability, loss of function (Janssen et al., 2002), and increased risk of falls (Szulc et al., 2004). Resistance exercise increases muscle mass (Bhasin et al., 1996; Abe et al., 2003; Verdijk et al., 2009) and improves strength outcomes (Pyka et al., 1994; Staron et al., 1994), but the mechanisms by which high load contractions regulate skeletal muscle fiber size are incompletely understood. In an attempt to elucidate these mechanisms, many resistance-based exercise models in mice have been developed (Cholewa et al., 2014), such as synergistic ablation (Goldberg, 1968), electrical stimulation (Baar and Esser, 1999), and chronic stretch (Goldspink, 1999). Although all valuable, they are invasive, cumbersome, and often do not mimic real life scenarios. Remarkably, many mouse strains voluntarily run large distances when given access to a running wheel (De Bono et al., 2005). Moreover, external resistance can be added to the wheel to increase muscle force production (Soffe et al., 2016). Therefore, as mouse handling and stress is minimal, the running wheel is considered an excellent model of physiological training with similar muscular adaptations as other well-accepted models such as synergistic ablation and electrical stimulation. Indeed, many groups have shown that voluntary resistance running leads to muscular hypertrophy in rodents (Legerlotz et al., 2008; Call et al., 2010; White et al., 2016; Mobley et al., 2018).

mTOR is a protein complex, which acts as a conductor in cell growth (Wolfson and Sabatini, 2017). In particular, mTOR complex 1 (mTORC1) integrates nutrient, growth, and stress signals to promote protein synthesis (Goodman et al., 2011; Huang and Fingar, 2014). Activation of mTOR is known to increase ribosomal biogenesis and protein translation (Mahajan, 1994; Thoreen et al., 2012; Figueiredo et al., 2015), two processes, which play a central role in the adaptation to resistance training or chronic overload (Bodine et al., 2001; Drummond et al., 2009; Ogasawara and Suginohara, 2018). Both a single bout or repeated bouts of resistance exercise can increase mTOR signaling in muscle (Baar and Esser, 1999; Kubica et al., 2005; Burd et al., 2010; Dreyer et al., 2010) and an enhancement in mTOR activation after resistance exercise is related to increased muscle mass (Baar and Esser, 1999). To confirm the role of mTOR on muscle hypertrophy, blocking mTOR signaling with compounds such as rapamycin or AZD8055 has been demonstrated to reduce protein synthesis and muscle growth (Bodine et al., 2001; Drummond et al., 2009; Ogasawara and Suginohara, 2018), underscoring the indispensable role of mTORC1 in muscular adaptations to resistance type exercise. Data on voluntary resistance running and mTOR activation are sparse, but one study showed no increase in mTOR activation after 8 months of resistance running in the m. quadriceps, despite hypertrophy in most of the hindlimb muscles, including the m. quadriceps (White et al., 2016). Interpretation of this data might be difficult since the mice were aged, samples were harvested several hours after exercise, no standardization of food intake before sample harvesting occurred, and - consistent with human data (Brook et al., 2015) - resistance training could have resulted in an attenuated activation of mTORC1 in response to resistance training. Additionally, other hindlimb muscles were not examined for downstream mTORC1 signaling (White et al., 2016). Thus, to date, the mechanisms behind resistance running-induced muscle hypertrophy are unclear.

Therefore, the aim of this study was to explore whether voluntary resistance running can be used as a non-invasive stress-free model to study and acutely modulate mTORC1 signaling *in vivo*.

MATERIALS AND METHODS

Animals

All experiments were performed on male C57BL/6 J mice. All mice used for the experiments were housed in individually ventilated cages (3–4 littermates per cage) at standard housing conditions (22°C, 12 h light/dark cycle, dark phase starting at 7 pm), with ad libitum access to chow (KlibaNafag, diet #3436 and diet #3437) and water. Health status of all mouse lines was regularly monitored according to FELASA guidelines.

Experimental Procedures

All animal procedures were approved by the Veterinary office of the Canton of Zürich (license nr. ZH254-16). During the intervention, mice were individually housed in open cages equipped with a running wheel device (TSE Systems). The running wheel device continuously records wheel movements out of which total distance (km), speed (m.s^{-1}), number of running bouts, and resistance on the wheel (N) can be extracted. Additionally, to increase the force needed to rotate the wheel, resistance (0–100%) can be added. To calculate total work, we used $W = Pt$, where W is work, P is power, and t is time. To calculate the power of the wheel at each braking resistance, we used the equation $P = 2\pi \times f \times M$, where f is the angular frequency of the wheel, and M is the torque at a given braking resistance. TSE Systems provided a torque braking resistance curve for which a braking resistance of 60% has a constant torque of 0.0125 N.m.

Experiment 1

An overview of the experimental procedures can be found in **Figure 1**. About 14 to 16-week-old male C57BL/6 J mice were randomly assigned to either the voluntary resistance-running group (VResRun) or sedentary (Sed) control group. VResRun mice were familiarized to the resistance running protocol for 1 week. During familiarization, VResRun mice had access to the wheel; with 0% braking resistance on the first night, with 20% braking resistance on the fourth night, and with 40% braking resistance on the seventh night. On the second, third, fifth, and sixth night, the running wheels were blocked. After the seventh night, mice remained in the resistance wheel cages without access to the running wheel for four nights to mitigate any potential

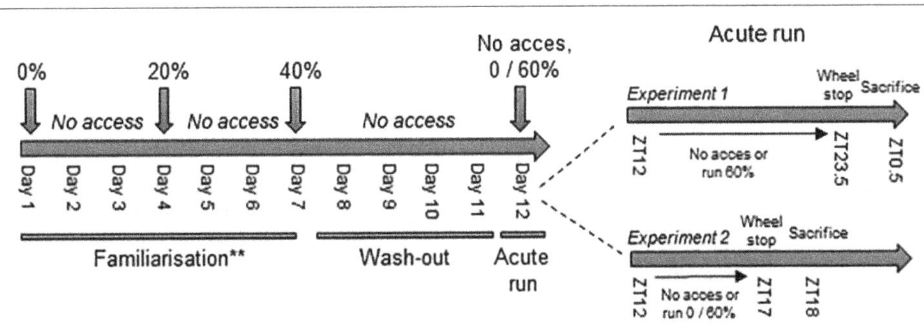

FIGURE 1 | Experimental set-up. ** In experiment 1, only the VResRun group was familiarized to the wheel. The Sed remained sedentary during the whole experiment. In experiment 2, all groups were familiarized to the wheel, including the Sed.

training effects. On the twelfth and final day of the intervention, mice had access to the running wheel at 60% braking resistance for the 12-h dark cycle (ZT12-ZT23.5). Sedentary mice did not undergo familiarization and were housed in a resistance running wheel cage with the wheel blocked. At ZT23.5, running wheels were blocked, mice were removed from running cages and fasted for 1 h. Muscle samples were collected 1 h after cessation of running, since at this time point, eccentric contraction induced activation of mTORC1 is maximal (O'Neil et al., 2009).

Experiment 2

Around 10–16-week-old male C57BL/6 mice were randomly allocated either to a Sed, voluntary run (VRun) or VResRun group. This time, Sed, VRun, and VResRun groups were all familiarized following the aforementioned familiarization protocol (**Figure 1**). Access to the running wheels was blocked for four nights. On the final night, VResRun mice ran at 60% braking resistance, Run mice ran at 0% braking resistance from ZT12 to ZT17 and Sed did not run (wheel blocked). Mice were removed from running cages at ZT17 am and fasted for 1 h prior to sample collection.

Sample Collection

Mice were fasted for 1 h at ZT23.5 (experiment 1) and ZT17 (experiment 2) and anesthetized using Ketamine/Xylazine 10 $\mu g.g^{-1}$ and acepromazine (2–5 $mg.kg^{-1}$) body weight *via* intraperitoneal injection. The depth of anesthesia was confirmed by testing pedal withdrawal reflex before tissue collection. Subsequently, the *m. gastrocnemius (GAS)*, *m. tibialis anterior (TA)*, *m. soleus (SOL)*, *m. plantaris (PLT)* and *m. triceps (TRI)* were dissected and snap frozen. One GAS was frozen in OCT embedding matrix (CellPath) in 2-Methylbutane (sigma Aldrich) on liquid nitrogen for histochemical analysis. After sample collection, animals were euthanized and major bleeding was induced to confirm death.

Protein Extraction and Western Blot

Sample Preparation

Between 10 and 25 mg of muscle sample was homogenized in ice cold lysis buffer (1:10, w/v) (50 mM Tris-HCl pH 7.0, 270 mM sucrose, 5 mM EGTA, 1 mM EDTA, 1 mM sodium orthovanadate, 50 mM glycerophosphate, 5 mM sodium pyrophosphate, 50 mM sodium fluoride, 1 mM DTT, 0.1% Triton-X 100 and 10% protease inhibitor) (20 µl per 1.8–2.5 of tissue sample) using an OMNI-THq Tissue homogenizer (OMNI International) for 20 s until a consistent homogenate was formed. Samples were centrifuged at 4°C at 10,000 g for 10 min and the supernatant with proteins collected. Protein concentration was determined using the DC assay protein method (Biorad Laboratories) to equalize the amount of protein.

Protein Transfer

Samples were prepared 3:4 with laemmli buffer containing 10% 2-mercaptoethanol (Bio-rad laboratories) and heated at 95° for 5 min. Proteins were run on a 4–20% Mini-PROTEAN TGX Stain Free Pre-Cast Gel (Biorad Laboratories) for 45 min at 120–140 V and subsequently transferred onto immuno-Blot PVDF Membranes (Biorad Laboratories) at 90 V for 100 min. Membranes were cut according to desired proteins, blocked for 1 h at room temperature in 5% milk in TBS-T, TBS (1:10, w/v) (24.23 g Trizma HCl, 80.06 g NaCl in 800 ml ultra-pure water pH 7.6, topped up to 1 L) with 1 ml of Tween, and incubated overnight with the following primary antibodies 1:1,000 (Cell Signaling); $pS6K1^{Thr389}$ (#9206), $pS6K1^{Thr421/Ser424}$ (#9204), $pRPS6^{Ser235/236}$ (#2211), $pSMAD2^{Ser245/250/255}$ (#3104), p4E-BP1Ser^{65} (#9451), and pSAPK/$JNK^{Thr183/Tyr185}$ (#9251). The membranes were washed for 10 min three times in TBS-T and subsequently incubated in secondary antibody 1:5,000 in TBS-T with 5% milk (Anti-rabbit IgG, HRP-linked Antibody #7074, Cell Signaling) for 1 h at room temperature. Proteins were washed for 10 min three times in TBS-T and incubated for 30 s in 1:1 Luminol/Enhancer solution and peroxide solution. Membranes were imaged with a Biorad Chemidoc Touch Imaging System (Biorad Laboratories).

Image Analysis

Images were quantified using Image Lab software (Biorad Laboratories) using the volume tools function with each band and lane quantified with the same volume or area. Total membrane protein or total gel loading was used as a loading control (Rivero-Gutiérrez et al., 2014) and a positive control sample was loaded to compare across gels. All quantified volumes were divided by the positive control and normalized to the control group.

Immunohistochemistry

Sample Preparation

P-RPS6

About 10 µm sections of muscle embedded in OCT were made using a cryostat (Leica CM 1950) and collected on Superfrost Ultra Plus slides (Thermo Scientific). Muscle samples were fixed with −20°C acetone for 10 min and subsequently incubated in PBS for 15 min. Slides were blocked for 1 h at room temperature in solution A (PBS with 5% normal goat serum and 0.3% CHAPS) and then incubated overnight at 4°C in solution B (PBS with 0.5% BSA and 0.3% CHAPS) containing primary antibody p-$RPS6^{Ser235/236}$ rabbit conjugated (1:200, cell signaling). The next day samples were washed three times with PBS and then incubated for 1 h at room temperature in solution A containing secondary antibodies Goat-anti rabbit IgG Alexa Fluor 488 (1:250, Invitrogen). Slides were once again washed two times for 5 min in PBS and then washed for 10 min with PBS containing WGA alexa fluor 647 (1:400, Invitrogen). Slides were mounted with immuno-mount (Thermo Scientific) and a glass coverslip and allowed to dry. A sample that followed the above procedure but was not incubated with primary antibodies was used as a negative control. Images were taken using an epifluorescence microscope (Zeiss Axio observer Z.1) at 20× using Zen Pro software. An image of a sedentary sample was used to define imaging settings and applied to all subsequent images.

Fiber Typing

About 10 µm sections were dried and washed for 5 min in PBS supplemented with 0.05% triton (PBST) and subsequently blocked for 60 min in PBST +10% goat serum (ThermoFisher

Scientific, 16200-064). Afterward, a primary antibody cocktail was applied for 120 min for myosin heavy chain I (1/50), IIa (1:200) (Developmental studies hybridoma bank) diluted in PBST +10% goat serum. After washing three times for 5 min, a secondary antibody cocktail, diluted in PBST +10% goat serum, was applied for goat anti-mouse Alexa Fluor 488, 350 and wheat germ agglutinin Alexa fluor 647 (1:250) for 60 min. Slides were mounted after a 3 × 5 min wash, sealed with glass cover slips and imaged with a epifluorescent microscope (Zeiss Axio observer Z.1) at 10×.

Statistical and Data Analyses

Results are presented as mean with standard error of the mean (SEM) bars and individual data points. An unpaired two-tailed Student's *t*-test was used for generating a p in experiment 1 when comparing two groups. Data in experiment 2 were subjected to a one-way analysis of variance (ANOVA) to generate a p value and *post hoc* tests were performed using Tukey's *post hoc* test using Graphpad Prism to compare between groups. Significance was set at $p < 0.05$.

RESULTS

Acute Resistance Running Activates the mTOR Signaling Pathway in Mouse Skeletal Muscle

To determine if resistance exercise activates mTOR signaling within skeletal muscle, we measured the phosphorylation of downstream mTORC1 target kinases 1 h after cessation of one night of resistance running. In mice, phosphorylation levels of pS6K1^{Thr389}, pS6K1$^{Thr421/Ser424}$, pRPS6$^{ser235/236}$, and p4EBP1^{ser65} were highly increased in SOL of VResRun compared to SED mice (**Figures 2A,C**). Furthermore, VResRun also lead to a strong increase pS6K1^{Thr389} in PLT and GAS (**Figure 2B**). Interestingly, there were no significant differences in phosphorylation of any mTOR targets in the TA muscle (**Figure 2B**) or TRI (data not shown). This data shows that VResRun activates downstream mTORC1 signaling.

The running activity over the night followed the pattern seen in **Figure 3**. Mice ran consistently and constantly between ZT12 and ZT18, after which they rested before recommencing running after ZT22. Interestingly, some mice did not restart at ZT22 for unknown reasons, a feature that could potentially induce variability in the signaling data. We therefore decided to further standardize the protocol by blocking the wheel at ZT17 and excise the muscles at ZT18 in experiment 2.

Acute Resistance Running Activates Mammalian Target of Rapamycin Complex 1 More Than Non-resistance Running

For the second experiment, we used the optimized protocol, and included an additional condition where no resistance was applied on the wheel (VRun). This would allow us to assess whether the observed increase in mTORC1 activity was caused by the increase in resistance applied on the wheel, rather than by running itself. Parameters from the free running and the resistance running bout are presented in **Table 1**. VResRun had to overcome 24 times more force per rotation of the wheel than the VRun, leading to 29 times more total work over the course

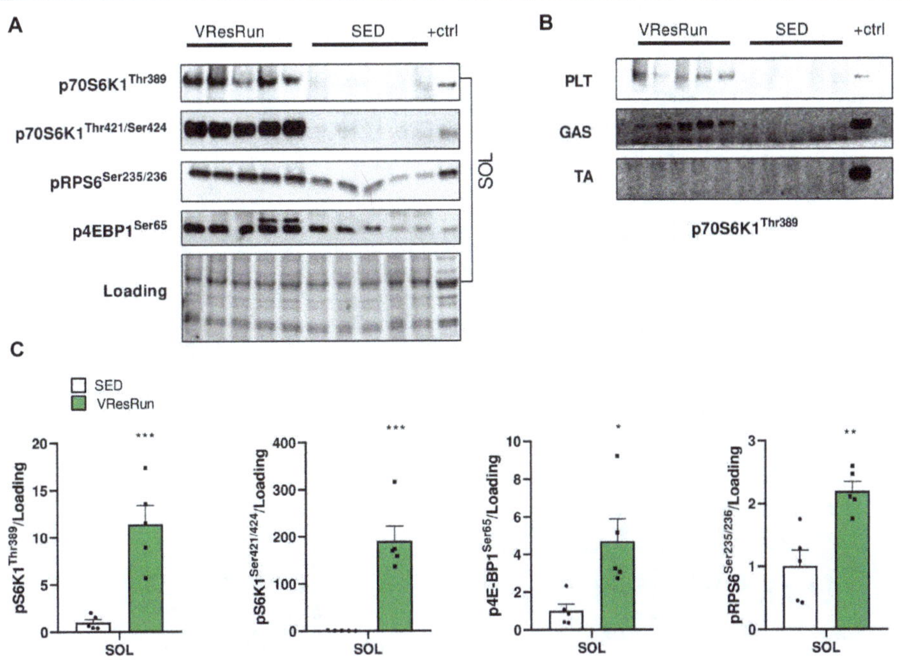

FIGURE 2 | The effect of one night of voluntary resistance running (VResRun, $n = 5$) on mTORC1 downstream signaling. **(A)** Representative blots of pS6K1^{Thr389}, pS6K1$^{Thr421/Ser424}$, pRPS6$^{Ser256/236}$, p4EBP1^{Ser65} in SOL. **(B)** Representative blots of pS6K1^{Thr389} in PLT, GAS, and TA. **(C)** Quantifications. (Sed; $n = 5$). $^{*}p < 0.05$ vs. SED, $^{**}p < 0.01$ vs. SED, $^{***}p < 0.001$ vs. SED.

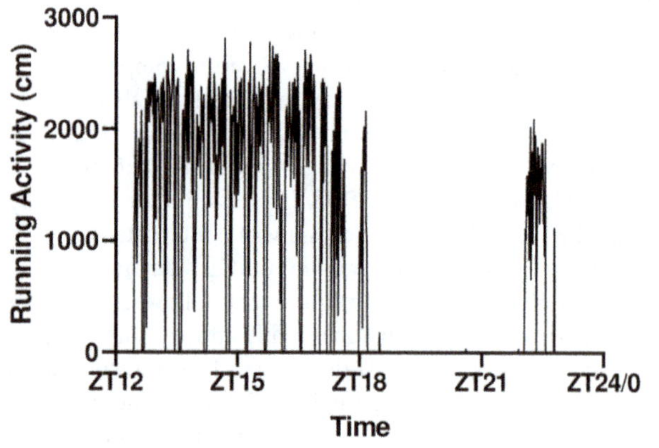

FIGURE 3 | Representative running pattern of a mouse during the active phase.

TABLE 1 | Running summary VRun vs. VResRun.

	VRun	VResRun
Distance (km)	3.46 ± 0.95	4.00 ± 0.40
Time (min)	129 ± 31	151 ± 12
Sum of all runs	1,014 ± 272	876 ± 278
Speed (m.s^{-1})	0.44 ± 0.05	0.44 ± 0.02
Work (J)	30 ± 8	867 ± 88***
Force (N)	0.009	0.22***

****Indicates p < 0.001 vs. VRun. VRun, n = 6; VResRun, n = 7.*

of the 5 h run time-window ($p < 0.001$, **Table 1**). Both acute VRun and VResRun increased downstream mTORC1 signaling in SOL and PLT as measured by pS6K1$^{Thr421/Ser424}$, pS6K1^{Thr389}, and pRPS6$^{ser235/236}$ (**Figures 4A–E**). Notably, VResRun augmented downstream mTORC1 signaling significantly more than VRun both in the SOL and PLT, indicating that load independently augments mTORC1 signaling in an *in vivo* setting (**Figures 4A–E**). Finally, total work was highly correlated with pS6K1$^{Thr421/Ser424}$ in both SOL ($r = 0.69$, $p < 0.05$) and PLT ($r = 0.63$, $p < 0.05$).

One of the proposed pathways of how high-load contractions regulate mTORC1 is *via* activation of the stress responsive mitogen-activated protein kinase (MAPK) pathway (Rahnert and Burkholder, 2013). More specifically, c-Jun N-terminal kinase (JNK), a member of the MAPK family, has been put forward as the molecular switch that, when active, promotes muscle hypertrophy and, when inhibited, allows endurance training adaptations such as enhanced aerobic capacity (Lessard et al., 2018). To investigate whether the increased mTORC1 signaling in VResRun muscle was related to increased JNK activation when compared to predominantly aerobic (VRun) or sedentary (SED) muscle, we measured pSAPK/JNK at Thr183/Tyr185 and its downstream target pSMAD2 at Ser245/250/255. VResRun increased pJNK and pSMAD2 modestly (~4 fold, $p < 0.05$) in SOL only, while PLT showed higher variation and was unaffected (**Figures 4A,B,F,G**). Thus, while we observed increased mTORC1 activation upon VRun, this seemed not to be dependent on increased JNK and SMAD2 phosphorylation (**Figures 4A,B,F,G**).

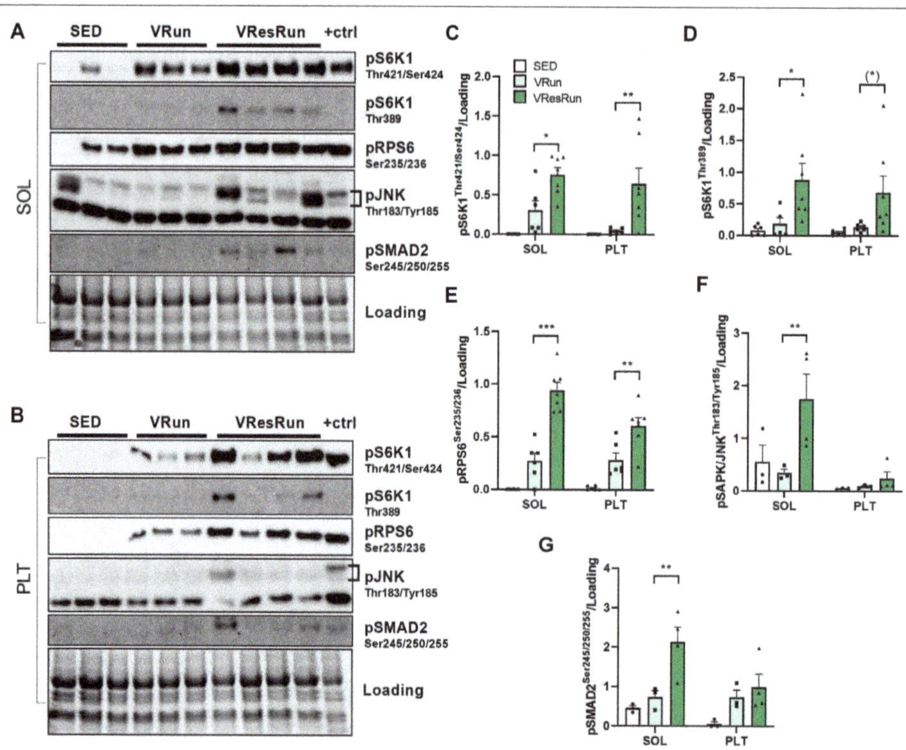

FIGURE 4 | The effect of 5 h of voluntary running (VRun, $n = 6$) and voluntary resistance running (VResRun, $n = 7$) on mTORC1 downstream signaling. **(A)** Representative blots in SOL. **(B)** Representative blots in PLT. **(C)** Quantification of pS6K1$^{Thr421/Ser424}$. **(D)** Quantification of pS6K1^{Thr389}. **(E)** Quantification of pRPS6$^{Ser235/236}$. **(F)** Quantification of pSAPK/JNK$^{Thr183/Tyr185}$. **(G)** Quantification of pSMAD2$^{Ser245/250/255}$. (Sed, $n = 6$). *$p < 0.05$ vs. SED, **$p < 0.01$ vs. SED, ***$p < 0.001$ vs. SED.

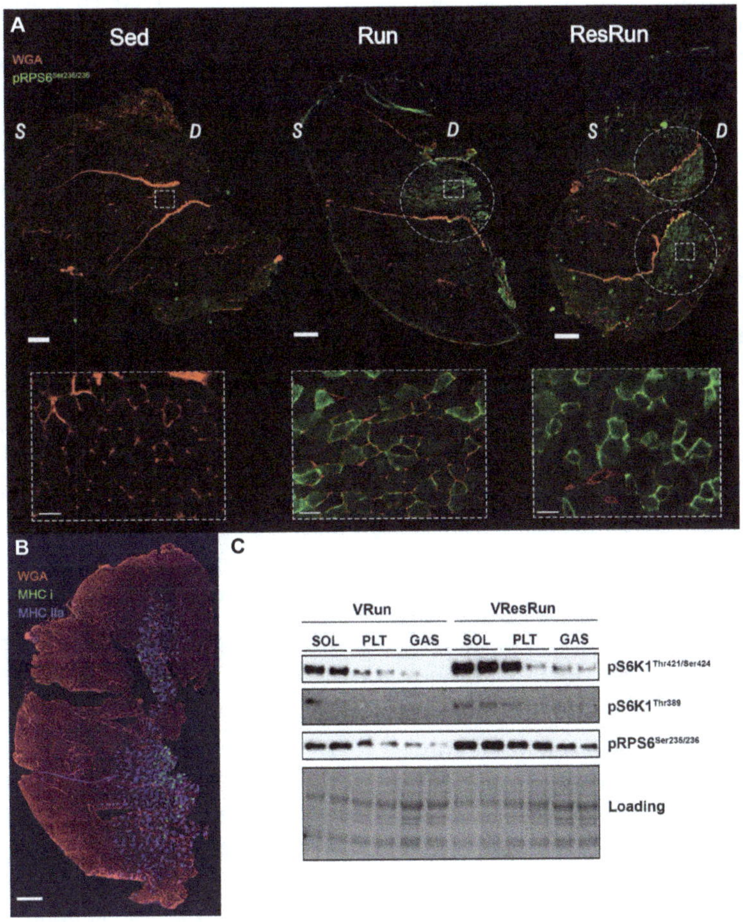

FIGURE 5 | (A) Representative immunofluorescence pictures of GAS in Sed, VRun, and VResRun with pPRS6$^{Ser235/236}$ in green and WGA in red. **(B)** Representative immunofluorescence staining of GAS with Myosin Heavy Chain type I in green, Myosin Heavy Chain type IIa in blue and Wheat Germ Agglutinin WGA in red. **(C)** Representative blots of downstream mTORC1 signaling (VRun and VResRun) in SOL, PLT, and GAS. Scale bar in tile scan represents 500 μm and scale bar in zoom-in represents 50 μm; WGA, wheat germ agglutinin; *S*, superficial part; *D*, deep part.

To visualize activation and distribution of mTORC1 in mouse skeletal muscle, we performed an immunohistochemical staining for phospho-RPS6$^{ser235/236}$ in GAS, a muscle that consists of both oxidative and glycolytic fibers, organized in specific regions. Interestingly, only a selected amount of fibers were phosphorylated in the VRun and VResRun (**Figure 5A**) and they were exclusively situated in the oxidative part (on the anterior side) of the GAS (**Figure 5B**; Sher and Cardasis, 1976). This also represented itself in a lesser activation of downstream mTORC1 after acute running when the phosphorylation of mTORC1 was measured in the whole GAS compared to the SOL and PLT (**Figure 5C**). These data suggest that voluntary running activates downstream mTORC1 signaling in a select amount of predominantly oxidative fibers.

DISCUSSION

This study aimed to validate acute resistance running as a model of resistance exercise-induced mTORC1 activation in mouse skeletal muscle. Previous research has shown muscle hypertrophy (Legerlotz et al., 2008; White et al., 2016) and increased strength (Roemers et al., 2017) following voluntary resistance running, and we aimed to link these models with a key molecular pathway, which regulates muscle protein synthesis. We show increased mTORC1 activity in the PLT, SOL, and GAS, whereas we did not detect enhanced activation in the TA or TRI muscle, suggesting muscle specific differences in mTORC1 activation upon acute resistance running, which might be determined by specific load applied on these muscles during running. To further study the involvement of mechanical load, we subjected mice to voluntary free and resistance running and found increased downstream mTORC1 signaling in SOL and PLT when resistance was applied to the wheel.

Numerous studies showed increased muscle mass after resistance running in mice. It has been reported that muscle mass is increased in the PLT (Legerlotz et al., 2008; Holland et al., 2016; Mobley et al., 2018), SOL (Konhilas et al., 2005; Legerlotz et al., 2008; Call et al., 2010; White et al., 2016),

GAS (Mobley et al., 2018), *m. quadriceps* (Soffe et al., 2016), and TRI (Call et al., 2010) after long term (>4 weeks) resistance running. Our findings provide evidence of a potential molecular basis for the above findings as we report increased mTORC1 activation after one night of resistance running in the aforementioned muscles. It has been reported before that during wheel running, the force shifts to the hindlimb (0.85:0.15) compared to overground running leading to a subsequent increase in hindlimb normal forces (Roach et al., 2012). It is therefore likely that the activation of mTORC1 after resistance running was load-dependent, as we did not find any, or minimal phosphorylation of its downstream kinases in the TRI of the forelimb. In agreement with this, we also failed to observe significant mTORC1 activation in TA, a dorsiflexor muscle that does not bear body weight, can produce less force than the plantar flexors (Ashton-Miller et al., 1992) and thus is likely recruited to a lower extent during (resistance) running when compared to muscles of the *m. triceps surae*.

At 60% resistance, the resistance we opted to put on the wheel in this study, the additional force needed to overcome the wheel resistance was 0.2 N. Plantar flexion strength of the *m. triceps surae* is much higher [3.3 N (Ashton-Miller et al., 1992)] indicating that maximal force production was not required to overcome the resistance imposed by the wheel. Thus, during a single contraction only a subset of motor units, likely the oxidative fibers which are recruited during submaximal force production (Henneman et al., 1965), needed to be activated. This was underscored by our observations that in the GAS, only the areas containing more oxidative fibers (the anterior part close to the bone) were highly positive for pRPS6, while the glycolytic part remained unaffected after VResRun and VRun. These findings are corroborated by the fact that nearly all aforementioned studies investigating hypertrophy after wheel running found significant hypertrophy in the SOL and/or PLT, while GAS and dorsiflexors were much less, or even not at all affected (Legerlotz et al., 2008; White et al., 2016). Nevertheless, future research needs to further evaluate whether load-dependent mTORC1-signaling directly affects hypertrophy in a muscle-specific way.

Besides to a large increase in downstream mTORC1 signaling after voluntary resistance running, we also observed a significant, albeit ~50% less potent increase in pS6K1 and pRPS6 in mice that acutely ran for a night without any resistance on the wheel. To the best of our knowledge, this is the first study that specifically alters load in an acute *in vivo* physiological training setting to modulate intra-muscular downstream mTORC1 signaling. The increase in mTORC1 activity after acute endurance exercise (VRun) was somewhat surprising as previous data has reported a decrease in mTORC1 activation 0.5, 3 and 6 h after a single bout of uphill treadmill running (18 $m.min^{-1}$ for 1 h at a 5° gradient) (Philp et al., 2015). On the other hand, studies using longer duration (and intensity) of running did indeed find higher downstream mTORC1 signaling immediately and 3 h after the running bout (Scribbans et al., 2014). In an attempt to elucidate the mechanisms that regulate muscular plasticity, a recent report showed JNK/SMAD2 to act as a major switch between muscle growth and endurance phenotype when the kinases were activated or inactivated, respectively (Lessard et al., 2018). We report an increase in pJNK1/2 and pSMAD2 in VResRun, while this effect was absent in the VRun condition. The absence of JNK activation and the induction of mTORC1 after VRun suggest that VRun is indeed a good model for endurance adaptations in skeletal muscle and that mechanisms other than the mechanosensitive MAPK signaling regulate mTORC1 upon endurance type training.

To conclude, we show that acute resistance running and acute free running increased activation of the mTORC1 pathway in mouse muscle. Our data suggest that this activation is dependent on load as the *m. triceps surae* muscles had higher activation compared to the hindlimb dorsi flexors and only a subset of oxidative fibers were activated in the GAS. Furthermore, resistance running, in which the force per contraction is increased compared to free wheel running, induced a more robust mTORC1 activation in both SOL and PLT. In this work, we present an easy-to-use, low stress, and time-efficient model to study mTORC1 signaling after resistance training in mice, which can be used in future studies to pin-down the molecular signaling events that determine muscle growth upon muscular contractions.

AUTHOR CONTRIBUTIONS

GD'H and AP designed the study, wrote the manuscript and performed all the experiments and data analysis. EM helped performing the experiments and edited the manuscript. OB-N helped in drafting and revising the m anuscript. K B designed the study and helped drafting and revising the manuscript.

ACKNOWLEDGMENTS

We would like to thank Nicola Bundschuh for her support and technical assistance in the lab.

REFERENCES

1. Abe, T., Kojima, K., and Kearns, C. F. (2003). Whole body muscle hypertrophy from resistance training: distribution and total mass. *Br. J. Sport. Med.* 37, 543–545. doi: 10.1136/bjsm.37.6.543
2. Ashton-Miller, J. A., He, Y., Kadhiresan, V. A., McCubbrey, D. A., and Faulkner, J. A. (1992). An apparatus to measure in vivo biomechanical behavior of dorsi- and plantarflexors of mouse ankle. *J. Appl. Physiol.* 72, 1205–1211. doi: 10.1152/jappl.1992.72.3.1205
3. Baar, K., and Esser, K. (1999). Phosphorylation of p70S6k correlates with increased skeletal muscle mass following resistance exercise. *Am. J. Physiol. Physiol.* 276, C120–C127. doi: 10.1152/ajpcell.1999.276.1.C120
4. Bhasin, S., Storer, T. W., Berman, N., Callegari, C., Clevenger, B., Phillips, J., et al. (1996). The effects of Supraphysiologic doses of testosterone on muscle size and strength in normal men. *N. Engl. J. Med.* 335, 1–7. doi: 10.1056/ NEJM199607043350101
5. Bodine, S. C., Stitt, T. N., Gonzalez, M., Kline, W. O., Stover, G. L., Bauerlein, R., et al. (2001). Akt/mTOR pathway is a crucial regulator of skeletal muscle hypertrophy and can prevent muscle atrophy *in vivo*. *Nat. Cell Biol.* 3, 1014–1019. doi: 10.1038/ncb1101-1014
6. Brook, M. S., Wilkinson, D. J., Mitchell, W. K., Lund, J. N., Szewczyk, N. J., Greenhaff, P. L., et al. (2015). Skeletal muscle hypertrophy adaptations predominate in the early stages of resistance exercise training, matching deuterium oxide- derived measures of muscle protein synthesis and mechanistic target of rapamycin complex 1 signaling. *FASEB J.* 29, 4485–4496. doi: 10.1096/fj.15-273755
7. Burd, N. A., Holwerda, A. M., Selby, K. C., West, D. W. D., Staples, A. W., Cain, N. E., et al. (2010). Resistance exercise volume affects myofibrillar protein synthesis and anabolic signalling molecule phosphorylation in young men. *J. Physiol.* 588, 3119–3130. doi: 10.1113/jphysiol.2010.192856
8. Call, J. A., McKeehen, J. N., Novotny, S. A., and Lowe, D. A. (2010). Progressive resistance voluntary wheel running in the mdx mouse. *Muscle Nerve* 42, 871–880. doi: 10.1002/mus.21764
9. Cholewa, J., Guimarães-Ferreira, L., da Silva Teixeira, T., Naimo, M. A., Zhi, X., de Sá, R. B. D. P., et al. (2014). Basic models modeling resistance training: an update for basic scientists interested in study skeletal muscle hypertrophy. *J. Cell. Physiol.* 229, 1148–1156. doi: 10.1002/jcp.24542
10. De Bono, J. P., Adlam, D., Paterson, D. J., and Channon, K. M. (2005). Novel quantitative phenotypes of exercise training in mouse models. *Am. J. Physiol. Integr. Comp. Physiol..* 290, R926–R934. doi: 10.1152/ajpregu.00694.2005
11. Dreyer, H. C., Fujita, S., Glynn, E. L., Drummond, M. J., Volpi, E., and Rasmussen, B. B. (2010). Resistance exercise increases leg muscle protein synthesis and mTOR signalling independent of sex. *Acta Physiol.* 199, 71–81. doi: 10.1111/j.1748-1716.2010.02074.x
12. Drummond, M. J., Fry, C. S., Glynn, E. L., Dreyer, H. C., Dhanani, S., Timmerman, K. L., et al. (2009). Rapamycin administration in humans blocks the contraction-induced increase in skeletal muscle protein synthesis. *J. Physiol.* 587, 1535–1546. doi: 10.1113/jphysiol.2008.163816
13. Figueiredo, V. C., Caldow, M. K., Massie, V., Markworth, J. F., Cameron-Smith, D., and Blazevich, A. J. (2015). Ribosome biogenesis adaptation in resistance training-induced human skeletal muscle hypertrophy. *Am. J. Physiol. Metab.* 309, E72–E83. doi: 10.1152/ajpendo.00050.2015
14. Goldberg, A. L. (1968). Protein synthesis during work-induced growth of skeletal muscle. *J. Cell Biol.* 36, 653–658.
15. Goldspink, G. (1999). Changes in muscle mass and phenotype and the expression of autocrine and systemic growth factors by muscle in response to stretch and overload. *J. Anat.* 194, 323–334. doi: 10.1046/J.1469-7580.1999.19430323.X
16. Goodman, C. A., Frey, J. W., Mabrey, D. M., Jacobs, B. L., Lincoln, H. C., You, J. S., et al. (2011). The role of skeletal muscle mTOR in the regulation of mechanical load-induced growth. *J. Physiol.* 589, 5485–5501. doi: 10.1113/ jphysiol.2011.218255
17. Henneman, E., Somjen, G., and Carpentier, D. (1965). Functional significance of cell size in spinal motor neurons. *J. Neurophysiol.* 28, 560–580. doi: 10.1152/ jn.1965.28.3.560
18. Holland, A. M., Kephart, W. C., Mumford, P. W., Mobley, C. B., Lowery, R. P., Shake, J. J., et al. (2016). Effects of a ketogenic diet on adipose tissue, liver, and serum biomarkers in sedentary rats and rats that exercised via resisted voluntary wheel running. *Am. J. Physiol. Integr. Comp. Physiol.* 311, R337–R351. doi: 10.1152/ajpregu.00156.2016
19. Huang, K., and Fingar, D. C. (2014). Growing knowledge of the mTOR signaling network. *Semin. Cell Dev. Biol.* 36, 79–90. doi: 10.1016/J.SEMCDB.2014.09.011 Janssen, I., Heymsfield, S. B., and Ross, R. (2002). Low relative skeletal muscle mass (sarcopenia) in older persons is associated with functional impairment and physical disability. *J. Am. Geriatr. Soc.* 50, 889–896. doi: 10.1046/j.1532-5415.2002.50216.x
20. Konhilas, J. P., Widegren, U., Allen, D. L., Paul, A. C., Cleary, A., and Leinwand, L. A. (2005). Loaded wheel running and muscle adaptation in the mouse. *Am. J. Physiol. Circ. Physiol.* 289, H455–H465. doi: 10.1152/ajpheart.00085.2005
21. Kubica, N., Bolster, D. E., Farrell, P. A., Kimball, S. E., and Jefferson, L. S. (2005). Resistance exercise increases muscle protein synthesis and translation of eukaryotic initiation factor 2Bε mRNA in a mammalian target of rapamycin- dependent manner. *J. Biol. Chem.* 280, 7570–7580. doi: 10.1074/jbc.M413732200
22. Legerlotz, K., Elliott, B., Guillemin, B., and Smith, H. K. (2008). Voluntary resistance running wheel activity pattern and skeletal muscle growth in rats. *Exp. Physiol.* 93, 754–762. doi: 10.1113/expphysiol.2007.041244
23. Lessard, S. J., MacDonald, T. L., Pathak, P., Han, M. S., Coffey, V. G., Edge, J., et al. (2018). JNK regulates muscle remodeling via myostatin/SMAD inhibition. *Nat. Commun.* 9:3030. doi: 10.1038/s41467-018-05439-3
24. Mahajan, P. B. (1994). Modulation of transcription of rRNA genes by rapamycin.*Int. J. Immunopharmacol.* 16, 711–721.
25. Mobley, C. B., Holland, A. M., Kephart, W. C., Mumford, P. W., Lowery, R. P., Kavazis, A. N., et al. (2018). Progressive resistance-loaded voluntary wheel running increases hypertrophy and differentially affects muscle protein synthesis, ribosome biogenesis, and proteolytic markers in rat muscle. *J. Anim. Physiol. Anim. Nutr.* 102, 317–329. doi: 10.1111/jpn.12691
26. O'Neil, T. K., Duffy, L. R., Frey, J. W., and Hornberger, T. A. (2009). The role of phosphoinositide 3-kinase and phosphatidic acid in the regulation of mammalian target of rapamycin following eccentric contractions. *J. Physiol.* 587, 3691–3701. doi: 10.1113/jphysiol.2009.173609
27. Ogasawara, R., and Suginohara, T. (2018). Rapamycin-insensitive mechanistic target of rapamycin regulates basal and resistance exercise-induced muscle protein synthesis. *FASEB J.* 32, 5824–5834. doi: 10.1096/fj.201701422R
28. Philp, A., Schenk, S., Perez-Schindler, J., Hamilton, D. L., Breen, L., Laverone, E., et al. (2015). Rapamycin does not prevent increases in myofibrillar or mitochondrial protein synthesis following endurance exercise. *J. Physiol.* 593, 4275–4284. doi: 10.1113/JP271219
29. Pyka, G., Lindenberger, E., Charette, S., and Marcus, R. (1994). Muscle strength and fiber adaptations to a year-long resistance training program in elderly men and women. *J. Gerontol.* 49, M22–M27. doi: 10.1093/geronj/49.1.M22
30. Rahnert, J. A., and Burkholder, T. J. (2013). High-frequency electrical stimulation reveals a p38-mTOR signaling module correlated with force-time integral. *J. Exp. Biol.* 216, 2619–2631. doi: 10.1242/jeb.080705
31. Rivero-Gutiérrez, B., Anzola, A., Martínez-Augustin, O., and De Medina, F. S. (2014). Stain-free detection as loading control alternative to Ponceau and housekeeping protein immunodetection in Western blotting. *Anal. Biochem.* 467, 1–3. doi: 10.1016/j.ab.2014.08.027
32. Roach, G. C., Edke, M., and Griffin, T. M. (2012). A novel mouse running wheel that senses individual limb forces: biomechanical validation and in vivo testing. *J. Appl. Physiol.* 113, 627–635. doi: 10.1152/japplphysiol.00272.2012 Roemers, P., Mazzola, P. N., De Deyn, P. P., Bossers, W. J., van Heuvelen, M. J., and van der Zee, E. A. (2017). Burrowing as a novel voluntary strength training method for mice: a comparison of various voluntary strength or resistance exercise methods. *J. Neurosci. Methods* 300, 112–126. doi: 10.1016/j. jneumeth.2017.05.027
33. Scribbans, T. D., Ma, J. K., Edgett, B. A., Vorobej, K. A., Mitchell, A. S., Zelt, J. G. E., et al. (2014). Resveratrol supplementation does not augment performance adaptations or fibre-type-specific responses to high-intensity interval training in humans. *Appl. Physiol. Nutr. Metab.* 39, 1305–1313. doi: 10.1139/apnm-2014-0070
34. Sher, J., and Cardasis, C. (1976). Skeletal muscle fiber types in the adult mouse. *Acta Neurol. Scand.* 54, 45–56. doi: 10.1111/j.1600-0404.1976.

tb07619.x Soffe, Z., Radley-Crabb, H. G., McMahon, C., Grounds, M. D., and Shavlakadze, T. (2016). Effects of loaded voluntary wheel exercise on performance and muscle hypertrophy in young and old male C57Bl/6J mice. *Scand. J. Med. Sci. Sports* 26, 172–188. doi: 10.1111/sms.12416

35. Staron, R. S., Karapondo, D. L., Kraemer, W. J., Fry, A. C., Gordon, S. E., Falkel, J. E., et al. (1994). Skeletal muscle adaptations during early phase of heavy-resistance training in men and women. *J. Appl. Physiol.* 76, 1247–1255. doi: 10.1152/jappl.1994.76.3.1247
36. Szulc, P., Beck, T. J., Marchand, F., and Delmas, P. D. (2004). Low skeletal muscle mass is associated with poor structural parameters of bone and impaired balance in elderly men-the MINOS study. *J. Bone Miner. Res.* 20, 721–729. doi: 10.1359/JBMR.041230
37. Szulc, P., Munoz, F., Marchand, F., Chapurlat, R., and Delmas, P. D. (2010). Rapid loss of appendicular skeletal muscle mass is associated with higher all-cause mortality in older men: the prospective MINOS study. *Am. J. Clin. Nutr.* 91, 1227–1236. doi: 10.3945/ajcn.2009.28256
38. Thoreen, C. C., Chantranupong, L., Keys, H. R., Wang, T., Gray, N. S., and Sabatini, D. M. (2012). A unifying model for mTORC1-mediated regulation of mRNA translation. *Nature* 485, 109–113. doi: 10.1038/nature11083
39. Verdijk, L. B., Gleeson, B. G., Jonkers, R. A. M., Meijer, K., Savelberg, H. H. C. M., Dendale, P., et al. (2009). Skeletal muscle hypertrophy following resistance training is accompanied by a fiber type-specific increase in satellite cell content in elderly men. *J. Gerontol. Ser. A Biol. Sci. Med. Sci.* 64A, 332–339. doi: 10.1093/gerona/gln050
40. White, Z., Terrill, J., White, R. B., McMahon, C., Sheard, P., Grounds, M. D., et al. (2016). Voluntary resistance wheel exercise from mid-life prevents sarcopenia and increases markers of mitochondrial function and autophagy in muscles of old male and female C57BL/6J mice. *Skelet. Muscle* 6, 1–21. doi: 10.1186/s13395-016-0117-3
41. Wolfson, R. L., and Sabatini, D. M. (2017). The dawn of the age of amino acid sensors for the mTORC1 pathway. *Cell Metab.* 26, 301–309. doi: 10.1016/j. cmet.2017.07.001

Whey Protein Supplementation Post-Resistance Exercise in Elderly Men Induces Changes in Muscle miRNA's Compared to Resistance Exercise Alone

*Randall F. D'Souza[1,2], Nina Zeng[1], James F. Markworth[1,3], Vandre C. Figueiredo[1,4], Christopher P. Hedges[5], Aaron C. Petersen[6], Paul A. Della Gatta[7], David Cameron-Smith[1,8,9] and Cameron J. Mitchell[1,10]**

[1] Liggins Institute, The University of Auckland, Auckland, New Zealand, [2] Discipline of Nutrition, The University of Auckland, Auckland, New Zealand, [3] Department of Molecular and Integrative Physiology, University of Michigan, Ann Arbor, MI, United States, [4] College of Health Sciences, University of Kentucky, Lexington, KY, United States, [5] Applied Surgery and Metabolism Laboratory, School of Biological Sciences, University of Auckland, Auckland, New Zealand, [6] Institute for Health and Sport (iHeS), Victoria University, Melbourne, VIC, Australia, [7] Institute for Physical Activity and Nutrition (IPAN), School of Exercise and Nutrition Sciences, Deakin University, Geelong, VIC, Australia, [8] Food and Bio-based Products, AgResearch Grasslands, Palmerston North, New Zealand, [9] The Riddet Institute, Massey University, Palmerston North, New Zealand, [10] School of Kinesiology, University of British Colombia, Vancouver, BC, Canada

***Correspondence:**
Cameron J. Mitchell
cameron.mitchell@ubc.ca

Progressive muscle loss with aging results in decreased physical function, frailty, and impaired metabolic health. Deficits in anabolic signaling contribute to an impaired ability for aged skeletal muscle to adapt in response to exercise and protein feeding. One potential contributing mechanism could be exerted by dysregulation of microRNAs (miRNAs). Therefore, the aim of this study was to determine if graded protein doses consumed after resistance exercise altered muscle miRNA expression in elderly men. Twenty-three senior men (67.9 ± 0.9 years) performed a bout of resistance exercise and were randomized to consume either a placebo, 20 or 40 g of whey protein ($n = 8$, $n = 7$, and $n = 8$, respectively). *Vastus lateralis* biopsies were collected before, 2 and 4 h after exercise. Expression of 19 miRNAs, previously identified to influence muscle phenotype, were measured via RT-PCR. Of these, miR-16-5p was altered with exercise in all groups ($p = 0.032$). Expression of miR-15a and-499a increased only in the placebo group 4 h after exercise and miR-451a expression increased following exercise only in the 40 g whey supplementation group. Changes in p-P70S6K^{Thr389} and p-Akt^{Ser473} following exercise were correlated with alterations in miR-208a and-499a and-206 expression, irrespective of protein dose, suggesting a possible role for miRNA in the regulation of acute phosphorylation events during early hours of exercise recovery.

Keywords: skeletal muscle, mTOR pathway, microRNA, older adults, resistance training, P70S6 K, protein dose

INTRODUCTION

Progressive muscle loss with aging results in decreases in physical function, frailty and metabolic health (1–3). Age-related impairment in the responses to anabolic stimuli such as protein ingestion and resistance exercise contribute to declining muscle mass (4, 5). Deficits in the activation of anabolic signaling proteins play a role in the anabolic resistance to protein feeding (6), however, the regulatory mechanisms are still unclear. MicroRNAs (miRNAs), small non-coding RNAs, regulate gene expression via promotion of transcript breakdown and inhibition of protein translation (7, 8). Recent evidence suggests that miRNA may play a role in the mechanism of anabolic resistance and regulation of cellular phosphorylation events (9, 10).

It is widely accepted that miRNAs regulate cellular control via transcriptional and translation inhibition. There is also emerging evidence that specific miRNAs including miR-499a,-208a, -206,-133a,-1,-99a, 99b,-100, and-149 are involved in controlling intramuscular signaling of key proteins including Akt, P70S6K, and RPS6. These proteins are critical mediators of anabolic signaling via the Akt-mTOR pathway and thus upstream regulators of muscle protein synthesis (MPS) (8–11). The ability of miRNAs to impact kinase phosphorylation *in vitro* has also been demonstrated (12). In cell models, miRNAs alter anabolic signaling, but it is unclear if this occurs as a result of direct regulation of kinase phosphorylation or indirectly via control of upstream gene expression influencing posttranslational modifications (12). As yet, no relationship *in-vivo* between the phosphorylation status of proteins such as Akt and P70S6K and the expression of these proposed miRNA regulators has been identified.

Zacharewicz et al. (9), identified via PCR validation of a microarray analysis, seven miRNAs that were differentially altered following exercise in young compared to old men while Rivas et al. identified 21 miRNAs regulated by exercise in young men but not old men (12). Only a single study (13) has assessed both the resting and post resistance exercise muscular miRNA abundances following protein supplementation in young and elderly males. In this study, Drummond et al. reported increased expression of miR-1 and the immature form of miR-133a (pri-miRNA) in elderly compared to young men at rest (13). Following exercise in combination with ingestion of 20 g essential amino acid (EAA), miR-1 was reduced in muscle of young but not elderly men (13). In young adults, protein but not placebo ingestion after concurrent exercise reportedly altered miRNA expression from rest at 4 h following exercise (14). Little is known about how protein ingestion might alter the acute response of miRNAs more recently identified as regulators of muscle growth to resistance exercise, especially in aged muscle.

The primary aim of the current study was to characterize muscular responses of putative miRNA regulators of muscle anabolism to acute resistance exercise in older men and whether graded amounts of whey protein ingestion alters that response. The secondary aim of the study was to identify whether changes in miRNA expression following exercise correlated with changes in Akt-mTOR pathway phosphorylation status in agreement with the relationships proposed by Margolis and Rivas (10). It is hypothesized that whey protein ingestion will alter miRNA expression patterns following exercise in a dose dependent fashion. Further, as suggested by Margolis and Rivas (10), a relationship between changes in Akt-mTOR phosphorylation status and miRNA expression will observed.

TABLE 1 | Participant characteristics.

	Placebo ($n = 8$)	20 g whey ($n = 7$)	40 g whey ($n = 8$)
Age (years)	67.3 ± 4.0	69.3 ± 3.7	67.4 ± 4.0
Height (cm)	180 ± 8	178 ± 11	181 ± 6
Weight (kg)	87.5 ± 14.7	90.5 ± 19.6	86.4 ± 12.2
BMI (kg/m^2)	27.2 ± 5.1	28.6 ± 5.3	26.5 ± 3.7
Thigh CSA (cm^2)	109.7 ± 16.7	120.6 ± 65.3	105.7 ± 44.6
1-RM Squat (kg)	73.9 ± 31.7	81.0 ± 27.0	91.9 ± 48.6
1-RM Leg Press (kg)	196.9 ± 80.0	211.9 ± 112.7	215.5 ± 71.3
1-RM Leg Ext.(kg)	49.5 ± 24.3	49.9 ± 29.9	64.2 ± 35.6

Values presented as means ± SD. 1-RM values were estimated via the Brzycki equation.

METHODS

Participants

Twenty-three elderly men (>60 years of age) from a larger clinical trial of sixty participants were included in the current study (**Table 1**) (15). Individuals who were undertaking any regular resistance exercise training or those with pre-existing metabolic or cardiovascular diseases were excluded. Participants who were taking anticoagulation or antihypertensive medications were not excluded from participation. All participants were recreationally active and completed at least 150 min per week of moderate intensity physical activity (walking, cycling, golf) and no more than 90 min a week of vigorous activity (jogging, faster cycling). Subjects taking aspirin/fish oil supplements were required to abstain from these medications throughout the duration of the trial. Prior to commencement of the study, participants were provided with written and oral information regarding the experimental protocols and potential risks involved and written consent to participate was obtained. All experimental procedures employed by this study were carried out in coherence with the Helsinki declaration and were formally approved by the Deakin University Human Research Ethics Committee.

Experimental Protocol

At least 1 week prior to the experimental trial day, a familiarization session which included one-repetition maximum (1RM) strength testing to determine the experimental exercise load (80% of 1RM) was conducted. The maximal weight that subjects could lift for 3–6 repetitions (3–6RM) of bilateral smith machine barbell squat, 45° leg press and seated leg extension exercises was determined and participants' 1RM was estimated using the Brzycki equation (16). In the week prior to the trial day, participants were instructed to abstain from any vigorous physical activity (>6 Mets). The evening before the trial, participants ingested a standard evening meal (2103 kJ, 54% carbohydrate, 29% fat, 17% protein) before 10 pm and were instructed to eat nothing afterward. The following morning, the subjects arrived (~7 a.m.) at the lab in a fasted state. Participants were randomly allocated into one of three treatment groups; non-caloric placebo ($n = 8$), 20 g whey ($n = 7$), and 40 g whey ($n = 8$).

Determination of Thigh CSA

Thigh CSA was determined via anthropometric measurement as described previously (17). The formula used for calculation was

$$A_M = 0.649 \times \left(\left[\frac{C_T}{\pi} - S_Q \right]^2 - (0.3 \times d_E)^2 \right)$$

where: A_M = Mid-thigh muscle cross sectional area (cm^2)
C_T = Thigh circumference (cm)
S_Q = Skinfold thickness of anterior quadriceps (cm)
d_E = distance across the medial and lateral femoral epicondyle (cm).

Resistance Exercise and Supplementation Trial

Upon arrival at the laboratory, individuals rested in a supine position for ~30 min prior to collection of resting muscle biopsy samples (see below). Participants then rested supine following collection of resting muscle biopsy for approximately ~10–15 min after which the exercise protocol commenced. The exercise protocol began with a 10-min warm-up involving light cycling on a bicycle ergometer and a single low load warm-up set for each of the three exercises. Participants then completed three sets of 8–10 repetitions of bilateral barbell smith rack squat, 45° leg press, and seated knee extensions at 80% of their predetermined 1RM. Exercises were performed in a circuit manner with 1 min rest between each exercise and 3 min rest between subsequent sets, the exercise protocol took ~20 min to complete. Following the exercise protocol, subjects were immediately provided with a beverage, containing a non-caloric placebo, or one of the two doses of whey protein concentrate (WPC instantized 8010, Hilmar Ingredients, Hilmar, CA, USA [20 g, or 40 g]) dissolved in 350 mL of water. All supplements were vanilla flavored and sweetened with aspartame. Amino acid composition of the protein supplement is presented in the **Table 2**. Subjects were instructed to ingest the beverage within 2 min following which they were rested in a supine position throughout the 4 h of post-exercise recovery with additional muscle biopsy samples collected at 2 and 4 h post exercise. A whey protein dose of 20 g was chosen because it has been shown to maximize post exercise anabolism in young men (18) while a 40 g group was included because this dose provokes a larger post exercise MPS and signaling response in older men (4, 15).

Muscle Biopsy Sampling

Muscle biopsies (~100 mg) were collected from the *vastus lateralis* muscle under local anesthesia (1% Xylocaine) using a Bergstrom needle modification of manual suction. All three biopsies were collected from the same limb starting distally and moving proximally. A gap of at least 2–3 cm between sequential biopsies was maintained to avoid potential confounding effects caused by repeated sampling from the same location. Biopsies were quickly frozen in liquid nitrogen and stored at -80°C until further analyses.

TABLE 2 | Amino acid profile of the whey protein supplement utilized in the current study.

Amino acids represented as g/100 g of product	
Alanine	4.2
Arginine	2.2
Aspartic Acid	8.7
Cystine	2.0
Glutamic Acid	14.0
Glycine	1.5
Histidine	1.5
Hydroxyproline	<0.1
Isoleucine*$	5.2
Leucine*$	8.5
Lysine*	7.8
Methionine*	1.8
Phenylalanine*	2.6
Proline	4.9
Serine	4.1
Threonine*	5.7
Tryptophan*	1.7
Tyrosine	2.5
Valine*$	4.5

*Essential Amino Acids.
$Branched-Chain Amino Acids (BCAA).

Muscle miRNA Isolation and RT/PCR

As previously described (8, 19) total RNA was extracted from ~20 mg of muscle tissue using the AllPrep® DNA/RNA/miRNA Universal Kit (QIAGEN GmbH, Hilden, Germany). Ten nanogram of total RNA from muscle was used for cDNA synthesis using TaqMan™ Advanced miRNA cDNA Synthesis Kit (Thermo Fisher Scientific, Carlsbad, CA, USA) and miRNA abundance were measured by RT-PCR on a QuantStudio 6 (Thermo Fisher Scientific, Carlsbad, CA, USA) using Applied Biosystems Fast Advanced Master Mix (Thermo Fisher Scientific, Carlsbad, CA, USA).

Target miRs are shown in **Table 3** (Thermo Fisher Scientific, Cat# A25576, Carlsbad, CA, USA). The geometric mean of three reference miRs (miR-361,-320a, and-186) for muscle (20) were used for normalization based on miRs that showed the least variation amongst the current sample set. The mean CTs ± CV% for each reference miRNA was 23.73 ± 4.23%, 23.63 ± 4.45%, and 24.40 ± 3.91%. RT-PCR data was analyzed using $2^{-\Delta\Delta CT}$ method (21). Fold changes are reflective of each participants response compared to their individual pre-exercise values.

Western Blotting

Approximately 50 mg of muscle tissue was homogenized in ice-cold RIPA containing protease and phosphatase inhibitors (15). Homogenates were agitated for 1 h at 4°C and centrifuged for 15 min at 13,000 g. Protein content was determined using a BCA-protein assay kit (Pierce, Rockford, IL) according to the manufacturer's instructions. Aliquots of protein homogenate containing 50 μg of total protein were prepared, mixed with

TABLE 3 | Catalog numbers for the miRNAs analyzed and housekeepers with Thermo Fisher Scientific independent miR assay IDs.

miR	ID Number
miR-15a-5p	477858_mir
miR-16-5p	477860_mir
miR-23a-3p	478532_mir
miR-23b-3p	478602_mir
miR-451a	477968_mir
miR-486-5p	478128_mir
miR-126-3p	477887_mir
miR-133a-3p	478511_mir
miR-206	477968_mir
miR-1-3p	477820_mir
miR-148b-3p	477806_mir
miR-30b-5p	478007_mir
miR-145-5p	477916_mir
miR-499a-3p	478948_mir
miR-100-5p	478224_mi
miR-99a-5p	478519_mir
miR-149-5p	477917_miR
miR-208a-3p	477819_mir
miR-186-5p	477940_mir
miR-320a	478594_mir
miR-361-5p	478056_mir

Laemmli buffer, boiled, and subjected to SDS/PAGE. Proteins were separated on an 8% gel and wet-transferred to a polyvinyl difluoride (PVDF) membrane. Following transfer, membranes were blocked in 5% bovine serum albumin (BSA)/Tris Buffered Saline/0.1% Tween 20 (TBST) for 1 h, followed by overnight incubation at 4°C with primary antibody against p-p70S6K (Thr389; 1:1,000, Cell Signaling, Danvers, MA) and p-Akt (Ser473, 1:1,000, cell signaling, Danvers, MA). p-AKT^{Ser473} was normalized to total Akt (Total Akt Cell Signaling 1:1,000). Due to large changes observed in the electrophoretic mobility of the Total p70S6K protein in highly phosphorylated postexercise and supplementation muscle samples it was difficult to accurately quantify total p70S6K. This large magnitude mobility shift in total p70S6K in samples with large degrees of p70S6K phosphorylation has been previously described (22). Total ERK2 (ERK1/2 Cell Signaling, 1:1,000) was thus used as a loading control because it did not change in any condition (15). Once normalized to a total, protein expression was also normalized to a pooled control sample loaded onto every gel so a correlation analysis could be performed.

Statistical Analysis

Two way repeated measures analysis of variance with time as a within subject factor and group as a between subject factor was conducted using SigmaPlot for Windows version 12.1 (Systat 218 Software Inc., San Jose, USA) to determine differences in miRNA expression. Where appropriate, group and time differences were assessed using Holm–Sidak *post hoc* tests. Based on putative relationships suggested by Margolis and Rivas (10), independent Pearson correlations were assessed between p-P70S6K^{Thr389} and miR-208a and miR-499a. Similarly, p-Akt^{Ser473} expression was correlated with miR-208a, 206,-133a,-499a, and-100. A Pearson correlation was assessed between resting miR-133a expression and thigh muscle CSA based on our previous findings where muscle mass and size measures were negatively related to miR-133a (23–25). Correlations were assessed using SigmaPlot for Windows version 12.1 (Systat 218 Software Inc., San Jose, USA). Data are shown as mean ± SD unless specified. Statistical significance was accepted at $p < 0.05$. Figures were drawn using GraphPad Prism 7 Software (GraphPad Software Inc., La Jolla, CA).

RESULTS

Expression of 19 miRNAs were assessed before, 2 and 4 h following the resistance exercise and feeding stimuli. Seven miRNAs (miR-1,-15a,-99a,-148b,-149,-451a, and-499a) demonstrated group by time interactions ($p = 0.048$, $p = 0.006$, $p = 0.025$, $p = 0.043$, $p = 0.039$, $p = 0.036$, and $p = 0.047$, respectively) (**Figure 1**). miR-15a was elevated at 4 h compared to rest ($p = 0.013$), a change that was attenuated in the 20 and 40 g protein groups ($p < 0.001$ and $p = 0.003$, respectively). Similarly, miR-499a was increased at 4 h after exercise in the placebo group ($p = 0.027$) and this response was suppressed in both the 20 and 40 g whey groups ($p = 0.001$ and $p = 0.002$, respectively). Also, at 4 h post-exercise miR-99a,-148b, and-149 exhibited lower expression in the 20 g protein group ($p = 0.019$, $p = 0.011$, and $p = 0.017$, respectively) and the 40 g protein group ($p = 0.041$, $p = 0.011$, and $p = 0.19$, respectively) when compared to the placebo group (**Figures 1C–E**). However, miR-99a,-148b, and -149 abundance were not altered following exercise in the placebo group ($p = 0.247$, $p = 0.166$, and $p = 0.222$). miR-1 was downregulated in the 40 g but not 20 g whey group when compared to the placebo group at 4 h following exercise ($p = 0.023$ and $p = 0.193$, respectively) (**Figure 1A**).

Muscle miR-451a appeared increase following exercise with only the 40 g whey group at both 2 and 4 h following exercise when compared to rest ($p = 0.0063$ and $p = 0.0191$, respectively) (**Figure 1F**). miR-16 demonstrated no group by time interaction however, there was a main effect of time $p = 0.0327$ (**Figure 1H**). Data and p-values for 10 additional miRNAs measured which did not exhibit significant group by time interaction effects are presented in **Table 4**.

p-P70S6K^{Thr389} has previously been reported for a larger cohort of participants including those in the present study (15). Immunoblotting demonstrated a group by time interaction for p-P70S6K^{Thr389} ($p < 0.001$) with only the 40 g whey group being elevated compared to the placebo group at 2 h post exercise ($p < 0.001$) (**Figures 2A,C**). At 2 h abundance of p-P70S6K^{Thr389} in the 20 and 40 g group was elevated and compared to pre-exercise ($p = 0.036$ and $p < 0.001$, respectively). This elevation was also evident in both groups at 4 h rfollowing exercise ($p = 0.046$ and $p = 0.008$, respectively). p-Akt^{Ser473} abundance demonstrated a main effect of time ($p = 0.001$) but no group by time interaction ($p = 0.745$). p-Akt^{Ser473} abundance was significantly elevated

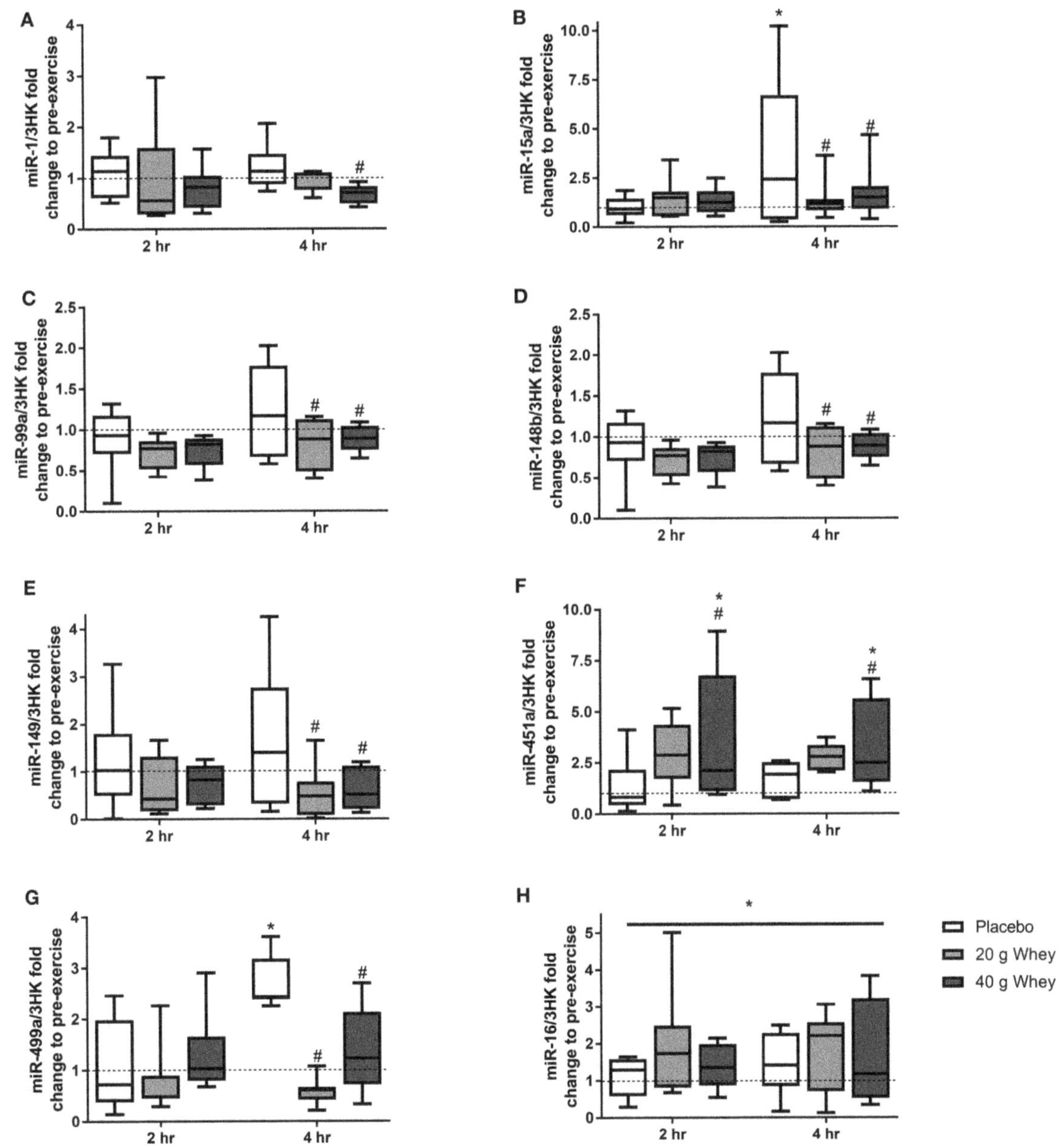

FIGURE 1 | miRNA expression. Fold changes of **(A)** miR-1, **(B)** miR-15a, **(C)** miR-99a, **(D)** miR-148b, **(E)** miR-149, **(F)** miR-451a, **(G)** miR-499a, and **(H)** miR-16 in placebo, 20 g and 40 g whey groups at 2 hr and 4 hr following exercise. *Difference between respective pre exercise expression $P < 0.05$. #Difference compared to placebo group at respective post-exercise time point, $P < 0.05$. Data are expressed as median ±1–99% confidence intervals as a fold change to respective pre-exercise expression. The boxes depict interquartile ranges. Dotted line reflects pre-exercise expression levels.

following exercise at 2 h and returned to pre-exercise levels by 4 h following exercise ($p < 0.001$ and $p = 0.574$) (**Figures 2B,C**). p-Akt^{Ser473} abundance at 2 h in all groups was also increased compared to abundance at 4 h ($p < 0.001$).

Fold change in p-P70S6K^{Thr389} expression at 4 h following exercise was positively correlated with the fold change in miR-208a and -499a expression at 4 h post-exercise ($p < 0.001$ and $R^2 = 0.680$ and $p < 0.001$ and $R^2 = 0.722$, respectively) (**Figures 3A,B**). p-Akt^{Ser473} expression at 4 h following exercise was positively correlated with miR-206 ($p = 0.001$ and $R^2 = 0.461$) and miR-208a ($p < 0.001$ and $R^2 = 0.628$) (**Figures 4A,B**). Inconsistent with Margolis and Rivas (10), no relationships between changes in p-Akt^{Ser473} and miR-133a,-499a, and -100 expression were identified ($p = 0.735$ and $R^2 = 0.008$, $p = 0.808$ and $R^2 < 0.001$, and $p = 0.634$ and $R^2 = 0.020$).

Furthermore, miR-133a, though unresponsive to exercise and feeding stimuli, demonstrated a negative correlation with thigh CSA ($p < 0.01$ and $R^2 = 0.485$) at rest (**Figure 5**).

TABLE 4 | Fold change of muscle miRNA expression in each group following exercise compared to respective resting values.

	Placebo		20 g Whey		40 g Whey		
miR	**2 h**	**4 h**	**2 h**	**4 h**	**2 h**	**4 h**	***p*-value**
miR-23a	0.92 ± 0.65	0.88 ± 0.48	1.49 ± 1.29	1.15 ± 0.58	1.23 ± 1.22	1.25 ± 1.16	0.858
miR-23b	0.95 ± 0.88	0.78 ± 0.40	1.11 ± 0.56	1.05 ± 0.85	1.25 ± 0.79	1.27 ± 0.71	0.915
miR-30b	1.20 ± 0.57	1.14 ± 0.54	1.16 ± 0.66	1.32 ± 1.03	1.05 ± 0.79	1.07 ± 0.51	0.968
miR-100	1.13 ± 0.71	1.15 ± 0.85	0.76 ± 0.11	1.20 ± 1.48	0.65 ± 0.23	1.33 ± 0.85	0.725
miR-126	1.29 ± 0.76	1.10 ± 0.88	1.40 ± 0.61	1.38 ± 0.98	1.17 ± 0.65	1.54 ± 0.71	0.762
miR-133a	1.55 ± 1.24	1.60 ± 1.84	1.90 ± 1.03	2.16 ± 2.14	1.65 ± 2.52	2.15 ± 1.64	0.979
miR-145	1.10 ± 0.65	0.95 ± 0.65	0.98 ± 0.48	1.10 ± 0.93	1.12 ± 0.71	1.32 ± 0.88	0.899
miR-206	1.39 ± 1.30	0.99 ± 0.68	1.48 ± 0.82	1.42 ± 0.85	1.14 ± 0.45	0.93 ± 0.57	0.829
miR-208a	1.46 ± 1.27	2.07 ± 2.12	1.23 ± 1.24	1.56 ± 2.01	1.17 ± 0.65	1.50 ± 0.82	0.969
miR-486	1.01 ± 0.34	1.35 ± 1.19	1.30 ± 0.85	1.32 ± 0.95	1.13 ± 0.48	1.26 ± 0.83	0.966

Values presented as means ± SD, n = 8 placebo, n = 7, 20 g whey, and n = 8, 40 g whey. p-values represent group by time interactions from two-way repeated measures ANOVA.

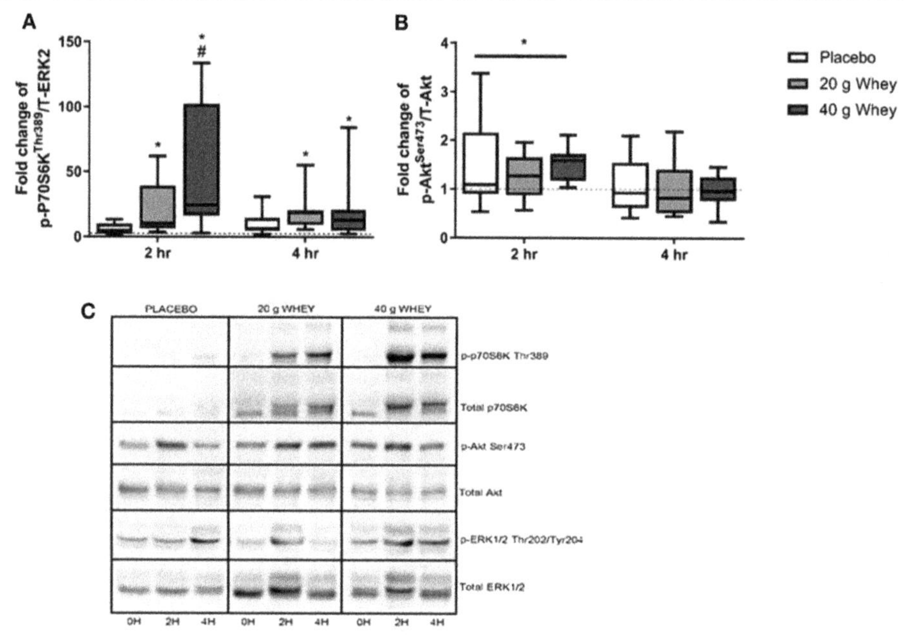

FIGURE 2 | Phosphoprotein expression. Fold changes of **(A)** p-P70S6k^{Thr389} and **(B)** p-Akt^{Ser473}in placebo, 20 g and 40 g whey groups at 2 h and 4 h following exercise. **(C)** Shows representative western blot images. *Difference between respective pre-exercise expression, $P < 0.05$. #Difference compared to placebo group at respective post-exercise time point, $P < 0.05$. Data are expressed as median ±1–99% confidence intervals as a fold change to respective pre-exercise expression. The boxes depict interquartile ranges. Dotted line reflects pre-exercise expression levels. Data for p-P70S6k^{Thr389} was originally published for a larger cohort (15).

DISCUSSION

Of the 19 miRNAs included in the current analyses, six miRNAs (miR-1,-15a,-99a,-148b,-149, and-499a) were differentially expressed between the placebo and increasing doses of 20 and 40 g whey protein supplementation immediately following resistance exercise. The general pattern of expression suggested that protein ingestion following resistance exercise in elderly individuals may result in a miRNA profile similar to what is previously reported in young men (12, 13). When correlation analysis of the changes in miRNA expression relative to the phosphorylation of key kinases required for anabolism was performed, it was observed that miR-208a and-100 both correlated positively with p-P70S6K^{Thr389}, whilst miR-206 and-208a expression was positively and negatively correlated with p-Akt^{Ser473}, respectively. These data are consistent with the hypotheses recently suggested by Margolis and Rivas (12). Together these findings demonstrate a potential involvement of specific miRNAs in the regulation of hypertrophic signaling events following resistance exercise in human muscle *in-vivo*.

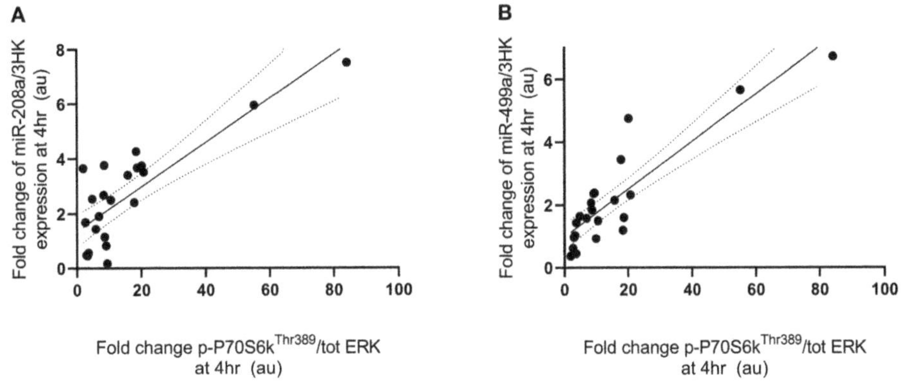

FIGURE 3 | miRNAs correlated with post-exercise P70S6K^{Thr389} phosphorylation. **(A)** miR-208a and **(B)** miR-499a. miRNAs are plotted as a fold change from pre-exercise on the y-axis with fold change of p-P70S6K^{Thr389}/ERK1/2 on the x-axis. The solid line represents the line of best fit as determined by linear regression with 95% confidence intervals.

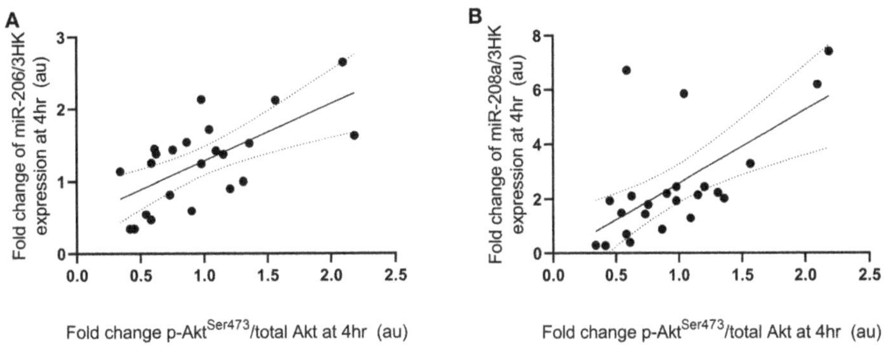

FIGURE 4 | miRNAs significantly correlated with post-exercise Akt^{Ser473} phosphorylation. **(A)** miR-206 and **(B)** miR-208a. miRNAs are plotted as a fold change from pre-exercise on the y-axis with fold change of p-Akt^{Ser473}/total Akt on the x-axis. The solid line represents the line of best fit as determined by linear regression with 95% confidence intervals.

The current study demonstrates a lower muscle miR-1 expression following the ingestion of 40 g whey (containing ~18 g of EAA) group compared to the placebo group at 4 h following exercise. miR-1 expression in the 40 g group however, was not significantly reduced compared to resting pre-exercise levels. The consumption of 20 g of EAA in combination with resistance exercise reportedly reduced miR-1 expression in young but not older individuals (13). These differences in findings between studies suggests that the current population may be more anabolically sensitive than the older participants reported by Drummond et al. (13). However, it has been previously reported that whey protein may be more effective than its constituent EAAs at stimulating an anabolic response (26, 27). The placebo in the present study was non-nutritive so it is not possible to separate the effects of protein *per se* from the energy content of the beverages. However, Drummond's (13) observed age difference in miR-1 following resistance exercise and EAA ingestions in conjunction with the known age-related decrease in anabolic sensitivity suggest protein is a more likely candidate to explain the observed response (6). Whereas, the placebo group appears most similar to the older adults in Drummond et al. Similarly, miR-499a was previously shown to increase 2 h following exercise in elderly but not young participants in the postabsorptive state (9), whilst no change was evident at 6 h following exercise (12). This is congruent with the present finding where miR-499a abundance increased within muscle of placebo treated individuals, a change that was attenuated at 4 h in both the protein supplemented groups when compared to the placebo group. From currently available research it is clear both participant age and feeding status alter the miRNA response to exercise. These findings suggest that whey protein feeding following resistance exercise may help to promote a more youthful post exercise muscle expression pattern of certain miRNAs in older adults. However, the findings are limited by the lack of young adult group and isoenergetic control in the present study.

miR-99a/100 family miRNAs particularly miR-99a and-149 demonstrated a similar pattern whereby expression at 4 h post-exercise was lower in the protein supplemented groups when compared to the placebo group. In trained young men, we

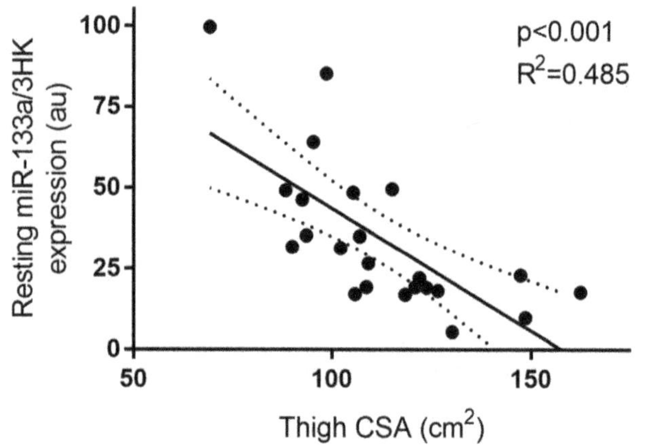

FIGURE 5 | Correlation between resting miR-133a and thigh muscle CSA. miRNA expression is plotted as $2^{-\Delta CT}$ on the y-axis with thigh CSA (cm^2) one the x-axis. The solid line represents the line of best fit as determined by linear regression with 95% confidence intervals.

previously observed no change in muscle miR-149 following exercise in the postabsorptive state (8). The relatively lower expression of both these miRNAs with protein supplementation in conjunction with a lack of change after fasted resistance exercise in previous studies (8, 9) suggest a role of protein ingestion in regulating miR -99a and -149 abundances. However, this cannot be completely confirmed as these miRNAs have not been measured following post-exercise feeding in a young cohort previously.

Previous *in vitro* work has demonstrated the ability for miRNAs to alter phosphorylation status of several proteins (11, 28, 29). The Akt-mTOR cascade has been extensively studied in response to feeding and resistance exercise with several miRNAs being implicated in the regulation of this pathway however it is unclear if miRNAs can directly modulate phosphorylation status of Akt-mTOR pathway targets (9, 10). In the present study the change in expression of miR-208a was positively correlated with changes in phosphorylation of $P70S6K^{Thr389}$ at 4 h following exercise, explaining ~68% of the observed variance. Expression of miR-499a was also positively correlated with phosphorylation of P70S6K ^{Thr389} at 4 h after exercise, explaining ~72% of participant variability. The positive relationships appear opposite to what is expected based on *in-vitro* models (9, 11). This can be interpreted to support the hypothesis that miRNA may be exerting regulation via negative feedback which is congruent with much of our previous work in muscle (8, 23, 30, 31) and has been proposed in other miRNA models (32–36). Whilst the quantification of $p\text{-}P70S6K^{Thr389}$ was limited by the inability to use total P70S6K for normalization, we strongly believe the utilization of total ERK is reflective of the expected pattern. Also, to the best of our knowledge we do not know of any reported changes in total P70S6K or total ERK2 expression upto 4 h following exercise.

miR-208a and-206 are also thought to inhibit Akt signaling upstream of mTOR (10). At 4 h post exercise, miR-206 and miR-208a were positively correlated with $p\text{-}AKT^{Ser473}$. These miRs explained ~46% and ~63% of the observed participant variance in $p\text{-}AKT^{Ser473}$, respectively. The identified relationships support a likely role of miRNAs in not just transcription and translational inhibition but also in understanding dysregulated signaling pathways that promote anabolic resistance in elderly individuals (9, 10). Although this is a novel finding in human muscle there is indirect evidence from *in vitro* models that miRNAs may be able to influence posttranslational modifications such as phosphorylation (11, 28, 29). It is possible that the relationship between miRNA and protein phosphorylation is the result of a direct interaction via an undescribed mechanism or perhaps more likely miRNAs may regulate protein translation of upstream mTOR effectors which in turn control downstream phosphorylation status. Alternatively, the design of the present study does not preclude the possibility of a simple correlative relationship with no direct mechanistic regulation of phosphorylation by miRNA.

Like miR-99a and-149, miR-148b was down regulated in the protein groups following resistance exercise in comparison with the placebo group. miR-148b is thought to promote Akt signaling via inhibition of PTEN. Further, chronic increases in miR-148b are evident in models of reduced physical activity in rats and humans (30, 37). The present findings suggest that the reduction in miR-148b expression in the protein supplemented groups may act as part of a negative feedback mechanism to promote PTEN dependent inhibition of Akt signaling upstream of P70S6K (38). However, further experiments are required using *in vitro* or transgenic animal models to test this hypothesis.

In agreement with several previous works from our lab and others, miR-133a was found to negatively correlate with thigh muscle CSA at rest (23–25, 30, 39). In the current cohort, a negative relationship was observed between anthropometrically determined thigh muscle CSA and miR-133a expression. The relationship explained ~49% of model variance. This finding is consistent with several studies in rested middle aged men (24, 25), healthy controls vs. competitive powerlifters (23), and the patterns seen with limb immobilization (30), as well as following overload induced hypertrophy via surgical ablation in rats (39). From our previous work, miR-133a in combination with miR-146a explained ~33% and ~34%, respectively, of participant variability in whole body and leg lean mass, respectively. The relationship observed in the current study was stronger than previously reported, which could be a random effect due to the smaller sample size or may reflect a greater importance of miR-133a in aged muscle.

The current study was limited by the differences in energy contents of the beverages provided to each group, making it impossible to conclusively attribute the results to whey protein *per se* rather than the small differences in energy intake associated with the protein. This is further pronounced in the placebo group who were asked to perform exercise following an overnight fast and not provided with any post exercise nutrition. However, given p-Akt abundances were not differentially regulated between supplement groups, it is unlikely that observed difference in miRNA response were related to insulin signaling (40) as might have been expected if energy intake was the dominant mechanism. The lack of a young control group prevents definitive conclusions about age related responses, thus any interpretation of the current results concerning the age-related differences in anabolic sensitivity can only be cautiously inferred from existing literature. Further, the lack of sufficient remaining muscle tissue prevented the measurement of targets regulating muscle catabolic processes which could have added additional depth to the results.

CONCLUSION

The present study identified a clear effect of large dose whey protein supplementation on post exercise muscular miRNA expression patterns. Additionally, the reported miR-206,-208a, and-499a expression changes demonstrated strong correlations with changes in expression of p-P70S6K^{Thr389} and p-Akt^{Ser473} at 4 h following exercise. These findings strongly implicate miR-206, 208a, and -499a in the regulation of phosphorylation of these proteins following exercise in elderly men. The pattern of expression suggests that whey protein ingestion in elderly men in combination with exercise more closely mimics the post-exercise microRNA response evident in younger adults. These results also for the first time demonstrate a relationship between changes in the abundances of p-P70S6K^{Thr389} and p-Akt^{Ser473} and alteration in miRNA expression following exercise *in-vivo*. The identified pattern suggests a potential role for miRNAs as negative feedback regulators of this key anabolic signaling cascade, which requires further study. The current findings suggest the need for more mechanistic knockout and *in-vitro* models to better understand the role miRNAs play in modulating the acute post-exercise anabolic response in the presence of whey protein and other nutrition sources. Furthermore, similar studies in individuals with low muscle function may also be required to better validate the ability of whey protein supplementation in improving anabolic signaling responses in elderly individuals. Lastly, the results presented also provided additional support for the role of resting miR-133a expression as a biomarker or possible causative agent in the control of muscle size.

AUTHOR CONTRIBUTIONS

RD, CM, and DC-S designed the study and wrote the manuscript. RD, NZ, JM, and VF performed experiments. JM, AP, and PD sample collection. RD, JM, NZ, CH, AP, PD, DC-S, and CM analyzed data. CM is responsible for the final content of the manuscript. All authors critically evaluated and approved of the final content of the manuscript.

FUNDING

The authors would like to acknowledge the participants for their time commitment. This study was funded by The National Dairy Council/DMI (Australia), Deakin University and the Liggins Institute.

REFERENCES

1. Janssen I, Heymsfield SB, Ross R. Low relative skeletal muscle mass (sarcopenia) in older persons is associated with functional impairment and physical disability. *J Am Geriatr Soc.* (2002) 50:889–96. doi: 10.1046/j.1532-5415.2002.50216.x
2. Narici MV, Maganaris CN, Reeves ND, Capodaglio P. Effect of aging on human muscle architecture. *J Appl Physiol.* (2003) 95:2229–34. doi: 10.1152/japplphysiol.00433.2003
3. Suetta C, Andersen JL, Dalgas U, Berget J, Koskinen S, Aagaard P, et al. Resistance training induces qualitative changes in muscle morphology, muscle architecture, and muscle function in elderly postoperative patients. *J Appl Physiol.* (2008) 105:180–6. doi: 10.1152/japplphysiol.01354.2007
4. Yang Y, Breen L, Burd NA, Hector AJ, Churchward-Venne TA, Josse AR, et al. Resistance exercise enhances myofibrillar protein synthesis with graded intakes of whey protein in older men. *Br J Nutr.* (2012) 108:1780–8. doi: 10.1017/S0007114511007422
5. Mitchell CJ, D'Souza RF, Mitchell SM, Figueiredo VC, Miller BF, Hamilton KL, et al. Impact of dairy protein during limb immobilization and recovery on muscle size and protein synthesis; a randomized controlled trial. *J Appl Physiol.* (2017) 124:717–28. doi: 10.1152/japplphysiol.00803.2017
6. Cuthbertson D, Smith K, Babraj J, Leese G, Waddell T, Atherton P, et al. Anabolic signaling deficits underlie amino acid resistance of wasting, aging muscle. *FASEB J.* (2005) 19:422–4. doi: 10.1096/fj.04-2640fje
7. Ebert MS, Sharp PA. Emerging roles for natural microRNA sponges. *Curr Biol.* (2010) 20:R858–R861. doi: 10.1016/j.cub.2010.08.052
8. D'Souza RF, Markworth JF, Aasen KM, Zeng N, Cameron-Smith D, Mitchell CJ. Acute resistance exercise modulates microRNA expression profiles: Combined tissue and circulatory targeted analyses. *PLoS ONE.* (2017) 12:e0181594. doi: 10.1371/journal.pone.0181594
9. Zacharewicz E, Della Gatta P, Reynolds J, Garnham A, Crowley T, Russell AP, et al. Identification of microRNAs linked to regulators of muscle protein synthesis and regeneration in young and old skeletal muscle. *PLoS ONE.* (2014) 9:e114009. doi: 10.1371/journal.pone.0114009
10. Margolis LM, Rivas DA. Potential role of microRNA in the anabolic capacity of skeletal muscle with aging. *Exerc Sport Sci Rev.* (2018) 46:86–91. doi: 10.1249/JES.0000000000000147
11. Elia L, Contu R, Quintavalle M, Varrone F, Chimenti C, Russo MA, et al. Reciprocal regulation of microRNA-1 and insulin-like growth factor-1 signal transduction cascade in cardiac and skeletal muscle in physiological and pathological conditions. *Circulation.* (2009) 120:2377–85. doi: 10.1161/CIRCULATIONAHA.109.879429
12. Rivas DA, Lessard SJ, Rice NP, Lustgarten MS, So K, Goodyear LJ, et al. Diminished skeletal muscle microRNA expression with aging is associated with attenuated muscle plasticity and inhibition of IGF-1 signaling. *FASEB J.* (2014) 28:4133–47. doi: 10.1096/fj.14-254490
13. Drummond MJ, McCarthy JJ, Fry CS, Esser KA, Rasmussen BB. Aging differentially affects human skeletal muscle microRNA expression at rest and after an anabolic stimulus of resistance exercise and essential amino acids. *Am J Physiol Endocrinol Metab.* (2008) 295:E1333–40. doi: 10.1152/ajpendo.90562.2008
14. Camera DM, Ong JN, Coffey VG, Hawley JA. Selective modulation of microRNA expression with protein ingestion following concurrent resistance and endurance exercise in human skeletal muscle. *Front Physiol.* (2016) 7:87. doi: 10.3389/fphys.2016.00087
15. D'Souza RF, Markworth JF, Figueiredo VC, Della Gatta PA, Petersen AC, Mitchell CJ, et al. Dose-dependent increases in p70S6K phosphorylation and intramuscular branched-chain amino acids in older men following resistance exercise and protein intake. *Physiol Rep.* (2014) 2:e12112. doi: 10.14814/phy2.12112

16. Reynolds JM, Gordon TJ, Robergs RA. Prediction of one repetition maximum strength from multiple repetition maximum testing and anthropometry. *J Strength Conditioning Res.* (2006) 20:584–92. doi: 10.1519/00124278-200608000-00020
17. Knapik JJ, Staab JS, Harman EA. Validity of an anthropometric estimate of thigh muscle cross-sectional area. *Med Sci Sports Exerc.* (1996) 28:1523–30. doi: 10.1097/00005768-199612000-00013
18. Witard OC, Jackman SR, Breen L, Smith K, Selby A, Tipton KD. Myofibrillar muscle protein synthesis rates subsequent to a meal in response to increasing doses of whey protein at rest and after resistance exercise. *Am J Clin Nutr.* (2014) 99:86–95. doi: 10.3945/ajcn.112.055517
19. Bjørnsen T, Wernbom M, Løvstad AT, Paulsen G, D'Souza RF, Cameron-Smith D, et al. Delayed myonuclear addition, myofiber hypertrophy and increases in strength with high-frequency low-load blood flow restricted training to volitional failure. *J Appl Physiol.* (2018) 126:578–92. doi: 10.1152/japplphysiol.00397.2018
20. Vandesompele J, De Preter K, Pattyn F, Poppe B, Van Roy N, De Paepe A, et al. Accurate normalization of real-time quantitative RT-PCR data by geometric averaging of multiple internal control genes. *Genome Biol.* (2002) 3:1. doi: 10.1186/gb-2002-3-7-research0034
21. Livak KJ, Schmittgen TD. Analysis of relative gene expression data using real-time quantitative PCR and the 2- ΔΔCT method. *Methods.* (2001) 25:402–8. doi: 10.1006/meth.2001.1262
22. Karlsson HK, Nilsson P-A, Nilsson J, Chibalin AV, Zierath JR, Blomstrand E. Branched-chain amino acids increase p70S6k phosphorylation in human skeletal muscle after resistance exercise. (2004). *Am J Physiol Endocrinol Metab.* 287:E1–7. doi: 10.1152/ajpendo.00430.2003
23. D'Souza RF, Bjørnsen T, Zeng N, Aasen KM, Raastad T, Cameron-Smith D, et al. MicroRNAs in muscle: characterizing the powerlifter phenotype. *Front Physiol.* (2017) 8:383. doi: 10.3389/fphys.2017.00383
24. Mitchell CJ, D'Souza RF, Schierding W, Zeng N, Ramzan F, O'Sullivan JM, et al. Identification of human skeletal muscle miRNA related to strength by high-throughput sequencing. *Physiol Genomics.* (2018) 50:416–24. doi: 10.1152/physiolgenomics.00112.2017
25. D'Souza RF, Zeng N, Poppitt SD, Cameron-Smith D, Mitchell CJ. Circulatory microRNAs are not effective biomarkers of muscle size and function in middle-aged men. *Am J Physiol Cell Physiol.* (2019) 316:C293–8. doi: 10.1152/ajpcell.00395.2018
26. Katsanos CS, Chinkes DL, Paddon-Jones D, Zhang XJ, Aarsland A, Wolfe RR. Whey protein ingestion in elderly persons results in greater muscle protein accrual than ingestion of its constituent essential amino acid content. *Nutr Res.* (2008) 28:651–8. doi: 10.1016/j.nutres.2008.06.007
27. Churchward-Venne TA, Burd NA, Mitchell CJ, West DW, Philp A, Marcotte GR, et al. Supplementation of a suboptimal protein dose with leucine or essential amino acids: effects on myofibrillar protein synthesis at rest and following resistance exercise in men. *J Physiol.* (2012) 590:2751–65. doi: 10.1113/jphysiol.2012.228833
28. Wang K-C, Garmire LX, Young A, Nguyen P, Trinh A, Subramaniam S, et al. Role of microRNA-23b in flow-regulation of Rb phosphorylation and endothelial cell growth. *Proc Natl Acad Sci USA.* (2010) 107:3234–9. doi: 10.1073/pnas.0914825107
29. Muddashetty RS, Nalavadi VC, Gross C, Yao X, Xing L, Laur O, et al. Reversible inhibition of PSD-95 mRNA translation by miR-125a, FMRP phosphorylation, and mGluR signaling. *Mol Cell.* (2011) 42:673–88. doi: 10.1016/j.molcel.2011.05.006
30. D'souza RF, Zeng N, Figueiredo VC, Markworth JF, Durainayagam BR, Mitchell SM, et al. Dairy protein supplementation modulates the human skeletal muscle microRNA response to lower limb immobilization. *Mol Nutr Food Res.* (2018) 62:e1701028. doi: 10.1002/mnfr.201701028
31. D'Souza RF, Zeng N, Markworth JF, Figueiredo VC, Roberts LA, Raastad T, et al. Divergent effects of cold water immersion versus active recovery on skeletal muscle fiber type and angiogenesis in young men. *Am J Physiol Regul Integr Comp Physiol.* (2018) 314:R824–33. doi: 10.1152/ajpregu.00421.2017
32. Yu Z, Wang C, Wang M, Li Z, Casimiro MC, Liu M, et al. A cyclin D1/microRNA 17/20 regulatory feedback loop in control of breast cancer cell proliferation. *J Cell Biol.* (2008) 182:509–17. doi: 10.1083/jcb.200801079
33. Hou J, Wang P, Lin L, Liu X, Ma F, An H, et al. MicroRNA-146a feedback inhibits RIG-I-dependent Type I IFN production in macrophages by targeting TRAF6, IRAK1, and IRAK2. *J Immunol.* (2009) 183:2150–8. doi: 10.4049/jimmunol.0900707
34. Zhao C, Sun G, Li S, Shi Y. A feedback regulatory loop involving microRNA-9 and nuclear receptor TLX in neural stem cell fate determination. *Nat Struct Mol Biol.* (2009) 16:365. doi: 10.1038/nsmb.1576
35. Liu N, Olson EN. MicroRNA regulatory networks in cardiovascular development. *Dev Cell.* (2010) 18:510–25. doi: 10.1016/j.devcel.2010.03.010
36. Pulikkan JA, Dengler V, Peramangalam PS, Zada AAP, Müller-Tidow C, Bohlander SK, et al. Cell-cycle regulator E2F1 and microRNA-223 comprise an autoregulatory negative feedback loop in acute myeloid leukemia. *Blood.* (2010) 115:1768–78. doi: 10.1182/blood-2009-08-240101
37. Gastebois C, Chanon S, Rome S, Durand C, Pelascini E, Jalabert A, et al. Transition from physical activity to inactivity increases skeletal muscle miR-148b content and triggers insulin resistance. *Physiol Rep.* (2016) 4:e12902. doi: 10.14814/phy2.12902
38. Wang Y, Li J, Kuang D, Wang X, Zhu Y, Xu S, et al. miR-148b-3p functions as a tumor suppressor in GISTs by directly targeting KIT. *Cell Commun Signal.* (2018) 16:16. doi: 10.1186/s12964-018-0228-z
39. Koltai E, Bori Z, Chabert C, Dubouchaud H, Naito H, Machida S, et al. SIRT1 may play a crucial role in overload-induced hypertrophy of skeletal muscle. *J Physiol.* (2017) 595:3361–76. doi: 10.1113/JP2 73774
40. Jensen J, Rustad PI, Kolnes AJ, Lai Y-C. The role of skeletal muscle glycogen breakdown for regulation of insulin sensitivity by exercise. *Front Physiol.* (2011) 2:112. doi: 10.3389/fphys.2011.00112

11

The Impact of Pre-Sleep Protein Ingestion on the Skeletal Muscle Adaptive Response to Exercise in Humans

Tim Snijders, Jorn Trommelen, Imre W. K. Kouw, Andrew M. Holwerda, Lex B. Verdijk and Luc J. C. van Loon*

Department of Human Biology, NUTRIM School of Nutrition and Translational Research in Metabolism, Maastricht University Medical Centre (MUMC+), Maastricht, Netherlands

***Correspondence:**
Tim Snijders
tim.snijders@maastrichtuniversity.nl

This review provides an update on recent research assessing the effect of pre-sleep protein ingestion on muscle protein synthesis rates during overnight sleep and the skeletal muscle adaptive response to exercise training. Protein ingested prior to sleep is effectively digested and absorbed during overnight sleep, thereby increasing overnight muscle protein synthesis rates. Protein consumption prior to sleep does not appear to reduce appetite during breakfast the following day and does not change resting energy expenditure. When applied over a prolonged period of resistance-type exercise training, pre-sleep protein supplementation has a beneficial effect on the increase in muscle mass and strength. Protein ingestion before sleep is hypothesized to represent an effective nutritional strategy to preserve muscle mass in the elderly, especially when combined with physical activity or muscle contraction by means of neuromuscular electrical stimulation. In conclusion, protein ingestion prior to sleep is an effective interventional strategy to increase muscle protein synthesis rates during overnight sleep and can be applied to support the skeletal muscle adaptive response to resistance-type exercise training.

Keywords: protein, exercise, satiety, amino acids, aging

INTRODUCTION

Resistance-type exercise training represents a potent stimulus to increase skeletal muscle mass and strength [see (1) for an extensive review]. Muscle protein synthesis as well as breakdown rates, are effectively stimulated following a single session of resistance type exercise, albeit breakdown rates are stimulated to a lesser extent (2, 3). However, in the absence of protein intake, the net muscle protein balance will remain negative (2, 3). Dietary protein intake shortly after exercise inhibits exercise-induced muscle protein breakdown and further augments the exercise-induced increase in muscle protein synthesis rate, resulting in a (more) positive post-exercise muscle protein balance. This synergistic effect between nutrition and exercise on the post-exercise muscle protein synthetic response has been well-established and forms an essential principle to enable the skeletal muscle adaptive response to more prolonged exercise training (4, 5). The muscle protein synthetic response following exercise has been observed to be modifiable to the type, amount, distribution, and timing of protein ingestion [see (6–8) for extensive reviews]. Recently, the concept of protein ingestion prior to sleep has been introduced as an additional meal moment to increase daily protein intake and increase overnight protein balance, which could further maximize the skeletal muscle adaptive response. In this review we will provide an update on the recent research investigating the impact of pre-sleep protein ingestion with and without exercise (training) on the muscle protein synthetic response in both young and older individuals.

PRE-SLEEP PROTEIN DIGESTION AND ABSORPTION

In recent years, food ingestion prior to sleep has received considerable media attention. It has previously been assumed that food intake should be limited or avoided in the hours close to night-time sleep as it would have a negative impact on body composition and overall health, increasing the risk for cardiovascular diseases, such as obesity and diabetes [see also (9) for an extensive review]. Although this may be true when food is ingested in large quantities at night, more recent studies investigating the impact of smaller and single macronutrient (i.e., protein) foods have demonstrated positive physiological outcomes in humans. In addition, the benefits of night-time supply of nutrients for overnight recovery have been suggested to support muscle reconditioning and improve physical performance in athletes. Over the past decade, we have performed a considerable number of *in vivo* human studies to provide insight on the impact of pre-sleep protein ingestion on (post-exercise) overnight muscle protein synthesis in both young and older adults (10–18). **Figure 1** provides a comprehensive overview of the studies performed in our laboratory, which will be discussed in more detail throughout this review.

In the study by Groen et al. (10) we demonstrated for the first time that administration of 40 g (intrinsically labeled) protein during sleep (via a nasogastric tube) is normally digested and absorbed in older adults, resulting in an increase in overnight muscle protein synthesis rates. This indicates that the gut functions appropriately at night and suggests that nocturnal protein administration may be applied as a nutritional strategy to increase muscle protein synthesis rates during overnight sleep. Although intragastric protein feeding during sleep may represent a feasible intervention strategy in certain clinical populations, it is far from being practical in a day-to-day situation in healthy individuals. In more recent studies by our laboratory, we have demonstrated that the ingestion of a single bolus of protein prior to sleep (ranging from 20 to 40 g protein) also leads to appropriate protein digestion and amino acid absorption during subsequent overnight sleep in both young (18) and healthy older adults (13, 16). In addition, our studies have shown no effect of pre-sleep protein ingestion on sleep onset latency, sleep quality, and/or next morning appetite in both young and older individuals (13, 18). As such, pre-sleep protein ingestion can be considered as an additional meal moment to increase total daily protein intake and improve overnight protein balance.

PRE-SLEEP PROTEIN AND OVERNIGHT RECOVERY

The concept of pre-sleep protein ingestion has been introduced as a way to increase overnight muscle protein synthesis rates when exercise is performed prior to bed-time. This is of particular relevance as previous research has shown that overnight muscle protein synthesis rates tend to be lower than those typically observed in the morning following an overnight fast (19). In the study by Res et al. (11) recreational athletes performed a single bout of resistance-type exercise in the evening. To maximize the immediate muscle protein synthetic response following exercise, all participants ingested 60 g of carbohydrates and 20 g of whey protein immediately after exercise. In addition, subjects were provided with either 40 g of casein protein or a placebo drink (water) immediately prior to sleep. Muscle protein synthesis rates were ~22% higher during overnight sleep when protein was consumed prior to sleep compared to participants ingesting the placebo drink (11). In contrast, in a more recent study from our laboratory we observed no significant increase in overnight myofibrillar protein synthesis rates in response to a single exercise session performed in the evening immediately followed by a post-exercise recovery drink (containing 20 g milk protein) and 30 g of casein protein with or without 2 g of crystalline leucine or placebo (water) prior to sleep (18). The apparent discrepancy between study outcomes may be explained by the more moderate amount of protein (30 g in the second study as opposed to 40 g protein in the first study) that was ingested prior to sleep. This may indicate that a dose-response relationship exists with pre-sleep protein ingestion, which is not in line with the immediate post-exercise recovery period (generally assessed over a relatively short 3–4 h recovery period as compared to a more prolonged 7.5 h overnight recovery period) during which 20 g has been reported to be sufficient to maximize muscle protein synthesis rates following a single bout of exercise in young healthy males (20, 21). Nevertheless, we have clearly shown that resistance-type exercise augments the overnight skeletal muscle adaptive response, with myofibrillar muscle protein synthesis rates being 37% higher when 30 g of pre-sleep protein (casein) ingestion is combined with a single session of resistance type exercise in the evening compared with pre-sleep protein ingestion only (14). Furthermore, the application of intrinsically labeled pre-sleep protein allowed us to demonstrate that 76% more of the pre-sleep protein derived amino acids were incorporated in myofibrillar protein when earlier that evening individuals engaged in a single resistance exercise session (14). Although the optimal dosage for pre-sleep protein ingestion remains to be determined, it has become clear that prior physical activity (e.g., resistance exercise) increases the efficiency by which pre-sleep protein derived amino acids are used in *de novo* muscle protein synthesis during overnight sleep.

Pre-sleep protein ingestion has been hypothesized to be a viable option to increase dietary protein intake to attenuate the loss of muscle mass with aging in older adults (5). In a recent study, we provided 40 g of casein protein prior to sleep in older adults and demonstrated and increase in overnight muscle protein synthesis rates (17). In this study, 40 g of casein ingested prior to sleep was compared with 20 g of casein with and without additional 1.5 g crystalline leucine, or a placebo. Ingestion of 20 g protein, as opposed to 40 g, did not result in a significant increase in overnight muscle protein synthesis rates when compared to the placebo condition. These results appear to be in line

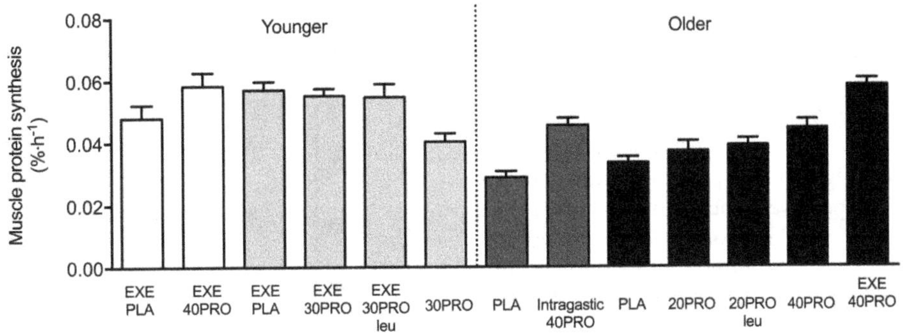

FIGURE 1 | Overview of previous published overnight muscle protein synthesis studies at Maastricht University. EXE, single bout of resistance exercise; PLA, placebo; PRO, protein; Intragastic, Protein ingestion via intragastric tube; Leu, enriched with free crystalline leucine. White [Res et al. (11)] and light gray [Trommelen et al. (14, 18)] bars indicate study results from healthy young men. Dark gray [Groen et al. (10)] and black [Kouw et al. (17) and Holwerda et al. (13)] bars indicate study results from healthy older men.

with studies performed during daytime demonstrating that the ingestion of a meal-like amount of protein (20 g) increases muscle protein synthesis rates by ~75% in healthy young individuals, whereas in an older population ~40 g protein is prerequisite to allow a similar rise in muscle protein synthesis rates during the postprandial period (17). Besides ingesting larger amounts of protein, fortifying lower amounts of protein with free leucine has been reported to further stimulate postprandial muscle protein synthesis rates in older adults (22–24). However, in the study by Kouw et al. (17), no differences in the post-prandial overnight muscle protein synthetic response were observed between 20 g casein protein ingested with or without additional free leucine (1.5 g). In this publication, we speculated that "*the absence of a stimulating effect after leucine co-ingestion could be attributed to the absence of a robust insulin response during the overnight period, the lack of sufficient amino acids as precursors for muscle protein synthesis during the relatively long overnight period, or simply that the stimulating properties of leucine are less evident during sleep*" (17). It is important to note that this study was performed in healthy older adults, whether more robust beneficial effects on overnight muscle protein synthesis can be observed when (small amounts of) protein is consumed prior to sleep by individuals with a relative low habitual dietary protein intake, like frail elderly, and/or more compromised clinical population, remains to be established. Furthermore, these studies were performed in the absence of performing physical activity or exercise in close proximity to the protein ingestion.

As already discussed, physical activity/exercise is known to further augment the postprandial rise in muscle protein synthesis in both young and older adults (25–27). In the study of Holwerda et al. (13) we showed that protein (40 g of casein) ingestion prior to sleep results in a positive overnight whole body protein balance in older adults. More importantly, overnight muscle protein synthesis rates were significantly higher when older adults performed a single exercise session earlier that evening. Overall, the existing studies suggest that pre-sleep protein consumption may represent an effective intervention to maintain muscle mass by increasing muscle protein synthesis rates during overnight sleep. In older and/or more clinically compromised populations the ingestion of a large bolus (40 g) of protein may not be feasible or practical, however, the study by Holwerda et al. (13) suggests that being physically active/performing exercise earlier that day may increase the beneficial effects when ingesting smaller amount of protein (<40 g) prior to sleep. During long periods of bed rest (e.g., due to illness or injury), however, physical activity can be severely restricted. The muscle protein synthetic response to protein ingestion is significantly reduced in response to physical inactivity (see (28) for extensive review). Neuromuscular electrical stimulation (NMES) represents an exercise mimetic that evokes muscle contractions and has been hypothesized to be an effective alternative to performing physical activity or exercise to attenuated disuse related anabolic resistance. Muscle protein synthesis rates have been reported to increase when NMES is performed in the morning after an overnight fast (29). More importantly, we have shown that NMES application prior to pre-sleep protein ingestion stimulates muscle protein synthesis during overnight sleep in healthy older adults (16). As such, the application of NMES with pre-sleep protein ingestion may represent a viable strategy to optimize overnight muscle protein balance and may be of significant clinical relevance to preserve skeletal muscle mass in bed-ridden, hospitalized patients.

In all our work in which we assessed the impact of pre-sleep protein ingestion on overnight muscle protein synthesis, participants received a pre-specified absolute amount of protein to ingest prior to sleep. However, total daily protein intake recommendations such as the Recommended Dietary Allowance (RDA) are often expressed relative to bodyweight, i.e., in g/kg. More recently, per-meal protein recommendations have also been expressed relative to bodyweight and lean body mass (30). Thus far, only one study has directly investigated the impact of lean body mass on the muscle protein synthetic response to protein ingestion. Macnaughton et al. (31) assessed the impact of whey protein ingestion (20 or 40 g) on (day-time) post-exercise muscle protein synthesis between young adults with a relative low compared with a high amount of fat free mass (~59 vs. 77 kg fat free mass, respectively). Interestingly, no differences in post-exercise muscle protein synthesis rates after the ingestion of 20 or

40 g of whey protein were observed between groups. These data suggest that lean body mass is not a strong modulator of protein requirements during the first couple of hours of post-exercise recovery. To provide further insight into the relation between relative protein intake (g/kg body weight) and the subsequent postprandial response, we have collapsed our data sets on previously performed overnight muscle protein synthesis studies ($n = 99$). Here we show a positive association between protein intake (g/kg body weight, or g/kg lean body mass) and overnight muscle protein synthesis rates (**Figures 2A,B**). This positive association with relative protein intake (g/kg) was also observed when only analyzing data from subjects who did not perform prior resistance-type exercise (**Supplemental Figure 1A**, $n = 56$), and those that did perform prior exercise (**Supplemental Figure 1B**, $n = 43$). Furthermore, similar trends were observed for both young (**Supplemental Figure 1C**, $n = 44$), and older (**Supplemental Figure 1D**, $n = 55$) adults separately. We speculate that pre-sleep protein requirements may be personalized based on bodyweight or lean body mass, however, more direct experimental comparisons are warranted to further corroborate this speculation.

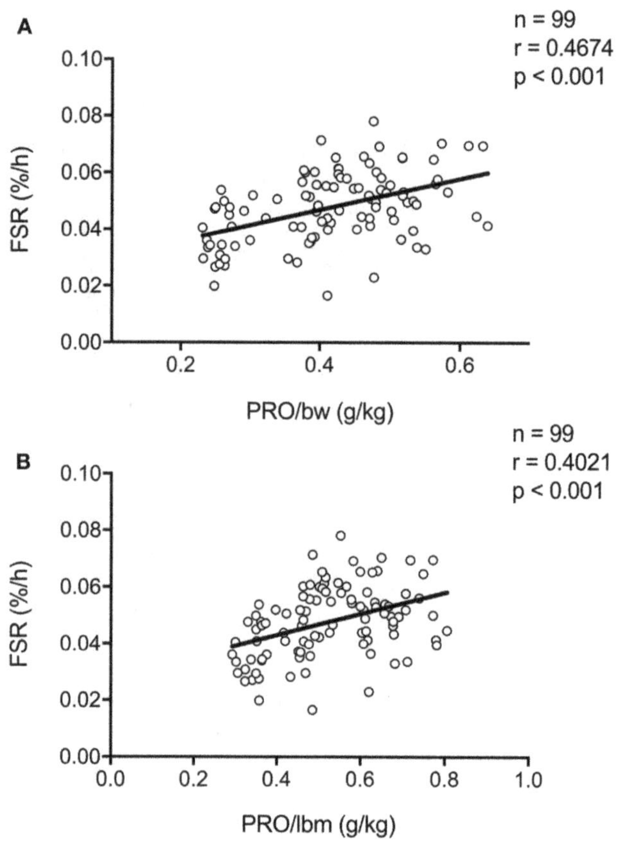

FIGURE 2 | Scatter plot of the correlation between overnight (mixed muscle or myofibrillar) protein fractional synthetic rate (FSR) as calculated based intravenous infusion of L-[ring-$^{2}H_{5}$]_phenylalanine and **(A)** protein ingested per kilogram bodyweight (BW) or **(B)** protein ingested per kilogram lean body mass (LBM) in humans. Collapsed data set from previously published studies (11, 13, 14, 17, 18).

PRE-SLEEP PROTEIN INGESTION AND APPETITE

A number of studies have recently assessed whether ingestion of a relative low-energy beverage prior to sleep could alter appetite, and/or cardio-metabolic risk factors the following morning in various populations. In a randomized, double-blind, cross-over study, Madzima et al. (32) compared the ingestion of various pre-sleep drinks containing different macronutrients (carbohydrate vs. protein) and different protein compositions (whey vs. casein vs. 50% blend) on satiety and resting energy expenditure on the following morning in healthy young men. In this study pre-sleep beverage consumption did not modulate satiety assessed the following morning (32). Interestingly, the authors did show that, irrespective of beverage composition, consumption of a pre-sleep caloric drink increased resting energy expenditure, without inhibiting fat oxidation, assessed the next morning when compared with a non-caloric placebo in healthy young men (32). These findings, together with an overnight increase in muscle protein synthesis rates following pre sleep protein ingestion (10, 11, 13, 14, 16–18), imply that protein ingestion prior to sleep does not appear to have negative effect on resting energy expenditure and fat metabolism the next morning and may be a viable option to support overnight muscle reconditioning and, as such, provide a competitive advantage to healthy young individuals/athletes. However, contrasting results have been reported by Kinsey et al. (33) applying the same research protocol and beverage composition in overweight and obese women. This study showed that the ingestion of a pre-sleep drink, irrespective of macronutrient composition, led to a greater subjective feeling of satiety the next morning. In addition, the morning following the nighttime ingestion of carbohydrate-only or protein-only pre-sleep beverages resulted in small but significant increases in resting insulin concentrations and subsequent an indicator of insulin resistance (assessed by Homeostatic Model Assessment of Insulin Resistance; HOMA-IR) (33). This indicates that in sedentary overweight and obese women ingestion of carbohydrate and/or protein beverages prior to sleep may elicit unfavorable metabolic effects. Interestingly though, the same research group has shown that these negative effects are completely abolished in overweight and obese subjects when protein and/or carbohydrate ingestion prior to sleep is combined with prolonged exercise training (34). But to truly assess whether the favorable (or absence of potential unfavorable) effects of pre-sleep protein ingestion *per se* on resting energy expenditure, glucose/fat metabolism and satiety the next morning, as observed in healthy young men (32), is also present in obese individuals, a comparison with a non-nutritive placebo would be prerequisite under well-standardized condition with regards to food intake during the day. Therefore, the same authors performed a cross-over follow-up study comparing pre-sleep protein ingestion (30 g protein) with a non-nutritive placebo in obese men during a period of well-controlled dietary intake. Here they showed that pre-sleep protein intake did not affect fat or glucose metabolism, resting energy expenditure, and did not suppress appetite the following morning in young obese men compared with a non-nutritive placebo. (35). Altogether, these studies indicate no direct negative effects on next morning appetite and resting energy metabolism when a low-energy, single nutrient/protein beverage is consumed prior to sleep. However, it is important to note that the impact of pre-sleep protein consumption on resting metabolic rate *during* overnight sleep remains to be established.

PROTEIN INTAKE DISTRIBUTION

Distribution of protein intake over the day has been showed to be an important factor to maximize daily muscle protein synthesis rates and, as such, to optimize muscle reconditioning. A balanced distribution of daily protein intake over three main meals has been shown to result in higher 24 h muscle protein synthesis rates when compared with an unbalanced distribution, in which most protein is consumed at dinner (36). In support, a more balanced pattern of protein intake during 12 h of post-exercise recovery has been reported to result in higher muscle protein synthesis rates when compared with "*the ingestion of the same total amount of protein provided in less frequent but larger amounts (40 g every 6 h), or in more frequent, smaller amounts (20 g every 1.5 h)*" (37). Based on such findings, it is currently recommended to consume with each main meal at least 20 g protein, with no more than 4–5 h between meals to support muscle protein synthesis (8). However, ingestion of an additional post-exercise and/or pre-sleep protein meal may modulate the anabolic response to ingestion of the main meals. For example, previous work has suggested that a continuous supply of exogenous amino acids via intravenous infusion may actually blunt the initial rise in muscle protein synthesis rates (38). However, whether protein ingestion following exercise and/or prior to sleep influences the muscle protein synthetic response to the ingestion of subsequent protein-rich meals remains largely ambiguous. We have started to address this issue in a recent study by investigating whether protein ingestion immediately following exercise and before subsequent sleep could influence the muscle protein synthetic response to the consumption of a meal-like amount of protein the following morning (15). In this study, we demonstrated that the consumption of ample amounts of protein (60 g whey) before sleep did not alter post-prandial muscle protein synthesis rates to the following morning (15). In other words, these data suggest that the protein ingested during every meal signifies an distinctive opportunity to stimulate muscle protein synthesis and that subsequent rises in post-prandial muscle protein synthesis to each meal may be additive. This is relevant for the athletic population who usually consume more than 1.2 g protein kg bodyweight^{-1} day^{-1}, with the majority of protein ingested during the three main meals, and only a small amount of protein ingested as an evening snack (39). Despite the relatively high amount of protein ingested earlier in the day, pre-sleep protein ingestion would presumably still provide an anabolic stimulus on overnight muscle protein synthesis rates, thereby enhancing daily muscle tissue re-conditioning (8).

LONG TERM EFFECT OF PRE-SLEEP PROTEIN INGESTION

The more long-term effects of pre-sleep protein ingestion on skeletal muscle conditioning has also been assessed in healthy young men during a 12-week resistance type exercise training program. In this study we showed a greater increase in skeletal muscle mass and strength when participants ingested 27.5 g protein (50% casein + 50% casein hydrolysate) compared with a non-protein placebo prior to sleep (on both training as well as non-training days) during 12 weeks resistance type exercise training in healthy young men (12). These results provide evidence that ingesting a moderate amount (~30 g) of protein prior to sleep represents an effective intervention strategy to augment gains in skeletal muscle mass and strength during a resistance-type exercise training program in young men. However, it is important to note that in this study the pre-sleep protein supplementation was compared with a non-protein placebo, and not to protein supplementation at other time points. Whether pre-sleep protein ingestion has surplus benefits compared with protein supplemented at other time points throughout the day remains to be established. It has been hypothesized that pre-sleep protein supplementation increases the gains in muscle mass during prolonged exercise training mainly as a function of increased total protein intake, rather than by its specific timing of protein intake thereby improving protein intake distribution (8, 40). As meta-analyses data are required to clearly demonstrate that protein supplementation can augment gains in lean tissue mass and strength during prolonged resistance-type exercise training (41), it appears unlikely that a differential effect of protein supplement timing on the gains in muscle mass and/or strength can be detected in a longitudinal study design. In support, a recent study reported no statistical significant difference in fat-free mass gains when whey protein was supplemented in the evening when compared to protein supplemented in the morning (42). Nonetheless, the observed increase in fat-free mass was numerically greater when protein was ingested in the evening compared with the morning (+1.2 kg vs. +0.4 kg, respectively), leading the authors to speculate that the study might have been underpowered to significantly detect a relevant difference. In line, Joy et al. (43) observed no differences in muscle mass gains following 10 wks of resistance type exercise training between nighttime or daytime casein protein supplementation (35 g) in healthy young men. Again, however, no firm conclusion can be drawn from this study due to its limited sample size, as also acknowledged by the authors. To obtain insight in the required sample size for such work, we performed an *a posteriori* sample size calculation based on our previous work (12). With an alpha level set at 0.05 and with a power of 80%, it would require 24 healthy young volunteers in both the placebo and pre-sleep protein treatment to detect a hypertrophic effect of additional pre-sleep protein ingestion. Our calculations reveal that it would require substantially more young adults in both groups to detect a potential superior hypertrophic effect of pre-sleep protein ingestion compared to protein ingestion earlier in the day.

Although pre-sleep protein ingestion has been demonstrated to enhance the gains in skeletal muscle mass and strength during resistance-type exercise training in young men (12), this does not appear the case in older adults (44). In a recently published study, we reported no beneficial effect of protein ingestion (20 g whey + 1 g leucine) immediately after exercise and prior to sleep on the increase in skeletal muscle mass and strength during 12 weeks of resistance-type exercise training in healthy older men (44). Age-related factors, like habitual physical activity level, lower absolute workload, and the prevalence of anabolic resistance may explain the discrepant findings on the surplus effect of pre-sleep protein consumption on the muscle mass and strength gains following resistance exercise training between young and older adults. Overall, more sufficiently powered studies are warranted to investigate whether pre-sleep protein intake can augment gains in muscle mass and strength in response to long-term exercise training in general and it would be of great interest to assess its efficacy in specifically more clinically compromised older populations. Thus, far only one study has assessed and showed a positive impact of pre-sleep protein ingestion outside the laboratory (45). Results from this study suggest an accelerated recovery in the first days after a soccer match when protein was ingested prior to sleep following an evening soccer match in young adults (45). Clearly more research is required to further establish the true impact pre-sleep protein ingestion may have on muscle reconditioning and recovery in more applied setting of sports performance. Finally, little is known on the short as well as long-term effects of pre-sleep protein intake on subsequent muscle reconditioning in response to more intermittent and endurance-type exercise training.

CONCLUSIONS

Protein ingested prior to sleep is effectively digested and absorbed during sleep, thereby increasing plasma amino acid availability and stimulating muscle protein synthesis during overnight sleep in both young and old. When pre-sleep protein intake is combined with exercise performed the same evening, overnight muscle protein synthesis rates will be further increased. Protein ingestion prior to sleep can be applied in combination with resistance type exercise training to further augment the gains in muscle mass and strength when compared to no protein supplementation. However, whether this beneficial effect on pre-sleep protein ingestion on muscle mass and strength gain during resistance-type exercise training are due to an increased total protein intake rather than by its specific timing remains elusive, and warrants further research. Protein ingestion before sleep has been hypothesized to represent an effective nutritional strategy to increase daily protein intake and, as such, to attenuate muscle mass loss in hospitalized older adults. In more clinically compromised older populations the combination with exercise or exercise mimetics (such as NMES) may further increase the efficacy of pre-sleep protein ingestion to improve overnight muscle protein balance.

AUTHOR CONTRIBUTIONS

TS, JT, and LvL drafted the manuscript. TS and JT prepared all the figures. IK, AH, and LV critically reviewed and revised the manuscript for important intellectual content. All authors contributed to manuscript revision, read, and approved the submitted version.

SUPPLEMENTARY MATERIAL

Supplemental Figure 1 | Pearson correlation between (mixed muscle or myofibrillar) overnight protein fractional synthetic rate (FSR) as calculated based upon intravenous infusion of L-[ring-$^2H_5$]-phenylalanine and protein consumption prior to sleep per kilogram bodyweight (BW) for **(A)** young and older adults in rest **(B)** young adults both in rest and following a single resistance exercise session **(C)** in young and older adults following a single resistance exercise session **(D)** older adults both in rest and following a single resistance exercise session. Collapsed data set from previously published studies (11, 13, 14, 17, 18).

REFERENCES

1. McGlory C, Phillips SM. Exercise and the regulation of skeletal muscle hypertrophy. *Prog Mol Biol Transl Sci.* (2015) 135:153–73. doi: 10.1016/bs.pmbts.2015.06.018
2. Biolo G, Maggi SP, Williams BD, Tipton KD, Wolfe RR. Increased rates of muscle protein turnover and amino acid transport after resistance exercise in humans. *Am J Physiol.* (1995) 268:E514–520. doi: 10.1152/ajpendo.1995.268.3.E514
3. Phillips SM, Tipton KD, Ferrando AA, Wolfe RR. Resistance training reduces the acute exercise-induced increase in muscle protein turnover. *Am J Physiol.* (1999) 276:E118–24. doi: 10.1152/ajpendo.1999.276.1.E118
4. Burd NA, Tang JE, Moore DR, Phillips SM. Exercise training and protein metabolism: influences of contraction, protein intake, and sex-based differences. *J Appl Physiol.* (2009) 106:1692–701. doi: 10.1152/japplphysiol.91351.2008
5. Wall BT, Cermak NM, van Loon LJ. Dietary protein considerations to support active aging. *Sports Med.* (2014) 44(Suppl. 2):S185–94. doi: 10.1007/s40279-014-0258-7
6. Morton RW, McGlory C, Phillips SM. Nutritional interventions to augment resistance training-induced skeletal muscle hypertrophy. *Front Physiol.* (2015) 6:245. doi: 10.3389/fphys.2015.00245
7. Wall BT, Morton JP, van Loon LJ. Strategies to maintain skeletal muscle mass in the injured athlete: nutritional considerations and exercise mimetics. *Eur J Sport Sci.* (2015) 15:53–62. doi: 10.1080/17461391.2014.936326
8. Trommelen J, van Loon LJ. Pre-sleep protein ingestion to improve the skeletal muscle adaptive response to exercise training. *Nutrients.* (2016) 8:E763. doi: 10.3390/nu8120763
9. Kinsey AW, Ormsbee MJ. The health impact of nighttime eating: old and new perspectives. *Nutrients.* (2015) 7:2648–62. doi: 10.3390/nu7042648
10. Groen BB, Res PT, Pennings B, Hertle E, Senden JM, Saris WH, et al. Intragastric protein administration stimulates overnight muscle protein synthesis in elderly men. *Am J Physiol Endocrinol Metab.* (2012) 302:E52–60. doi: 10.1152/ajpendo.00321.2011
11. Res PT, Groen B, Pennings B, Beelen M, Wallis GA, Gijsen AP, et al. Protein ingestion before sleep improves postexercise overnight recovery.

Med Sci Sports Exerc. (2012) 44:1560–9. doi: 10.1249/MSS.0b013e31824cc363
12. Snijders T, Res PT, Smeets JS, van Vliet S, van Kranenburg J, Maase K, et al. Protein ingestion before sleep increases muscle mass and strength gains during prolonged resistance-type exercise training in healthy young men. *J Nutr.* (2015) 145:1178–84. doi: 10.3945/jn.114.208371
13. Holwerda AM, Kouw IW, Trommelen J, Halson SL, Wodzig WK, Verdijk LB, et al. Physical activity performed in the evening increases the overnight muscle protein synthetic response to presleep protein ingestion in older men. *J Nutr.* (2016) 146:1307–14. doi: 10.3945/jn.116.230086
14. Trommelen J, Holwerda AM, Kouw IW, Langer H, Halson SL, Rollo I, et al. Resistance exercise augments postprandial overnight muscle protein synthesis rates. *Med Sci Sports Exerc.* (2016) 48:2517–25. doi: 10.1249/MSS.0000000000001045
15. Wall BT, Burd NA, Franssen R, Gorissen SH, Snijders T, Senden JM, et al. Presleep protein ingestion does not compromise the muscle protein synthetic response to protein ingested the following morning. *Am J Physiol Endocrinol Metab.* (2016) 311:E964–73. doi: 10.1152/ajpendo.00325.2016
16. Dirks ML, Groen BB, Franssen R, van Kranenburg J, van Loon LJ. Neuromuscular electrical stimulation prior to presleep protein feeding stimulates the use of protein-derived amino acids for overnight muscle protein synthesis. *J Appl Physiol.* (2017) 122:20–7. doi: 10.1152/japplphysiol.00331.2016
17. Kouw IW, Holwerda AM, Trommelen J, Kramer IF, Bastiaanse J, Halson SL, et al. Protein ingestion before sleep increases overnight muscle protein synthesis rates in healthy older men: a randomized controlled trial. *J Nutr.* (2017) 147:2252–61. doi: 10.3945/jn.117.254532
18. Trommelen J, Kouw IWK, Holwerda AM, Snijders T, Halson SL, Rollo I, et al. Pre-sleep dietary protein-derived amino acids are incorporated in myofibrillar protein during post-exercise overnight recovery. *Am J Physiol Endocrinol Metab.* (2017) 273:2016. doi: 10.1152/ajpendo.00273.2016
19. Beelen M, Tieland M, Gijsen AP, Vandereyt H, Kies AK, Kuipers H, et al. Coingestion of carbohydrate and protein hydrolysate stimulates muscle protein synthesis during exercise in young men, with no further increase during subsequent overnight recovery. *J Nutr.* (2008) 138:2198–204. doi: 10.3945/jn.108.092924
20. Moore DR, Robinson MJ, Fry JL, Tang JE, Glover EI, Wilkinson SB, et al. Ingested protein dose response of muscle and albumin protein synthesis after resistance exercise in young men. *Am J Clin Nutr.* (2009) 89:161–8. doi: 10.3945/ajcn.2008.26401
21. Witard OC, Jackman SR, Breen L, Smith K, Selby A, Tipton KD. Myofibrillar muscle protein synthesis rates subsequent to a meal in response to increasing doses of whey protein at rest and after resistance exercise. *Am J Clin Nutr.* (2014) 99:86–95. doi: 10.3945/ajcn.112.055517
22. Katsanos CS, Kobayashi H, Sheffield-Moore M, Aarsland A, Wolfe RR. A high proportion of leucine is required for optimal stimulation of the rate of muscle protein synthesis by essential amino acids in the elderly. *Am J Physiol Endocrinol Metab.* (2006) 291:E381–387. doi: 10.1152/ajpendo.00488.2005
23. Rieu I, Balage M, Sornet C, Giraudet C, Pujos E, Grizard J, et al. Leucine supplementation improves muscle protein synthesis in elderly men independently of hyperaminoacidaemia. *J Physiol.* (2006) 575:305–15. doi: 10.1113/jphysiol.2006.110742
24. Wall BT, Hamer HM, de Lange A, Kiskini A, Groen BB, Senden JM, et al. Leucine co-ingestion improves post-prandial muscle protein accretion in elderly men. *Clin Nutr.* (2013) 32:412–9. doi: 10.1016/j.clnu.2012.09.002
25. Pennings B, Koopman R, Beelen M, Senden JM, Saris WH, van Loon LJ. Exercising before protein intake allows for greater use of dietary protein-derived amino acids for de novo muscle protein synthesis in both young and elderly men. *Am J Clin Nutr.* (2011) 93:322–31. doi: 10.3945/ajcn.2010.29649
26. Yang Y, Breen L, Burd NA, Hector AJ, Churchward-Venne TA, Josse AR, et al. Resistance exercise enhances myofibrillar protein synthesis with graded intakes of whey protein in older men. *Br J Nutr.* (2012) 108:1780–8. doi: 10.1017/S0007114511007422
27. Yang Y, Churchward-Venne TA, Burd NA, Breen L, Tarnopolsky MA, Phillips SM. Myofibrillar protein synthesis following ingestion of soy protein isolate at rest and after resistance exercise in elderly men. *Nutr Metab.* (2012) 9:57. doi: 10.1186/1743-7075-9-57
28. Wall BT, Dirks ML, van Loon LJ. Skeletal muscle atrophy during short-term disuse: implications for age-related sarcopenia. *Ageing Res Rev.* (2013) 12:898–906. doi: 10.1016/j.arr.2013.07.003
29. Wall BT, Dirks ML, Verdijk LB, Snijders T, Hansen D, Vranckx P, et al. Neuromuscular electrical stimulation increases muscle protein synthesis in elderly type 2 diabetic men. *Am J Physiol Endocrinol Metab.* (2012) 303:E614–23. doi: 10.1152/ajpendo.00138.2012
30. Moore DR, Churchward-Venne TA, Witard O, Breen L, Burd NA, Tipton KD, et al. Protein ingestion to stimulate myofibrillar protein synthesis requires greater relative protein intakes in healthy older versus younger men. *J Gerontol A Biol Sci Med Sci.* (2015) 70:57–62. doi: 10.1093/gerona/glu103
31. Macnaughton LS, Wardle SL, Witard OC, McGlory C, Hamilton DL, Jeromson S, et al. The response of muscle protein synthesis following whole-body resistance exercise is greater following 40 g than 20 g of ingested whey protein. *Physiol Rep.* (2016) 4:e12893. doi: 10.14814/phy2.12893
32. Madzima TA, Panton LB, Fretti SK, Kinsey AW, Ormsbee MJ. Night-time consumption of protein or carbohydrate results in increased morning resting energy expenditure in active college-aged men. *Br J Nutr.* (2014) 111:71–7. doi: 10.1017/S000711451300192x
33. Kinsey AW, Eddy WR, Madzima TA, Panton LB, Arciero PJ, Kim JS, et al. Influence of night-time protein and carbohydrate intake on appetite and cardiometabolic risk in sedentary overweight and obese women. *Br J Nutr.* (2014) 112:320–7. doi: 10.1017/S0007114514001068
34. Ormsbee MJ, Kinsey AW, Eddy WR, Madzima TA, Arciero PJ, Figueroa A, et al. The influence of nighttime feeding of carbohydrate or protein combined with exercise training on appetite and cardiometabolic risk in young obese women. *Appl Physiol Nutr Metab.* (2015) 40:37–45. doi: 10.1139/apnm-2014-0256
35. Kinsey AW, Cappadona SR, Panton LB, Allman BR, Contreras RJ, Hickner RC, et al. The effect of casein protein prior to sleep on fat metabolism in obese men. *Nutrients.* (2016) 8:E452. doi: 10.3390/nu8080452
36. Mamerow MM, Mettler JA, English KL, Casperson SL, Arentson-Lantz E, Sheffield-Moore M, et al. Dietary protein distribution positively influences 24-h muscle protein synthesis in healthy adults. *J Nutr.* (2014) 144:876–80. doi: 10.3945/jn.113.185280
37. Areta JL, Burke LM, Ross ML, Camera DM, West DW, Broad EM, et al. Timing and distribution of protein ingestion during prolonged recovery from resistance exercise alters myofibrillar protein synthesis. *J Physiol.* (2013) 591:2319–31. doi: 10.1113/jphysiol.2012.244897
38. Bohe J, Low JF, Wolfe RR, Rennie MJ. Latency and duration of stimulation of human muscle protein synthesis during continuous infusion of amino acids. *J Physiol.* (2001) 532:575–9. doi: 10.1111/j.1469-7793.2001.0575f.x
39. Gillen JB, Trommelen J, Wardenaar FC, Brinkmans NY, Versteegen JJ, Jonvik KL, et al. Dietary protein intake and distribution patterns of well-trained dutch athletes. *Int. J. Sport Nutr. Exerc. Metab.* (2016) 27:105–14. doi: 10.1123/ijsnem.2016-0154
40. Reidy PT, Rasmussen BB. Role of ingested amino acids and protein in the promotion of resistance exercise-induced muscle protein anabolism. *J Nutr.* (2016) 146:155–83. doi: 10.3945/jn.114.203208
41. Cermak NM, Res PT, de Groot LC, Saris WH, van Loon LJ. Protein supplementation augments the adaptive response of skeletal muscle to resistance-type exercise training: a meta-analysis. *Am J Clin Nutr.* (2012) 96:1454–64. doi: 10.3945/ajcn.112.037556

42. Antonio J, Ellerbroek A, Peacock C, Silver T. Casein protein supplementation in trained men and women: morning versus evening. *Int J Exerc Sci.* (2017) 10:479–86.
43. Joy JM, Vogel RM, Shane Broughton K, Kudla U, Kerr NY, Davison JM, et al. Daytime and nighttime casein supplements similarly increase muscle size and strength in response to resistance training earlier in the day: a preliminary investigation. *J Int Soc Sports Nutr.* (2018) 15:24. doi: 10.1186/s12970-018-0228-9
44. Holwerda AM, Overkamp M, Paulussen KJM, Smeets JSJ, van Kranenburg J, Backx EMP, et al. Protein supplementation after exercise and before sleep does not further augment muscle mass and strength gains during resistance exercise training in active older men. *J Nutr.* (2018) 148:1723–32. doi: 10.1093/jn/nxy169
45. Abbott W, Brett A, Cockburn E, Clifford T. Presleep casein protein ingestion: acceleration of functional recovery in professional soccer players. *Int J Sports Physiol Perform.* (2018) 11:1–24. doi: 10.1123/ijspp. 2018-0385

12

The Influence of Omega-3 Fatty Acids on Skeletal Muscle Protein Turnover in Health, Disuse and Disease

Chris McGlory[1*], *Philip C. Calder*[2,3] *and Everson A. Nunes*[4]

[1] *School of Kinesiology and Health Studies, Queen's University, Kingston, ON, Canada,* [2] *Human Development and Health, Faculty of Medicine, University of Southampton, Southampton, United Kingdom,* [3] *NIHR Southampton Biomedical Research Centre, University Hospital Southampton NHS Foundation Trust and University of Southampton, Southampton, United Kingdom,* [4] *Department of Physiological Sciences, Federal University of Santa Catarina, Florianópolis, Brazil*

Correspondence:
Chris McGlory
chris.mcglory@queensu.ca

Ingestion of omega-3 fatty acids is known to exert favorable health effects on a number of biological processes such as improved immune profile, enhanced cognition, and optimized neuromuscular function. Recently, data have emerged demonstrating a positive influence of omega-3 fatty acid intake on skeletal muscle. For instance, there are reports of clinically-relevant gains in muscle size and strength in healthy older persons with omega-3 fatty acid intake as well as evidence that omega-3 fatty acid ingestion alleviates the loss of muscle mass and prevents decrements in mitochondrial respiration during periods of muscle-disuse. Cancer cachexia that is characterized by a rapid involuntary loss of lean mass may also be attenuated by omega-3 fatty acid provision. The primary means by which omega-3 fatty acids positively impact skeletal muscle mass is via incorporation of eicosapentaenoic acid (EPA; 20:5*n*−3) and docosahexaenoic acid (DHA; 22:6*n*−3) into membrane phospholipids of the sarcolemma and intracellular organelles. Enrichment of EPA and DHA in these membrane phospholipids is linked to enhanced rates of muscle protein synthesis, decreased expression of factors that regulate muscle protein breakdown, and improved mitochondrial respiration kinetics. However, exactly how incorporation of EPA and DHA into phospholipid membranes alters these processes remains unknown. In this review, we discuss the interaction between omega-3 fatty acid ingestion and skeletal muscle protein turnover in response to nutrient provision in younger and older adults. Additionally, we examine the role of omega-3 fatty acid supplementation in protecting muscle loss during muscle-disuse and in cancer cachexia, and critically evaluate the molecular mechanisms that underpin the phenotypic changes observed in skeletal muscle with omega-3 fatty acid intake.

Keywords: Omega-3 fatty acid, protein synthesis, protein breakdown, skeletal muscle, inflammation

INTRODUCTION

Omega-3 (n-3) polyunsaturated fatty acids are a class of long chain fatty acids reported to have a range of beneficial effects on human health such as improved immune profile, enhanced cognition, blood lipid regulation, and optimized neuromuscular function (1–3). The beneficial impact of omega-3 fatty acid ingestion on health markers is often related to increases in the omega-3 fatty acid content of phospholipids in membranes at the expense of omega-6 fatty acids (1). This shift in the omega-3: omega-6 fatty acid ratio in cell membranes has been shown to induce changes in a multitude of biological processes including the expression of pro- and anti-inflammatory lipid mediators and cytokines (1), gene expression (4), and mitochondrial respiration kinetics (5, 6). As dysregulation of these processes is closely linked with impaired metabolic health (1, 7), omega-3 fatty acid intake could be considered a viable strategy to combat metabolic dysfunction in a variety of settings.

Eicosapentaenoic acid (EPA; 20:5$n-3$) and docosahexaenoic acid (DHA; 22:6$n-3$) are the most studied omega-3 fatty acids and can be found in oily fish and many dietary supplements. EPA and DHA serve as the necessary substrates for the production of anti-inflammatory and inflammation resolving mediators (resolvins, protectins, and maresins) whilst simultaneously inhibiting the transcription of pro-inflammatory genes (1, 4). Current population recommendations for EPA and DHA intake for general health vary from country to country but are typically 250–500 mg/day as a combination of both fatty acids (8). Although humans can endogenously synthesize EPA and DHA from dietary alpha linolenic acid they are considered conditionally essential as the synthesis of EPA and DHA from alpha linolenic acid is limited in humans. Indeed, the conversion of alpha linolenic acid to EPA and DHA in men is estimated to be as low as <8% and <4% respectively, whilst in women it is slightly higher at 21 and 9%, respectively (9). Therefore, dietary or supplemental intake of preformed EPA and DHA intake is necessary to significantly enhance the EPA and DHA content of biological tissues in humans with known significant inter-individual variability (10).

In recent years, there have been a number of reports in cell systems (11, 12), pre-clinical mammalian models (13–15) as well as humans (16–18) demonstrating a positive influence of EPA and DHA intake on skeletal muscle. The notion that EPA and DHA intake may affect skeletal muscle has garnered much attention not only because skeletal muscle mass and strength are important in promoting metabolic health (19) and longevity (20), but are also critical determinants of recovery from situations of accelerated muscle loss (e.g., surgery/intensive care) (21). Yet, the underlying mechanisms by which EPA and DHA intake confer a positive effect on skeletal muscle remain unclear. In this review, we address data related to the interaction between omega-3 fatty acid ingestion and skeletal muscle anabolism with a specific emphasis on muscle protein turnover kinetics and translational control. Additionally, we examine the potential efficacy of omega-3 fatty acid supplementation to counteract muscle loss during periods of muscle-disuse, cancer cachexia, as well as the relevance of inflammatory signaling events. Given the focused nature of this review we apologize in advance to respected colleagues whose work we were unable to address and instead refer the interested reader to excellent commentaries on this topic (22–24).

Regulation of Skeletal Muscle Mass

In healthy, normal-weight individuals, skeletal muscle comprises ~45% of body mass and plays a fundamental role in locomotion, respiration, amino acid storage, glycemic control, and the ability to sustain independent living with aging (19). Understanding the factors that regulate skeletal muscle mass is therefore critical for the development of strategies to support optimal health across the lifespan. The size and composition of skeletal muscle is determined by changes in rates of muscle protein synthesis (MPS) relative to those of muscle protein breakdown. In the rested, fasted-state, the rate of MPS is lower than that of muscle protein breakdown resulting in a negative state of protein balance (25). The ingestion of high-quality protein, rich in essential amino acids stimulates a transient increase in the rate of MPS resulting in a positive state of muscle protein balance (26, 27). It is also known that a single bout of resistance exercise performed in the fasted-state will induce a rise in both MPS and breakdown; however, the rate of MPS is elevated 48 h post-exercise whereas the rate of breakdown is returned to baseline at 48 h post-exercise (28). Critically, protein feeding and resistance exercise impart additive effects on MPS and net protein balance (26, 29) so when repeated bouts of resistance exercise are coupled with adequate protein feeding there is a protracted state of positive muscle protein balance leading to a gradual increase in skeletal muscle size (30).

Omega-3 Fatty Acids and Skeletal Muscle Lipid Profiles

Omega-3 fatty acid status is often assessed using either venous or fingerpick blood samples followed by analysis for fatty acid composition of membrane phospholipids with a number of basic mathematical calculations based on the relative abundance of omega-3 fatty acids to other fatty acids employed to determine risk of either disease or deficiency (31, 32). Changes in the omega-3 fatty acid composition of human blood membrane phospholipids with omega-3 fatty acid intake occurs rapidly (days) in a dose-dependent manner (33, 34) with washout kinetics exhibiting comparable declines following the cessation of intake (35). Due to slower turnover rates compared to blood, changes in omega-3 fatty acid composition of whole skeletal muscle phospholipid profiles even with high doses of omega-3 fatty acid intake (~3 g/d EPA and ~2 g/d DHA) require at least 2 weeks of supplementation in young men before detectable changes are observed (33). Recent work in young women using a similar dose of EPA + DHA has also demonstrated increases in the omega-3 fatty acid content of skeletal muscle phospholipids that plateaued somewhere between 6 and 8 weeks of supplementation (36). Interestingly, work in human blood has shown that there are sex-dependent effects in the change in the ratio of EPA:DHA with omega-3 fatty acid supplementation (35); however, no study has directly compared changes in omega-3 fatty acid skeletal muscle phospholipid profiles between men and women with omega-3 fatty acid intake. Moreover, unlike blood (35), no study has established a dose-response and washout of skeletal muscle phospholipid omega-3 fatty acid content with omega-3 fatty acid supplementation. Another important consideration is that the rate of incorporation of omega-3 fatty acids into skeletal muscle phospholipid membranes may differ depending on the fraction assessed (e.g., whole muscle vs.

sarcolemmal vs. mitochondrial) (37). As both the sarcolemmal and mitochondrial membranes serve as major sites of protein interactions and substrate transport, understanding how omega-3 fatty acid intake alters the lipid composition of distinct cellular organelles would provide key insights into the impact of compartmental lipid shifts on skeletal muscle physiology.

OMEGA 3 FATTY ACIDS AND MUSCLE PROTEIN TURNOVER

One of the first reports suggesting that omega-3 fatty acid intake alters muscle protein turnover *in vivo* was conducted in growing steers. In that study, Gingras et al. (38) examined the impact of omega-3 fatty acid-enriched menhaden oil infusion (13.5% EPA and 14.4% DHA) on whole-body protein kinetics using isotopically-labeled phenylalanine coupled with infusion of amino acids and insulin. The primary finding was that following omega-3 fatty acid provision, there was a doubling in the amount of amino acids required to prevent a state of hypo-aminoacidemia during a hyper-insulinemic clamp; indicative of increased whole-body protein anabolism. The authors speculated that the increased rate of amino acid clearance from the systemic circulation following omega-3 fatty acid provision was likely a function of either greater amino acid uptake into peripheral tissues, increased amino acid oxidation, and/or a reduction in the rate of protein breakdown. As neither direct rates of protein synthesis nor protein breakdown were measured it was not possible to delineate the relative contribution of protein synthesis vs. breakdown to the whole-body response. Moreover, tissue-specific (i.e., skeletal muscle vs. gut) turnover rates were not measured. This point is particularly relevant as the rate of gut protein turnover can be significantly higher than that of skeletal muscle (39) rendering it difficult to draw any conclusions as to whether the altered whole-body protein kinetics were a function of changes in amino acid handling at the level of skeletal muscle. What the authors did show was that omega-3 fatty acid supplementation increased the omega-3 fatty acid composition of skeletal muscle membrane phospholipids that coincided with enhanced phosphorylation of mechanistic target of rapamycin (mTOR)^{Ser2448} and ribosomal protein of 70 kDa S6 (p70S6K1)^{Thr389}, two key proteins known to regulate skeletal MPS (40).

Building on the early work of Gingras et al. (38) Smith and colleagues conducted two studies in younger (17) and older (16) human adults that assessed the influence of 8 weeks of omega-3 fatty acid supplementation (1.86 g/d of EPA and 1.50 g/d DHA) on rates of mixed skeletal MPS in the fasted-state, and in response to a hyper-aminoacidemic-hyper-insulinemic infusion. These studies (16, 17) demonstrated that whilst EPA and DHA supplementation and subsequent incorporation into membrane phospholipids had no impact on fasted rates of mixed MPS, in response to the hyper-aminoacidemic-hyper-insulinemic infusion, there was a potentiation of mixed MPS compared to before supplementation. Additionally, the potentiation of mixed MPS by EPA and DHA feeding was associated with enhanced mTOR^{Ser2448} and p70S6K1^{Thr389} phosphorylation in skeletal muscle, corroborating the previous observations of Gingras et al. (38). A separate study (18), showed that 6 months of 1.86 g/d of EPA and 1.50 g/d DHA supplementation lead to a significant increase in lean mass and clinically-relevant gains in muscle volume and muscle strength in older adults in a free-living environment. When taken together with the animal work of Gingras et al. (38), these human studies (16, 17) indicated that omega-3 fatty acid intake increased the omega-3 fatty acid composition of skeletal muscle phospholipids that is linked to enhanced rates of mixed MPS supporting gains in skeletal muscle mass and size over time (18). Given that the age-related loss of skeletal muscle mass and strength with advancing age, termed sarcopenia, is now recognized as an independent condition (International Classification of Disease, ICD-10-CM) (41), the use of omega-3 fatty acids to promote skeletal muscle anabolism may soon prove to have important utility in geriatric populations.

Since the seminal investigations of Gingras et al. (38) and Smith et al. (16–18) there have been other studies examining the role of omega-3 fatty acids on skeletal muscle protein metabolism. For instance, omega-3 fatty acids have been shown to alter protein turnover in C_2C_{12} cells (11, 12), as well as augmenting anabolic signaling in skeletal muscle of both rodents (15) and humans (33). There are also reports that supplementation with omega-3 fatty acids enhances resistance exercise-induced gains in skeletal muscle strength (42), an effect that appears to be particularly potent in older women (43). However, not all studies support the notion that omega-3 fatty acids enhance muscle anabolism. One study by McGlory et al. (44) failed to show any measurable effect of 8 weeks of 5 g/d EPA and DHA feeding on changes in myofibrillar MPS following either ingestion of 30 g protein or when protein feeding was combined with a bout of unilateral resistance exercise in young men. Additionally, Da Boit et al. (43) failed to demonstrate any effect of 2.1 g EPA/d and 0.6 g DHA/d supplementation on integrated rates of myofibrillar MPS or muscle size in older adults undergoing 18 weeks of resistance exercise training.

The conflicting reports regarding the efficacy of omega-3 fatty acid supplementation on MPS in humans could be underpinned by a number of factors, not least differences in experimental design. Unlike the repeated measures design of Smith et al. (16, 17) there was no pre-post supplementation measurement of myofibrillar MPS in the work of Da Boit et al. (43) and McGlory et al. (44) thus reducing statistical power. Furthermore, the 30 g dose of protein used by McGlory et al. (44) is a dose known to maximize rates of myofibrillar MPS in younger persons (45), whereas in the studies of Smith et al. (16, 17) amino acids were infused at a rate to elicit a state of aminoacidemia that is suboptimal for the stimulation of myofibrillar MPS. Thus, it is entirely possible that in the study of McGlory et al. (44) maximal rates of myofibrillar MPS had already been achieved and leaving no further capacity for omega-3 fatty acids to confer anabolic influence. As older adults require a greater relative per dose of protein to optimally stimulate rates of myofibrillar MPS than younger adults (0.40 vs. 0.24 g/kg body mass) (45), this contention may explain the greater relative increase in rates of mixed MPS in response to aminoacidemia in older compared to younger adults following omega-3 fatty acid feeding (16,

17). It could also provide some explanation as to the marked gains in muscle size with omega-3 fatty acid feeding in older adults in a free-living setting (18) during which dietary intake was not controlled and protein consumption likely suboptimal. Conversely, older adults who are already consuming adequate dietary protein may not receive the same benefit with omega-3 fatty acid supplementation compared to those who do not, at least with respect to changes in rates of MPS.

COUNTERACTING SKELETAL MUSCLE LOSS WITH OMEGA-3 FATTY ACIDS

Skeletal Muscle-Disuse Atrophy

Although resistance exercise enhances rates of MPS in response to amino acid ingestion (29), periods of muscle-disuse (i.e., immobilization) result in decreased rates of MPS in both the fed and fasted state (46, 47). This reduction induces an aggregate negative state of protein balance leading to a decline in muscle mass and size over time (36). Physically active younger women also appear to be more susceptible to periods of muscle-disuse as they are ~3 times more likely to sustain anterior cruciate ligament tears in select sporting activities requiring surgical intervention compared to their male counterparts (48). Whilst younger adults recover muscle mass and size from such periods, older adults display an impaired regenerative capacity in response to episodes of muscle-disuse (49, 50). When superimposed onto the natural biological decline in muscle mass with advancing age, these periods of muscle-disuse in older adults give rise to the "catabolic crisis model" of accelerated muscle loss, rendering older persons at greater risk of premature entry to a state of functional disability (51). Strategies such as resistance exercise (52) and neuromuscular electrical stimulation (53) are effective means to attenuate muscle-disuse atrophy. However, in situations in which patients are immobilized due to surgery/injury, resistance exercise, and neuromuscular electrical stimulation may not be the most practical approaches due to associated contraindications (e.g., pain/inflammation) as well as the necessity for qualified supervision, particularly in an institutionalized setting.

Given that omega-3 fatty acid supplementation enhances amino acid and insulin-mediated increases in rates of MPS (16, 17), it is possible that omega-3 fatty acid intake may serve to attenuate disuse-induced declines in MPS and thus attenuate muscle loss. Supplementation of rodents undergoing hindlimb suspension with fish oils rich in omega-3 fatty acids has been shown to alleviate soleus atrophy, which was associated with partial preservation of myosin heavy chain content and p70S6K1^{Thr389} phosphorylation (14). Moreover, others recently demonstrated that 6-weeks of ~3 g/d EPA and ~2 g/d DHA attenuated declines in muscle volume and muscle mass during 2-weeks of unilateral leg immobilization in young women (36). A key finding of this work (36) was that following 2-weeks of free-living recovery participants in the omega-3 fatty acid group recovered the losses in muscle volume whereas those in the control group did not. The attenuation of muscle-disuse atrophy by omega-3 fatty acids also coincided with increased daily rates of integrated myofibrillar MPS. These findings (36) complement previous reports using amino acid and insulin infusions (16, 17) and highlight the efficacy of omega-3 fatty acid feeding to protect the loss of skeletal muscle in response to, and recovery from, periods of muscle-disuse in young women. It is important to note that this study (36) was conducted in the context of simple muscle-disuse atrophy and in the absence of factors that likely accompany injury/recovery from surgery such as excessive inflammation/hypercortisolemia. It is also unknown whether omega-3 fatty acid feeding protects muscle loss during periods of muscle-disuse in older men and women or younger men. Further work in situations that recapitulate real-life clinical scenarios of muscle-disuse in both younger and older adults would add to these findings.

Cancer Cachexia

As omega-3 fatty acid intake has been shown to confer anabolic influence in ostensibly healthy individuals, it is entirely possible that omega-3 fatty acid intake may also positively impact skeletal muscle in situations of disease (**Figure 1**). Cancer cachexia is a multifactorial syndrome characterized by a marked involuntary loss of skeletal muscle mass that has a negative impact on muscle function, and is highly predictive of poor survival (54). Treatment of cancer cachexia continues to be one of the most prominent challenges faced by clinicians and scientists since the beginning of modern cancer therapy (55). The lack of adequate energy and nutrient ingestion, high concentration of plasma pro-inflammatory factors, tumoral factors, chemo/radiotherapy, and low-physical activity all contribute to the loss of muscle mass seen with cancer cachexia (55–58). As such, in the clinical setting a multifactorial approach that includes increased physical activity and targeted nutritional strategies is often employed to combat cancer cachexia.

Most nutritional guidelines targeted at attenuating cancer cachexia focus on reaching energy requirements of 25–30 kcal/kg/day and protein ingestion of 1.2–1.5 g/kg body mass/day (59, 60). Due to complications associated with some types of cancers (e.g., esophageal) and related surgeries resulting in dysphagia, achieving these guidelines in a real-world scenario can be problematic. Omega-3 fatty acids, mainly EPA (at 2–2.5 g/day) (59, 60) have been given as part of the anti-inflammatory and anti-catabolic nutritional therapy to combat the pro-inflammatory burden of cancer cachexia (58). The use of omega-3 fatty acids to counteract cancer cachexia came to practice following studies in rodents with various types of cancer showing that ingestion of fish oils rich in EPA and DHA (61–63) or increasing the omega-3 to omega-6 fatty acid ratio in the diet (64) were effective in decreasing tumor growth and cachexia development. After these initial studies (61–63), further reports were published in humans corroborating the positive effects of omega-3 fatty acids seen in rodent models. For example, there is evidence that low skeletal muscle mass is associated with reduced plasma fatty acid EPA status in cancer patients (65). Provision of 2.2 g/d EPA for 5 d pre-operatively and 21 d postoperatively in patients undergoing esophageal cancer surgery has been shown to preserve lean body mass as assessed by bioelectrical impedance (66). Furthermore, others have shown

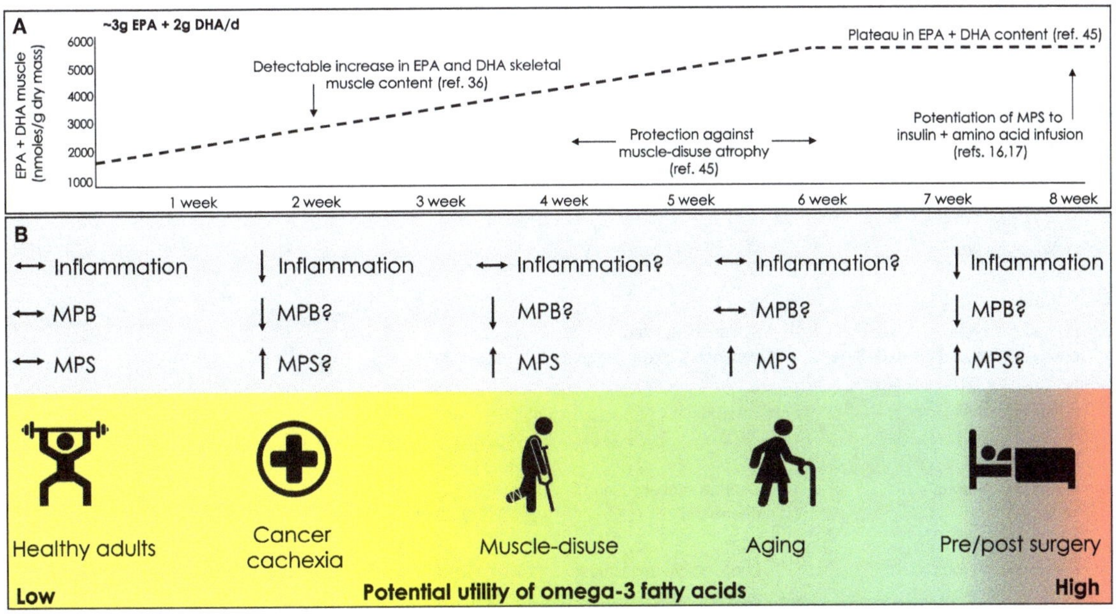

FIGURE 1 | (A) Time course change in skeletal muscle lipid content with omega-3 fatty acid supplementation. **(B)** Potential clinical scenarios for the use of omega-3 fatty acid supplementation to promote and/or mitigate losses in skeletal muscle mass; eicosapentaenoic acid (EPA), docosahexaenoic acid (DHA), muscle protein synthesis (MPS), muscle protein breakdown (MPB).

in patients with mixed-stage non-small cell lung cancer that 2.5 g/d of EPA + DHA resulted in a significant gain in lean body mass and a corresponding decrease in fat mass (67). However, the experimental evidence supporting the use of omega-3 fatty acids in the treatment of cancer cachexia is far from conclusive. A recent systematic review of studies published from 2000 to 2015 examining the impact of omega-3 fatty acids on cancer cachexia identified that out of 140 studies only 7 reached the quality threshold of inclusion according to the Delphi list (68). Out of those 7 studies, only one study in pre-cachexic cancer patients demonstrated a statistically positive effect of omega-3 fatty acids (69, 70). The fact that only 5% of available studies reached the required threshold of quality in this systematic review (68), highlights the challenges faced by scientists and clinicians in conducting high-quality, statistically-powered, randomized controlled trials in this specialized population.

Unlike periods of uncomplicated muscle-disuse in which the declines in skeletal muscle mass are primarily driven by a decrement in rates of MPS (71), it is generally assumed that cachexia is underpinned by both a diminished rate of MPS and an elevated rate of protein breakdown induced by a hyper-inflammatory state (**Table 1**). Given the anti-inflammatory effects of omega-3 fatty acids (see section Anti-inflammatory Effects of Omega-3 Fatty Acids) taken together with the stimulatory influence of omega-3 fatty acids on MPS (16, 17), it is likely that any impact of omega-3 fatty acids on lean body mass in cancer cachexia is a result of the dual action on both MPS and protein breakdown. To our knowledge, no study has directly assessed the impact of omega-3 fatty acids in isolation on changes in rates of MPS or protein breakdown in human cancer patients. One study in patients with various types of cancer (i.e., lung, colorectal, breast, esophagus, b-cell lymphoma) demonstrated that ingestion of a multi nutritional supplement containing 11 g whey protein, 4 g leucine, and 2.2 g EPA and 1.1 g DHA increased MPS above control (75). Whether the inclusion of omega-3 fatty acids in this formula was additive toward rates of MPS is unknown. However, it is unlikely that omega-3 fatty acids contributed to the enhanced MPS response given that MPS was measured 5 h post supplement ingestion and omega-3 fatty acids at the dose provided, would not have been incorporated into skeletal muscle within such a time-frame (33). Due to ethical limitations associated with multi-biopsy sampling in cancer cachexic patients, data related to muscle protein turnover in this clinical population are sparse. The introduction of the "virtual biopsy" procedure in which the synthetic rate of plasma proteins is used as a proxy of muscle proteins (79), may serve to circumvent ethical issues related to biopsy sampling and contribute to the development of nutritional interventions to combat cancer cachexia. However, more work is needed to validate this approach in compromised populations particularly during conditions of inactivity and muscle atrophy.

MECHANISMS OF ACTION OF OMEGA-3 FATTY ACIDS

Traditional thought is that their anti-inflammatory properties are primarily responsible for many of the reported health benefits of omega-3 fatty acids (1). In diseased states that are often accompanied by a state of excessive inflammation, the production of anti-inflammatory molecules and corresponding suppression of pro-inflammatory agents induced by omega-3 fatty acids is

TABLE 1 | Skeletal muscle protein synthesis and breakdown rates in patients with cancer cahchexia.

References	Methods	Basal MPS controls	Type of cancer	Basal MPS cancer	Postprandial MPS cancer	Basal MPB cancer	Nutritional intervention
Emery et al. (72)	Primed infusion [$^{13}C_2$]-Leu and ^{13}C labeled sodium bicarbonate and continuous [$^{13}C_2$]-Leu	0.198 ± 0.020 (%h)	Kidney and lung cancer (pre-treatment)	0.030 ± 0.007 (%/h)	–	–	–
Dworzak et al. (73)	Primed L-[$^2H_5$] phenylalanine and L[$^2H_4$] Tyrosine and continuous -[$^2H_5$] phenylalanine	0.048 ± 0.013 (%/h)	Advanced gastric carcinoma (pre-treatment)	0.021 ± 0.004 (%/h)	–	–	–
Dillon et al. (74)	Primed continuous infusion L-[ring-$^2H_5$]-Phe	–	Ovarian cancer (during treatment)	0.052 ± 0.009 (%/h)	0.120 ± 0.008 (%h)	–	Amino acid supplement
Deutz et al. (75)	Primed continuous infusion L-[ring-$^{13}C_6$]-Phe	–	Lung, colorectal, Breast, Esophagus, b-cell Lymphoma (no treatment for 4 weeks before the study)	0.073 ± 0.023 (%/h) 0.073 ± 0.022 (%/h)	0.065 ± 0.028 (%h) 0.097 ± 0.033 (%h)	– –	Conventional medical food Re-designed medical food
Dillon et al. (76)	Pulse bolus injection L-[ring-$^{13}C_6$]-Phe and 15N-Phe	–	Recurrent cervical carcinoma (case study)	0.07 (%/h)	–	0.03 (%/h)	–
Williams et al. (77)	Primed continuous infusion [1,2-$^{13}C_2$]-Leu and ring-D5-Phe	0.038 (%h)	Colonic adenocarcinoma booked for curative resection	0.028 ± 0.004 (%/h)	0.038 ± 0.004 (%/h)	–	Intravenous mixed amino acids
MacDonald et al. (78)	Single dose Deuterium oxide 133 g (70 Atom %)	37.2 [34.0–45.4] (g/day)	Upper gastrointestinal cancer	41.1 [38.2–41.8] (g/day)		42.4 [39.1–42–8] (g/day)[a]	–

MPS, muscle protein synthesis; MPB, muscle protein breakdown; Leu, leucine; Phe, phenylalanine.
[a]Calculated indirectly based on muscle mass loss.

thought to underpin improved health status (1). However, in healthy adults, reports of enhanced MPS (16) and increased muscle mass (18) with omega-3 fatty acid feeding occurred in the absence of any corresponding change in the concentration of putative circulating inflammatory markers. These findings (16, 18) suggest that in non-pathological states, omega-3 fatty acids do not confer anabolic influence via an anti-inflammatory mechanism. A schematic illustration of the potential actions of omega-3 fatty acids in skeletal muscle addressed in the following sections can be seen in **Figure 2**.

EPA vs. DHA

Whilst studies often provide EPA and DHA in combination, both fatty acids are known to exert independent biological actions. Reports have shown that EPA may have a greater influence on muscle protein turnover (11, 12) whereas DHA, likely owing to its higher content in neuromuscular tissues [~50 times higher than EPA in brain (80)], is heavily involved in neuromuscular function (81). Work in C_2C_{12} myotubes has demonstrated that treatment with 50 μM EPA but not 50 μM DHA stimulated an increase in protein synthesis (11) and a decrease in protein breakdown (11). Others, again in C_2C_{12} myotubes, have shown that 24 h incubation with 50 μM EPA resulted in protein accretion, an effect likely driven by decreased protein breakdown, with no effect of 50 μM DHA. Although delineating the differential effects of EPA and DHA on muscle protein turnover *in vitro* is interesting, the concentration of fatty acids used in each experiment may have a direct bearing on the outcome (23, 82). Indeed, in one report, treatment of C_2C_{12} myotubes with 400–600 μM of EPA resulted in a decrease in protein degradation; however, a similar effect on protein degradation was also achieved across a range of 300–700 μM DHA (82). Importantly, the concentrations of EPA and DHA used in many *in vitro* studies are higher than would typically be seen in the human bloodstream even after high-dose supplementation (83). To our knowledge, no study has directly compared the effect of physiological doses

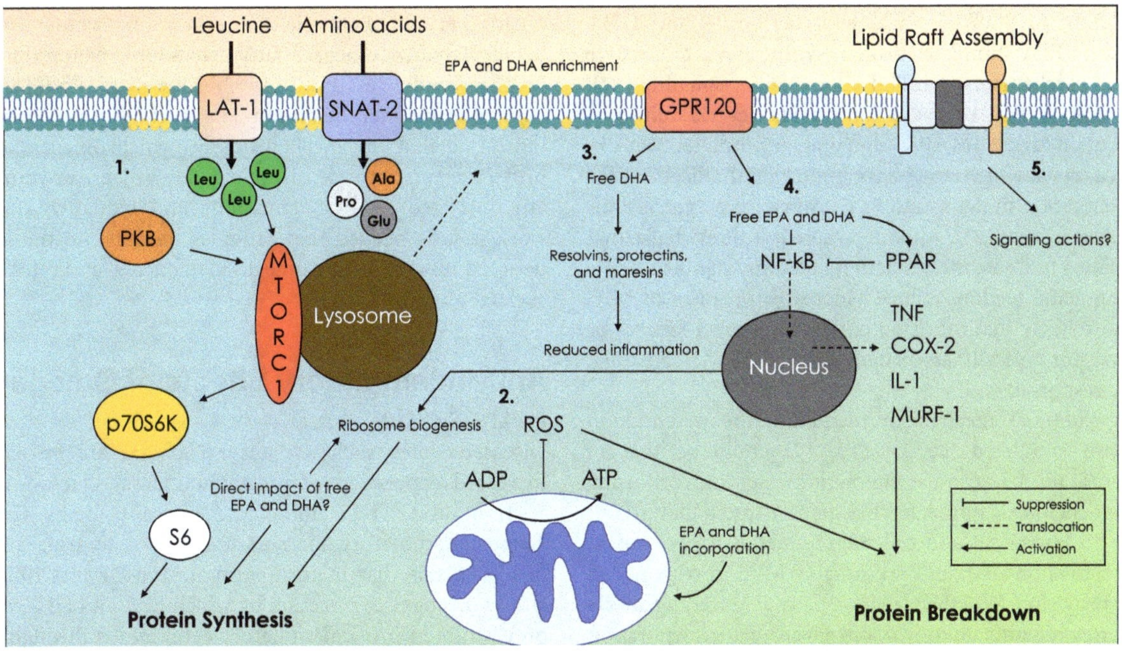

FIGURE 2 | Schematic illustration of molecular mechanisms of action of omega-3 fatty acids in skeletal muscle. 1. Translocation of the mechanistic target of rapamycin complex-1 (mTORC-1) with the lysosome to the membrane in close proximity to amino acid transporters. 2. Enhanced adenosine diphosphate (ADP) sensitivity and altered reactive oxygen species emissions (ROS). 3. G-coupled protein receptor 120 (GPR120) and free docosahexaenoic acid (DHA)-mediated production of resolvins, protectins, and maresins. 4. Cystolic retention of nuclear factor kappa B (NF-κB) preventing upregulation of proteolytic and pro-inflammatory agents. 5. Altered lipid raft formation that acts as signaling platforms for unknown signaling agents; eicosapentaenoic acid (EPA), docosahexaenoic acid (DHA).

of EPA vs. DHA ingestion on rates of MPS or protein breakdown in humans. Given that EPA and DHA serve as the substrates for the production of different pro-and anti-inflammatory mediators (e.g., resolvins) each with their own specialized function (1), defining the mechanisms underpinning how EPA and DHA alter muscle protein turnover in an *in vivo* setting is an interesting area worthy of future work.

Amino Acid Transport

As omega-3 fatty acids appear to promote anabolism via enhanced feeding-induced increases in MPS (16, 17), one potential mechanism by which omega-3 fatty acids alter rates of MPS could be that of enhanced amino acid transport. One study in pigs (84) identified an increase in the mRNA expression of the system L-amino acid transporter (LAT-1) following the ingestion of a diet rich in omega-3 fatty acids. As LAT-1 is known to transport the amino acid leucine, which is a key agonist of MPS, it could be contended that omega-3 fatty acid modulation of the phospholipid membrane somehow enhances LAT-1 expression thus facilitating leucine-mediated stimulation of MPS. This theory may, in part, explain the observation of enhanced rates of MPS in response to a hyper-aminoacidemic hyper-insulinemic infusion (16, 17). There is some experimental evidence for this thesis in humans, as in response to immobilization omega-3 fatty acid feeding has been shown to increase the LAT-1 mRNA expression in young women, which was linked to higher integrated rates of MPS (6). However, the change in LAT-1 mRNA expression in that study (36) did not translate into a detectable increase in LAT-1 protein content. Whether omega-3 fatty acid feeding alters the expression and/or function of other amino acid transporters remains unknown.

Protein Kinase Activity

Many studies that have shown a positive influence of omega-3 fatty acids on skeletal muscle anabolism also detect increases in the phosphorylation status of kinases related to the mTORC-1 signaling axis (e.g., protein kinase B (PKB)$^{Thr308/Ser473}$, mTOR^{Ser2448}, p70S6K1^{Thr389}) (11, 15–17). There is also evidence that omega-3 fatty acid supplementation increases the content of mechanically-sensitive protein kinases upstream of mTORC-1 (33). These findings would be expected as the mTORC-1 signaling axis is important for acute nutrient- and contraction-mediated increases in rates of MPS in humans (40, 85). However, using radiolabelled (γ-^{32}P) ATP, providing as a gold-standard measurement of protein-kinase activity *in vitro*, we identified a suppression of p70S6K1 activity in response to protein feeding and resistance exercise following 8 weeks of omega-3 fatty acid intake in young men (86). There was even a downregulation in the activity of PKB in response to omega-3 fatty acid supplementation alone. One consideration is the *in vitro* kinase assay is a V_{max} measure of kinase activity and does not necessarily reflect *in vivo* kinase function, nor single-residue phosphorylation status. It is also entirely possible that omega-3 fatty acids influence muscle anabolism via mTORC-1 independent mechanisms. Indeed, the study in which 50 μM EPA but not 50 μM DHA stimulated an increase in protein synthesis in C_2C_{12} myotubes also identified an increase in the phosphorylation of p70S6K1^{Thr389} with both EPA and DHA (11) suggesting EPA stimulates protein synthesis via alternative or additional mechanisms to mTORC1-p70S6K1 signaling (87). There is evidence that omega-3 fatty acids act via mitogen-activated protein kinase (MAPK) signaling and/or alterations in satellite cell activity, which could have important implications for muscle regeneration in aging and in recovery from exercise; for an extended review see (23). Although there is little evidence that MAPK signaling and satellite cell activity play any significant role in mediating acute feeding-induced increases on rates of MPS and it is more likely that other, potentially unknown kinases or at least those not typically associated with mTORC-1 signaling, mediate the response.

Another potential mechanism mediating the potentiation of MPS with simulated feeding (16, 17) could be that of changes in mTORC1-lysosomal interactions. Recent work using immunohistochemical approaches has demonstrated that mTOR localization to lysosomal and cell membranes is a key step in mTORC-1 activation (88), and presumably MPS in response to amino acid provision. Whether omega-3 fatty acid feeding affects these processes remains unknown, but given that incorporation of omega-3 fatty acids into lipid membranes alters membrane-associated proteomic profiles (12), future work utilizing a combination of immunohistochemical and immunoprecipitation approaches coupled with direct measurement of muscle protein turnover would provide further insight.

Mitochondrial Function

In addition to the sarcolemma, mitochondrial membranes are known to be sensitive to omega-3 fatty acid intake (37). One study has demonstrated that 12 weeks of omega-3 fatty acid supplementation (3 g EPA + 2 g DHA daily) increased mitochondrial EPA and DHA content in young men that was concordant with improved ADP sensitivity (5). Similarly, others have shown that 8 weeks of omega-3 fatty acid-rich tuna supplementation reduced whole-body oxygen consumption during steady-state exercise (89). Although improved respiration kinetics with omega-3 fatty acids are unlikely to explain previous reports of enhanced rates of MPS in response to feeding (16, 17), there is evidence that omega-3 fatty acid-mediated changes in mitochondrial function may play a role in mitigating muscle loss during aging and periods of muscle-disuse. Indeed, in the work of Smith et al. (18) in which 6 months of 1.86 g/d of EPA and 1.50 g/d DHA supplementation promoted gains in muscle size in older adults, there was also a corresponding increase in the expression of mitochondrial-related transcripts (90). Moreover, it was recently shown that the alleviation of muscle loss during 2 weeks of unilateral limb immobilization in young women undergoing omega-3 fatty acid supplementation (36) was linked to the preservation of maximal and submaximal ADP sensitivity as well as mitochondrial protein content (6). This is an important point, as ADP-stimulated oxidative phosphorylation reduces reactive oxygen species (ROS) emission, and aberrant ROS have been implicated in the pathology of muscle-disuse atrophy (91). Thus, collectively, these data (6, 36) suggest that the preservation of mitochondrial function plays a key role in the regulation of muscle size during periods of muscle-disuse in young women, which may be alleviated by omega-3 fatty acid supplementation. However, in that study (6, 36), immobilization did not alter H_2O_2 emissions in either the omega-3 fatty acid group or control group indicating that the mechanisms by which omega-3 fatty acids protect against muscle disuse atrophy at least in young women are unrelated to ROS emissions and oxidative stress. More work is now needed that provides insight into the interaction between mitochondria, omega-3 fatty acids, and rates of MPS in skeletal muscle.

Anti-inflammatory Effects of Omega-3 Fatty Acids

Diseased states such as cancer cachexia are associated with increased expression of pro-inflammatory cytokines (e.g., IL-1, IL-6, and TNF) and acute phase proteins (e.g., CRP). These inflammatory markers are known to trigger regulators of proteolysis that in turn promote muscle loss (92, 93). The classic mechanism of action by which EPA and DHA modify the production of pro-inflammatory cytokines is through alteration in the synthesis of lipid mediators, principally derivatives of the omega-6 fatty acid arachidonic acid (ARA) and of EPA and DHA themselves. These lipid mediators are biologically active and include prostaglandins and leukotrienes as well as specialized pro-resolution mediators. The fatty acid substrate (e.g., ARA, EPA or DHA) for production of lipid mediators is released from cell membrane phospholipids through the action of phospholipase enzymes, in particular phospholipase A2. Typically, ARA is more abundant than EPA or DHA [i.e., it is reported to comprise 10.5% of fatty acids in skeletal muscle lipids (33) and 17.2% of fatty acids in skeletal muscle phospholipids (17), and therefore it is the dominant substrate]. ARA is metabolized by cyclooxygenase (COX) enzymes (e.g., COX-2) to 2-series prostaglandins and by 5-lipoxygenase (LOX) to 4-series leukotrienes. These mediators are closely involved in inflammatory processes, acting through specific G-protein coupled receptors. Enrichment of EPA in cell membranes is partly at the expense of ARA, thus altering the balance of substrates available. This is seen in both inflammatory cells (94) and in skeletal muscle (17, 33). EPA is also metabolized by COX and LOX enzymes but gives rise to metabolites with a slightly different structure from those produced from ARA, typically resulting in lower affinity for receptors (95) and lower bioactivity (94). As a result, EPA enrichment is linked with lower concentrations of potent ARA-derived mediators being produced and higher concentrations of less potent EPA-derived mediators being produced. EPA and DHA can also decrease COX-2 gene and protein expression (62, 96), which has the effect of lowering lipid mediator production due to less available enzyme.

The mechanism behind the omega-3 fatty acid-induced lowering of COX-2 gene expression seems to be inhibition of the nuclear factor kappa B (NF-κB) pathway. NF-κB is a transcription factor that acts to up-regulate inflammatory gene expression (97). NF-κB exists as an inactive trimer in the cytosol of cells. In the presence of an inflammatory trigger or stimulus, a signaling pathway results in phosphorylation of the inhibitory subunit of the NF-κB trimer which then dissociates and is degraded. This leaves the remaining dimer free to translocate to the nucleus and bind to response elements in target genes altering their transcription. Through inhibiting the signaling pathway that activates NF-κB, EPA, and DHA not only down-regulate COX-2 gene expression but also the expression of genes encoding common pro-inflammatory cytokines like TNF and IL-1, genes encoding important chemokines like monocyte chemotactic protein-1, and genes encoding adhesion molecules responsible for leukocyte infiltration (94). The inhibition of NF-κB activation by EPA and DHA is linked to changes in cell membranes (98, 99) suggesting omega-3 fatty acid induces alterations in very early signaling events. In addition, EPA and DHA and some of their lipid mediator derivatives can activate peroxisome proliferator-activated receptor (PPAR) γ (100, 101), which physically interferes with NF-κB translocation to the nucleus (102). Consistent with the importance of this interaction, knockdown of PPARγ significantly reduced the effect of EPA on NF-κB signaling (103). Another target for NF-κB is the muscle ring finger-1 (MuRF-1) gene (103) linking this pro-inflammatory pathway directly with muscle protein breakdown as MuRF-1 aids protein degradation through the ubiquitination pathway (104).

It appears that EPA and DHA can down-regulate NF-κB activation through several mechanisms, one being through activation of PPARγ (100), a second being action via a G-protein coupled receptor GPR120 (105), and a third being through effects within the cell membrane (98, 99). GPR120 was first identified to be expressed on inflammatory macrophages and adipocytes, but has more recently been described on skeletal muscle cells (106). DHA appears to be the major endogenous ligand for GPR120 and DHA was shown to inhibit NF-κB activation and expression of NF-κB target genes and proteins via GPR120 (105). GPR120 was also involved in beneficial metabolic effects of DHA in adipocytes (105) and skeletal muscle (106), but whether GPR120 mediates anti-inflammatory effects of DHA in skeletal muscle has not been reported.

The effects of DHA on NF-κB activation and NF-κB mediated events have been shown to involve modifications to cell membrane structures termed lipid rafts (99). Lipid rafts are cell membrane regions that are rich in sphingolipids, saturated fatty acids, cholesterol and signaling proteins. They form in response to certain stimuli and act to bring together different proteins involved in common signaling pathways, essentially forming signaling platforms. Lipid rafts are well described in immune cells, cancer cells and neurones. They are also described in skeletal muscle (107) and intriguingly they are disrupted by short term muscle disuse in the rat (108). Some saturated fatty acids have been shown to promote lipid raft formation and inflammatory signaling (98, 99) while DHA was shown to inhibit lipid raft formation in response to inflammatory stimuli, including saturated fatty acids, and this was linked to reduced activation of the NF-κB pathway (98, 99). It is not known if omega-3 fatty acids affect lipid raft formation in skeletal muscle cells and whether such an effect might be linked to reduced inflammation and the expression of molecules that regulate muscle protein turnover.

The effects of EPA and DHA on production of prostaglandins and leukotrienes and on pathways that reduce NF-κB activation and subsequent production of pro-inflammatory cytokines, chemokines and adhesion molecules are generally regarded as being anti-inflammatory (1, 94). It is now known that EPA and DHA are substrates for lipid mediators that actively turn-off (i.e., resolve) inflammation (109–111). These so-called specialized pro-resolution mediators include resolvins produced from EPA (E-series) and DHA (D-series) and protectins and maresins produced from DHA. The synthesis of resolvins, protectins, and maresins involves the COX and LOX pathways, with different epimers being produced in the presence and absence of aspirin (109–111). As might be expected, resolvin synthesis is increased by feeding laboratory rodent diets rich in EPA and DHA (112) and there are reports of increased levels of various resolvins in human serum and plasma following daily intake of omega-3 fatty acid supplements for a period of weeks (113, 114). The biological effects of resolvins, protectins and maresins have been examined extensively in cell culture and animal models of inflammation, and they have been demonstrated to be anti-inflammatory and inflammation resolving, preventing leukocyte infiltration into tissue and decreasing production of cytokines like TNF and IL-1β (109–111). A recent study (115) mapped the lipid mediator signature during a murine model of muscle injury and regeneration and identified a temporal pattern of production of classic pro-inflammatory mediators like prostaglandins/leukotrienes and pro-resolving mediators like resolvins. These mediators were produced by infiltrating leukocytes (neutrophils and macrophages) and the temporal change was linked to a change in phenotype of these leukocytes. The resolution phase was associated with the emergence of an anti-inflammatory phenotype of macrophage. The role of such lipid mediators in muscle protein turnover and how this may be optimized by managing omega-3 fatty acid exposure is not currently known.

FUTURE DIRECTIONS AND CONCLUSION

In summary, the available evidence would suggest that omega-3 fatty acid intake has the potential to enhance skeletal muscle anabolism, but the magnitude of the effect may be dependent upon a number of factors. These factors include, but are not limited to, the daily dose of protein intake, measurement technique, as well as age and metabolic status of participants. One particular area of promise is the potential for omega-3 fatty acids to counteract muscle atrophy, and promote recovery, from periods of muscle-disuse induced by surgery and subsequent bedrest/inactivity. However, before firm conclusions can be drawn as to the efficacy of omega-3 fatty acid intake on musculoskeletal health and subsequent translation to the clinical setting there remains many unanswered questions that require experimental attention. For instance, what are the molecular mechanisms that mediate improved skeletal muscle protein turnover and functionality with omega-3 fatty acid intake? Is there a dose-response relationship between omega-3 fatty acid intake and physiological outcomes, and is the efficacy of omega-3 fatty acid intake on skeletal muscle influenced by sex? Given their independent biological actions, it will also be vitally important to discern the independent roles of EPA and DHA in mediating changes in skeletal muscle plasticity. Another important but often overlooked factor is what are the off-target effects of increasing omega-3 fatty acid intake and are there any negative consequences in other vitally important processes. The answers to such questions will inevitably require the application of a range of invasive and non-invasive methodologies in pre-clinical models as well as humans. We hope that such work will provide important information for the development of omega-3 fatty acid therapies to promote musculoskeletal health in a variety of settings and populations.

AUTHOR CONTRIBUTIONS

CM, PC, and EN contributed to the writing and critical evaluation of the manuscript. All authors approved the final version of the manuscript for submission.

ACKNOWLEDGMENTS

The authors would like to thank Jonathan McLeod and Raveen Bahniwal for their critical comments during the drafting of this manuscript. CM would like to thank Dr. Stuart M. Phillips for facilitating insightful discussion related to scientific concepts addressed in this work. EN was a research productivity fellow for the National Council for Scientific and Technological Development (CNPq) of Brazil (grant number 302692/2016-9).

REFERENCES

1. Calder PC. Omega-3 fatty acids and inflammatory processes: from molecules to man. *Biochem Soc Trans.* (2017) 45:1105–15. doi: 10.1042/BST20160474
2. Engler MB, Engler MM. Docosahexaenoic acid–induced vasorelaxation in hypertensive rats: mechanisms of action. *Biol Res Nurs.* (2000) 2:85–95. doi: 10.1177/109980040000200202
3. Cardoso C, Afonso C, Bandarra NM. Dietary DHA and health: cognitive function ageing. *Nutr Res Rev.* (2016) 29:281–94. doi: 10.1017/S0954422416000184
4. Kliewer SA, Sundseth SS, Jones SA, Brown PJ, Wisely GB, Koble CS, et al. Fatty acids and eicosanoids regulate gene expression through direct interactions with peroxisome proliferator-activated receptors alpha and gamma. *Proc Natl Acad Sci USA.* (1997) 94:4318–23. doi: 10.1073/pnas.94.9.4318
5. Herbst EA, Paglialunga S, Gerling C, Whitfield J, Mukai K, Chabowski A, et al. Omega-3 supplementation alters mitochondrial membrane composition and respiration kinetics in human skeletal muscle. *J Physiol.* (2014) 592:1341–52. doi: 10.1113/jphysiol.2013.267336
6. Miotto PM, McGlory C, Bahniwal R, Kamal M, Phillips SM, Holloway GP. Supplementation with dietary ω-3 mitigates immobilization-induced reductions in skeletal muscle mitochondrial respiration in young women. *FASEB J.* (2019) 33:8232–40. doi: 10.1096/fj.201900095R
7. Stephenson EJ, Hawley JA. Mitochondrial function in metabolic health: a genetic and environmental tug of war. *Biochim Biophys Acta.* (2014) 1840:1285–94. doi: 10.1016/j.bbagen.2013.12.004
8. Thompson M, Hein N, Hanson C, Smith LM, Anderson-Berry A, Richter CK, et al. Omega-3 fatty acid intake by age, gender, and pregnancy status in the United States: National Health and Nutrition Examination Survey 2003(-)2014. *Nutrients.* (2019) 11:E177. doi: 10.3390/nu11010177
9. Arterburn LM, Hall EB, Oken H. Distribution, interconversion, and dose response of n-3 fatty acids in humans. *Am J Clin Nutr.* (2006) 83:1467–76S. doi: 10.1093/ajcn/83.6.1467S
10. Nording ML, Yang J, Georgi K, Hegedus Karbowski C, German JB, Weiss RH, et al. Individual variation in lipidomic profiles of healthy subjects in response to omega-3 Fatty acids. *PLoS ONE.* (2013) 8:e76575. doi: 10.1371/journal.pone.0076575
11. Kamolrat T, Gray SR. The effect of eicosapentaenoic and docosahexaenoic acid on protein synthesis and breakdown in murine C2C12 myotubes. *Biochem BiophysRes Commun.* (2013) 432:593–8. doi: 10.1016/j.bbrc.2013.02.041
12. Jeromson S, Mackenzie I, Doherty MK, Whitfield PD, Bell G, Dick J, et al. Lipid remodeling and an altered membrane-associated proteome may drive the differential effects of EPA and DHA treatment on skeletal muscle glucose uptake and protein accretion. *Am J Physiol Endocrinol Metab.* (2018) 314:E605–19. doi: 10.1152/ajpendo.00438.2015
13. You JS, Park MN, Lee YS. Dietary fish oil inhibits the early stage of recovery of atrophied soleus muscle in rats via Akt-p70s6k signaling and PGF2α. *J Nutr Biochem.* (2010) 21:929–34. doi: 10.1016/j.jnutbio.2009.07.007
14. You JS, Park MN, Song W, Lee YS. Dietary fish oil alleviates soleus atrophy during immobilization in association with Akt signaling to p70s6k and E3 ubiquitin ligases in rats. *Appl Physiol NutrMetab.* (2010) 35:310–8. doi: 10.1139/H10-022
15. Kamolrat T, Gray SR, Thivierge MC. Fish oil positively regulates anabolic signalling alongside an increase in whole-body gluconeogenesis in ageing skeletal muscle. *Eur J Nutr.* (2013) 52:647–57. doi: 10.1007/s00394-012-0368-7
16. Smith GI, Atherton P, Reeds DN, Mohammed BS, Rankin D, Rennie MJ, et al. Dietary omega-3 fatty acid supplementation increases the rate of muscle protein synthesis in older adults: a randomized controlled trial. *Am J Clin Nutr.* (2010) 93:402–12. doi: 10.3945/ajcn.110.005611
17. Smith GI, Atherton P, Reeds DN, Mohammed BS, Rankin D, Rennie MJ, et al. Omega-3 polyunsaturated fatty acids augment the muscle protein anabolic response to hyperinsulinaemia-hyperaminoacidaemia in healthy young and middle-aged men and women. *Clin Sci.* (2011) 121:267–78. doi: 10.1042/CS20100597
18. Smith GI, Julliand S, Reeds DN, Sinacore DR, Klein S, Mittendorfer B. Fish oil-derived n-3 PUFA therapy increases muscle mass and function in healthy older adults. *Am J Clin Nutr.* (2015) 102:115–22. doi: 10.3945/ajcn.114.105833
19. Wolfe RR. The underappreciated role of muscle in health and disease. *Am J Clin Nutr.* (2006) 84:475–82. doi: 10.1093/ajcn/84.3.475
20. Newman AB, Kupelian V, Visser M, Simonsick EM, Goodpaster BH, Kritchevsky SB, et al. Strength, but not muscle mass, is associated with mortality in the health, aging and body composition study cohort. *J Gerontol A Biol Sci Med Sci.* (2006) 61:72–7. doi: 10.1093/gerona/61.1.72
21. Wischmeyer PE, Puthucheary Z, San Millan I, Butz D, Grocott MPW. Muscle mass and physical recovery in ICU: innovations for targeting of nutrition and exercise. *Curr Opin Crit Care.* (2017) 23:269–78. doi: 10.1097/MCC.0000000000000431
22. Rossato LT, Schoenfeld BJ, de Oliveira EP. Is there sufficient evidence to supplement omega-3 fatty acids to increase muscle mass and strength in young and older adults? *Clin Nutr.* (2019). doi: 10.1016/j.clnu.2019.01.001. [Epub ahead of print].
23. Tachtsis B, Camera D, Lacham-Kaplan O. Potential Roles of n-3 PUFAs during skeletal muscle growth and regeneration. *Nutrients.* (2018) 10:E309. doi: 10.3390/nu10030309
24. Witard OC, Combet E, Gray SR. Long-chain n-3 fatty acids as an essential link between musculoskeletal and cardio-metabolic health in older adults. *Proc Nutr Soc.* (2019):1–9. doi: 10.1017/S0029665119000922. [Epub ahead of print].
25. Biolo G, Maggi SP, Williams BD, Tipton KD, Wolfe RR. Increased rates of muscle protein turnover and amino acid transport after

resistance exercise in humans. *Am J Physiol.* (1995) 268:E514–20. doi: 10.1152/ajpendo.1995.268.3.E514

26. Biolo G, Tipton KD, Klein S, Wolfe RR. An abundant supply of amino acids enhances the metabolic effect of exercise on muscle protein. *Am J Physiol.* (1997) 273:E122–9. doi: 10.1152/ajpendo.1997.273.1.E122
27. Greenhaff PL, Karagounis L, Peirce N, Simpson EJ, Hazell M, Layfield R, et al. Disassociation between the effects of amino acids and insulin on signalling, ubiquitin-ligases and protein turnover in human muscle. *Am J Physiol Endocrinol Metab.* (2008) 295:E595–604. doi: 10.1152/ajpendo.90411.2008
28. Phillips S, Tipton K, Aarsland A, Wolf S, Wolfe R. Mixed muscle protein synthesis and breakdown after resistance exercise in humans. *Am J Physiol Endocrinol Metab.* (1997) 273:E99–107. doi: 10.1152/ajpendo.1997.273.1.E99
29. Witard OC, Tieland M, Beelen M, Tipton KD, van Loon LJ, Koopman R. Resistance exercise increases postprandial muscle protein synthesis in humans. *Med Sci Sports Exerc.* (2009) 41:144–54. doi: 10.1249/MSS.0b013e3181844e79
30. Morton RW, Murphy KT, McKellar SR, Schoenfeld BJ, Henselmans M, Helms E, et al. A systematic review, meta-analysis and meta-regression of the effect of protein supplementation on resistance training-induced gains in muscle mass and strength in healthy adults. *Br J Sports Med.* (2018) 52:376–84.. doi: 10.1136/bjsports-2017-097608
31. Harris WS, Von Schacky C. The Omega-3 Index: a new risk factor for death from coronary heart disease? *Prev Med.* (2004) 39:212–20. doi: 10.1016/j.ypmed.2004.02.030
32. Bell JG, Mackinlay EE, Dick JR, Younger I, Lands B, Gilhooly T. Using a fingertip whole blood sample for rapid fatty acid measurement: method validation and correlation with erythrocyte polar lipid compositions in UK subjects. *Br J Nutr.* (2011) 106:1408–15. doi: 10.1017/S0007114511001978
33. McGlory C, Galloway SD, Hamilton DL, McClintock C, Breen L, Dick JR, et al. Temporal changes in human skeletal muscle and blood lipid composition with fish oil supplementation. *Prostaglandins Leukot Essent Fatty Acids.* (2014) 90:199–206. doi: 10.1016/j.plefa.2014.03.001
34. Browning LM, Walker CG, Mander AP, West AL, Madden J, Gambell JM, et al. Incorporation of eicosapentaenoic and docosahexaenoic acids into lipid pools when given as supplements providing doses equivalent to typical intakes of oily fish. *Am J Clin Nutr.* (2012) 96:748–58. doi: 10.3945/ajcn.112.041343
35. Metherel AH, Armstrong JM, Patterson AC, Stark KD. Assessment of blood measures of n-3 polyunsaturated fatty acids with acute fish oil supplementation and washout in men and women. *Prostaglandins Leukot Essent Fatty Acids.* (2009) 81:23–9. doi: 10.1016/j.plefa.2009.05.018
36. McGlory C, Gorissen SHM, Kamal M, Bahniwal R, Hector AJ, Baker SK, et al. Omega-3 fatty acid supplementation attenuates skeletal muscle disuse atrophy during two weeks of unilateral leg immobilization in healthy young women. *FASEB J.* (2019) 33:4586–97. doi: 10.1096/fj.201801857RRR
37. Gerling CJ, Mukai K, Chabowski A, Heigenhauser GJF, Holloway GP, Spriet LL, et al. Incorporation of Omega-3 Fatty Acids Into Human Skeletal Muscle Sarcolemmal and mitochondrial membranes following 12 weeks of fish oil supplementation. *Front Physiol.* (2019) 10:348. doi: 10.3389/fphys.2019.00348
38. Gingras AA, White PJ, Chouinard PY, Julien P, Davis TA, Dombrowski L, et al. Long-chain omega-3 fatty acids regulate bovine whole-body protein metabolism by promoting muscle insulin signalling to the Akt-mTOR-S6K1 pathway and insulin sensitivity. *J Physiol.* (2007) 579:269–84. doi: 10.1113/jphysiol.2006.121079
39. Nakshabendi IM, McKee R, Downie S, Russell RI, Rennie MJ. Rates of small intestinal mucosal protein synthesis in human jejunum and ileum. *Am J Physiol.* (1999) 277(6Pt 1):E1028-E31. doi: 10.1152/ajpendo.1999.277.6.E1028
40. Dickinson JM, Fry CS, Drummond MJ, Gundermann DM, Walker DK, Glynn EL, et al. Mammalian target of rapamycin complex 1 activation is required for the stimulation of human skeletal muscle protein synthesis by essential amino acids. *J Nutr.* (2011) 141:856–62. doi: 10.3945/jn.111.139485
41. Cao L, Morley JE. Sarcopenia Is Recognized as an Independent Condition by an International Classification of Disease, Tenth Revision, Clinical Modification (ICD-10-CM) code. *J Am Med Dir Assoc.* (2016) 17:675–7. doi: 10.1016/j.jamda.2016.06.001
42. Rodacki CL, Rodacki AL, Pereira G, Naliwaiko K, Coelho I, Pequito D, et al. Fish-oil supplementation enhances the effects of strength training in elderly women. *Am J Clin Nutr.* (2012) 95:428–36. doi: 10.3945/ajcn.111.021915
43. Da Boit M, Sibson R, Sivasubramaniam S, Meakin JR, Greig CA, Aspden RM, et al. Sex differences in the effect of fish-oil supplementation on the adaptive response to resistance exercise training in older people: a randomized controlled trial. *Am J Clin Nutr.* (2017) 105:151–8. doi: 10.3945/ajcn.116.140780
44. McGlory C, Wardle SL, Macnaughton LS, Witard OC, Scott F, Dick J, et al. Fish oil supplementation suppresses resistance exercise and feeding-induced increases in anabolic signaling without affecting myofibrillar protein synthesis in young men. *Physiol Rep.* (2016) 4:e12715. doi: 10.14814/phy2.12715
45. Moore DR, Churchward-Venne TA, Witard O, Breen L, Burd NA, Tipton KD, et al. Protein ingestion to stimulate myofibrillar protein synthesis requires greater relative protein intakes in healthy older versus younger men. *J Gerontol A Biol Sci Med Sci.* (2015) 70:57–62. doi: 10.1093/gerona/glu103
46. Glover EI, Phillips SM, Oates BR, Tang JE, Tarnopolsky MA, Selby A, et al. Immobilization induces anabolic resistance in human myofibrillar protein synthesis with low and high dose amino acid infusion. *J Physiol.* (2009) 586:6049–61. doi: 10.1113/jphysiol.2008.160333
47. Wall BT, Dirks ML, Snijders T, van Dijk JW, Fritsch M, Verdijk LB, et al. Short-term muscle disuse lowers myofibrillar protein synthesis rates and induces anabolic resistance to protein ingestion. *Am J Physiol Endocrinol Metab.* (2016) 310:E137–47. doi: 10.1152/ajpendo.00227.2015
48. Prodromos CC, Han Y, Rogowski J, Joyce B, Shi K. A meta-analysis of the incidence of anterior cruciate ligament tears as a function of gender, sport, and a knee injury-reduction regimen. *Arthroscopy.* (2007) 23:1320–5 e6. doi: 10.1016/j.arthro.2007.07.003
49. Suetta C, Frandsen U, Mackey AL, Jensen L, Hvid LG, Bayer ML, et al. Ageing is associated with diminished muscle re-growth and myogenic precursor cell expansion early after immobility-induced atrophy in human skeletal muscle. *J Physiol.* (2013) 591:3789–804. doi: 10.1113/jphysiol.2013.257121
50. McGlory C, von Allmen MT, Stokes T, Morton RW, Hector AJ, Lago BA, et al. Failed recovery of glycemic control and myofibrillar protein synthesis with 2 wk of physical inactivity in overweight, prediabetic older adults. *J Gerontol A Biol Sci Med Sci.* (2018) 73:1070–7. doi: 10.1093/gerona/glx203
51. English KL, Paddon-Jones D. Protecting muscle mass and function in older adults during bed rest. *Curr Opin Clin Nutr Metab Care.* (2010) 13:34–9. doi: 10.1097/MCO.0b013e328333aa66
52. Oates BR, Glover EI, West DW, Fry JL, Tarnopolsky MA, Phillips SM. Low-volume resistance exercise attenuates the decline in strength and muscle mass associated with immobilization. *Muscle Nerve.* (2010) 42:539–46. doi: 10.1002/mus.21721
53. Dirks ML, Wall BT, Snijders T, Ottenbros CL, Verdijk LB, van Loon LJ. Neuromuscular electrical stimulation prevents muscle disuse atrophy during leg immobilization in humans. *Acta Physiol.* (2014) 210:628–41. doi: 10.1111/apha.12200
54. Blauwhoff-Buskermolen S, Versteeg KS, de van der Schueren MA, den Braver NR, Berkhof J, Langius JA, et al. Loss of muscle mass during chemotherapy is predictive for poor survival of patients with metastatic colorectal cancer. *J Clin Oncol.* (2016) 34:1339–44. doi: 10.1200/JCO.2015.63.6043
55. Ryan AM, Power DG, Daly L, Cushen SJ, Ni Bhuachalla E, Prado CM. Cancer-associated malnutrition, cachexia and sarcopenia: the skeleton in the hospital closet 40 years later. *Proc Nutr Soc.* (2016) 75:199–211. doi: 10.1017/S002966511500419X
56. Aguiar JPS, Fabre MES, Waitzberg DL. Omega-3 supplements for patients in chemotherapy and/or radiotherapy: a systematic review. *Clin Nutr.* (2015) 34:359–66. doi: 10.1016/j.clnu.2014.11.005
57. Camargo CQ, Borges DS, de Oliveira PF, Chagas TR, Del Moral JA, Durigon GS, et al. Individuals with hematological malignancies before undergoing chemotherapy present oxidative stress parameters and acute phase proteins correlated with nutritional status. *Nutr Cancer.* (2015) 67:463–71. doi: 10.1080/01635581.2015.1004732
58. Gorjao R, Dos Santos CMM, Serdan TDA, Diniz VLS, Alba-Loureiro TC, Cury-Boaventura MF, et al. New insights on the regulation of cancer cachexia by N-3 polyunsaturated fatty acids. *Pharmacol Ther.* (2019) 196:117–34. doi: 10.1016/j.pharmthera.2018.12.001

59. Huhmann MB, August DA. Review of American Society for Parenteral and Enteral Nutrition (ASPEN) Clinical Guidelines for Nutrition Support in Cancer Patients: nutrition screening and assessment. *Nutr Clin Pract*. (2008) 23:182–8. doi: 10.1177/0884533608314530
60. Arends J, Baracos V, Bertz H, Bozzetti F, Calder PC, Deutz NEP, et al. ESPEN expert group recommendations for action against cancer-related malnutrition. *Clin Nutr*. (2017) 36:1187–96. doi: 10.1016/j.clnu.2017.06.017
61. Whitehouse AS, Smith HJ, Drake JL, Tisdale MJ. Mechanism of attenuation of skeletal muscle protein catabolism in cancer cachexia by eicosapentaenoic acid. *Cancer Res*. (2001) 61:3604–9.
62. Mund RC, Pizato N, Bonatto S, Nunes EA, Vicenzi T, Tanhoffer R, et al. Decreased tumor growth in Walker 256 tumor-bearing rats chronically supplemented with fish oil involves COX-2 and PGE2 reduction associated with apoptosis and increased peroxidation. *Prostaglandins Leukot Essent Fatty Acids*. (2007) 76:113–20. doi: 10.1016/j.plefa.2006.11.008
63. Iagher F, de Brito Belo SR, Souza WM, Nunes JR, Naliwaiko K, Sassaki GL, et al. Antitumor and anti-cachectic effects of shark liver oil and fish oil: comparison between independent or associative chronic supplementation in Walker 256 tumor-bearing rats. *Lipids Health Dis*. (2013) 12:146. doi: 10.1186/1476-511X-12-146
64. Pizato N, Bonatto S, Yamazaki RK, Aikawa J, Nogata C, Mund RC, et al. Ratio of n6 to n-3 fatty acids in the diet affects tumor growth and cachexia in Walker 256 tumor-bearing rats. *Nutr Cancer*. (2005) 53:194–201. doi: 10.1207/s15327914nc5302_8
65. Murphy RA, Mourtzakis M, Chu QS, Reiman T, Mazurak VC. Skeletal muscle depletion is associated with reduced plasma (n-3) fatty acids in non-small cell lung cancer patients. *J Nutr*. (2010) 140:1602–6. doi: 10.3945/jn.110.123521
66. Ryan AM, Reynolds JV, Healy L, Byrne M, Moore J, Brannelly N, et al. Enteral nutrition enriched with eicosapentaenoic acid (EPA) preserves lean body mass following esophageal cancer surgery: results of a double-blinded randomized controlled trial. *Ann Surg*. (2009) 249:355–63. doi: 10.1097/SLA.0b013e31819a4789
67. Murphy RA, Mourtzakis M, Chu QS, Baracos VE, Reiman T, Mazurak VC. Nutritional intervention with fish oil provides a benefit over standard of care for weight and skeletal muscle mass in patients with nonsmall cell lung cancer receiving chemotherapy. *Cancer*. (2011) 117:1775–82. doi: 10.1002/cncr.25709
68. Lavriv DS, Neves PM, Ravasco P. Should omega-3 fatty acids be used for adjuvant treatment of cancer cachexia? *Clin Nutr ESPEN*. (2018) 25:18–25. doi: 10.1016/j.clnesp.2018.02.006
69. van der Meij BS, Langius JA, Smit EF, Spreeuwenberg MD, von Blomberg BM, Heijboer AC, et al. Oral nutritional supplements containing (n-3) polyunsaturated fatty acids affect the nutritional status of patients with stage III non-small cell lung cancer during multimodality treatment. *J Nutr*. (2010) 140:1774–80. doi: 10.3945/jn.110.121202
70. van der Meij BS, Langius JA, Spreeuwenberg MD, Slootmaker SM, Paul MA, Smit EF, et al. Oral nutritional supplements containing n-3 polyunsaturated fatty acids affect quality of life and functional status in lung cancer patients during multimodality treatment: an RCT. *Eur J Clin Nutr*. (2012) 66:399–404. doi: 10.1038/ejcn.2011.214
71. Phillips SM, Glover EI, Rennie MJ. Alterations of protein turnover underlying disuse atrophy in human skeletal muscle. *J Appl Physiol*. (2009) 107:643–54. doi: 10.1152/japplphysiol.00452.2009
72. Emery PW, Edwards RH, Rennie MJ, Souhami RL, Halliday D. Protein synthesis in muscle measured *in vivo* in cachectic patients with cancer. *Br Med J*. (1984) 289:584–6. doi: 10.1136/bmj.289.6445.584
73. Dworzak F, Ferrari P, Gavazzi C, Maiorana C, Bozzetti F. Effects of cachexia due to cancer on whole body and skeletal muscle protein turnover. *Cancer*. (1998) 82:42–8.
74. Dillon EL, Volpi E, Wolfe RR, Sinha S, Sanford AP, Arrastia CD, et al. Amino acid metabolism and inflammatory burden in ovarian cancer patients undergoing intense oncological therapy. *Clin Nutr*. (2007) 26:736–43. doi: 10.1016/j.clnu.2007.07.004
75. Deutz NE, Safar A, Schutzler S, Memelink R, Ferrando A, Spencer H, et al. Muscle protein synthesis in cancer patients can be stimulated with a specially formulated medical food. *Clin Nutr*. (2011) 30:759–68. doi: 10.1016/j.clnu.2011.05.008
76. Dillon EL, Basra G, Horstman AM, Casperson SL, Randolph KM, Durham WJ, et al. Cancer cachexia and anabolic interventions: a case report. *J Cachexia Sarcopenia Muscle*. (2012) 3:253–63. doi: 10.1007/s13539-012-0066-6
77. Williams JP, Phillips BE, Smith K, Atherton PJ, Rankin D, Selby AL, et al. Effect of tumor burden and subsequent surgical resection on skeletal muscle mass and protein turnover in colorectal cancer patients. *Am J Clin Nutr*. (2012) 96:1064–70. doi: 10.3945/ajcn.112.045708
78. MacDonald AJ, Johns N, Stephens N, Greig C, Ross JA, Small AC, et al. Habitual myofibrillar protein synthesis is normal in patients with upper GI cancer cachexia. *Clin Cancer Res*. (2015) 21:1734–40. doi: 10.1158/1078-0432.CCR-14-2004
79. Shankaran M, King CL, Angel TE, Holmes WE, Li KW, Colangelo M, et al. Circulating protein synthesis rates reveal skeletal muscle proteome dynamics. *J Clin Invest*. (2016) 126:288–302. doi: 10.1172/JCI79639
80. Igarashi M, Ma K, Gao F, Kim HW, Greenstein D, Rapoport SI, et al. Brain lipid concentrations in bipolar disorder. *J Psychiatr Res*. (2010) 44:177–82. doi: 10.1016/j.jpsychires.2009.08.001
81. Salem N, Jr, Litman B, Kim HY, Gawrisch K. Mechanisms of action of docosahexaenoic acid in the nervous system. *Lipids*. (2001) 36:945–59. doi: 10.1007/s11745-001-0805-6
82. Wang Y, Lin QW, Zheng PP, Zhang JS, Huang FR. DHA inhibits protein degradation more efficiently than EPA by regulating the PPARgamma/NFkappaB pathway in C2C12 myotubes. *Biomed Res Int*. (2013) 2013:318981. doi: 10.1155/2013/318981
83. Calder PC. Docosahexaenoic acid. *Ann Nutr Metab*. (2016) 69 (Suppl. 1):7–21. doi: 10.1159/000448262
84. Li F, Duan Y, Li Y, Tang Y, Geng M, Oladele OA, et al. Effects of dietary n-6:n-3 PUFA ratio on fatty acid composition, free amino acid profile and gene expression of transporters in finishing pigs. *Br J Nutr*. (2015) 113:739–48. doi: 10.1017/S0007114514004346
85. Drummond MJ, Fry CS, Glynn EL, Dreyer HC, Dhanani S, Timmerman KL, et al. Rapamycin administration in humans blocks the contraction-induced increase in skeletal muscle protein synthesis. *J Physiol*. (2009) 587:1535–46. doi: 10.1113/jphysiol.2008.163816
86. McGlory C, White A, Treins C, Drust B, Close GL, Maclaren DP, et al. Application of the [γ-^{32}P] ATP kinase assay to study anabolic signaling in human skeletal muscle. *J Appl Physiol*. (2014) 116:504–13. doi: 10.1152/japplphysiol.01072.2013
87. You JS, McNally RM, Jacobs BL, Privett RE, Gundermann DM, Lin KH, et al. The role of raptor in the mechanical load-induced regulation of mTOR signaling, protein synthesis, and skeletal muscle hypertrophy. *FASEB J*. (2019) 33:4021–34. doi: 10.1096/fj.201801653RR
88. Hodson N, McGlory C, Oikawa SY, Jeromson S, Song Z, Ruegg MA, et al. Differential localization and anabolic responsiveness of mTOR complexes in human skeletal muscle in response to feeding and exercise. *Am J Physiol Cell Physiol*. (2017) 313:C604–11. doi: 10.1152/ajpcell.00176.2017
89. Peoples GE, McLennan PL, Howe PR, Groeller H. Fish oil reduces heart rate and oxygen consumption during exercise. *J Cardiovasc Pharmacol*. (2008) 52:540–7. doi: 10.1097/FJC.0b013e3181911913
90. Yoshino J, Smith GI, Kelly SC, Julliand S, Reeds DN, Mittendorfer B. Effect of dietary n-3 PUFA supplementation on the muscle transcriptome in older adults. *Physiol Rep*. (2016) 4:e12785. doi: 10.14814/phy2.12785
91. Powers SK, Smuder AJ, Criswell DS. Mechanistic links between oxidative stress and disuse muscle atrophy. *Antioxid Redox Signal*. (2011) 15:2519–28. doi: 10.1089/ars.2011.3973
92. Crossland H, Skirrow S, Puthucheary ZA, Constantin-Teodosiu D, Greenhaff PL. The impact of immobilisation and inflammation on the regulation of muscle mass and insulin resistance: different routes to similar end-points. *J Physiol*. (2019) 597:1259–70. doi: 10.1113/JP275444
93. Frost RA, Lang CH. Skeletal muscle cytokines: regulation by pathogen-associated molecules and catabolic hormones. *Curr Opin Clin Nutr Metab Care*. (2005) 8:255–63. doi: 10.1097/01.mco.0000165003.16578.2d
94. Calder PC. Marine omega-3 fatty acids and inflammatory processes: effects, mechanisms and clinical relevance. *Biochim Biophys Acta*. (2015) 1851:469–84. doi: 10.1016/j.bbalip.2014.08.010

95. Wada M, DeLong CJ, Hong YH, Rieke CJ, Song I, Sidhu RS, et al. Enzymes and receptors of prostaglandin pathways with arachidonic acid-derived versus eicosapentaenoic acid-derived substrates and products. *J Biol Chem.* (2007) 282:22254–66. doi: 10.1074/jbc.M703169200
96. Li X, Yu Y, Funk CD. Cyclooxygenase-2 induction in macrophages is modulated by docosahexaenoic acid via interactions with free fatty acid receptor 4 (FFA4). *FASEB J.* (2013) 27:4987–97. doi: 10.1096/fj.13-235333
97. Sigal LH. Basic science for the clinician 39: NF-kappaB-function, activation, control, and consequences. *J Clin Rheumatol.* (2006) 12:207–11. doi: 10.1097/01.rhu.0000231385.94784.e4
98. Lee JY, Sohn KH, Rhee SH, Hwang D. Saturated fatty acids, but not unsaturated fatty acids, induce the expression of cyclooxygenase-2 mediated through Toll-like receptor 4. *J Biol Chem.* (2001) 276:16683–9. doi: 10.1074/jbc.M011695200
99. Wong SW, Kwon MJ, Choi AM, Kim HP, Nakahira K, Hwang DH. Fatty acids modulate Toll-like receptor 4 activation through regulation of receptor dimerization and recruitment into lipid rafts in a reactive oxygen species-dependent manner. *J Biol Chem.* (2009) 284:27384–92. doi: 10.1074/jbc.M109.044065
100. Krey G, Braissant O, L'Horset F, Kalkhoven E, Perroud M, Parker MG, et al. Fatty acids, eicosanoids, and hypolipidemic agents identified as ligands of peroxisome proliferator-activated receptors by coactivator-dependent receptor ligand assay. *Mol Endocrinol.* (1997) 11:779–91. doi: 10.1210/mend.11.6.0007
101. Zapata-Gonzalez F, Rueda F, Petriz J, Domingo P, Villarroya F, Diaz-Delfin J, et al. Human dendritic cell activities are modulated by the omega-3 fatty acid, docosahexaenoic acid, mainly through PPAR(gamma):RXR heterodimers: comparison with other polyunsaturated fatty acids. *J Leukoc Biol.* (2008) 84:1172–82. doi: 10.1189/jlb.1007688
102. Vanden Berghe W, Vermeulen L, Delerive P, De Bosscher K, Staels B, Haegeman G. A paradigm for gene regulation: inflammation, NF-kappaB and PPAR. *Adv Exp Med Biol.* (2003) 544:181–96. doi: 10.1007/978-1-4419-9072-3_22
103. Huang F, Wei H, Luo H, Jiang S, Peng J. EPA inhibits the inhibitor of kappaBalpha (IkappaBalpha)/NF-kappaB/muscle RING finger 1 pathway in C2C12 myotubes in a PPARgamma-dependent manner. *Br J Nutr.* (2011) 105:348–56. doi: 10.1017/S0007114510003703
104. Li H, Malhotra S, Kumar A. Nuclear factor-kappa B signaling in skeletal muscle atrophy. *J Mol Med.* (2008) 86:1113–26. doi: 10.1007/s00109-008-0373-8
105. Oh DY, Talukdar S, Bae EJ, Imamura T, Morinaga H, Fan W, et al. GPR120 is an omega-3 fatty acid receptor mediating potent anti-inflammatory and insulin-sensitizing effects. *Cell.* (2010) 142:687–98. doi: 10.1016/j.cell.2010.07.041
106. Kim N, Lee JO, Lee HJ, Kim HI, Kim JK, Lee YW, et al. Endogenous ligand for GPR120, docosahexaenoic acid, exerts benign metabolic effects on the skeletal muscles via AMP-activated protein kinase pathway. *J Biol Chem.* (2015) 290:20438–47. doi: 10.1074/jbc.M115.657379
107. Zhou Y, Wong CO, Cho KJ, van der Hoeven D, Liang H, Thakur DP, et al. SIGNAL TRANSDUCTION. Membrane potential modulates plasma membrane phospholipid dynamics and K-Ras signaling. *Science.* (2015) 349:873–6. doi: 10.1126/science.aaa5619
108. Petrov AM, Kravtsova VV, Matchkov VV, Vasiliev AN, Zefirov AL, Chibalin AV, et al. Membrane lipid rafts are disturbed in the response of rat skeletal muscle to short-term disuse. *Am J Physiol Cell Physiol.* (2017) 312:C627–37. doi: 10.1152/ajpcell.00365.2016
109. Bannenberg G, Serhan CN. Specialized pro-resolving lipid mediators in the inflammatory response: an update. *Biochim Biophys Acta.* (2010) 1801:1260–73. doi: 10.1016/j.bbalip.2010.08.002
110. Serhan CN, Chiang N, Van Dyke TE. Resolving inflammation: dual anti-inflammatory and pro-resolution lipid mediators. *Nat Rev Immunol.* (2008) 8:349–61. doi: 10.1038/nri2294
111. Serhan CN, Chiang N. Resolution phase lipid mediators of inflammation: agonists of resolution. *Curr Opin Pharmacol.* (2013) 13:632–40. doi: 10.1016/j.coph.2013.05.012
112. Hong S, Gronert K, Devchand PR, Moussignac RL, Serhan CN. Novel docosatrienes and 17S-resolvins generated from docosahexaenoic acid in murine brain, human blood, and glial cells. Autacoids in anti-inflammation. *J Biol Chem.* (2003) 278:14677–87. doi: 10.1074/jbc.M300218200
113. Mas E, Croft KD, Zahra P, Barden A, Mori TA. Resolvins D1, D2, and other mediators of self-limited resolution of inflammation in human blood following n-3 fatty acid supplementation. *Clin Chem.* (2012) 58:1476–84. doi: 10.1373/clinchem.2012.190199
114. Polus A, Zapala B, Razny U, Gielicz A, Kiec-Wilk B, Malczewska-Malec M, et al. Omega-3 fatty acid supplementation influences the whole blood transcriptome in women with obesity, associated with pro-resolving lipid mediator production. *Biochim Biophys Acta.* (2016) 1861:1746–55. doi: 10.1016/j.bbalip.2016.08.005
115. Giannakis N, Sansbury BE, Patsalos A, Hays TT, Riley CO, Han X, et al. Dynamic changes to lipid mediators support transitions among macrophage subtypes during muscle regeneration. *Nat Immunol.* (2019) 20:626–36. doi: 10.1038/s41590-019-0356-7

13

Glycine Protects Muscle Cells from Wasting *in vitro* via mTORC1 Signaling

*Marissa K. Caldow, Daniel J. Ham†, Jennifer Trieu, Jin Dylan Chung, Gordon S. Lynch and René Koopman**

Centre for Muscle Research, Department of Physiology, The University of Melbourne, Melbourne, VIC, Australia

***Correspondence:**
René Koopman
rkoopman@unimelb.edu.au

†Present address:
Daniel J. Ham,
The Center for Molecular Life Sciences, Biozentrum University of Basel, Basel, Switzerland

Glycine supplementation can protect skeletal muscles of mice from cancer-induced wasting, but the mechanisms underlying this protection are not well-understood. The aim of this study was to determine whether exogenous glycine directly protects skeletal muscle cells from wasting. C2C12 muscle cells were exposed to non-inflammatory catabolic stimuli via two models: serum withdrawal (SF) for 48 h; or incubation in HEPES buffered saline (HBS) for up to 5 h. Cells were supplemented with glycine or equimolar concentrations of L-alanine. SF- and HBS-treated myotubes (with or without L-alanine) were ~20% and ~30% smaller than control myotubes. Glycine-treated myotubes were up to 20% larger ($P < 0.01$) compared to cells treated with L-alanine in both models of muscle cell atrophy. The mTORC1 inhibitor rapamycin prevented the glycine-stimulated protection of myotube diameter, and glycine-stimulated S6 phosphorylation, suggesting that mTORC1 signaling may be necessary for glycine's protective effects *in vitro*. Increasing glycine availability may be beneficial for muscle wasting conditions associated with inadequate nutrient intake.

Keywords: atrophy, amino acids, muscle wasting, starvation, C2C12, protein synthesis

INTRODUCTION

The non-essential amino acid glycine is often considered biologically neutral, and not required for the regulation of protein synthesis under normal healthy conditions. However, reduced intracellular levels of glycine have been reported in older individuals (1) and in mouse models of diabetes and muscular dystrophy (2, 3), suggesting that either glycine metabolism is increased during these conditions, or tissue demand exceeds dietary intake. Our observations in several mouse models of muscle wasting showed that supplementation with glycine preserved muscle mass and metabolic function in a range of conditions where the anabolic response to nutrition was altered (4–6). Glycine administration attenuated skeletal muscle wasting and loss of physical function in a mouse model of cancer cachexia, which was associated with a reduction in protein breakdown and skeletal muscle markers of inflammation and ROS (4). In a mouse model of acute (LPS-induced) inflammation, glycine administration preserved the skeletal muscle anabolic response to leucine, through upregulation of mTORC1 signaling and preservation of protein synthesis. Glycine can affect cell homeostasis via glycine receptor mediated signaling and via its metabolism (7). Indeed, previous reports have linked glycine receptor-mediated signaling, via its scaffolding protein gephyrin, to mTORC1 activation in other tissues (8). In the *in vivo* LPS model we also showed a reduction in oxidative stress (DHE) but not mRNA expression of pro-inflammatory cytokines and chemokines in skeletal muscle (6). Dietary glycine supplementation in a mouse model of caloric restriction reduced adiposity (whole-body and epididymal fat mass) and preserved lean mass and muscle mass (5). Together, these data revealed a positive effect of glycine treatment on skeletal muscle protein metabolism, mass and function during muscle wasting conditions. However, it is currently unclear whether the beneficial effects of glycine on skeletal muscle are entirely the result of inflammatory cell inactivation, or whether glycine has muscle cell-specific effects. We tested the hypothesis that glycine would directly attenuate myotube wasting in an mTORC1-dependent manner.

We aimed to determine whether exogenous glycine protects muscle cells from cachectic stimuli. To investigate the effect of glycine on myotube wasting mature C2C12 myotubes were supplemented with glycine or equimolar concentrations of L-alanine and atrophy induced via 2 different approaches: serum withdrawal for 48 h; or incubation in HEPES buffered saline for up to 5 h.

METHODS

Cell Culture

Murine C2C12 myoblasts (Cryosite distribution, NSW, Australia) were cultured in DMEM (Life Technologies, Australia) containing 10% (v/v) fetal calf serum (Life Technologies), 1% L-glutamine (v/v) (Life Technologies), and 1% (v/v) antibiotic solution (100 unit/ml penicillin/streptomycin, Life Technologies) at 37°C in an atmosphere of 5% CO_2. Upon confluency, the media was changed to differentiation media [DMEM containing 2% (v/v) horse serum, 1% L-glutamine and 1% antibiotic solution (Life Technologies)] for 5 days to promote formation of mature multinucleated myotubes (9).

Wasting Conditions

To induce wasting via growth factor deprivation, cells were washed once in serum free DMEM (Life Technologies, Australia) and then incubated in DMEM (i.e., standard amino acid composition) containing 1% L-glutamine and 1% antibiotic solution (Life Technologies) but lacking 2% horse serum for 48 h (SF) (9). SF was supplemented with an additional 2.5 mM glycine (Sigma-Aldrich, Castle Hill, NSW, Australia) or L-alanine (Sigma-Aldrich). To induce wasting via nutrient starvation, cells were washed once in HEPES buffered saline (HBS; 20 mM HEPES/Na pH 7.4, 140 mM NaCl, 2.5 mM $MgSO_4$, 5 mM KCl, and 1 mM $CaCl_2$, no amino acids present), then incubated in HBS (9, 10) with glycine or equimolar concentrations of L-alanine for up to 5 h. L-alanine serves as an isonitrogenous control as it does not modulate cell size and protein turnover in cell and animal models (4–6, 9, 10).

Rapamycin (100 nM, Sigma-Aldrich) was used to inhibit mTORC1 activation (10). We have previously reported that these atrophy models are not associated with altered myotube viability as assessed by Trypan Blue staining (9).

Glycine Withdrawal

DMEM media was formulated without glycine (Life Technologies). Basal levels (0.4 mM) or additional amounts (2.5 mM) of glycine (Sigma-Aldrich) were added when appropriate to serum free or differentiation media, as specified.

Myotube Diameter

Cells were washed 2 × 5 min in phosphate buffered saline (PBS) and then fixed with 4% paraformaldehyde/PBS for 15 min. Cells were then washed in PBS (3 × 5 min), permeated with 0.1% TritonX-100/PBS, washed in PBS (3 × 5 min) and then incubated in 3% bovine serum albumin (BSA)/PBS for 2 h. Cells were incubated with primary antibody overnight at 4°C. MF20 (1:50; Developmental Studies Hybridoma Bank, University of Iowa, Department of Biology, Iowa City, IA, USA) in 3% BSA/PBS was used to stain myosin heavy chain (MHC). Cells were then washed with PBS (3 × 5 min) and incubated in goat-anti-mouse IgG2b Alexa555 secondary antibody (1:500, Life Technologies) and DAPI (1:1,000) for 2 h in 3% BSA/PBS. Cells were washed in PBS (3 × 5 min) and then imaged on a Zeiss Axiovert 40 CFL inverted microscope using a 10X objective. Four images were taken in each well from pre-defined locations within each quadrant. Myotube diameter was measured using AxioVision software (AxioVision AC Rel. 4.8.2, Carl Zeiss Imaging Solutions, Wrek, Göttingen; Germany). A total of ~50–80 myotubes were measured per well and the average diameter of each well was used for statistical analysis as described previously (6, 9, 10).

Protein Synthesis

Myotubes were grown and treated as described previously. To determine the rate of protein synthesis we utilized SUnSET methodology, as described (10, 11). Briefly, puromycin (Sigma-Aldrich) was administered to the media at a final concentration of 1 μM exactly 30 min before cells were collected in ice-cold homogenizing buffer. Anti-puromycin was purchased from Millipore (Kilsyth, Victoria, Australia) and immunoblotting was used to detect changes in puromycin incorporation as described (9, 10).

Protein Extraction and Immunoblotting

Cell lysates were prepared using RIPA lysis buffer (Merck Millipore, VIC, Australia) including protease and phosphatase inhibitor cocktails (Sigma-Aldrich). Lysates were rotated end over end at 4°C for 30 min, then centrifuged at 13,000 RPM at 4°C for 10 min to collect the supernatant. Protein content was determined via Bio-Rad DC protein assay as per manufacturer's instructions (Bio-Rad Laboratories, NSW, Australia). Briefly, samples were separated by SDS-PAGE using Criterion™ TGX Stain-Free™ Precast Gels (Bio-Rad) and proteins were transferred to 0.45 mm PVDF via Trans-Blot® Turbo™ transfer system (Bio-Rad). Gels were visualized using a ChemiDoc™ imaging system (Bio-Rad) and images were captured prior to and following transfer. Membranes were blocked for 2 h at room temperature (RT) in 5% (w/v) bovine serum albumin (BSA, Sigma-Aldrich) or 5% Skim Milk (for puromycin) in Tris-buffered saline-Tween 20 (TBST). Membranes were incubated overnight at 4°C with primary antibodies. The following day membranes were incubated for 1 h at RT in horseradish peroxidise-conjugated secondary antibodies. Membranes were treated with enhanced chemiluminescence (Super Signal West Femto; Thermo Scientific) and proteins were visualized using ChemiDoc™ imaging system (Bio-Rad). Blots were quantified using ImageLab® software (Bio-Rad), and normalized to total protein as quantified from the Stain Free Gel imaging (**Figure 3**) or by BLOT FastStain™ as per manufacturer's instructions (G-Biosciences, St. Louis, MO; **Figure 2**).

Antibodies

pAkt (S473), Akt, pmTOR (S2448), mTOR, pp70S6K (Thr389), p70S6K, pS6 (S235/236), S6, p4EBP1 (T37/46), 4EBP1, pSTAT3 (Tyr705), and STAT3 were purchased from Cell Signaling Technologies (Beverly, MA, USA) and diluted 1:1,000 in 5% BSA/TBST. Secondary antibodies (donkey anti-rabbit HRP immunoglobulins, GE Healthcare Life Sciences, Australia) were diluted in 5% BSA/TBST.

To assess whether protein expression of key structural protein were affected by glycine in the wasting models, MF20 (Developmental Studies Hybridoma Bank) was diluted 1:50 in 5% BSA/TBST. α-actin (Sigma-Aldrich) was diluted 1/3,000 in 5% BSA/TBST. Secondary antibodies (sheep anti-mouse HRP immunoglobulins GE Healthcare Life Sciences) were diluted in 5% BSA/TBST.

Anti-puromycin (Clone 12D10; Millipore) was diluted 1:5,000 in 1% BSA/TBST. Secondary antibodies (goat anti-mouse IgG Fc 2a, Jackson ImmunoResearch Laboratories Inc., West Grove, PA, USA) were diluted 1:50,000 in 5% milk/TBST.

Statistics

All values were expressed as mean ± SD. Data were normalized to the appropriate control group for ease of visualization, unless otherwise stated. Two-way ANOVAs (time and treatment) were used to compare between groups for dose-response, time-course, and rapamycin experiment, while one-way ANOVAs were used for all other comparisons. Tukey's *post hoc* test was used to determine significant differences between individual groups and P values reported in figures. For transparency, we report both significant differences ($P < 0.05$) and trends ($P < 0.1$) are reported where appropriate.

RESULTS

Glycine Reduces Muscle Wasting in a Dose-Dependent Manner During Growth Factor Deprivation

Growth factor deprivation (48 h) significantly reduced myotube diameter (SF, −13%; $P < 0.05$; **Figure 1A**). The addition of glycine to SF media attenuated muscle wasting in a dose-dependent manner, reaching significance at a concentration of 0.5, 1, and 2.5 mM. Importantly, equimolar concentrations of L-alanine did not attenuate myotube wasting, compared to SF alone. Serum starved glycine-treated myotubes were larger (0.5 mM, 18%; 1 mM, 16%; 2.5 mM, 22%; $P < 0.01$) compared with SF containing L-alanine-treated myotubes (SF ALA$^+$). We have not further investigated why the beneficial effects of glycine were lost at a concentration of 5 mM as we used the dose-response studies to select the most appropriate and effective dose. All further experiments in SFM were performed using 2.5 mM glycine or L-alanine.

We also removed glycine from SF to determine if basal glycine contributed to any effects on myotube diameter. The removal of glycine (0.4 mM) from SF (SF GLY$^-$) did not augment the effects of SF alone (**Figure 1B**).

Glycine Is Important for Myotube Size Under Normal Growth Conditions

Removal of glycine from DM (48 h) induced myotube wasting similar to that caused by nutrient deprivation (SF). Differentiation media without basal glycine reduced myotube diameter by 17% compared to DM ($P < 0.001$; **Figure 1C**).

Glycine Reduces Muscle Wasting in a Dose-Dependent Manner During Nutrient Starvation

Nutrient starvation (5 h) reduced myotube diameter (HBS, −29%; $P < 0.05$; **Figure 2A**). The addition of glycine to HBS attenuated muscle wasting in a dose-dependent manner, reaching significance at a concentration of 1 and 2.5 mM. Importantly, equimolar concentrations of L-alanine did not increase myotube diameter, compared to HBS alone. Nutrient deprived (HBS) glycine-treated myotubes were larger (1 mM, 18%; 2.5 mM 14%; $P < 0.01$) than myotubes treated with L-alanine (HBS ALA$^+$). The beneficial effects of glycine were lost at a concentration of 5 mM. All further experiments in HBS were performed using 2.5 mM glycine or L-alanine.

Glycine Maintains Protein Synthesis During Nutrient Starvation

Protein synthesis was improved by the presence of 2.5 mM glycine during 4 h of nutrient starvation. At each time point, puromycin incorporation was greater in glycine treated cells, compared to L-alanine treated cells ($P < 0.01$, **Figure 2B**).

Glycine Protects From Muscle Wasting During Nutrient Starvation and Growth Factor Deprivation via mTORC1

Myotubes were incubated with the mTORC1 inhibitor rapamycin to determine the involvement of mTORC1 in the protective effect of glycine in the nutrient starvation and growth factor deprivation models. We measured the effects of rapamycin on myotube diameter and the phosphorylation

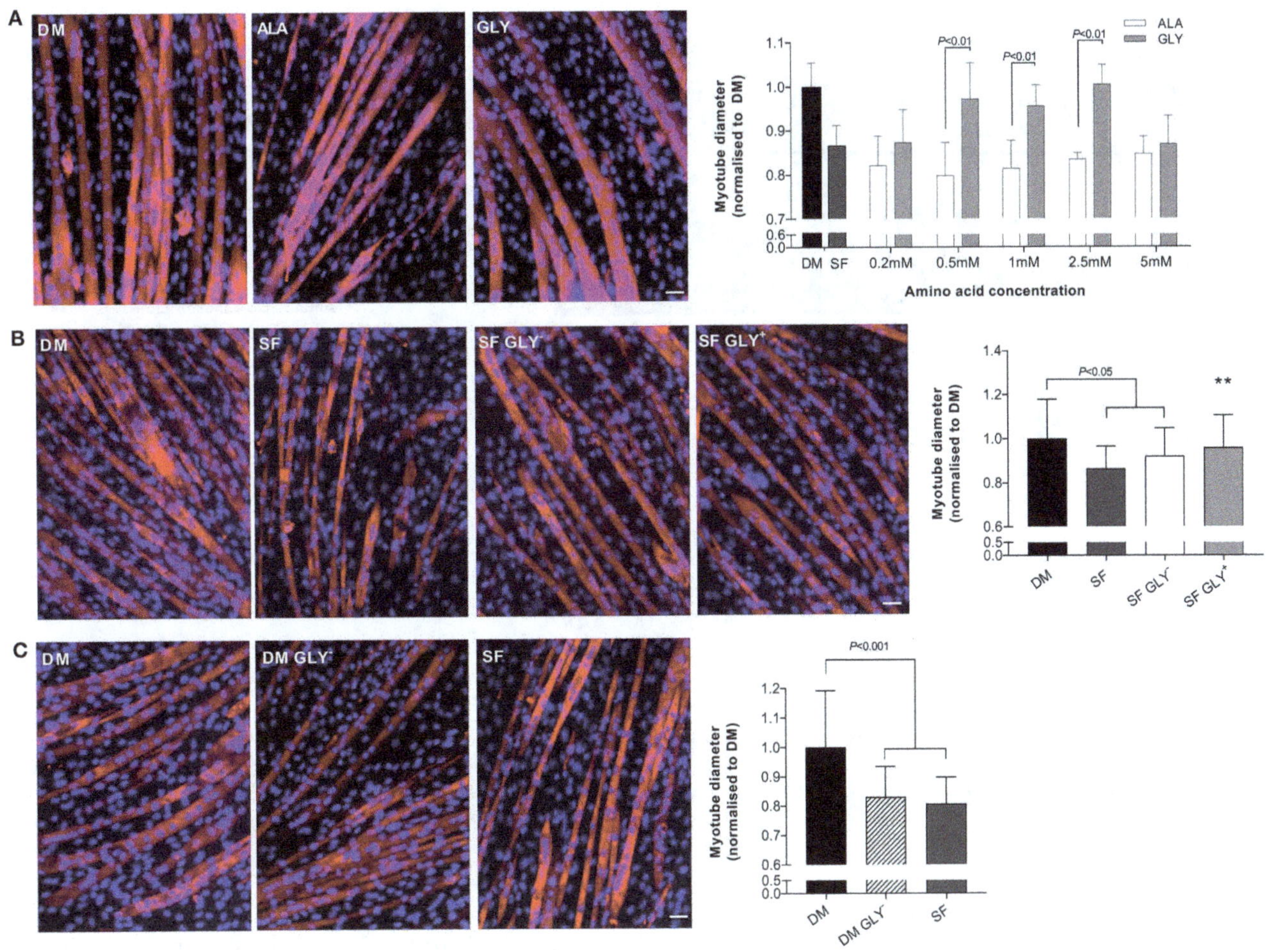

FIGURE 1 | Glycine attenuates muscle wasting during growth factor deprivation. Myotube diameter for cells incubated in differentiation media (DM) or serum free (SF) media for 48 h with increasing concentrations of glycine or isomolar concentrations of L-alanine, and representative images at the optimal dose of 2.5 mM **(A)**. Removal of glycine from SF (SF GLY$^-$) did not further impact myotube size compared to SF **(B)**. Removal of glycine from DM for 48 h induced myotube wasting like that in SF media **(C)**. Scale bar represents 50 μm. This applies to all images. Values are means ± SD, n = 4–6 per group. Significant differences are displayed where appropriate. ** Significantly different to SF, $P < 0.01$.

status of downstream targets of mTORC1. In a model of 4 h nutrient starvation (HBS), rapamycin attenuated the protective effects of glycine by 13% ($P < 0.01$). There were no significant effects of rapamycin on myotube diameter in L-alanine treated cells (**Figure 3A**). Rapamycin also prevented the glycine-induced S6 phosphorylation ($P < 0.001$, **Figure 3C**). Similarly, when cells were treated acutely with amino acids and rapamycin in the growth factor deprivation model (4 h, SF), rapamycin prevented the maintenance of S6 phosphorylation ($P < 0.001$, **Figure 3E**). In L-alanine-treated cells, rapamycin also reduced S6 phosphorylation in both the deprivation (4 h HBS, $P < 0.05$) and starvation models (4 h SF, $P < 0.01$). No changes in AKT, mTOR, p70S6K or 4EBP1 phosphorylation were observed under any treatment condition (**Figures 3B,D**). Similarly, there were no changes in pSTAT3 phosphorylation or MF20 and α-actin protein abundance between the treatment groups (**Supplementary Figure 1**).

DISCUSSION

Calorie restriction is a common lifestyle intervention effective in combating obesity and the associated risk of metabolic diseases. Although glycine supplementation helps preserve lean mass in a mouse model of calorie restriction (5), the mechanisms for the protective effect have not been resolved. In the present study, we demonstrated that glycine protects against myotube wasting in an mTORC signaling-dependent manner in two *in vitro* models of nutrient/growth factor restriction.

Our model of nutrient starvation (HBS) has been shown previously to dramatically reduce protein synthesis and mTORC1 signaling and reduce myotube diameter (10). Similarly, 48 h of nutrient deprivation (SF) induced myotube atrophy. We observed a dose-dependent protection from myotube wasting in glycine treated C2C12 cells, in both HBS and SF models. The applied dose (2.5 mM) of glycine is ~10-fold higher than basal plasma concentrations, but only 40% higher than basal

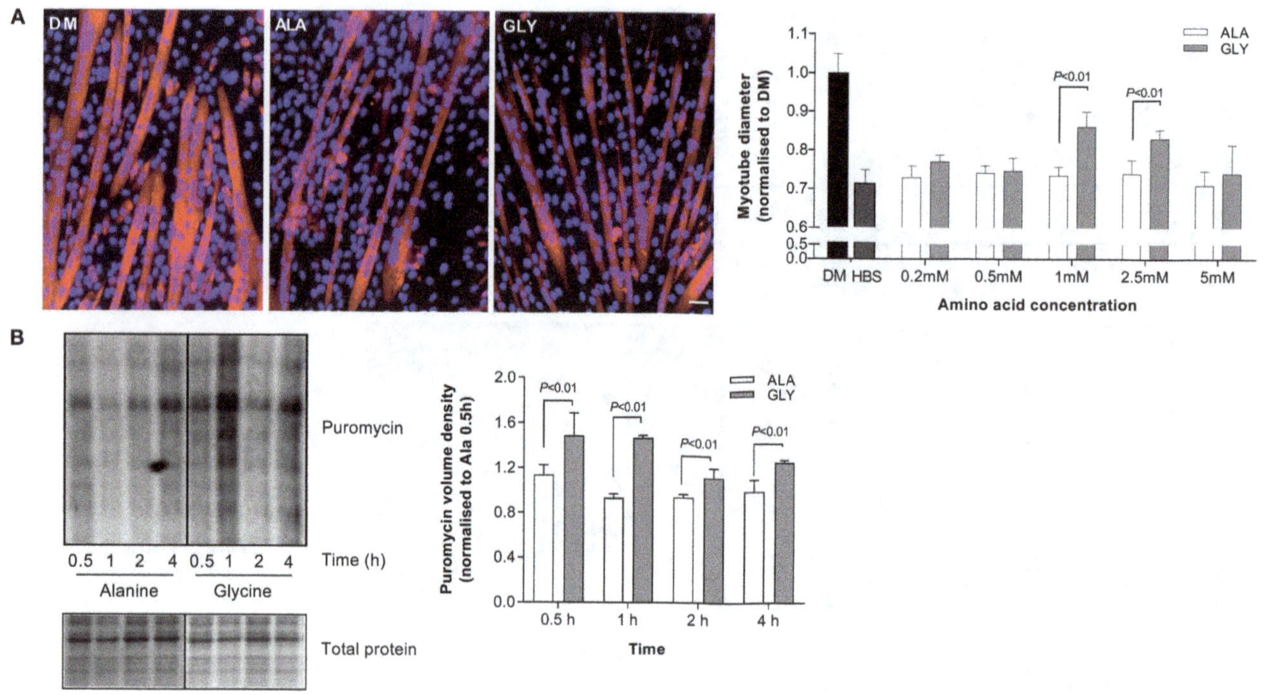

FIGURE 2 | Glycine attenuates muscle wasting and preserves rates of protein synthesis during nutrient starvation. Myotube diameter for cells incubated in differentiation media (DM) or HEPES buffered saline (HBS) for 5 h with increasing concentrations of glycine or isomolar concentrations of L-alanine, and representative images at the optimal dose of 2.5 mM **(A)**. Glycine supplementation improves protein synthesis as assessed using puromycin after incubation in HBS for up to 4 h **(B)**. Scale bar represents 50 μm. This applies to all images. Values are means ± SD, $n = 4–6$ per group. Significant differences are displayed where appropriate.

concentration in muscle and comparable to that seen after ingestion of a protein rich meal (12). Removal of glycine from SF media did not aggravate nutrient deprivation-induced atrophy. Interestingly, removal of glycine from differentiation media for 48 h induced atrophy, comparable to that of cells incubated in SF media. This may be attributed to a disruption in one-carbon metabolism by the loss of exogenous glycine availability and a subsequent inability to maintain cellular homeostasis (13, 14). The observation that glycine did not modulate STAT3 phosphorylation in HBS treated cells is in accordance with our previous studies demonstrating that glycine did not affect LPS-induced increases in cytokine production (6). For these reasons we did not pursue studying inflammatory pathways but focused instead on mTORC1 associated signaling.

In C2C12 myotubes incubated in HBS, glycine supplementation attenuated myotube wasting, maintained protein synthesis and promoted S6 phosphorylation. In both wasting models, the glycine-induced increases in S6 phosphorylation were completely prevented by rapamycin. Likewise, rapamycin inhibited the glycine-stimulated protection of myotube diameter, indicating that mTORC1 signaling is necessary for glycine's protective effects on myotube size in both growth factor deprivation and nutrient starvation models. These results are consistent with the effect of glycine on C2C12 myoblasts where acute exposure (30 min–6 h) promoted proliferation, cell viability and protein synthesis in the absence of serum, in an mTORC1-dependent manner (15). However, in myoblasts isolated from neonatal chicks, there was no effect of glycine supplementation on mTOR expression (16). The meaning of these observations is unclear since this study measured mTOR and S6K1 mRNA expression rather than the phosphorylation status of these signaling molecules as a measure of mTOR activity. Importantly for the present study, although rapamycin treatment reduced myotube diameter and S6 phosphorylation in L-alanine and glycine treated myotubes, L-alanine did not provide protection from atrophy during wasting conditions.

Upon activation, mTORC1 phosphorylates and activates two parallel signaling pathways. S6 kinase 1 phosphorylation leads to activation of the ribosomal protein S6, while phosphorylation of the eukaryotic initiation factor 4E (eIF4E)-binding protein (4EBP1) ultimately allows for the synthesis of new proteins. Despite inhibition of S6 phosphorylation by rapamycin in glycine treated cells, there was no alteration in phosphorylation of mTOR, P70S6K and 4EBP1 in either of the nutritional wasting models after 4 h of treatment suggesting that upstream signaling occurs earlier. Divergence in signaling between S6 and 4EBP1 has been described previously in glycine treated C2C12 myoblasts (15), and myotubes treated with other amino acids (10) and the reason for these discrepancies remain to be established.

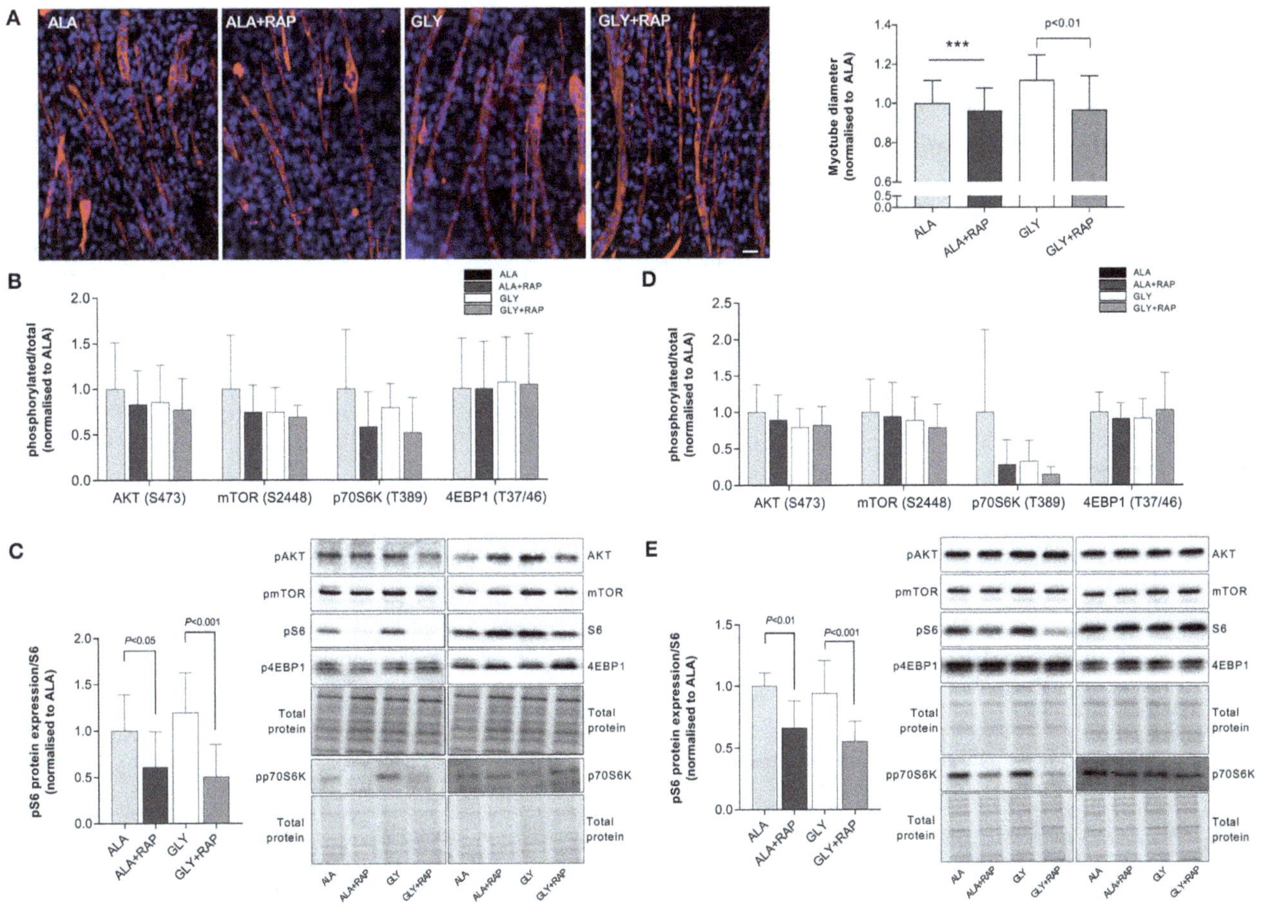

FIGURE 3 | Glycine attenuates muscle wasting in an mTORC dependent manner. Representative images and myotube diameter for cells incubated in HBS for 5 h with 2.5 mM glycine or L-alanine co-treated with the mTORC1 inhibitor rapamycin (100 nM) **(A)**. Phosphorylation status of AKT, mTOR, p70S6K, 4EBP1 **(B)** and S6 **(C)** was measured following 4 h of HBS treatment with amino acids and rapamycin (100 nM). Phosphorylation status of AKT, mTOR, p70S6K, 4EBP1 **(D)**, and S6 **(E)** was measured following 4 h of SF treatment with amino acids and rapamycin (100 nM). Scale bar represents 50 μm. This applies to all images. Values are means ± SD, $n = 4$–8 per group. Significant differences are displayed where appropriate. *** Significantly different to GLY (treatment effect), $P < 0.001$.

The way in which many amino acids signal to mTORC1 is still relatively unknown. It is possible glycine may signal to mTORC1 via a non-canonical mechanism using Vps34 (17–19). However, it remains to be established whether glycine can mediate Vps34 expression in skeletal muscle. Alternatively, glycine may signal to mTORC1 via its receptor, GlyR (7). GlyRs are inhibitory Cl^- channels composed of three different subunits: (1) the ligand binding α subunits (GLRA1, GLRA2, GLRA3, or GLRA4); (2) a structural β subunit (GLRB); and (3) a cytoplasmic anchoring protein known as gephyrin (GPHN). GlyR mediated cell-cell communication is enabled by gephyrin, an anchoring protein that provides the scaffolding needed for cytoplasmic GlyRβ binding (20). Interestingly, it has been suggested gephyrin is required for mTORC1 signaling and contributes to the intracellular localization of mTORC1 and downstream signaling in a variety of cell types (8, 21). Although a functional GlyR is still to be identified in skeletal muscle, its presence in cardiac and smooth muscle suggests it is highly likely (22–24). Further studies are required to confirm GlyR-mTORC signaling in skeletal muscle.

In summary our results in C2C12 myotubes demonstrate a role for glycine in the protection of skeletal muscle wasting *in vitro*. Rapamycin inhibited the glycine-stimulated protection of myotube diameter, and the glycine-stimulated S6 phosphorylation, indicating that mTORC1 signaling is necessary for glycine's protective effects *in vitro*. The removal of glycine from differentiation media for 48 h highlights that glycine is required to maintain cellular homeostasis under normal differentiation conditions. Our results suggest that increasing glycine availability may be beneficial for muscle wasting conditions associated with inadequate nutrient intake.

AUTHOR CONTRIBUTIONS

MC, DH, GL, and RK interpreted results, conception and design of research, edited and revised manuscript, and approved final version of manuscript. MC, DH, JC, and JT performed experiments. MC and DH analyzed data. MC drafted manuscript.

FUNDING

MC was supported by a McKenzie Fellowship from the University of Melbourne. DH and MC were funded by an ESPEN Fellowship. This work was supported in part by the National Health and Medical Research Council, Australia (GNT1103571; RK, GL).

ACKNOWLEDGMENTS

The authors wish to thank Audrey Chan for technical assistance.

SUPPLEMENTARY MATERIAL

Supplementary Figure 1 | Phosphorylation of STAT3 and MF20 and α-actin protein abundance was measured following 4 h of HBS **(A)** or SFM **(B)** treatment with amino acids and rapamycin (100 nM). Values are means ± SD, $n = 4$ per group.

REFERENCES

1. Fazelzadeh P, Hangelbroek RW, Tieland M, de Groot LC, Verdijk LB, van Loon LJ, et al. The muscle metabolome differs between healthy and frail older adults. *J Proteome Res.* (2016) 15:499–509. doi: 10.1021/acs.jproteome.5b00840
2. Martins-Bach AB, Bloise AC, Vainzof M, Rahnamaye Rabbani S. Metabolic profile of dystrophic mdx mouse muscles analyzed with *in vitro* magnetic resonance spectroscopy (MRS). *Magn Reson Imaging.* (2012) 30:1167–76. doi: 10.1016/j.mri.2012.04.003
3. Giesbertz P, Padberg I, Rein D, Ecker J, Hofle AS, Spanier B, et al. Metabolite profiling in plasma and tissues of ob/ob and db/db mice identifies novel markers of obesity and type 2 diabetes. *Diabetologia.* (2015) 58:2133–43. doi: 10.1007/s00125-015-3656-y
4. Ham DJ, Murphy KT, Chee A, Lynch GS, Koopman R. Glycine administration attenuates skeletal muscle wasting in a mouse model of cancer cachexia. *Clin Nutr.* (2014) 33:448–58. doi: 10.1016/j.clnu.2013.06.013
5. Caldow MK, Ham DJ, Godeassi DP, Chee A, Lynch GS, Koopman R. Glycine supplementation during calorie restriction accelerates fat loss and protects against further muscle loss in obese mice. *Clin Nutr.* (2015) 35:1118–26. doi: 10.1016/j.clnu.2015.08.013
6. Ham DJ, Caldow MK, Chhen V, Chee A, Wang X, Proud CG, et al. Glycine restores the anabolic response to leucine in a mouse model of acute inflammation. *Am J Physiol Endocrinol Metab.* (2016) 310:E970–81. doi: 10.1152/ajpendo.00468.2015
7. Koopman R, Caldow MK, Ham DJ, Lynch GS. Glycine metabolism in skeletal muscle: implications for metabolic homeostasis. *Curr Opin Clin Nutr Metab Care.* (2017) 20:237–42. doi: 10.1097/MCO.0000000000000383
8. Sabatini DM, Barrow RK, Blackshaw S, Burnett PE, Lai MM, Field ME, et al. Interaction of RAFT1 with gephyrin required for rapamycin-sensitive signaling. *Science.* (1999) 284:1161–4. doi: 10.1126/science.284.5417.1161
9. Ham DJ, Gleeson BG, Chee A, Baum DM, Caldow MK, Lynch GS, et al. L-Citrulline protects skeletal muscle cells from cachectic stimuli through an iNOS-dependent mechanism. *PLoS ONE.* (2015) 10:e0141572. doi: 10.1371/journal.pone.0141572
10. Ham DJ, Caldow MK, Lynch GS, Koopman R. Arginine protects muscle cells from wasting *in vitro* in an mTORC1-dependent and NO-independent manner. *Amino Acids.* (2014) 46:2643–52. doi: 10.1007/s00726-014-1815-y
11. Goodman CA, Hornberger TA. Measuring protein synthesis with SUnSET: a valid alternative to traditional techniques? *Exerc Sport Sci Rev.* (2013) 41:107–15. doi: 10.1097/JES.0b013e3182798a95
12. Bergstrom J, Furst P, Vinnars E. Effect of a test meal, without and with protein, on muscle and plasma free amino acids. *Clin Sci (Lond).* (1990) 79:331–7. doi: 10.1042/cs0790331
13. Maddocks OD, Berkers CR, Mason SM, Zheng L, Blyth K, Gottlieb E, et al. Serine starvation induces stress and p53-dependent metabolic remodelling in cancer cells. *Nature.* (2013) 493:542–6. doi: 10.1038/nature11743
14. Maddocks ODK, Athineos D, Cheung EC, Lee P, Zhang T, van den Broek NJF, et al. Modulating the therapeutic response of tumours to dietary serine and glycine starvation. *Nature.* (2017) 544:372–6. doi: 10.1038/nature22056
15. Sun K, Wu Z, Ji Y, Wu G. Glycine regulates protein turnover by activating protein kinase B/mammalian target of rapamycin and by inhibiting MuRF1 and atrogin-1 gene expression in C2C12 myoblasts. *J Nutr.* (2016) 146:2461–7. doi: 10.3945/jn.116.231266
16. She Y, Deng H, Cai H, Liu G. Regulation of the expression of key signalling molecules in mTOR pathway of skeletal muscle satellite cells in neonatal chicks: effects of leucine and glycine-leucine peptide. *J Anim Physiol Anim Nutr (Berl).* (2019) 103:786–90. doi: 10.1111/jpn.13090
17. Nobukuni T, Joaquin M, Roccio M, Dann SG, Kim SY, Gulati P, et al. Amino acids mediate mTOR/raptor signaling through activation of class 3 phosphatidylinositol 3OH-kinase. *Proc Natl Acad Sci USA.* (2005) 102:14238–43. doi: 10.1073/pnas.0506925102
18. Nobukuni T, Kozma SC, Thomas G. hvps34, an ancient player, enters a growing game: mTOR Complex1/S6K1 signaling. *Curr Opin Cell Biol.* (2007) 19:135–41. doi: 10.1016/j.ceb.2007.02.019
19. Yoon MS, Chen J. Distinct amino acid-sensing mTOR pathways regulate skeletal myogenesis. *Mol Biol Cell.* (2013) 24:3754–63. doi: 10.1091/mbc.e13-06-0353
20. Fritschy JM, Harvey RJ, Schwarz G. Gephyrin: where do we stand, where do we go? *Trends Neurosci.* (2008) 31:257–64. doi: 10.1016/j.tins.2008.02.006
21. Wuchter J, Beuter S, Treindl F, Herrmann T, Zeck G, Templin MF, et al. A comprehensive small interfering RNA screen identifies signaling pathways required for gephyrin clustering. *J Neurosci.* (2012) 32:14821–34. doi: 10.1523/JNEUROSCI.1261-12.2012
22. Qi RB, Zhang JY, Lu DX, Wang HD, Wang HH, Li CJ. Glycine receptors contribute to cytoprotection of glycine in myocardial cells. *Chin Med J (Engl).* (2007) 120:915–21. doi: 10.1097/00029330-200705020-00012
23. Yim PD, Gallos G, Xu D, Zhang Y, Emala CW. Novel expression of a functional glycine receptor chloride channel that attenuates contraction in airway smooth muscle. *FASEB J.* (2011) 25:1706–17. doi: 10.1096/fj.10-170530
24. Jose Alburquerque-Bejar J, Barba I, Valls-Lacalle L, Ruiz-Meana M, Pecoraro M, Rodriguez-Sinovas A, et al. Remote ischemic conditioning provides humoural cross-species cardioprotection through glycine receptor activation. *Cardiovasc Res.* (2017) 113:52–60. doi: 10.1093/cvr/cvw242

14

mTORC1 Signaling in Individual Human Muscle Fibers Following Resistance Exercise in Combination with Intake of Essential Amino Acids

Sebastian Edman[1], Karin Söderlund[1], Marcus Moberg[1], William Apró[1] and Eva Blomstrand[1,2]*

[1] *The Åstrand Laboratory, the Swedish School of Sport and Health Sciences, Stockholm, Sweden,*

[2] *Department of Physiology and Pharmacology, Karolinska Institutet, Stockholm, Sweden*

***Correspondence:**
Sebastian Edman
sebastian.edman@gih.se

Human muscles contain a mixture of type I and type II fibers with different contractile and metabolic properties. Little is presently known about the effect of anabolic stimuli, in particular nutrition, on the molecular responses of these different fiber types. Here, we examine the effect of resistance exercise in combination with intake of essential amino acids (EAA) on mTORC1 signaling in individual type I and type II human muscle fibers. Five strength-trained men performed two sessions of heavy leg press exercise. During exercise and recovery, the subjects ingested an aqueous solution of EAA (290 mg/kg) or flavored water (placebo). Muscle biopsies were taken from the vastus lateralis before and 90 min after exercise. The biopsies were freeze-dried and single fibers dissected out and weighed (range 0.95–8.1 μg). The fibers were homogenized individually and identified as type I or II by incubation with antibodies against the different isoforms of myosin. They were also analyzed for both the levels of protein as well as phosphorylation of proteins in the mTORC1 pathway using Western blotting. The levels of the S6K1 and eEF2 proteins were ~50% higher in type II than in type I fibers ($P < 0.05$), but no difference was found between fiber types with respect to the level of mTOR protein. Resistance exercise led to non-significant increases (2–3-fold) in mTOR and S6K1 phosphorylation as well as a 50% decrease ($P < 0.05$) in eEF2 phosphorylation in both fiber types. Intake of EAA caused a 2 and 6-fold higher ($P < 0.05$) elevation of mTOR and S6K1 phosphorylation, respectively, in both type I and type II fibers compared to placebo, with no effect on phosphorylation of eEF2. In conclusion, protein levels of S6K1 and eEF2 were significantly higher in type II than type I fibers suggesting higher capacity of the mTOR pathway in type II fibers. Ingestion of EAA enhanced the effect of resistance exercise on phosphorylation of mTOR and S6K1 in both fiber types, but with considerable variation between single fibers of both types.

Keywords: muscle fiber type, protein expression, S6K1, single muscle fiber, EAA

INTRODUCTION

Human skeletal muscle contains a mixture of fibers with different contractile and metabolic properties, these fibers also differ with respect to adaptability to training. Slow twitch type I fibers have, in general, more mitochondria and a higher oxidative capacity (1, 2). In contrast, type II fibers are more able to produce energy rapidly due to their elevated intracellular level of phosphocreatine and higher glycolytic capacity (3–5).

Resistance exercise enhances the size of individual muscle fibers, in particular fast-twitch fibers (6, 7). Another strong activator of muscle protein synthesis is dietary intake of protein or amino acids (8, 9). The anabolic response evoked by both of these factors is mediated through changes in phosphorylation of proteins in the mechanistic target of rapamycin complex 1 (mTORC1) pathway, including p70 ribosomal protein S6 kinase 1 (S6K1) and eukaryotic elongation factor 2 (eEF2) (10, 11). Furthermore, the extent of phosphorylation levels of these enzymes is an indicator of skeletal muscle hypertrophy and strength adaptation (12, 13). Resistance exercise and intake of protein or amino acids also act synergistically, with the latter potentiating stimulation of mTORC1 signaling (14, 15), as well as protein synthesis by resistance exercise (16).

In an earlier study, we demonstrated that maximal eccentric contractions evoked dissimilar responses in type I and type II fibers: phosphorylation of S6K1 and of ribosomal protein (rp) S6 was elevated 3-4-fold and 6–9-fold, respectively, in type II fibers, with no change in the type I fibers (17). In this study, protein phosphorylation was measured in pools (100–600 fibers) of type I and type II fibers (17). Furthermore, when subjects are provided nutritional supplement shortly before and after resistance exercise, the responses of type I and II fibers appear to be similar (18). Koopman and colleagues, who employed immunohistochemical evaluation of cross-sections of muscle fibers, detected similar elevations in rpS6 phosphorylation in type I and type II fibers during the recovery phase following resistance exercise when protein was administered together with carbohydrates. However, the variation within the different fiber types was not taken into consideration in these studies.

Accordingly, in the present study, the subjects performed a session of heavy resistance exercise in combination with intake of essential amino acids (EAA) or placebo. Muscle biopsies were taken before and after exercise for analysis of individual type I and type II fibers with respect to both the levels of protein and the degrees of phosphorylation of proteins of the mTORC1 pathway. For this purpose, we employed a novel application of the Western blotting technique, an approach similar to that described by Murphy (19). This procedure provides us with a unique insight into muscle adaptation, as well as variations in intracellular signaling within the same type of fiber. We hypothesize that both exercise and intake of EAA will elicit a larger response in the type II than in type I fibers.

MATERIALS AND METHODS

Subjects

Five healthy men who had been performing resistance training for at least 1 year gave both their oral and written consent to participate after being fully informed about the procedure and possible risks involved. Their mean age was 25 ± 3 years, height 179 ± 4 cm, weight 85 ± 4 kg, and maximal one repetition leg press (1RM) 442 ± 18 kg. These subjects were a sub-group from our earlier study (20). The present investigation was approved by the Regional Ethical Review Board in Stockholm.

Experimental Trial

Following a 9 h fast, subjects reported to the laboratory in the morning. A baseline biopsy was taken from the vastus lateralis muscle with a Weil-Bakesley conchotome (AB Wisex, Mölndal, Sweden) (21) under local anesthesia (Carbocain® 20 mg/ml AstraZeneca AB, Södertälje, Sweden). Thereafter, the subjects performed 10 sets of 8–12 repetitions starting at a load of 85% of 1RM and gradually decreasing with 3 min rests between sets. Muscle biopsies were taken repeatedly during recovery (20), although in the present study only the biopsy taken 90 min after exercise was analyzed since the response was most pronounced at this time point (20). All biopsies were rapidly freed from blood and frozen in liquid nitrogen for storage at −80°C.

At nine time points during the experiment (immediately before and after the warm-up exercise, after the fourth and eighth sets, and following 15, 30, 60, 90, and 120 min of recovery), the participants consumed 150 ml of either an aqueous solution of EAA or placebo (flavored water) in a double-blind, counterbalanced order (20). The EAA mixture consisted of 17.8% L-lysine, 17.1% L-leucine, 14.3% L-phenylalanine, 13.6% L-histidine, 13.6% L-threonine, 11.4% L-valine, 9.5% L-isoleucine, and 2.9% L-methionine (Ajinomoto, Kanagawa, Japan). The total amount of EAA supplied to each subject was 290 mg/kg body weight. Both solutions contained salts and artificial sweetener.

Tissue Processing

The biopsies were freeze-dried and single fibers dissected out under a light microscope (Nikon, Japan) and each fiber weighed using a quartz-fiber fish pole balance, spectrophotometrically calibrated with p-nitrophenol (22). Fibers weighing <0.95 μg were found to produce Western blots of unreliable quality and were therefore discarded. A total of 684 muscle fibers were analyzed. The number of fibers analyzed for each subject is presented in **Table 1** and the average fiber weight is presented in **Table 2**.

Homogenization

Each muscle fiber was dissolved in 5 μl homogenization solution consisting of 2 mM Hepes, 1 mM EDTA, 5 mM EGTA, 10 mM $MgCl_2$, 1% Triton X-100, 50 mM β-glycero-P, 1 mM sodium ortovanadate, 1% Phosphatase Inhibitor Cocktail 3 (Sigma-Aldrich), 1% Halt™ Protease Inhibitor Cocktail (Thermo Scientific), and 2 mM 4,4′-DDT at pH 7.4. The samples were stored on ice for approximately 1 h throughout homogenization followed by addition of 5 μl 2X Laemmli sample buffer (Bio Rad). The samples were then heated at 95°C for 5 min and stored at −20°C. The procedure is modified from the method originally described by Murphy (19).

Immunoblotting

The entire 10 μl containing each dissolved muscle fiber was loaded onto a 26 well Criterion TGX gradient gel (4–20% acrylamide; Bio Rad). A supernatant from a whole muscle homogenate of a post-exercise muscle biopsy was also loaded onto each gel to control for between membrane differences in protein phosphorylation and expression. The Western blotting protocol employed has been described in detail previously (20).

In brief, electrophoresis was run for 30 min at 300 V in Tris buffer (25 mM Tris base, 192 mM glycine, and 3.5 mM SDS) on an ice bed in a cold room at 4°C. The gels were subsequently incubated in transfer buffer (25 mM Tris base and 192 mM glycine in 90% dH_2O–10% methanol) for 30 min at 4°C and the proteins transferred to polyvinylidine fluoride membranes (Biorad) at 300 mA for 180 min at 4°C. The membranes were subsequently stained using Pierce® Reversible Stain Kit (Thermo Scientific).

Prior to incubation with primary antibodies, the membranes were blocked for 1 h at room temperature using 5% milk in Tris buffer-saline (TBS) (20 mM Tris base and 137 mM NaCl). Incubation with primary antibodies targeting the phosphorylated proteins was carried out over-night at 4°C, the membranes were then washed prior to incubation with secondary antibodies for 1 h at room temperature, and then washed once again prior to visualization with SuperSignal® West Femto Maximum Sensitivity Substrate (Thermo Scientific). The Molecular Imager ChemiDoc™ XRS system was used to detect protein bands and the Quantity One® software, version 4.6.3 (Bio-Rad Laboratories) for quantification.

The membranes were subsequently washed thoroughly with dH_2O (5 × 1 min) and TBS (3 × 3 min) and thereafter stripped for 30 min at 50°C utilizing Restore™ PLUS Western Blot Stripping Buffer (Thermo Scientific). After being washed once again with dH_2O (5 × 1 min) and TBS (3 × 3 min), the membranes were incubated with primary antibodies for detection of total protein as described above. The levels of phosphorylated and total protein are expressed in relation to the weight of the fiber.

TABLE 1 | Number of fibers analyzed in biopsies from the five subjects (S).

Subject	Type I				Type II			
	Placebo Pre	Placebo 90	EAA Pre	EAA 90	Placebo Pre	Placebo 90	EAA Pre	EAA 90
S 1	9	10	7	4	12	10	9–10	14
S 2	10–11	9	13	7–9	7	12	9	12
S 3	13–22	4–11	9–15	5–12	9–21	29–30	20	14–28
S 4	9–18	12–15	4–9	3–6	29–38	29–38	36–52	36–49
S 5	11	9–12	8	11–12	26	30	29–30	25–26

A different number of fibers was in some cases analyzed for the three proteins (indicated by range).
Pre indicates before exercise and 90 indicates 90 min after exercise.

Fiber Typing

The membranes were again stripped twice prior to exposure of antibodies targeting myosin heavy chain I (MHC I) and then myosin heavy chain II (MHC II). On the basis of visual inspection of the MHC I and MHC II staining, fibers were categorized either as type I, type II, or hybrid fibers (staining for both MHC I and II). The hybrid fibers were discarded; only 22 fibers (about 3% of the fibers) were classified as hybrid fibers, which is too small to give a valuable result.

Antibodies

Both primary and secondary antibodies were diluted with TBS containing 2.5% milk. The primary antibodies used were Mouse Anti-Slow Skeletal Myosin Heavy Chain (Abcam #ab11083, diluted 1:10,000), Rabbit Anti-Fast Myosin Skeletal Heavy Chain (Abcam #ab91506, diluted 1:10,000), total mTOR (Cell Signaling #2983S, diluted 1:1,000), phosphorylated mTOR Ser^{2448} (Cell Signaling #5536S, diluted 1:1,000), total S6K1 (Cell Signaling #2708S, diluted 1:1,000), phosphorylated S6K1 Thr^{389} (Cell Signaling #9234S, diluted 1:1,000), total eEF2 (Cell Signaling #2332S, diluted 1:1,000), and phosphorylated eEF2 Thr^{56} (Cell Signaling #2331S, diluted 1:1,000). The secondary antibodies, anti-rabbit HRP-linked (#7074S) and anti-mouse HRP-linked (#7076S), were both purchased from Cell Signaling and diluted 1:10,000.

Statistical Analysis

A repeated measures three-way ANOVA (supplement, fiber type, and time) was applied to compare changes in mean levels of

TABLE 2 | Weight of the fibers (μg) analyzed in the different conditions.

	Type I				Type II			
	Placebo Pre	Placebo 90	EAA Pre	EAA 90	Placebo Pre	Placebo 90	EAA Pre	EAA 90
mTOR	2.54 (0.95–5.73)	2.38 (1.09–8.10)	2.18 (0.95–4.37)	2.18 (1.09–6.00)	3.03 (1.09–6.00)	2.86 (1.09–7.09)	2.56 (1.23–5.87)	2.46 (1.09–5.73)
S6K1	2.55 (0.95–5.73)	2.26 (1.09–8.10)	2.12 (0.95–4.23)	2.26 (1.09–6.00)	2.99 (1.09–6.00)	2.82 (1.09–7.09)	2.52 (1.23–5.87)	2.32 (1.09–5.46)
eEF2	2.54 (0.95–5.73)	2.43 (1.09–8.10)	2.13 (0.95–4.37)	2.18 (1.09–6.00)	3.03 (1.09–6.00)	2.85 (1.09–7.09)	2.53 (1.23–5.87)	2.37 (1.09–5.73)

The values are presented as means (range).
Pre indicates before exercise and 90 indicates 90 min after exercise.

protein expression and phosphorylation in the type I and type II fibers in the two conditions. When a main or interaction effect was detected, planned comparisons was performed to identify where the differences occurred. The level of statistical significance was set at $P < 0.05$. Statistical analysis was carried out with Statistica software (version 12.0, Statsoft, Tulsa, OK).

RESULTS

Protein Levels

Figure 1 shows a representative picture of fiber type identification as well as protein levels of mTOR, S6K1, and eEF2 in type I and type II fibers. The levels of both the S6K1 and eEF2 proteins were significantly higher in type II than type I fibers (50% for both proteins, $P < 0.05$), whereas no difference was observed with respect to the mTOR protein (**Table 3**). With the exception of a significant increase in the level of mTOR following exercise, no main effect of time or supplementation was observed. The variability in protein levels between single muscle fibers within and between subjects is illustrated in **Figure 2**.

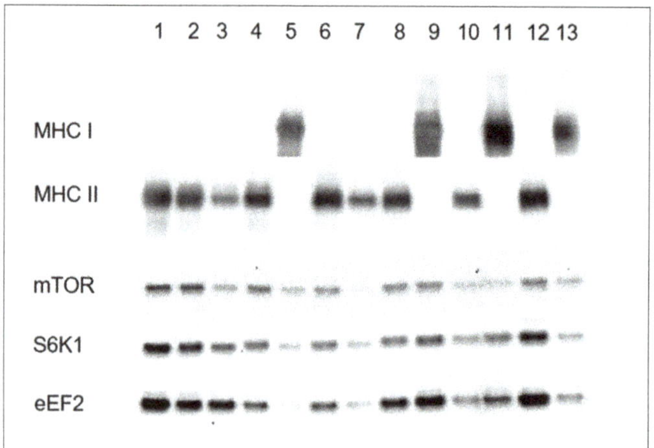

FIGURE 1 | Identification of type I and type II fibers following incubation with antibodies targeting MHCI and MHCII. Lower bands represent protein levels of mTOR, S6K1, and eEF2 in individual fibers. Proteins were separated on 4–20% acrylamide gels and transferred to PVDF membranes.

TABLE 3 | Protein levels of mTOR, S6K1 and eEF2 in type I and type II muscle fibers.

Protein		Type I		Type II	
		Pre	90	Pre	90
mTOR	Placebo	965 ± 161	1115 ± 164*	962 ± 133	1027 ± 146*
	EAA	868 ± 184	1106 ± 201*	939 ± 159	1177 ± 176*
S6K1	Placebo	1181 ± 174	1055 ± 156	1828 ± 154$^{\$}$	1669 ± 136$^{\$}$
	EAA	1084 ± 171	1272 ± 155	1647 ± 173$^{\$}$	1558 ± 113$^{\$}$
eEF2	Placebo	564 ± 93	629 ± 99	995 ± 92$^{\$}$	912 ± 124$^{\$}$
	EAA	586 ± 131	596 ± 130	926 ± 110$^{\$}$	818 ± 97$^{\$}$

*The values presented (arbitrary units) are means ± SE for five subjects. *$P < 0.05$ vs. Pre (main effect of time), and $^{\$}P < 0.05$ vs. type I fibers (main effect of fiber type). Pre indicates before exercise and 90 indicates 90 min after exercise.*

Protein Phosphorylation

A main effect of time was found for phosphorylation of both $mTOR^{Ser2448}$ and $S6K1^{Thr389}$, in addition to an interaction between time and supplement. The planned comparison analysis revealed an increase in both fiber types 90 min after exercise in the EAA condition only, despite a 2–3-fold increase in the levels of phosphorylated mTOR ($P = 0.085$) and S6K1, in the placebo condition (**Figures 3A,D**). However, when phosphorylation was normalized to the level of the corresponding protein, the

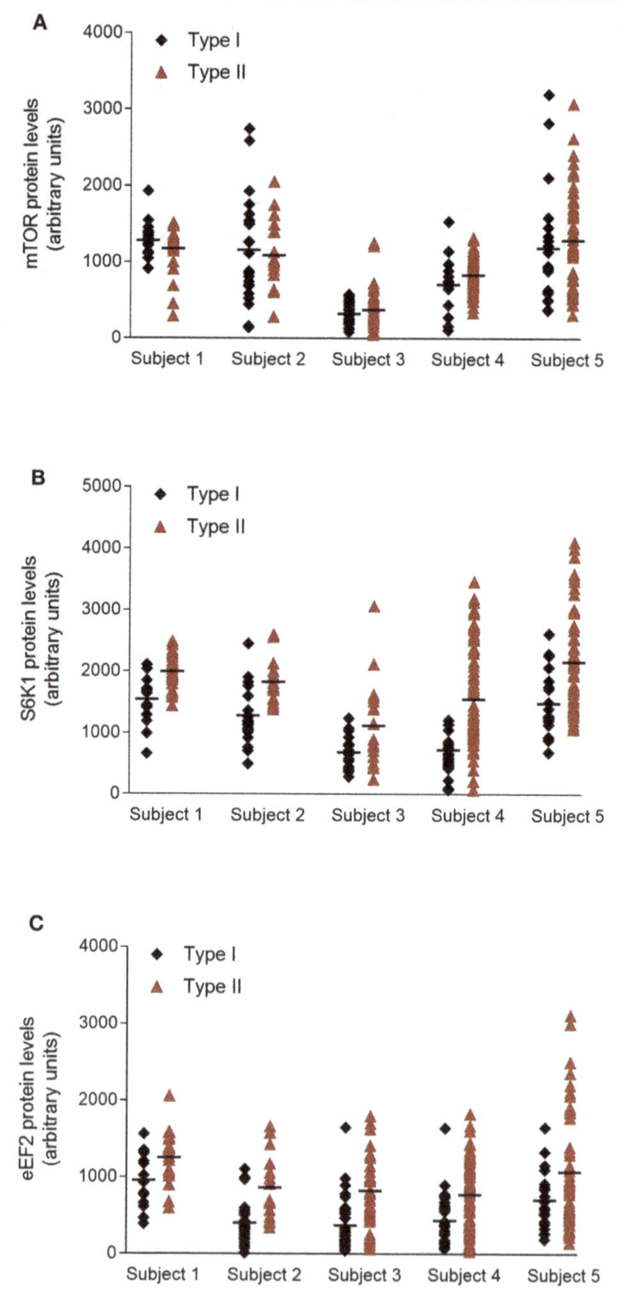

FIGURE 2 | Protein levels in individual type I and type II fibers before exercise from the five subjects. **(A)** mTOR, **(B)** S6K1, and **(C)** eEF2. Horizontal lines illustrate the average values.

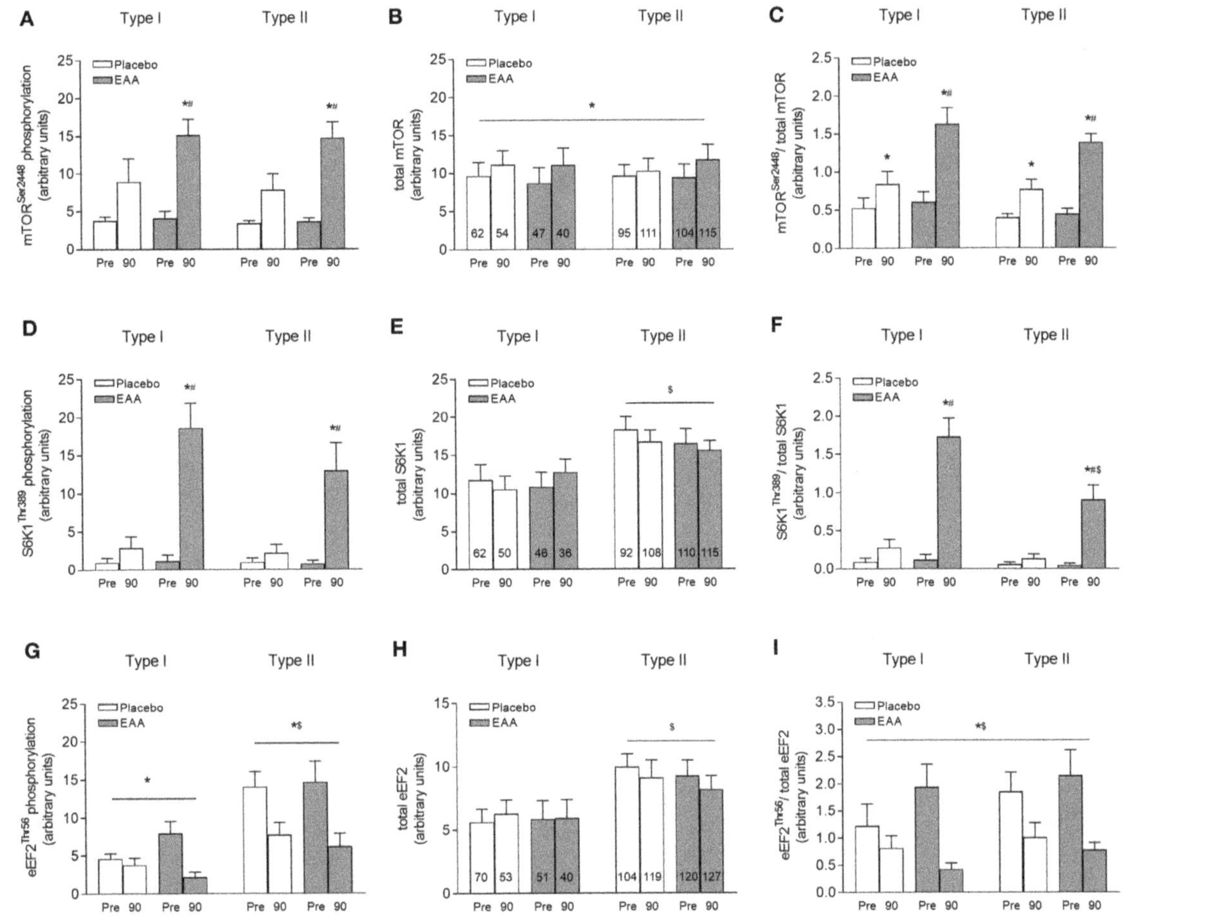

FIGURE 3 | (A) Phosphorylation of mTOR at Ser^{2448}, **(B)** total protein level of mTOR, **(C)** phosphorylation of mTOR/total protein, **(D)** phosphorylation of S6K1 at Thr^{389}, **(E)** total protein level of S6K1, **(F)** phosphorylation of S6K1/total protein, **(G)** phosphorylation of eEF2 at Thr^{56}, **(H)** total protein level of eEF2, and **(I)** phosphorylation of eEF2/total protein. Pre indicates before exercise and 90 indicates 90 min after exercise. Figures within bars indicate the number of fibers analyzed. The values presented (arbitrary units/100) are means ± SE for the five subjects. $^*P < 0.05$ vs. Pre, $^{\#}P < 0.05$ vs. placebo, and $^{\$}P < 0.05$ vs. type I fibers.

increase in mTOR phosphorylation proved to be significant (**Figure 3C**). There were no differences between fiber types and no interaction involving fiber type with respect to mTOR or S6K1 phosphorylation, other than when the S6K1 phosphorylation was normalized to the total level of corresponding protein. In this case phosphorylation of S6K1 was higher in type I than in type II fibers 90 min after exercise (interaction between fiber type and supplement; $P < 0.05$, **Figure 3F**).

Phosphorylation of eEF2 at Thr^{56} was associated with a main effect of both time and fiber type. An interaction between time and fiber type was also found, with no main or interaction effects involving supplement. At rest, phosphorylation of eEF2 at Thr^{56} was 128% higher in type II than type I fibers ($P < 0.05$, **Figure 3G**). Following exercise, the phosphorylation was reduced by 53% in both types of fiber ($P < 0.05$ compared to Pre, **Figure 3G**). When the level of phosphorylation was normalized to the level of protein, the ANOVA did not reveal a significant interaction between fiber type and time. Hence, an overall higher phosphorylation in type II than in type I fibers, including both resting and exercised levels, was detected (**Figure 3I**).

Figure 4 illustrates the variability in phosphorylation status of S6K1 between individual fibers within and between subjects before and 90 min after exercise in both conditions.

DISCUSSION

It is well-known that human skeletal muscle contains fiber types with different metabolic properties and the vast majority of studies in this area have examined whole muscle. In the present study, we have isolated and analyzed individual muscle fibers with respect to protein components of the mTORC1 signaling pathway. The major findings are (1) type II fibers express higher levels of the S6K1 and eEF2 proteins than type I fibers, (2) type I and type II fibers respond similarly to intake of EAA in combination with resistance exercise, and (3) there is a large variation in this response between individual fibers within each subject as well as between subjects.

Type II muscle fibers had approximately 50% higher levels of both S6K1 and eEF2, signal transduction proteins downstream of mTOR. These findings are in agreement with a previous

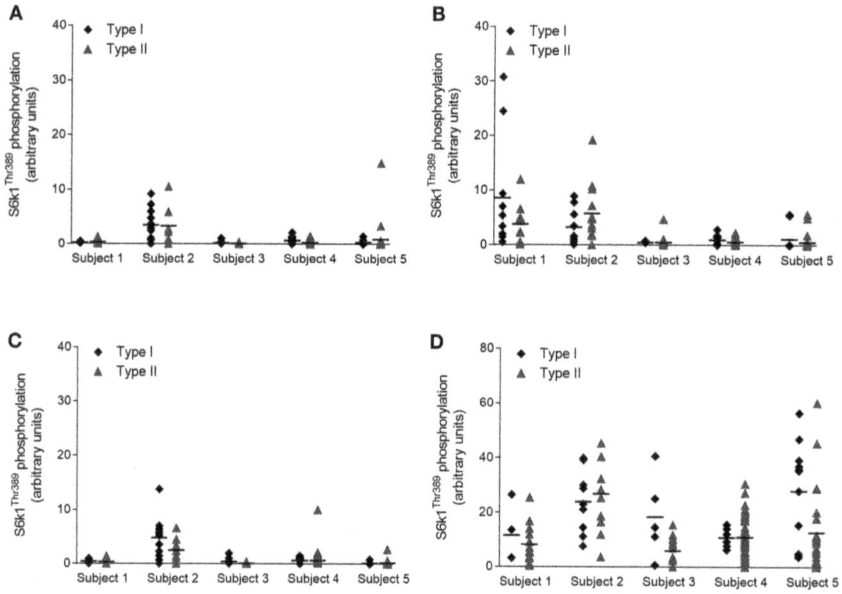

FIGURE 4 | Phosphorylation of S6K1 at Thr^{389} in individual fibers of five subject. **(A,C)** Levels at rest prior to exercise and supplementation. **(B)** Levels following exercise in placebo condition, and **(D)** levels following exercise and supplementation with EAA. Horizontal lines illustrate the average values. Y-axis in **(D)** (0–80) is different from **(A–C)** (0–40).

report on rat muscle where the levels of S6K1 and protein kinase B (Akt/PKB) are higher in the fast EDL than in the slow soleus muscle (23). These proteins are known to be involved in regulating translation initiation or elongation processes in skeletal muscle (24), but the functional consequences of the elevated protein levels of S6K1 and eEF2 in type II human muscle fibers are not entirely clear. However, it may suggest a larger capacity of the mTORC1 pathway, i.e., a higher activity of key enzymes in the pathway provided that anabolic stimuli induce similar degree of phosphorylation of these enzymes, which may explain why hypertrophy can be stimulated to greater extent in type II fibers (6, 7).

Resistance exercise alone did not increase the phosphorylation of mTOR and S6K1 significantly, although the levels were elevated by 2–3-fold 90 min after exercise. This differs from our previous observation that maximal eccentric contractions markedly elevated phosphorylation of S6K1 and reduced phosphorylation of eEF2 in type II fibers only (17). The failure to detect such a difference here is most probably due to the differences between the exercise protocols utilized. Maximal eccentric contractions impose a pronounced strain on the muscle, the force is ~30% higher than maximal concentric contractions (25) together with the lengthening and stretching of the muscle fiber. The latter phenomenon is an important component of the training response, as well as for activation of S6K1 (26, 27). Despite the heavy work performed by our subjects, the leg press exercise involves both eccentric and concentric movements. The initial exercise at 85% of 1RM, gradually reducing the load to 65% of 1RM, entails a relatively low contribution from the eccentric phase to force development, as well as less strain during the lengthening and stretching of the muscle fibers. In addition, repeated sets of resistance exercise with short rest periods between sets have been suggested to fatigue primarily the type II fibers (28). This may imply that the type of exercise employed here could have fatigued the type II fibers, and hence, explaining the larger involvement of type I fibers as compared to maximal eccentric contractions.

When the subjects ingested a mixture of EAA, mTOR, and S6K1 were stimulated considerably in both type I and type II fibers following resistance exercise (**Figure 3**). Interestingly, but in contrast to our hypothesis, when normalized to the total level of protein, S6K1 was significantly more phosphorylated in type I than type II fibers, suggesting that amino acid-induced stimulation of translation initiation is more responsive in type I fibers. This finding implies that type I fibers may have a higher growth potential following amino acid ingestion, given the positive associations between S6K1 phosphorylation and muscle hypertrophy (12, 13). However, this notion is difficult to reconcile with previous reports showing that fiber type enlargement following resistance exercise occurs primarily in type II fibers (6, 7). While it is generally accepted that the protein synthetic response is the major determinant of muscle growth (10), it should be emphasized that for muscle accretion to occur, both acutely and in the long term, accumulated increases in muscle protein synthesis must be higher than those of muscle breakdown. Consequently, measurements pertaining only to one side of the protein balance equation may not fully reflect the growth potential of muscle (29). We did not measure fiber type-specific protein synthesis in the present study, but the close agreement generally found between S6K1 phosphorylation and muscle protein synthesis (30–32) suggests that the higher degree of S6K1 phosphorylation found in the type I fibers may be reflective of elevated rates of protein synthesis compared to the type II fibers. This notion is supported by a previous study showing slightly higher rates of muscle protein synthesis in isolated type I compared to type II fibers following resistance exercise in a postprandial state (33).

However, data on resting muscle do not support a larger responsiveness in type I fibers (34, 35). Infusion of a mixture of EAA induced similar increases in the rate of muscle protein synthesis (in both the myofibrillar and sarcoplasmatic fractions) in the soleus, vastus lateralis, and triceps muscles (35). The proportion of type I fibers in these three muscles ranged from 20 to 80% and there was no correlation between the fractional synthetic rate (FSR) and percentage of type I fibers, indicating that type I and type II fibers are equally responsive to hyperaminoacidemia in a resting condition.

Our observations of elevated phosphorylation of eEF2 in type II fibers in resting muscle are in accordance with previous findings (36). Here, the level of eEF2 protein was also higher in type II fibers (**Table 3**, **Figure 3H**). The potential consequences of these differences are unclear; it has been suggested that they may reflect a higher resting FSR in type I fibers, which is supported by measurements on pools of fibers revealing a 30% higher rate in type I fibers at rest (37). Further support for this opinion can be found in a study on different human muscles with varying proportions of type I and type II fibers (35), but not in others (34, 38). However, such differences may be more difficult to detect in whole muscle due to the content of both type I and type II fibers as well as hybrid fibers.

We observed here considerable variation in the levels of both protein and phosphorylation between individual fibers of both type I and type II. The large variation in signaling response indicates that some fibers are not recruited, despite the heavy work load. Similar large variations in substrate levels (glycogen) and ATP within fibers of the same type have been reported following endurance exercise or electrical stimulation of the muscle (39, 40), further supporting that only certain fibers are recruited and contribute to force development during muscle contraction. The even larger variation when EAA were ingested is likely caused by the enhancing effect such intake has on fibers that are actually recruited than on inactive fibers (14, 15). The large variation also in protein concentration within the same fiber type (**Figure 2**) is in line with previous studies showing that both ATP (40) and glycogen (39) vary greatly within fibers of the same type. Although valuable, mean values fail to describe the entire picture within skeletal muscle. Adding single fiber analysis to the otherwise more common whole muscle analysis should add another dimension in understanding the complexity of skeletal muscle adaptation.

In the present study, the number of type II fibers dissected out and analyzed was more than double the number of type I fibers (**Table 1**). Similar observations have been made previously (5, 41), but we have no explanation to this phenomenon. It could of course reflect the subjects' fiber composition, however, this is unlikely. A more likely explanation is that type II fibers are more robust and easier to dissect without breaking the fibers, meaning that a great amount of fibers need to be dissected out to ensure that a sufficient number of type I fibers is obtained. Dissecting and analyzing single fibers is time consuming, an advantage with the present methodology is that fiber typing and protein analyses are carried out on the same fiber fragment, which shortens the analysis time.

In summary, the levels of both S6K1 and eEF2 proteins were higher in type II than type I muscle fibers, suggesting that in the former the mTORC1 pathway has a greater capacity. Heavy resistance exercise in combination with consumption of EAA elevates phosphorylation of both mTOR and S6K1 in both fiber types above the levels seen at rest and following resistance exercise alone. The only minor differences in the response to intake of EAA was that when normalized to protein content, S6K1 was slightly more phosphorylated in type I fibers. Large variations in the responses of individual fibers to the different stimuli were observed, with some fibers demonstrating high levels of phosphorylation following exercise and others no stimulation at all. Future studies exploring possible relationship between signaling response, on one hand, and substrate levels or metabolic changes, on the other, within individual type I and type II fibers may help to understand the mechanism involved in training adaptation.

AUTHOR CONTRIBUTIONS

SE, KS, and EB designed the study. MM and WA carried out the experiment. SE dissected and analyzed muscle fibers and performed statistical analyses. SE and EB wrote the manuscript. KS, MM, and WA edited the manuscript. All authors approved the final version of the manuscript.

FUNDING

The study was supported by grants from The Swedish Research Council for Sport Science (P2017-0168). The amino acids were kindly provided by Ajinomoto, Japan.

ACKNOWLEDGMENTS

The authors thank Elisabeth Berg from the Department of Learning, Informatics, Management and Ethics (LIME), unit for Medical Statistics, Karolinska Institutet, Stockholm, Sweden for valuable statistical advice.

REFERENCES

1. Essen B, Jansson E, Henriksson J, Taylor AW, Saltin B. Metabolic characteristics of fibre types in human skeletal muscle. *Acta Physiol Scand.* (1975) 95:153–65. doi: 10.1111/j.1748-1716.1975.tb10038.x
2. Howald H, Hoppeler H, Claassen H, Mathieu O, Straub R. Influences of endurance training on the ultrastructural composition of the different muscle fiber types in humans. *Pflugers Arch.* (1985) 403:369–76. doi: 10.1007/BF00589248
3. Soderlund K, Greenhaff PL, Hultman E. Energy metabolism in type I and type II human muscle fibres during short term electrical stimulation at different frequencies. *Acta Physiol Scand.* (1992) 144:15–22. doi: 10.1111/j.1748-1716.1992.tb09262.x

4. Greenhaff PL, Nevill ME, Soderlund K, Bodin K, Boobis LH, Williams C, et al. The metabolic responses of human type I and II muscle fibres during maximal treadmill sprinting. *J Physiol.* (1994) 478(Pt 1):149–55. doi: 10.1113/jphysiol.1994.sp020238
5. Gray SR, Soderlund K, Watson M, Ferguson RA. Skeletal muscle ATP turnover and single fibre ATP and PCr content during intense exercise at different muscle temperatures in humans. *Pflugers Archiv.* (2011) 462:885–93. doi: 10.1007/s00424-011-1032-4
6. Tesch PA. Skeletal muscle adaptations consequent to long-term heavy resistance exercise. *Med Sci Sports Exerc.* (1988) 20(5 Suppl.):S132–4. doi: 10.1249/00005768-198810001-00008
7. Fry AC. The role of resistance exercise intensity on muscle fibre adaptations. *Sports Med.* (2004) 34:663–79. doi: 10.2165/00007256-200434100-00004
8. Rennie MJ, Edwards RH, Halliday D, Matthews DE, Wolman SL, Millward DJ. Muscle protein synthesis measured by stable isotope techniques in man: the effects of feeding and fasting. *Clin Sci (Lond).* (1982) 63:519–23. doi: 10.1042/cs0630519
9. Tipton KD, Ferrando AA, Phillips SM, Doyle D Jr., Wolfe RR. Postexercise net protein synthesis in human muscle from orally administered amino acids. *Am J Physiol Endocrinol Metab.* (1999) 276:E628–34. doi: 10.1152/ajpendo.1999.276.4.E628
10. Rasmussen BB, Phillips SM. Contractile and nutritional regulation of human muscle growth. *Exerc Sport Sci Rev.* (2003) 31:127–31. doi: 10.1097/00003677-200307000-00005
11. Dickinson JM, Fry CS, Drummond MJ, Gundermann DM, Walker DK, Glynn EL, et al. Mammalian target of rapamycin complex 1 activation is required for the stimulation of human skeletal muscle protein synthesis by essential amino acids. *J Nutr.* (2011) 141:856–62. doi: 10.3945/jn.111.139485
12. Baar K, Esser K. Phosphorylation of p70(S6k) correlates with increased skeletal muscle mass following resistance exercise. *Am J Physiol.* (1999) 276(1 Pt 1):C120–7. doi: 10.1152/ajpcell.1999.276.1.C120
13. Terzis G, Georgiadis G, Stratakos G, Vogiatzis I, Kavouras S, Manta P, et al. Resistance exercise-induced increase in muscle mass correlates with p70S6 kinase phosphorylation in human subjects. *Eur J Appl Physiol.* (2008) 102:145–52. doi: 10.1007/s00421-007-0564-y
14. Apro W, Blomstrand E. Influence of supplementation with branched-chain amino acids in combination with resistance exercise on p70S6 kinase phosphorylation in resting and exercising human skeletal muscle. *Acta Physiol.* (2010) 200:237–48. doi: 10.1111/j.1748-1716.2010.02151.x
15. Moore DR, Atherton PJ, Rennie MJ, Tarnopolsky MA, Phillips SM. Resistance exercise enhances mTOR and MAPK signalling in human muscle over that seen at rest after bolus protein ingestion. *Acta Physiol.* (2011) 201:365–72. doi: 10.1111/j.1748-1716.2010.02187.x
16. Tang JE, Moore DR, Kujbida GW, Tarnopolsky MA, Phillips SM. Ingestion of whey hydrolysate, casein, or soy protein isolate: effects on mixed muscle protein synthesis at rest and following resistance exercise in young men. *J Appl Physiol.* (2009) 107:987–92. doi: 10.1152/japplphysiol.00076.2009
17. Tannerstedt J, Apro W, Blomstrand E. Maximal lengthening contractions induce different signaling responses in the type I and type II fibers of human skeletal muscle. *J Appl Physiol.* (2009) 106:1412–8. doi: 10.1152/japplphysiol.91243.2008
18. Koopman R, Pennings B, Zorenc AH, van Loon LJ. Protein ingestion further augments S6K1 phosphorylation in skeletal muscle following resistance type exercise in males. *J Nutr.* (2007) 137:1880–6. doi: 10.1093/jn/137.8.1880
19. Murphy RM. Enhanced technique to measure proteins in single segments of human skeletal muscle fibers: fiber-type dependence of AMPK-alpha1 and -beta1. *J Appl Physiol.* (2011) 110:820–5. doi: 10.1152/japplphysiol.01082.2010
20. Moberg M, Apro W, Ekblom B, van Hall G, Holmberg HC, Blomstrand E. Activation of mTORC1 by leucine is potentiated by branched-chain amino acids and even more so by essential amino acids following resistance exercise. *Am J Physiol Cell Physiol.* (2016) 310:C874–84. doi: 10.1152/ajpcell.00374.2015
21. Henriksson KG. "Semi-open" muscle biopsy technique. A simple outpatient procedure. *Acta Neurol Scand.* (1979) 59:317–23. doi: 10.1111/j.1600-0404.1979.tb02942.x
22. Lowry O, Passonneau J. *A Flexible System of Enzymatic Analysis.* New York, NY: Academic Press (1972).
23. Atherton PJ, Higginson JM, Singh J, Wackerhage H. Concentrations of signal transduction proteins exercise and insulin responses in rat extensor digitorum longus and soleus muscles. *Mol Cell Biochem.* (2004) 261:111–6. doi: 10.1023/B:MCBI.0000028745.58567.81
24. Rommel C, Bodine SC, Clarke BA, Rossman R, Nunez L, Stitt TN, et al. Mediation of IGF-1-induced skeletal myotube hypertrophy by PI(3)K/Akt/mTOR and PI(3)K/Akt/GSK3 pathways. *Nat Cell Biol.* (2001) 3:1009–13. doi: 10.1038/ncb1101-1009
25. Eliasson J, Elfegoun T, Nilsson J, Kohnke R, Ekblom B, Blomstrand E. Maximal lengthening contractions increase p70 S6 kinase phosphorylation in human skeletal muscle in the absence of nutritional supply. *Am J Physiol Endocrinol Metab.* (2006) 291:E1197–205. doi: 10.1152/ajpendo.00141.2006
26. Hornberger TA, Sukhija KB, Wang XR, Chien S. mTOR is the rapamycin-sensitive kinase that confers mechanically-induced phosphorylation of the hydrophobic motif site Thr(389) in p70(S6k). *FEBS Lett.* (2007) 581:4562–6. doi: 10.1016/j.febslet.2007.08.045
27. Jacobs BL, You JS, Frey JW, Goodman CA, Gundermann DM, Hornberger TA. Eccentric contractions increase the phosphorylation of tuberous sclerosis complex-2 (TSC2) and alter the targeting of TSC2 and the mechanistic target of rapamycin to the lysosome. *J Physiol.* (2013) 591:4611–20. doi: 10.1113/jphysiol.2013.256339
28. Burd NA, Holwerda AM, Selby KC, West DW, Staples AW, Cain NE, et al. Resistance exercise volume affects myofibrillar protein synthesis and anabolic signalling molecule phosphorylation in young men. *J Physiol.* (2010) 588(Pt 16):3119–30. doi: 10.1113/jphysiol.2010.192856
29. Mitchell CJ, Churchward-Venne TA, Parise G, Bellamy L, Baker SK, Smith K, et al. Acute post-exercise myofibrillar protein synthesis is not correlated with resistance training-induced muscle hypertrophy in young men. *PLoS ONE.* (2014) 9:e89431. doi: 10.1371/journal.pone.0089431
30. Atherton PJ, Etheridge T, Watt PW, Wilkinson D, Selby A, Rankin D, et al. Muscle full effect after oral protein: time-dependent concordance and discordance between human muscle protein synthesis and mTORC1 signaling. *Am J Clin Nutr.* (2010) 92:1080–8. doi: 10.3945/ajcn.2010.29819
31. Wilkinson SB, Phillips SM, Atherton PJ, Patel R, Yarasheski KE, Tarnopolsky MA, et al. Differential effects of resistance and endurance exercise in the fed state on signalling molecule phosphorylation and protein synthesis in human muscle. *J Physiol.* (2008) 586:3701–17. doi: 10.1113/jphysiol.2008.153916
32. Kumar V, Selby A, Rankin D, Patel R, Atherton P, Hildebrandt W, et al. Age-related differences in the dose-response relationship of muscle protein synthesis to resistance exercise in young and old men. *J Physiol.* (2009) 587:211–7. doi: 10.1113/jphysiol.2008.164483
33. Koopman R, Gleeson BG, Gijsen AP, Groen B, Senden JM, Rennie MJ, et al. Post-exercise protein synthesis rates are only marginally higher in type I compared with type II muscle fibres following resistance-type exercise. *Eur J Appl Physiol.* (2011) 111:1871–8. doi: 10.1007/s00421-010-1808-9
34. Carroll CC, Fluckey JD, Williams RH, Sullivan DH, Trappe TA. Human soleus and vastus lateralis muscle protein metabolism with an amino acid infusion. *Am J Physiol Endocrinol Metab.* (2005) 288:E479–85. doi: 10.1152/ajpendo.00393.2004
35. Mittendorfer B, Andersen JL, Plomgaard P, Saltin B, Babraj JA, Smith K, et al. Protein synthesis rates in human muscles: neither anatomical location nor fibre-type composition are major determinants. *J Physiol.* (2005) 563(Pt 1):203–11. doi: 10.1113/jphysiol.2004.077180
36. Rose AJ, Bisiani B, Vistisen B, Kiens B, Richter EA. Skeletal muscle eEF2 and 4EBP1 phosphorylation during endurance exercise is dependent on intensity and muscle fiber type. *Am J Physiol Regul Integr Comp Physiol.* (2009) 296:R326–33. doi: 10.1152/ajpregu.90806.2008
37. Dickinson JM, Lee JD, Sullivan BE, Harber MP, Trappe SW, Trappe TA. A new method to study *in vivo* protein synthesis in slow- and fast-twitch muscle fibers and initial measurements in humans. *J Appl Physiol.* (2010) 108:1410–6. doi: 10.1152/japplphysiol.00905.2009
38. Harber MP, Dickinson JM, Crane JD, Trappe SW, Trappe TA. Influence of tracer selection on protein synthesis rates at rest and postexercise in multiple human muscles. *Metabolism.* (2011) 60:689–97. doi: 10.1016/j.metabol.2010.07.003
39. Essen B, Henriksson J. Glycogen content of individual muscle fibres in man. *Acta Physiol Scand.* (1974) 90:645–7. doi: 10.1111/j.1748-1716.1974.tb05629.x

40. Soderlund K, Hultman E. ATP content in single fibres from human skeletal muscle after electrical stimulation and during recovery. *Acta Physiol Scand.* (1990) 139:459–66. doi: 10.1111/j.1748-1716.1990.tb 08947.x

41. Gray SR, Soderlund K, Ferguson RA. ATP and phosphocreatine utilization in single human muscle fibres during the development of maximal power output at elevated muscle temperatures. *J Sports Sci.* (2008) 26:701–7. doi: 10.1080/02640410701744438

15

Greek Yogurt and 12 Weeks of Exercise Training on Strength, Muscle Thickness and Body Composition in Lean, Untrained, University-Aged Males

*Aaron Bridge[1], Joseph Brown[1], Hayden Snider[2], Matthew Nasato[1], Wendy E. Ward[1,3], Brian D. Roy[1,3] and Andrea R. Josse[1,2,3]**

[1] *Department of Kinesiology, Faculty of Applied Health Sciences, Brock University, St. Catharines, ON, Canada,*

[2] *School of Kinesiology and Health Science, Faculty of Health, York University, Toronto, ON, Canada,*

[3] *Centre for Bone and Muscle Health, Faculty of Applied Health Sciences, Brock University, St. Catharines, ON, Canada*

***Correspondence:**
Andrea R. Josse
ajosse@yorku.ca

Milk and/or whey protein plus resistance exercise (RT) increase strength and muscle size, and optimize body composition in adult males and females. Greek yogurt (GY) contains similar muscle-supporting nutrients as milk yet it is different in several ways including being a semi-solid food, containing bacterial cultures and having a higher protein content (mostly casein) per serving. GY has yet to be investigated in the context of a RT program. The purpose of this study was to assess the effects of GY consumption plus RT on strength, muscle thickness and body composition in lean, untrained, university-aged males. Thirty untrained, university-aged (20.6 ± 2.2 years) males were randomized to 2 groups (n = 15/group): fat-free, plain GY or a Placebo Pudding (PP; isoenergetic carbohydrate-based pudding) and underwent a combined RT/plyometric training program 3 days/week for 12 weeks. They consumed either GY (20 g protein/dose) or PP (0 g protein/dose) daily, 3 times on training days and 2 times on non-training days. After 12 weeks, both groups significantly increased strength, muscle thickness and fat-free mass (FFM) ($p < 0.05$). The GY group gained more total strength (GY; 98 ± 37 kg, PP; 57 ± 15 kg), more biceps brachii muscular thickness (GY; 0.46 ± 0.3 cm, PP; 0.12 ± 0.2 cm), more FFM (GY; 2.4 ± 1.5 kg, PP; 1.3 ± 1.3 kg), and reduced % body fat (GY; −1.1 ± 2.2%, PP; 0.1 ± 2.6%) than PP group ($p < 0.05$ expressed as absolute change). Thus, consumption of GY during a training program resulted in improved strength, muscle thickness and body composition over a carbohydrate-based placebo. Given the results of our study, the general benefits of consuming GY and its distinctiveness from milk, GY can be a plausible, post-exercise, nutrient-rich alternative for positive strength, muscle, and body composition adaptations.

Keywords: Greek yogurt, muscular strength, body composition, young males, muscle thickness, protein nutrition, intervention study, resistance training program

INTRODUCTION

The use of protein supplements to facilitate resistance training (RT) adaptations has long been documented in human populations (1–3). Dairy protein, which is comprised mostly of casein and whey, is a beneficial muscle building protein due to the complete essential amino acid (AA) profile and adequate leucine levels, which is primarily responsible for muscle protein synthesis (MPS) (4–6). Dairy products may also promote fat loss, possibly due to their increased content of bioavailable calcium (7), and effect on appetite suppression (8). Whey, which is a rapidly absorbed protein, is able to provide essential AAs to the exercised muscle to begin MPS soon after consumption (1, 9). Casein, which constitutes 80% of dairy protein, is a more slowly absorbed protein, and is able to prolong elevated levels of plasma-AAs and enhance whole-body protein turnover (10). This unique characteristic of casein protein may act to attenuate muscle protein breakdown (MPB), however further research is required to specifically determine this. Nevertheless, both proteins allow for a net positive protein balance (or a less negative balance) over a prolonged period time (11). Because of this (and other important features), dairy protein, and especially milk, which has garnered the majority of research, has been shown to be an effective beverage for facilitating adaptations to RT (12, 13). This poses the question; would other dairy products elicit the same positive adaptations to RT as milk?

There is strong support for the use of isolated protein supplements, such as whey for increasing strength, muscle size, and lean mass while undergoing RT (1, 9, 14). However, research regarding whole food protein-sources is limited. It is important to study whole-food protein sources as they contain additional components such as micronutrients, antioxidants, and bacterial cultures that are beneficial to overall health, and that may improve the digestibility and absorption of nutrients such as protein from the food (15). Moreover, whole food products are more accessible and are consumed more readily by the population. In terms of milk research, Hartman et al. (12) in males, and Josse et al. (13) in females, have shown that milk consumption following RT for 12 weeks was able to produce significant strength and body composition improvements compared to isoenergetic carbohydrate (CHO)-based placebos (12, 16). However, research by Rankin et al. (17), found no benefit of chocolate milk post-RT on these outcomes compared to CHO (17). Similar to milk, GY contains important nutrients for musculoskeletal health such as calcium, phosphorus and protein, however the consistency and composition of GY is different. GY possesses unique properties including its solidity and the provision of bacterial cultures, that may provide additional health benefits (8). Solid foods are more satiating than liquid foods and can delay gastric emptying (18), and probiotic/fermented foods improve digestion, increase bioavailability of nutrients, and enhance immunity (8, 19–23). Yogurt can also serve as a vehicle for the consumption of other healthful foods such as cereals, nuts and fruits to form a complete meal, thus also improving overall diet quality (24). Due to its potential benefits and unique characteristics, GY warrants further investigation.

Greek Yogurt (GY), also draws attention as a potential post-exercise health food due to its high protein content (mostly casein) which is created during the manufacturing and condensing process in which GY is made from regular yogurt (25). To date, only regular yogurt but not GY has been studied in combination with exercise for strength, muscle and body composition. One study in young, normal weight, untrained females indicated no further benefit of regular yogurt (5 g protein/serving, 3x/day) plus RT on increasing strength and lean mass compared to a protein-matched control and a CHO control (26). In addition, only 2 studies using regular yogurt (5 g protein/serving, 2–3 servings/day) in a weight loss context have been conducted, and results on body composition were inconclusive (23). These studies were conducted in overweight, predominantly female populations, and only one included an exercise (RT) component (27, 28). In most of these studies, the amount of protein provided by the regular yogurt [5 g × 3 servings per day (27) and 5 g × 2 servings per day (28)] was likely insufficient to enhance adaptive remodeling favoring the yogurt groups. Previous research in young individuals determined that an isolated dose of 20 g of protein was superior in stimulating MPS as compared to lower isolated doses of 5 and 10 g (29, 30). GY contains 3 to 4-fold the amount of protein as regular yogurt. One serving of plain GY (175 g) provides 17 g protein (31). The same amount of protein can be consumed from ~500 ml of milk (2 servings) (32). Given the effectiveness of milk in this context (12, 13) and noting the additional potential benefits of yogurt consumption (15, 33–35), interventions assessing similar effects on body composition, strength and other related health outcomes using GY are warranted.

Thus, the aim of our study was to assess whether the consumption of GY will increase strength and muscle thickness, and improve body composition more than a semi-solid, CHO-based placebo pudding (PP) following a 12-week exercise (RT and plyometric [PLY]) training intervention in untrained, university-aged males. Although both groups should experience favorable training adaptations, we hypothesized that GY supplementation would facilitate significantly greater increases in strength, muscle thickness, and fat free mass (FFM) while reducing fat mass (FM) compared to the PP group.

METHODS

Participants

Thirty healthy, university-aged (18–25 y) males were recruited for the study from the Brock University (Ontario, Canada) student population. Following a general screening protocol, subjects that were free of medical conditions were eligible to participate in the study. Screening ensured participants were untrained (RT <0–2 times/week for last 6 months), of normal body fatness (<25% fat), and had not been consuming dietary supplements (e.g., vitamins, minerals, protein supplements, creatine) in the last 6 months prior to entering the study. Once all inclusion criteria were met, subjects were informed of potential study risks, and written informed consent was obtained. The protocol was approved by the Brock University Research Ethics

Board and conformed to all standards of Canada's Interagency Panel on Research Ethics for conducting human research.

Supplement Protocol

This study was a parallel randomized controlled trial (clinical trial registration #: NCT03196856). Subjects were randomized to one of two groups; GY group (GY; $n = 15$) or placebo pudding group (PP; $n = 15$). Participants randomized to the GY group consumed 200 g of Oikos 0% fat, plain GY (~110 Kcals, 20 g protein, 8 g CHO; Danone Canada Inc., Boucherville, Quebec) 3 times/day on training days (immediately post-exercise, 1 h post-exercise and before bed) and 150 g, 2 times/day on non-training days (breakfast and before bed). To encourage compliance, participants could flavor the GY with calorie-free sweeteners or syrups if they preferred. The control group consumed 47 g of a placebo pudding (PP), which was an isoenergetic, chocolate flavored, CHO-based semi-solid food (~110 Kcals, 0 g protein, 28 g CHO) on the same supplement schedule as the GY group. The PP was comprised of maltodextrin (2 parts), chocolate pudding powder (1 part), and water, and was designed to resemble the consistency and texture of GY. The PP was made by the same researcher during the entire duration of the study. To ensure anonymity of the PP, it was termed the "*study-designed supplement*" and its contents were kept discreet to participants and other study personnel (e.g., exercise trainers). In fact, many subjects (and trainers) within the PP group believed that this supplement was the "test product" and that it may have contained muscle-supporting nutrients such as protein. Both groups had their respective supplements divided into individual serving containers and labeled by study personnel. On training days, the post-exercise doses were consumed in the research lab following training with study personnel present, whereas on non-training days and before bed, doses were consumed away from the laboratory and/or at home. These supplements were given to the participants to take home on a weekly basis. During the study, both groups were encouraged to maintain their habitual diets, except for the intervention food. Participants were provided with the same information and advice to help them compensate for the added calories consumed from the supplements.

Training Protocol

Both intervention groups underwent 12 weeks of exercise training, 3 days/week, at the campus gym or in other equipped research laboratories at Brock University. All training was facilitated by certified trainers and/or trained senior kinesiology students to ensure proper lifting form and to provide motivation to the subjects. Each formal training session (~60 min) consisted of either full-body RT (2 d/week) which included exercises such as leg press, bench press and seated row (at ~2% 1-RM, 8–10 total exercises, 3–4 sets/exercise, 8–12 reps/set), or PLY training (1 d/week) which included exercises such as box jumps and frog jumps (150–250 total jumps/impacts per session). The training sessions followed the principles of undulated periodization (36), varying intensity and/or volume throughout the intervention. Within this training paradigm, most RT exercises were taken to voluntary failure (or close).

Dietary Analysis

Participants recorded their habitual food and drink intake prior to beginning the study and again during the 12th week of training using a 7 and 3-days food diary, respectively. The 3-days food diary consisted of 2 weekdays and 1 weekend day. Instructions on how to fill out a food diary were thoroughly explained to each participant in advance. Upon completion, food diaries were examined, and any uncertainties were clarified with the subject by the research personnel. Dietary intake was inputted and analyzed using a diet analysis program (Food Processor, ESHA Inc., Salem, OR). All food diaries were inputted and analyzed by the same researcher.

Strength Assessment

Muscular strength was evaluated via voluntary 1 repetition maximum (1-RM) testing of four exercises at baseline and following week 12 of the intervention. Participants arrived hydrated and fed on testing days and did not participate in any structured exercise for a minimum of 48 h prior to testing. 1-RMs were determined for the following exercises: chest press, seated row, leg extension, and hamstring curl. Participants were made familiar with the exercises and testing protocol by doing light (estimated 40–50% 1-RM), practice repetitions (8–12) before the actual assessments began. During the assessment, weight was progressively added to each exercise until 1-RM was determined. Rests of 2–3 min were given between each set. Failure was determined when participants were unable to complete the full range of motion of a repetition without compensation. If 1-RM was not determined after 4 consecutive sets, it was estimated using the O'Connor calculation [1-RM= weight × (1+ (0.025 × reps))] (37, 38) from the set with the lowest number of completed reps. The use of a predictive equation for estimating 1-RM has been previously validated in a young, untrained male population (38, 39). Weight was adjusted so that most participants experienced voluntary failure at 4 or less repetitions. All pre and post-testing for all outcome variables (strength, muscle thickness, and body composition) were completed by the same researcher.

Muscle Thickness Assessment

Muscle thickness was measured via ultrasonography (GE Medical Systems, Ultrasound Vivid I portable, Milwaukee, WI, USA.). Muscle thickness was measured at 2 locations: the biceps brachii and the quadriceps femoris (rectus femoris + vastus intermedius). Muscle thickness for the quadriceps was measured at 50% between the greater trochanter and lateral epicondyle of the femur. For the biceps, muscle size was measured at 40% from the proximal end between the greater tubercle and the lateral epicondyle of the humerus. These sites correspond to where the muscle belly is the thickest. Subjects laid in a supine position, relaxed, with palms facing into their body. A thin layer of gel was applied to each muscle site and the ultrasound probe was placed on the site without depressing the skin. The measurement was obtained by pressing the probe gently on skin and moving it over the muscle. Muscle thickness was measured from the bone to the outer/superficial sarcolemma. Three images were obtained for each site and then averaged to obtain a final value.

Ultrasound tests were completed 48–72 h following exercise. All testing occurred in the morning, with subjects fasted (10–12 h).

Body Composition Assessment

Body composition was assessed using air-displacement plethysmography via the bod pod (COSMED USA Inc., BODPOD, Chicago, Il.). On testing days, subjects arrived at the laboratory in the morning, fasted (10–12 h), changed into compression shorts and put on a swim cap (the same outfit for each participant was used for the pre- and post-intervention measures). The testing procedure began with calibration of the empty chamber with a known volume. Participants then stepped into the bod pod and sat inside the unit for 45 s where their raw body volume is determined as the volume of air displaced (the difference between the volume of the empty vessel and the volume of the vessel with the participant inside). Body volume was entered into a pre-set equation accounting for body weight (measured on a scale before they entered the bod pod), height (measured on a stadiometer before they entered the bod pod), age, and ethnicity. Thoracic volume was predicted based on the Siri density model. Two tests were completed for each participant and compared, if the variation between the two tests was large (as assessed directly by the bod pod), a third test was completed. FFM, FM, and % body fat were then estimated via calculations.

Statistics

Data were analyzed using SPSS (IBM Corp. Released 2013. IBM SPSS Statistics for Windows, Version 22.0. Armonk, NY: IBM Corp.). Data were checked, and normality was confirmed by assessing measures of central tendency and homogeneity of variances, and sphericity. Data points that were more than +/−2 SD from the mean were categorized as outliers and removed. Missing data points (1 GY participant for all post-strength measures, 1 GY and 1 PP participant for post-ultrasound measures, 2 GY participants and 1 PP participant for post-dietary data) were replaced with the series mean for that timepoint. Repeated measures ANOVA (RMANOVA) was used to analyze time (pre and post), intervention (GY vs. PP), and interaction effects (intervention x time). Independent t-tests were used to analyze baseline data and percent change data between the groups. An ANCOVA design was used to assess changes over time while controlling for baseline % body fat differences.

RESULTS

Baseline Characteristics

Thirty participants were randomized, and 27 participants completed 12 weeks of the intervention. One GY participant stopped exercise after 6 weeks due to injury (unrelated to the study). Two participants (1 PP and 1 GY) ended the study early (after 6 weeks of training) because they moved away from the university area. Post-testing was completed on all three of these subjects and their data were included in the analysis, except for the injured participant who did not complete the 1-RM post-testing.

There were no differences at baseline for any variable between groups except for % body fat, with PP being higher than GY ($p = 0.049$). This was also reflected in the fat mass measure although the difference did not reach statistical significance ($p = 0.066$).

Adherence to the Study Supplements and Exercise Program

Trainers and study personnel ensured that the post-exercise supplement doses (of either GY or PP) were consumed in the laboratory, following training. This produced a 100% adherence rate for the post-exercise supplements. Bedtime and non-training day supplement doses were consumed without direct supervision. Food diaries completed at week 12 indicated a 97 and 99% adherence rate for the intake of the unsupervised supplements for the GY and PP groups, respectively. Training was well-tolerated, and attendance was 31.6 and 30.1 out of 36 sessions for the GY and PP groups equating to an 88 and 84% adherence rate, respectively, which was not significantly different between groups.

Strength (Table 1; Figure 1)

There was a significant main time effect for all 1-RM strength exercises ($p < 0.001$). Significant interaction effects for the chest press ($p = 0.026$), seated row ($p < 0.001$), leg extension ($p = 0.004$), and 1-RM total ($p < 0.001$) indicated that the GY group gained more strength over time for these exercises than the PP group.

Muscle Thickness (Table 2)

Main time effects were present for muscle thickness of the biceps and the quadriceps ($p < 0.001$). A significant interaction effect for muscle thickness of the biceps indicated that the GY group increased their average muscle thickness to a greater extent compared to the PP group ($p = 0.004$). Intra-operator variability (%CV) was 0.94% (95% CI = 0.5, 1.38) and 0.83% (95% CI = 0.6, 1.05) for biceps and quadriceps measures of muscle thickness, respectively. The change in biceps thickness correlated with the change in total strength across all participants ($R = 0.61$, $P = 0.001$).

Body Composition (Table 3; Figures 2–4)

A significant main effect of time was observed for FFM ($p < 0.001$). A significant interaction effect for FFM indicated that the GY group increased FFM more than the PP group ($p = 0.046$). There was a significant main effect of group for FM ($p = 0.035$), with GY subjects having a lower FM than PP subjects regardless of timepoint. There was a significant main effect of group for % body fat ($p = 0.022$), with GY subjects having less % body fat than PP subjects. Because there was a significant difference in % body fat between groups at baseline, an ANCOVA was used with baseline % body fat as a covariate, to assess the change in % body fat between groups. The ANCOVA indicated that the GY group reduced % body fat significantly more than the PP group ($p = 0.048$). **Figure 4** expresses the mean lean and fat mass changes as a percent of the total weight change over 12 weeks per group. The GY group appears to have a more favorable body

TABLE 1 | 1-RM Strength measurements pre- and post-training.

	Greek yogurt				Placebo pudding				RM-ANOVA		
	n	Pre kg	Post kg	Change Δ	*n*	Pre kg	Post kg	Change Δ	Time *p*-value	Group *p*-value	Interaction *p*-value
Chest press	14	81 ± 23	103 ± 20	22 [13.1–24.6]	15	87 ± 18	100 ± 20	13 [9.3, 16.9]	<0.001	0.82	0.026
Seated row	15	84 ± 21	105 ± 23	21 [15.1, 23.5]	15	83 ± 17	93 ± 17	10 [6.9, 16.9]	<0.001	0.34	<0.001
Leg extension	15	111 ± 24	150 ± 21	39 [29.4, 45.1]	15	124 ± 22	148 ± 27	24 [21.1, 30.7]	<0.001	0.51	0.004
Leg curl	15	79 ± 16	92 ± 15	13 [7.3, 14.8]	15	85 ± 15	94 ± 17	9 [6.1, 14.8]	<0.001	0.42	0.22
1-RM total	15	357 ± 80	455 ± 79	98 [72.6, 110.6]	15	379 ± 67	435 ± 76	57 [48, 65.3]	<0.001	0.96	<0.001

Strength values (absolute values displayed as mean ± SD, change values displayed as mean [95% CI]). Statistical analysis was by RM-ANOVA with time (pre and post) as the within factor and group (GY and PP) as the between factor. Significance was set at p < 0.05.

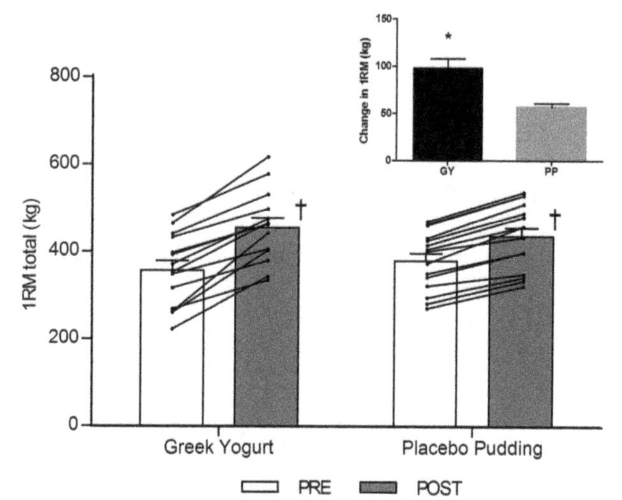

FIGURE 1 | Total 1-RM strength before and 12 weeks after RT and PLY in GY ($n = 14$) and PP ($n = 15$) groups. Individual pre and post-responses are represented by the lines over the bars. The inset graph shows the change in total 1-RM strength from baseline. †Significantly different from Pre within the same group ($p < 0.05$). *Significantly different from PP in the change from baseline in inset ($p < 0.001$). Values are presented as mean ± SE. RM = Repetition maximum.

composition change (i.e., increase in FFM and decrease in FM) than the PP group. That is, all body mass the GY group gained was FFM and they lost fat mass (100 and −26%, respectively), whereas the PP group gained both FFM and fat mass (76 and 24%, respectively).

Nutrition (Table 4)

Main time effects were present for energy ($p = 0.022$), protein (absolute and relative to body weight; $p < 0.001$), carbohydrate (absolute; $p = 0.003$, and relative; $p = 0.009$), and calcium ($p = 0.007$) intake throughout the intervention. Significant Interactions for protein intake (absolute and relative) and calcium intake indicated that the GY group had greater intakes than the PP group (<0.001). A significant interaction for carbohydrate intake (absolute and relative) indicated that the PP group had greater intakes than the GY group ($p = 0.002$). There were no significant differences in fat intake throughout the intervention.

Percent Change Analyses (Table 5)

Percent change was calculated for each variable using the equation: [(post-pre)/pre) × 100]. Independent *T*-Tests revealed a greater percent change decrease in FM and % body fat in the GY group compared to the PP group ($p = 0.042$ and $p = 0.038$, respectively). Similar to the RM-ANOVA results, percent change for the biceps muscle thickness and 1-RM strength measures (except the leg curl) were greater for the GY group compared to the PP group.

DISCUSSION

Our data demonstrate that the consumption of plain 0% fat GY (600 g on training days, 300 g on non-training days) following resistance and plyometric exercise as part of a 12-week training program increased most measures of strength, biceps muscle thickness and fat free mass while reducing FM more than an isoenergetic, CHO-based placebo pudding consumed at the same timepoints. This study is the first to use GY in this context and demonstrate such an effect with resistance exercise.

Strength was one of our main outcome measures. Strength is an important functional measure and can be used as a surrogate for muscle size and lean mass as these variables are highly correlated (40). Although strength increased in both groups following the intervention, our data revealed a significant time by group interaction effect for the chest press, seated row, and leg extension exercises as well as the composite measure of 1-RM total (**Table 1**; **Figure 1**), indicating that the GY group increased strength more than the PP group. Our research supports previous findings in young, untrained adults where milk and RT was shown to increase strength greater than a CHO placebo (12, 13). However, some training studies that utilize different whole dairy foods like chocolate milk (17) or regular yogurt (26) showed no additional strength increases compared to a CHO placebo. This may be because the amount of protein provided in the aforementioned studies was insufficient to see divergent strength adaptations between the groups. For example, both dairy groups, after supplementation, were habitually consuming only 1.3 g/kg/day (17) and 1.0 g/kg/day

TABLE 2 | Muscle thickness measurements analyzed using ultrasonography of the biceps and quadriceps muscles pre- and post-training.

	Greek yogurt				Placebo pudding				RM-ANOVA		
	n	Pre cm	Post cm	Change Δ	*n*	Pre cm	Post cm	Change Δ	Time *p*-value	Group *p*-value	Interaction *p*-value
Biceps	13	2.64 ± 0.4	3.1 ± 0.4	0.46 [0.23, 0.51]	14	2.75 ± 0.4	2.87 ± 0.5	0.12 [0.01, 0.25]	<0.001	0.70	0.004
Quadriceps	14	3.81 ± 0.8	4.47 ± 0.8	0.66 [0.34, 0.8]	14	3.65 ± 0.7	4.06 ± 0.7	0.41 [0.21, 0.65]	<0.001	0.27	0.14

Muscle thickness values (absolute values displayed as mean ± SD, change values displayed as mean [95% CI]). Statistical analysis was by RM-ANOVA with time (pre and post) as the within factor and group (GY and PP) as the between factor. Significance was set at $p < 0.05$.

TABLE 3 | Body composition measurements as assessed by Bod Pod pre- and post-training.

	Greek yogurt				Placebo pudding				RM-ANOVA		
	n	Pre	Post	Change Δ	*n*	Pre	Post	Change Δ	Time *p*-value	Group *p*-value	Interaction *p*-value
Body mass (kg)	14	69.9 ± 9.6	71.8 ± 9.5	1.9 [0.3, 3.1]	15	69.7 ± 10.4	71.4 ± 10.4	1.7 [0.4, 2.3]	<0.001	0.935	0.776
Fat-free mass (kg)	14	60.1 ± 7.9	62.5 ± 7.6	2.4 [1.5, 3.2]	15	57.5 ± 6.9	58.8 ± 6.5	1.3 [0.5, 2]	<0.001	0.25	0.046
Fat mass (kg)	14	8.6 ± 4.0	8.1 ± 4.4	−0.5 [−1.4, 0.6]	15	12.2 ± 6.0	12.6 ± 5.4	0.4 [−0.9, 1.6]	0.918	0.035	0.296
Body fat (%)	14	12.3 ± 4.5	11.2 ± 5.1	−1.1 [2.2, 0.2]	15	16.9 ± 7.2	17.0 ± 6.1	0.1 [1.3, 1.6]	0.35	0.022	0.205

Body composition values (absolute values displayed as mean ± SD, change values displayed as mean [95% CI]). Statistical analysis was by RM-ANOVA with time (pre and post) as the within factor and group (GY and PP) as the between factor. Significance was set at $p < 0.05$.

(26) of protein, which not only was close to the amount of protein consumed by their respective placebo groups, but also below the recommended threshold of protein intake for novice exercisers. Research suggests protein intakes of approximately 1.6 g/kg/day are necessary for individuals new to RT to facilitate optimal strength adaptations (2, 41, 42). The justification for the increased protein recommendation of 1.6 g/kg/day is due to a higher rate of MPS in novices (43) and a reduced efficiency of protein utilization compared to trained individuals (44). In our study, GY supplementation enabled subjects to increase their protein intake to 1.74 g/kg/day (whereas PP subjects consumed 1.22 g/kg/day of protein). This could explain why significantly greater strength gains were observed in this group. Our research is consistent with other chronic (minimum 10 weeks) training studies in young, untrained males which demonstrate that increased protein intakes optimize strength adaptations during a RT program (12, 45–47).

Initially, during a RT program strength gains are typically the result of neurological adaptations (48). However, to continue to develop muscular strength, morphological adaptations are necessary. These adaptations include increasing muscle cross sectional area (CSA) by increasing contractile proteins, altering tendon and connective tissue, changes in fiber type and hyperplasia, all of which require additional dietary protein (48). RT causes metabolic and mechanical stress to the muscle which signals MPS (49, 50). Once this stimulus has occurred, hyperaminoacidemia is required to facilitate the incorporation of amino acids (AAs) into the muscle to make new myofibrillar proteins (51). If this process is consistently repeated, like our study design intended, total muscle CSA can increase (52). Therefore, another outcome measure in our study was muscle thickness, a surrogate for muscle CSA, via ultrasonography (53).

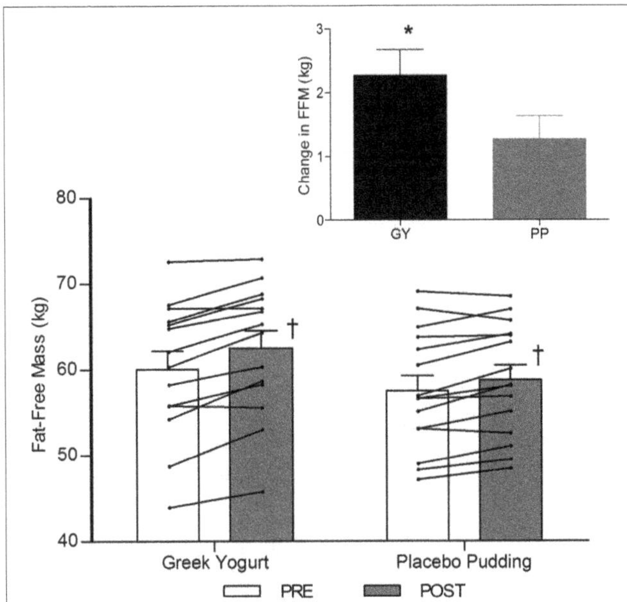

FIGURE 2 | Fat-free mass before and 12 weeks after RT and PLY in GY (n = 14) and PP (n = 15). Individual pre and post-responses are represented by the lines over the bars. The inset graph shows the change in total fat-free mass from baseline. †Significantly different from Pre within the same group ($p < 0.05$). *Significantly different from PP in the change from baseline in inset ($p < 0.05$). Bars are presented as mean ± SE.

Ultrasonography has been shown to be reliable and valid for this measure when compared to MRI (54, 55). Our study revealed a significant main effect of time for biceps and quadriceps muscle thickness following the intervention (**Table 2**). This can

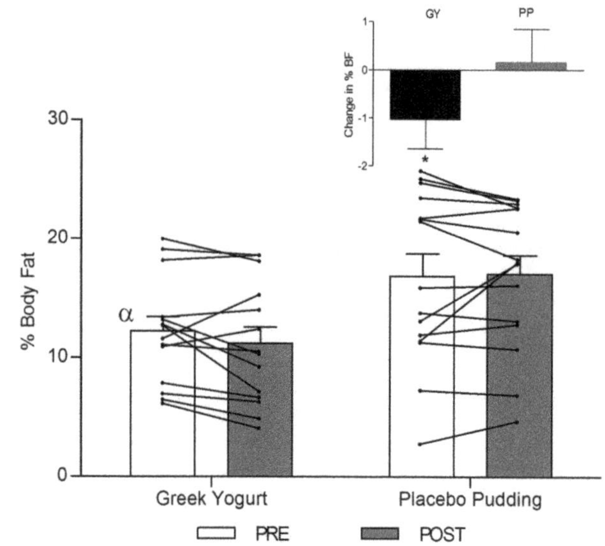

FIGURE 3 | Total fat-free mass before and 12 weeks after RT and PLY in GY ($n = 14$) and PP ($n = 15$). Individual pre and post-responses are represented by the lines over the bars. The inset graph shows the change in total fat-free mass from baseline. α Significantly different at baseline between groups ($p < 0.05$). *Significantly different from PP in the change from baseline in inset as assessed by ANCOVA ($p < 0.05$). Bars are presented as mean ± SE.

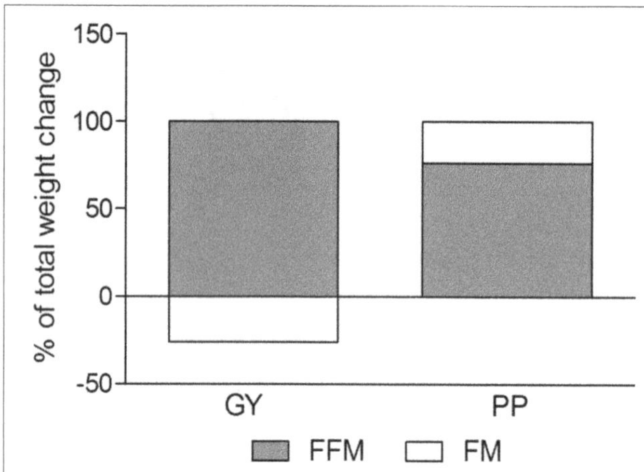

FIGURE 4 | Fat mass and Fat-free mass visually expressed as a percent of total mass change during the intervention for the GY and PP groups (GY = 14, PP = 15).

likely be attributed to the effectiveness of the RT program in stimulating muscle hypertrophy (56). Our data also indicated that habitual consumption of GY yielded greater increases in biceps brachii muscle thickness compared to the consumption of the PP. These findings are supported by similar research in milk (12, 16) and isolated dairy proteins (e.g., whey and casein) (45, 47, 57) where greater increases in muscle size were seen in these groups compared to a placebo following RT in untrained, young, adult subjects.

Our data also demonstrated a favorable change in body composition for the GY group compared to the PP group. GY subjects gained significantly more FFM and reduced FM and % fat greater than PP subjects (**Figures 2**, **3** and **Tables 2**, **5**). Although both groups gained significantly more body mass, all the body mass gained in the GY group was FFM and they were able to lose FM (100 and −26%, respectively). Whereas, the PP group gained both FFM and FM (76 and 24%, respectively). This represents a more favorable body compositional change in the GY group (**Figures 2–4**). Reductions in fat mass and increases in lean mass with GY are likely also due to other characteristics and nutrients in GY aside from protein. GY, as a semi-solid food, is satiating (58, 59) which can reduce hunger and delay subsequent energy intake (60), and it contains calcium which has been shown to inhibit intracellular lipogenesis, promote lipolysis and increase lipid oxidation (7, 61).

The current study provided subjects with 2 × 20 g doses of dairy protein from GY within 1 h post-exercise. This was done to ensure protein was provided to the working muscles in close temporal proximity to exercise and was designed to mimic similar research done in milk (12, 13). Research in young adults indicates 20 g of protein is just as effective at stimulating MPS as 40 g (29, 30), and, expressed relative to body weight and per meal, that 0.24 g/kg/meal is sufficient to stimulate myofibrillar protein synthesis (62). A recent review by Schoenfeld and Aragon (42) proposed a greater protein dose to maximize anabolism of 0.4 g/kg/meal, especially when the protein source is slower digesting (potentially like semi-solid Greek yogurt) and when consumed in the presence of other macronutrients which may further delay AA absorption (42). Based on these two dosing recommendations, for a 70 kg male (like those in our study), this corresponds to 16.8 and 28 g of protein per bolus, respectively. Our dose was within these recommendations and thus likely contributed to the greater training adaptations incurred with GY over time. Although participants in our study experienced increases in muscle thickness, fat-free mass and strength, it is important to note that myofibrillar muscle protein synthesis (mMPS) was not directly measured. It, therefore, cannot be directly concluded that our intervention lead to increases in mMPS, nor that only muscle tissue changes are primarily responsible for the observed effects (63).

Our participants also consumed GY prior to sleep in efforts to attenuate the rise in MPB and maintain a positive net protein balance during sleep, since sleep tends to be a fasted period in which protein balance naturally favors breakdown (64, 65). Interestingly, an acute study demonstrated that casein supplementation (40 g) prior to sleep was able to increase blood AA levels during sleep (7.5 h) and significantly increase whole body protein synthesis and net protein balance vs. the placebo (66). A training study subsequently confirmed that 28 g of casein given prior to sleep as part of a 12 week RT program (3 times/week) produced greater muscle mass and strength gains compared to a non-caloric placebo (flavored water) (45). Since GY primarily consists of casein protein, a similar mechanism of inhibiting or attenuating MPB may have occurred in our study resulting in greater cumulative strength, size and FFM gains.

Compared to milk, GY likely has a greater ratio of casein to whey [based on the manufacturing process of removing the liquid-whey from GY (23, 67)], it is more acidic (68), and it exists in a semi-solid food matrix (18). All these factors could attenuate digestion and subsequent absorption rates such that

TABLE 4 | Total daily nutrient intakes from food diaries for each group, at baseline and week 12.

Nutrient intake per day	Greek yogurt			Placebo pudding			RM-ANOVA		
	n	Baseline	Week 12	*n*	Baseline	Week 12	Time	Group	Interaction *p*-value
Energy (kcal)	14	2146 ± 407	2207 ± 345	15	1989 ± 398	2303 ± 588	0.022	0.83	0.11
Protein (g)	13	90.6 ± 15.2	124.8 ± 13.4	15	85.7 ± 14.6	85.9 ± 19.9	<0.001	<0.001	<0.001
Protein (g/Kg)	13	1.31 ± 0.32	1.74 ± 0.31	15	1.25 ± 0.26	1.22 ± 0.27	<0.001	0.007	<0.001
CHO (g)	15	246.1 ± 52.2	242.2 ± 55.2	14	225.0 ± 54.9	283.3 ± 55.2	0.006	0.57	0.002
CHO (g/Kg)	13	3.46 ± 0.87	3.38 ± 0.71	14	3.3 ± 0.89	4.04 ± 0.9	0.013	0.416	0.002
Fat (g)	15	79.2 ± 18.0	78.4 ± 18.6	15	79.9 ± 27.5	84.9 ± 35.7	0.57	0.68	0.43
Fat (g/Kg)	15	1.18 ± 0.27	1.11 ± 0.26	15	1.15 ± 0.37	1.19 ± 0.46	0.81	0.84	0.32
Calcium (mg)	14	699 ± 267	1069 ± 243	14	678 ± 225	585 ± 211	0.007	0.003	<0.001

Nutrient intake values (displayed as mean ± SD). Nutrient intakes include daily diet and GY or PP supplementation. Statistical analysis was by RM-ANOVA with time as the within factor (week 0 and week 12) and group as the between factor. Significance was set at $p < 0.05$.

TABLE 5 | Percent (%) change for both groups, from pre to post-intervention.

Variable	Greek yogurt		Placebo pudding		Independent *T*-test
	n	%	*n*	%	*p*-value
Body mass (Kg)	15	2.4	14	2.0	0.77
Fat-free mass (Kg)	15	3.9	15	2.3	0.11
Fat mass (Kg)	14	−11.1	14	5.8	0.042
Body fat (%)	14	−13.2	13	−1.1	0.038
Biceps muscle thickness (cm)	14	16.4	13	7.1	0.026
Quadriceps muscle thickness (cm)	14	15.0	14	13.0	0.67
Chest press (Kg)	13	28.3	15	15.4	0.030
Seated row (Kg)	13	23.7	14	11.7	0.002
Leg extension (Kg)	14	11.7	14	20.9	0.006
Leg curl (Kg)	13	14.6	14	12.8	0.62
1-RM total (Kg)	13	26.8	15	15.1	0.003

% change values (displayed as means). Statistical analysis was by independent t-test between groups (GY and PP). Significance was set at $p < 0.05$.

GY would elevate blood-AA concentrations for a longer duration than milk. Despite the plausibility of this hypothesis, no research exists on the post-prandial absorption rate and plasma AA response of GY compared to other dairy products, like milk. Research with intrinsically labeled casein protein indicates that absorption is even slower when consumed in a whole food matrix vs. isolated casein (69, 70). This research also demonstrated that a higher proportion of labeled casein consumed from milk was incorporated into skeletal muscle than when consumed as isolated casein, suggesting that the presence of other nutrients within the whole food may positively influence the utilization of AAs by muscle tissue (70). For this reason, GY may be at least as, or even more, beneficial at promoting a positive protein balance than milk or casein alone. On the other hand, it may also be possible that the presence of other factors within the GY food matrix (that are not present in milk) or the fact that it is a solid food could act to suppress the release of AAs too much and inhibit them from providing a sufficient trigger for MPS. Nonetheless, we did see positive adaptations with GY, so it may be possible that GY (a predominantly casein-based, semi-solid dairy product containing different nutrient compounds) may act to promote muscle adaptations via different mechanisms. More research on this using yogurt and other dairy and whole foods needs to be done.

High protein GY has demonstrated the ability to reduce appetite and energy intake in subsequent meals compared to lower protein snacks and snack-skipping (8). The GY and PP supplementation in our study was energy-matched and provided each group with 330 calories per training day (3 doses of supplement) and 165 calories per non-training day (1.5 doses of supplement). Our data show that both groups did not completely compensate their habitual diets for the added supplementation which caused them to significantly increase their energy intake from baseline. The GY group only increased their habitual energy intake, on average, by 61 calories at week 12, compared to 314 calories in the PP group. Although this increase in energy was not statistically different between the groups, the consumption of 300+ kcals/day over time is arguably more physiologically significant and can lead to an increase in fat mass compared to an increase of 61 kcals/day (71). For example, a 6 month study that replaced caloric beverages with non-caloric beverages, a straight-forward strategy to reduce energy intake, resulted in 2.5% weight loss (71). This likely contributed to the PP group gaining fat mass, and, on the other hand, the GY may have been more satiating resulting in less of an increase in energy intake in this group.

Our study had several strengths. The use of only one tester for all subject pre- and post-testing was a strength that minimized inter-tester variation. All supplementation was prepared by the same individual to ensure consistency. We kept the contents of the PP discreet and called it the "study-designed supplement," which we believe may have facilitated our high supplement adherence rates (because the participants may have thought the PP contained different beneficial bioactives). Also, trainers involved in the study were unaware of the contents of the PP to prevent bias. Our study also had limitations. Subjects were not blinded to which supplement group they were in. Blinding is notoriously difficult to achieve in nutrition studies (72–74). However, we did conceal the contents of the PP from our subjects (and trainers). We also did not use state-of-the-art measurement tools, such as DXA or MRI, for body composition determination (75–77). We used the Bod Pod which is unable to give a specific measure of muscle mass. However, the Bod Pod is considered a reliable method for measuring body fat in normal weight populations compared to DXA (78, 79). Lastly, since subjects were initially untrained, they may have experienced a learning effect on the 1-RM exercises which may partly explain the increased strength during the post-testing. However, this would have been consistent for all participants regardless of group and cannot explain the divergent results in favor of GY.

In summary, the consumption of fat-free, plain GY during a 12-week exercise program promoted greater improvements in strength, muscle thickness and body composition than a CHO pudding placebo in untrained, university-aged males. Our study is the first to report a positive effect of GY with exercise on a comprehensive set of muscle-related outcome variables, which allows us to robustly assert GY's favorable role within this context. Thus, given our specific results, GY should be considered as a viable post-exercise, whole food, protein source for individuals beginning a RT program with the goal of increasing strength and lean mass and decreasing fat mass. Furthermore, the beneficial characteristics of GY beyond protein, such as its satiating effect, probiotic cultures and micronutrient content may offer additional benefits, above other dairy products, to digestive (80–82) and bone (83–85) health, and may have further implications in different age groups including the elderly. Future research is needed to elucidate the multiple health effects of GY as part of a healthy diet (with or without exercise) that extend beyond muscular benefit in different contexts.

AUTHOR CONTRIBUTIONS

AJ conceptualized the idea. AB and AJ designed research project with critical input from BR and WW. AB, HS, JB, and MN provided a critical role in data collection and analysis. AB and AJ carried out the statistical analysis. AB wrote initial version of the manuscript. All authors contributed to the final version of the manuscript.

FUNDING

Funding for this study was provided by AJ's unrestricted research grant from Brock University.

ACKNOWLEDGMENTS

Greek yogurt was kindly provided by Danone Inc.

REFERENCES

1. Devries M, Phillips S. Supplemental protein in support of muscle mass and health: advantage whey. *J Food Sci.* (2015) 1:8–15. doi: 10.1111/1750-3841.12802
2. Morton RW, Murphy KT, McKellar SR, Schoenfeld BJ, Henselmans M, Helms E, et al. A systematic review, meta-analysis and meta-regression of the effect of protein supplementation on resistance training-induced gains in muscle mass and strength in healthy adults. *Br J Sports Med.* (2017) 52:376–84. doi: 10.1136/bjsports-2017-097608
3. Cermak NM, Res PT, De Groot LCPGM, Saris WHM, Van Loon LJC. Protein supplementation augments the adaptive response of skeletal muscle to resistance-type exercise training: a meta-analysis. *Am J Clin Nutr.* (2012) 96:1454–64. doi: 10.3945/ajcn.112.037556
4. Anthony JC, Anthony TG, Kimball SR, Jefferson LS. Signaling pathways involved in translational control of protein synthesis in skeletal muscle by leucine. *J Nutr.* (2001) 131:856–60. doi: 10.1093/jn/131.3.856S
5. Layman DK, Anthony TG, Rasmussen BB, Adams SH, Lynch CJ, Brinkworth GD, et al. Defining meal requirements for protein to optimize metabolic roles of amino acids. *Am J Clin Nutr.* (2015) 101:1330S–8S. doi: 10.3945/ajcn.114.084053
6. Norton LE, Layman DK. Leucine regulates translation initiation of protein synthesis in skeletal muscle after exercise. *J Nutr.* (2006) 136:533S–7S. doi: 10.1093/jn/136.2.533S
7. Christensen R, Lorenzen JK, Svith CR, Bartels EM, Melanson EL, Saris WH, et al. Effect of calcium from dairy and dietary supplements on faecal fat excretion: A meta-analysis of randomized controlled trials. *Obes Rev.* (2009) 10:475–86. doi: 10.1111/j.1467-789X.2009.00599.x
8. Panahi S, Tremblay A. The potential role of yogurt in weight management and prevention of type 2 diabetes. *J Am Coll Nutr.* (2016) 35:717–31. doi: 10.1080/07315724.2015.1102103
9. Miller PE, Alexander DD, Perez V. Effects of whey protein and resistance exercise on body composition: a meta-analysis of randomized controlled trials. *J Am Coll Nutr.* (2014) 33:163–75. doi: 10.1080/07315724.2013.875365
10. Boirie Y, Dangin M, Gachon P, Vasson MP, Maubois JL, Beaufrere B. Slow and fast dietary proteins differently modulate postprandial protein

accretion. *Proc Natl Acad Sci USA.* (1997) 94:14930–5. doi: 10.1073/pnas.94.26.14930

11. Reitelseder S, Agergaard J, Doessing S, Helmark IC, Lund P, Kristensen NB, et al. Whey and casein labeled with L-[1-13C]leucine and muscle protein synthesis: effect of resistance exercise and protein ingestion. *Am J Physiol Endocrinol Metab.* (2011) 300:E231–42. doi: 10.1152/ajpendo.00513.2010
12. Hartman JW, Tang JE, Wilkinson SB, Tarnopolsky MA, Lawrence RL, Fullerton AV, et al. Phillips SM. Consumption of fat-free fluid milk after resistance exercise promotes greater lean mass accretion than does consumption of soy or carbohydrate in young, novice, male weightlifters. *Am J Clin Nutr.* (2007) 86:373–81. doi: 10.1093/ajcn/86.2.373
13. Josse AR, Tang JE, Tarnopolsky MA, Phillips SM. Body composition and strength changes in women with milk and resistance exercise. *Med Sci Sports Exerc.* (2010) 42:1122–30. doi: 10.1249/MSS.0b013e3181c854f6
14. Naclerio F, Larumbe-Zabala E. Effects of whey protein alone or as part of a multi-ingredient formulation on strength, fat-free mass, or lean body mass in resistance-trained individuals: a meta-analysis. *Sports Med.* (2016) 2016:125–37. doi: 10.1007/s40279-015-0403-y
15. Thorning TK, Bertram HC, Bonjour JP, De Groot L, Dupont D, Feeney E, et al. Whole dairy matrix or single nutrients in assessment of health effects: current evidence and knowledge gaps. *Am J Clin Nutr.* (2017) 105:1033–45. doi: 10.3945/ajcn.116.151548
16. Josse AR, Phillips SM. Impact of milk consumption and resistance training on body composition of female athletes. *Med Sport Sci.* (2013) 59:94–103. doi: 10.1159/000341968
17. Rankin JW, Goldman LP, Puglisi MJ, Nickols-Richardson SM, Earthman CP, Gwazdauskas FC. Effect of post-exercise supplement consumption on adaptations to resistance training. *J Am Coll Nutr.* (2004) 23:322–30. doi: 10.1080/07315724.2004.10719375
18. Zhu Y, Hsu WH, Hollis JH. The impact of food viscosity on eating rate, subjective appetite, glycemic response and gastric emptying rate. *PLoS ONE.* (2013) 8:e67482. doi: 10.1371/journal.pone.0067482
19. Beena Divya J, Kulangara Varsha K, Madhavan Nampoothiri K, Ismail B, Pandey A. Probiotic fermented foods for health benefits. *Eng Life Sci.* (2012) 12:377–90. doi: 10.1002/elsc.201100179
20. Ismail MM, Ibrahim MM, Youssef EF, El Shorbagy KM. Plyometric training versus resistive exercises after acute lateral ankle sprain. *Foot Ankle Int.* (2010) 31:523–30. doi: 10.3113/FAI.2010.0523
21. Marco ML, Heeney D, Binda S, Cifelli CJ, Cotter PD, Foligne B, et al. Health benefits of fermented foods: microbiota and beyond. *Curr Opin Biotechnol.* (2017) 44:94–102. doi: 10.1016/j.copbio.2016.11.010
22. Tamang JP, Shin DH, Jung SJ, Chae SW. Functional properties of microorganisms in fermented foods. *Front Microbiol.* (2016) 7:578. doi: 10.3389/fmicb.2016.00578
23. Jacques PF, Wang H. Yogurt and weight management. *Am J Clin Nutr.* (2014) 99:1229S–34S. doi: 10.3945/ajcn.113.073031
24. Fernandez MA, Marette A. Potential health benefits of combining yogurt and fruits based on their probiotic and prebiotic properties. *Adv Nutr An Int Rev J.* (2017) 8:155–64. doi: 10.3945/an.115.011114
25. Chandan RC. An overview of yogurt production and composition. *Yogurt Health Dis Prev.* (2017) 2017:31–47. doi: 10.1016/B978-0-12-805134-4.00002-X
26. White KM, Bauer SJ, Hartz KK, Baldridge M. Changes in body composition with yogurt consumption during resistance training in women. *Int J Sport Nutr Exerc Metab.* (2009) 19:18–33. doi: 10.1123/ijsnem.19.1.18
27. Zemel MB, Richards J, Mathis S, Milstead A, Gebhardt L, Silva E. Dairy augmentation of total and central fat loss in obese subjects. *Int J Obes.* (2005) 29:391–7. doi: 10.1038/sj.ijo.0802880
28. Thomas DT, Wideman L, Lovelady CA. Effects of a dairy supplement and resistance training on lean mass and insulin-like growth factor in women. *Int J Sport Nutr Exerc Metab.* (2011) 21:181–8. doi: 10.1123/ijsnem.21.3.181
29. Moore DR, Robinson MJ, Fry JL, Tang JE, Glover EI, Wilkinson SB, et al. Ingested protein dose response of muscle and albumin protein synthesis after resistance exercise in young men. *Am J Clin Nutr.* (2009) 89:161–8. doi: 10.3945/ajcn.2008.26401
30. Witard OC, Jackman SR, Breen L, Smith K, Selby A, Tipton KD. Myofibrillar muscle protein synthesis rates subsequent to a meal in response to increasing doses of whey protein at rest and after resistance exercise. *Am J Clin Nutr.* (2014) 99:86–95. doi: 10.3945/ajcn.112.055517
31. Danone (2019). Available online at: https://oikos.ca/en/oikos/plain-0 (accessed February 1, 2019).
32. Natrel (2019). Available online at: https://www.natrel.ca/en/products/fine-filtered-milks/fine-filtered-skim-milk (accessed February 1, 2019).
33. Fisberg M, Machado R. History of yogurt and current patterns of consumption. *Nutr Rev.* (2015) 73:4–7. doi: 10.1093/nutrit/nuv020
34. Wu L, Sun D. Consumption of yogurt and the incident risk of cardiovascular disease: A meta-analysis of nine cohort studies. *Nutrients.* (2017) 9:315. doi: 10.3390/nu9030315
35. Dehghan M, Mente A, Rangarajan S, Sheridan P, Mohan V, Iqbal R, et al. Association of dairy intake with cardiovascular disease and mortality in 21 countries from five continents (PURE): a prospective cohort study. *Lancet.* (2018) 392: 2288–2297. doi: 10.1016/S0140-6736(18)31812-9
36. Haff G, Haff E. *Training Integration and Periodization. NSCA's Guide to Program Design.* Windsor, ON: Human Kinetics, Inc. (2012).
37. Mayhew JL, Johnson BD, Lamonte MJ, Lauber D, Kemmler W. Accuracy of prediction equations for determining one repetition maximum bench press in women before and after resistance training. *J Strength Cond Res.* (2008) 22:1570–7. doi: 10.1519/JSC.0b013e31817b02ad
38. LeSuer DA, McCormick JH, Mayhew JL, Wasserstein RL, Arnold MD. The accuracy of prediction equations for estimating 1-rm performance in the bench press, squat, and deadlift. *J Strength Cond Res.* (1997) 11:211.
39. Dohoney P, Chromiak JA, Lemire D, Abadie BR, Kovacs C. Prediction of one repetition maximum (1-RM) strength from a 4-6 RM and a7-10 RM submaximal strength test in healthy young adult males. *J Exerc Physiol.* (2002) 5:54–9. Available online at: https://www.scopus.com/record/display.uri?eid=2-s2.0-3242766756&origin=inward&txGid=785e48d262ae7a8a189d38c91f688115
40. Bamman MM, Newcomer BR, Larson-Meyer DE, Weinsier RL, Hunter GR. Evaluation of the strength-size relationship *in vivo* using various muscle size indices. *Med Sci Sports Exerc.* (2000) 32:1307–13. doi: 10.1097/00005768-200007000-00019
41. Lemon PW. Beyond the zone: protein needs of active individuals. *J Am Coll Nutr.* (2000) 19:513S–21S. doi: 10.1080/07315724.2000.10718974
42. Schoenfeld BJ, Aragon AA. How much protein can the body use in a single meal for muscle-building? Implications for daily protein distribution. *J Int Soc Sports Nutr.* (2018) 15:10. doi: 10.1186/s12970-018-0215-1
43. Hakkinen K, Pakarinen A, Alen M, Kauhanen H, Komi PV. Neuromuscular and hormonal adaptations in athletes to strength training in two years. *J Appl Physiol.* (1988) 65:2406–12. doi: 10.1152/jappl.1988.65.6.2406
44. Phillips SM. Protein requirements and supplementation in strength sports. *Nutrition.* (2004) 20:689–95. doi: 10.1016/j.nut.2004.04.009
45. Snijders T, Res PT, Smeets JSJ, Vliet SV, Kranenburg JV, Maase K, et al. Protein ingestion before sleep increases muscle mass and strength gains during prolonged resistance-type exercise training in healthy young men. *J Nutr.* (2015) 145:1178–84. doi: 10.3945/jn.114.208371
46. Willoughby DS, Stout JR, Wilborn CD. Effects of resistance training and protein plus amino acid supplementation on muscle anabolism, mass, and strength. *Amino Acids.* (2007) 32:467–77. doi: 10.1007/s00726-006-0398-7
47. Andersen LL, Tufekovic G, Zebis MK, Crameri RM, Verlaan G, Kjaer M, et al. The effect of resistance training combined with timed ingestion of protein on muscle fiber size and muscle strength. *Metabolism.* (2005) 54:151–6. doi: 10.1016/j.metabol.2004.07.012
48. Folland JP, Williams AG. The adaptations to strength training: morphological and neurological contributions to increased strength. *Sport Med.* (2007) 37:145–68. doi: 10.2165/00007256-200737020-00004
49. Schoenfeld BJ. The mechanisms of muscle hypertrophy and their application to resistance training. *J Strength Cond Res.* (2010) 24:2857–72. doi: 10.1519/JSC.0b013e3181e840f3
50. Schoenfeld BJ. Potential mechanisms for a role of metabolic stress in hypertrophic adaptations to resistance training. *Sport Med.* (2013) 43:179–94. doi: 10.1007/s40279-013-0017-1
51. Phillips SM, Hartman JW, Wilkinson SB. Dietary protein to support anabolism with resistance exercise in young men. *J Am Coll Nutr.* (2005) 24:134S–9S. doi: 10.1080/07315724.2005.10719454

52. Hulmi JJ, Lockwood CM, Stout JR. Effect of protein/essential amino acids and resistance training on skeletal muscle hypertrophy: a case for whey protein. *Nutr Metab.* (2010) 7:51. doi: 10.1186/1743-7075-7-51
53. Ahtiainen JP, Hoffren M, Hulmi JJ, Pietikäinen M, Mero AA, Avela J, et al. Panoramic ultrasonography is a valid method to measure changes in skeletal muscle cross-sectional area. *Eur J Appl Physiol.* (2010) 108:273-9. doi: 10.1007/s00421-009-1211-6
54. Ishida Y, Carroll JF, Pollock ML, Graves JE, Leggett SH. Reliability of B-mode ultrasound for the measurement of body fat and muscle thickness. *Am J Hum Biol.* (1992) 4:511–20. doi: 10.1002/ajhb.1310040410
55. Reeves ND, Maganaris CN, Narici MV. Ultrasonographic assessment of human skeletal muscle size. *Eur J Appl Physiol.* (2004) 91:116-8. doi: 10.1007/s00421-003-0961-9
56. Phillips SM, Tipton KD, Aarsland A, Wolf SE, Wolfe RR. Mixed muscle protein synthesis and breakdown after resistance exercise in humans. *Am J Physiol Metab.* (1997) 273:99–107. doi: 10.1152/ajpendo.1997.273.1.E99
57. Hulmi JJ, Tannerstedt J, Selänne H, Kainulainen H, Kovanen V, Mero AA. Resistance exercise with whey protein ingestion affects mTOR signaling pathway and myostatin in men. *J Appl Physiol.* (2009) 106:1720-9. doi: 10.1152/japplphysiol.00087.2009
58. Tsuchiya A, Almiron-Roig E, Lluch A, Guyonnet D, Drewnowski A. Higher satiety ratings following yogurt consumption relative to fruit drink or dairy fruit drink. *J Am Diet Assoc.* (2006) 106:550–7. doi: 10.1016/j.jada.2006.01.004
59. Tremblay A, Doyon C, Sanchez M. Impact of yogurt on appetite control, energy balance, and body composition. *Nutr Rev.* (2015) 73:23-7. doi: 10.1093/nutrit/nuv015
60. Douglas SM, Ortinau LC, Hoertel HA, Leidy HJ. Low, moderate, or high protein yogurt snacks on appetite control and subsequent eating in healthy women. *Appetite.* (2013) 60:117–22. doi: 10.1016/j.appet.2012.09.012
61. Zemel MB, Thompson W, Milstead A, Morris K, Campbell P. Calcium and dairy acceleration of weight and fat loss during energy restriction in obese adults. *Obes Res.* (2004) 12:582–90. doi: 10.1038/oby.2004.67
62. Moore DR, Churchward-Venne TA, Witard O, Breen L, Burd NA, Tipton KD, et al. Protein ingestion to stimulate myofibrillar protein synthesis requires greater relative protein intakes in healthy older versus younger men. *J Gerontol A Biol Sci Med Sci.* (2015) 70:57–62. doi: 10.1093/gerona/glu103
63. Roberts MD, Haun CT, Mobley CB, Mumford PW, Romero MA, Roberson PA, et al. Physiological differences between low versus high skeletal muscle hypertrophic responders to resistance exercise training: current perspectives and future research directions. *Front Physiol.* (2018) 9:834. doi: 10.3389/fphys.2018.00834
64. Trommelen J, Loon L. Pre-sleep protein ingestion to improve the skeletal muscle adaptive response to exercise training. *Nutrients.* (2016) 8:763. doi: 10.3390/nu8120763
65. Trommelen J, Holwerda AM, Kouw IWK, Langer H, Halson SL, Rollo I, et al. Resistance exercise augments postprandial overnight muscle protein synthesis rates. *Med Sci Sports Exerc.* (2016) 48:2517–25. doi: 10.1249/MSS.0000000000001045
66. Res PT, Groen B, Pennings B, Beelen M, Wallis GA, Gijsen AP, et al. Protein ingestion before sleep improves postexercise overnight recovery. *Med Sci Sports Exerc.* (2012) 44:1560–9. doi: 10.1249/MSS.0b013e31824cc363
67. Bong DD, Moraru CI. Use of micellar casein concentrate for Greek-style yogurt manufacturing: effects on processing and product properties. *J Dairy Sci.* (2014) 97:1259–69. doi: 10.3168/jds.2013-7488
68. Liljeberg H, Björck I. Delayed gastric emptying rate may explain improved glycaemia in healthy subjects to a starchy meal with added vinegar. *Eur J Clin Nutr.* (1998) 52:368–71. doi: 10.1038/sj.ejcn.1600572
69. Churchward-Venne TA, Snijders T, Linkens AM, Hamer HM, van Kranenburg J, van Loon LJ. Ingestion of casein in a milk matrix modulates dietary protein digestion and absorption kinetics but does not modulate postprandial muscle protein synthesis in older men. *J Nutr.* (2015) 145:1438-45. doi: 10.3945/jn.115.213710
70. Soop M, Nehra V, Henderson GC, Boirie Y, Ford GC, Nair KS. Coingestion of whey protein and casein in a mixed meal: demonstration of a more sustained anabolic effect of casein. *AJP Endocrinol Metab.* (2012) 1:152-62. doi: 10.1152/ajpendo.00106.2012
71. Tate DF, Turner-McGrievy G, Lyons E, Stevens J, Erickson K, Polzien K, et al. Replacing caloric beverages with water or diet beverages for weight loss in adults: main results of the choose healthy options consciously everyday (CHOICE) randomized clinical trial. *Am J Clin Nutr.* (2012) 95:555–63. doi: 10.3945/ajcn.111.026278
72. Weaver CM, Miller JW. Challenges in conducting clinical nutrition research. *Nutr Rev.* (2017) 75:491–9. doi: 10.1093/nutrit/nux026
73. Staudacher HM, Irving PM, Lomer MCE, Whelan K. The challenges of control groups, placebos and blinding in clinical trials of dietary interventions. *Proc Nutr Soc.* (2017) 76:628. doi: 10.1017/S0029665117 002816
74. Hébert JR, Frongillo EA, Adams SA, Turner-McGrievy GM, Hurley TG, Miller DR, et al. Perspective: Randomized controlled trials are not a panacea for diet-related research. *Adv Nutr.* (2016) 7:423–32. doi: 10.3945/an.115.011023
75. Thibault R, Pichard C. The evaluation of body composition: a useful tool for clinical practice. *Ann Nutr Metab.* (2012) 60:6–16. doi: 10.1159/0003 34879
76. Hangartner TN, Warner S, Braillon P, Jankowski L, Shepherd J. The official positions of the international society for clinical densitometry: acquisition of dual-energy x-ray absorptiometry body composition and considerations regarding analysis and repeatability of measures. *J Clin Densitom.* (2013) 16:520–36. doi: 10.1016/j.jocd.2013.08.007
77. Salamat MR, Shanei A, Khoshhali M, Salamat AH, Siavash M, Asgari M. Use of conventional regional DXA scans for estimating whole body composition. *Arch Iran Med.* (2014) 17:674–8. doi: 0141710/AIM.007
78. Lowry DW, Tomiyama AJ. Air displacement plethysmography versus dual-energy X-ray absorptiometry in underweight, normal-weight, and overweight/obese individuals. *PLoS ONE.* (2015) 10:e0115086. doi: 10.1371/journal.pone.0115086
79. Fields DA, Goran MI, McCrory MA. Body-composition assessment via air-displacement plethysmography in adults and children: a review. *Am J Clin Nutr.* (2002) 75:453–67. doi: 10.1093/ajcn/75.3.453
80. Morelli L. Yogurt, living cultures, and gut health. *Am J Clin Nutr.* (2014) 99: 1248S—50S. doi: 10.3945/ajcn.113.073072
81. Adolfsson O, Meydani SN, Russell RM. Yogurt and gut function. *Am J Clin Nutr.* (2004) 80:245–56. doi: 10.1093/ajcn/ 80.2.245
82. Pei R, Martin DA, DiMarco DM, Bolling BW. Evidence for the effects of yogurt on gut health and obesity. *Crit Rev Food Sci Nutr.* (2017) 57:1569-83. doi: 10.1080/10408398.2014.883356
83. Rizzoli R. Dairy products, yogurts, and bone health. *Am J Clin Nutr.* (2014) 99: 1256S—2S. doi: 10.3945/ajcn.113.073056
84. Rizzoli R, Biver E. Effects of fermented milk products on bone. *Calcif Tissue Int.* (2018) 102:489–500. doi: 10.1007/s00223-017-0317-9
85. Sahni S, Tucker KL, Kiel DP, Quach L, Casey VA, Hannan MT. Milk and yogurt consumption are linked with higher bone mineral density but not with hip fracture: the framingham offspring study. *Arch Osteoporos.* (2013) 8:119. doi: 10.1007/s11657-013-0119-2

Effects of Graded Whey Supplementation During Extreme-Volume Resistance Training

Cody T. Haun[1†], Christopher G. Vann[1], Christopher B. Mobley[1], Paul A. Roberson[1], Shelby C. Osburn[1], Hudson M. Holmes[1], Petey M. Mumford[1], Matthew A. Romero[1], Kaelin C. Young[1,2], Jordan R. Moon[3], L. Bruce Gladden[1], Robert D. Arnold[4], Michael A. Israetel[5], Annie N. Kirby[2] and Michael D. Roberts[1,2†]*

[1] School of Kinesiology, Auburn University, Auburn, AL, United States, [2] Department of Cell Biology and Physiology, Edward Via College of Osteopathic Medicine-Auburn Campus, Auburn, AL, United States, [3] Impedimed Inc., Carlsbad, CA, United States, [4] Harrison School of Pharmacy, Auburn University, Auburn, AL, United States, [5] Renaissance Periodization, Charlotte, NC, United States

***Correspondence:**
Michael D. Roberts
mdr0024@auburn.edu

†Co-principal investigators

We examined hypertrophic outcomes of weekly graded whey protein dosing (GWP) vs. whey protein (WP) or maltodextrin (MALTO) dosed once daily during 6 weeks of high-volume resistance training (RT). College-aged resistance-trained males (training age = 5 ± 3 years; mean ± SD) performed 6 weeks of RT wherein frequency was 3 d/week and each session involved 2 upper- and 2 lower-body exercises (10 repetitions/set). Volume increased from 10 sets/exercise (week 1) to 32 sets/exercise (week 6), which is the highest volume investigated in this timeframe. Participants were assigned to WP (25 g/d; $n = 10$), MALTO (30 g/d; $n = 10$), or GWP (25–150 g/d from weeks 1–6; $n = 11$), and supplementation occurred throughout training. Dual-energy x-ray absorptiometry (DXA), vastus lateralis (VL), and biceps brachii ultrasounds for muscle thicknesses, and bioelectrical impedance spectroscopy (BIS) were performed prior to training (PRE) and after weeks 3 (MID) and 6 (POST). VL biopsies were also collected for immunohistochemical staining. The GWP group experienced the greatest PRE to POST reduction in DXA fat mass (FM) (−1.00 kg, $p < 0.05$), and a robust increase in DXA fat- and bone-free mass [termed lean body mass (LBM) throughout] (+2.93 kg, $p < 0.05$). However, the MALTO group also experienced a PRE to POST increase in DXA LBM (+2.35 kg, $p < 0.05$), and the GWP and MALTO groups experienced similar PRE to POST increases in type II muscle fiber cross-sectional area (~+300 μm^2). When examining the effects of training on LBM increases (ΔLBM) in all participants combined, PRE to MID (+1.34 kg, $p < 0.001$) and MID to POST (+0.85 kg, $p < 0.001$) increases were observed. However, when adjusting ΔLBM for extracellular water (ECW) changes, intending to remove the confounder of edema, a significant increase was observed from PRE to MID (+1.18 kg, $p < 0.001$) but not MID to POST (+0.25 kg; $p = 0.131$). Based upon DXA data, GWP supplementation may be a viable strategy to improve body composition during high-volume RT. However, large LBM increases observed in the MALTO group preclude us from suggesting that GWP supplementation is clearly superior in facilitating skeletal muscle hypertrophy. With regard to the implemented RT program, ECW-corrected ΔLBM gains were largely dampened, but still positive, in resistance-trained participants when RT exceeded ~20 sets/exercise/wk.

Keywords: muscle hypertrophy, resistance training, recovery, adaptation, graded whey protein

INTRODUCTION

Resistance training (RT) is well documented to enhance skeletal muscle hypertrophy, and greater RT volume (e.g., 1 set vs. 3 sets) is associated with higher muscle protein turnover (1). Numerous studies indicate post-exercise protein ingestion, particularly whey protein, acutely stimulates significant increases in post-exercise muscle protein synthesis (MPS) [reviewed in (2)]. Moreover, significantly greater acute post-exercise MPS responses have been shown to occur with the ingestion of moderate whey protein doses (≥35 g) compared to lower doses (e.g., ≤20 g) (3, 4). It has been argued that the consumption of very high protein doses (e.g., 60+ g) do not further stimulate post-exercise MPS levels relative to moderate doses (e.g., 30–40 g). For instance, recent meta-analytical data from Morton et al. (5) suggests a plateau in hypertrophic benefits of protein intake when combined with RT beyond doses of ~1.60 g/kg/day based on data from 49 studies with 1,863 participants combined. Furthermore, Moore et al. (6) reported via breakpoint analysis that protein doses of ~0.30 g/kg maximally stimulated myofibrillar fractional synthesis rates at rest. However, considering that greater RT volumes induce higher rates of muscle protein turnover (7), a potential confounding variable in the analysis by Morton et al. is the heterogeneity in RT volume completed in the studies analyzed. Additionally, the analysis by Moore et al. was completed on data derived from resting subjects whom consumed varying doses of protein and not based on data derived from subjects consuming protein after RT. As argued by Wolfe (8), the highest net muscle protein balances have been observed after both RT and ingestion of protein compared to one or the other. Moreover, higher RT volumes may increase the need for protein to optimize the hypertrophic response.

Indeed, evidence suggests high-dose whey protein supplementation combined with supervised RT enhances skeletal muscle hypertrophy. For instance, four studies in previously-trained subjects have reported that high-dose (~80–120 g/d) supplementation with whey protein (or a protein blend containing whey protein) significantly increases fat free mass following 6–12 weeks of RT (9–12). However, Lockwood et al. (13) reported that 60 g/d of whey protein concentrate or hydrolyzed whey protein supplementation over an 8-week period did not further increase fat free mass in previously-trained subjects compared to counterparts supplementing with maltodextrin. Along with the above, two additional lines of evidence suggest that graded intakes of whey protein concurrent to graded increases in RT volume could enhance a short-term hypertrophic response to RT. As stated previously, Burd et al. (1) reported significantly higher MPS rates after 3 sets of leg extensions compared to 1 set of leg extensions with the same relative load, indicating that higher volumes of RT result in greater acute increases in MPS, at least to a point. This acute data agrees with recent meta-analytical data from Schoenfeld et al. (14) suggesting greater hypertrophy in response to 10 or more sets of RT per muscle per week compared to 5 or less sets.

It stands to reason that concurrently increasing the dosage of whey protein consumption and RT volume could enhance short-term muscle hypertrophy given that: (a) there have been observed increases in MPS in response to graded amounts of whey protein consumption, and (b) higher protein intakes as well as higher RT volumes generally result in greater hypertrophic outcomes. However, no studies to date have investigated if incrementally dosing whey protein in a proportional manner to RT volume is a viable strategy for enhancing skeletal muscle hypertrophy in well-trained subjects. Therefore, the purpose of this study was to investigate the potential hypertrophic effects of graded whey protein supplementation dosing during unaccustomed and extremely voluminous RT. To accomplish this aim, participants in this study were instructed to consume either: (a) a single 25 g supplemental dose of whey protein per day (WP), (b) a graded dose of protein throughout the study for which the dose per day was increased by 25 g each week [GWP (25–150 g from week 1 to week 6)], or (c) a single 30 g supplemental dose of a maltodextrin-based carbohydrate supplement per day (MALTO). As a secondary aim, we sought to examine the effects of RT volumes higher than previously investigated during a 6-week timeframe on hypertrophic outcomes in all participants independent of supplementation. Given the exploratory nature of this work, we adopted a null hypothesis for all independent and dependent variable relationships.

MATERIALS AND METHODS

Ethical Approval and Participant Screening

This study was approved by the Institutional Review Board at Auburn University and conformed to the standards set by the latest revision of the Declaration of Helsinki (IRB approval #: 17-425 MR 1710). Resistance-trained young men from the local community were recruited to participate in this study. Participants provided both verbal and written informed consent, and completed a medical history form prior to screening. Two primary criteria were used to establish training status: (a) self-reported >1.0 years of RT, and (b) back squat 1RM ≥1.5 × body mass [estimated from a three-repetition maximum (3RM) test conducted for each participant with strict criteria (e.g., crease of the hip below the top of the knee joint at the bottom of the squat)]. After screening, 34 participants were counterbalanced among groups to ensure no significant differences existed between groups in DXA fat- and bone-free mass (termed lean body mass [LBM] throughout) and 3RM squat at baseline. One participant withdrew from the study during week 1 for personal reasons, and 2 others missed more than 3 sessions over the course of the first 4 weeks and we did not feel comfortable with making up this volume during other days/weeks so these participants were removed from the study. Hence, 31 participants completed the study and were partitioned to one of three groups: (1) daily single dose of whey protein (WP, 25 g/d; $n = 10$), (2) daily single dose of maltodextrin (MALTO, 30 g/d; $n = 10$), or (3) graded dose of WP (GWP, 25–150 g/d from weeks 1 to 6; $n = 11$). Descriptive characteristics are provided in **Table 1** below and in **Supplementary Table 1**. Notably, participants were instructed to refrain from ergogenic aids throughout the duration of the study (particularly pre-workout supplements, amino acid, or protein supplements), but were not restricted from using the following (if chronically consumed prior to the study): (a) multivitamin-mineral supplement, (b) creatine monohydrate, or (c) caffeine in the form of coffee.

Study Design

Figure 1 provides a visual representation of the study design. Briefly, a battery of tests was performed prior to week 1 (PRE), after week 3 (MID), and after week 6 (POST). These tests will be further described below following an explanation of the resistance training program, supplementation paradigm, and nutritional recommendations.

Resistance Training

Participants were familiarized with the design of training and technical parameters during testing of 3RMs which occurred 3–7 days prior to PRE testing and training initiation. Strict technical parameters were employed for testing to ensure accurate reflections of strength under direct supervision of research staff holding the Certified Strength and Conditioning Specialist Certification from the National Strength and Conditioning Association.

Following the PRE testing battery and 3RM testing, RT occurred 3 days per week and was progressed according to **Figure 1B**. Loads corresponding to 60% 1RM, based on 3RM testing, were programmed for each set of each exercise. Sets of 10 repetitions were programmed for each set of each exercise throughout the study. Prior to beginning each training session, participants were instructed to perform a general warm-up involving 25 jumping jacks, 10 bodyweight squats, 10 push-ups, and 10 bodyweight standing reaches mimicking the kinematics of the stiff-legged deadlift (SLDL) for 2 rounds. Next, participants were instructed to perform the following specific warm-up for each exercise: 50% of working set weight for 10 repetitions, 75% for 3 repetitions, and 95–100% for 1 repetition. Exercises were completed one set at a time, in the following order during each training session: Days 1 and 3—barbell (BB) back squat, BB bench press, BB SLDL, and an underhand grip cable machine pulldown exercise designed to target the elbow flexors and latissimus dorsi muscles (Lat Pulldown); Day 2—BB back squat, BB overhead (OH) press, BB SLDL, and Lat Pulldown. A single set of one exercise was completed, followed by a set of each of the succeeding exercises before starting back at the first exercise of the session (e.g., compound sets or rounds). Participants were recommended to take 2 min of rest between each exercise of the compound set. Additionally, participants were recommended to take 2 min of rest between each compound set. However, if participants felt prepared to execute exercises with appropriate technique under investigator supervision they were allowed to proceed to the next exercise without 2 min of rest. Additionally, if participants desired slightly longer than 2 min of rest, this was allowed with intention for the participant to execute the programmed training volume in <2 h each training session. This design was based on evidence indicating that total volume load (sum of the total repetitions x weight for each individual exercise) for a week of training is primarily related to hypertrophic outcomes, with specific rest intervals between sets being less important. In the interest of ecological validity, we elected a more self-regulated pace of the training session in which participants could be somewhat autonomous while under direct supervision of research staff ensuring technical execution of exercises. Both the extremely high training volumes planned for this investigation and pilot testing of this design led to the implementation of this rest scheme paradigm.

TABLE 1 | Pre-study body composition and strength descriptive measurements.

Variable	WP ($n = 10$)	GWP ($n = 11$)	MALTO ($n = 10$)	Total ($n = 31$)
Age (years)	21.20 ± 2.39	20.60 ± 1.51	22.10 ± 2.28	21.48 ± 2.13
Height (cm)	177.85 ± 5.60	177.75 ± 9.56	184.00 ± 7.55	179.81 ± 7.91
Weight (kg)	82.19 ± 8.69	84.51 ± 14.34	81.35 ± 10.72	82.74 ± 11.29
Total lean mass (kg)	63.73 ± 7.11	67.15 ± 10.90	62.06 ± 8.44	64.45 ± 9.08
Total fat mass (kg)	15.18 ± 4.15	13.82 ± 4.74	16.10 ± 3.55	14.94 ± 4.12
Squat 3RM (kg)	134.53 ± 21.36	135.70 ± 15.18	126.13 ± 17.25	132.24 ± 17.93
Bench press 3RM (kg)	106.85 ± 19.47	99.82 ± 24.79	89.61 ± 11.43	98.79 ± 20.20
Stiff-legged deadlift 3RM (kg)	129.31 ± 33.00	140.45 ± 28.29	118.42 ± 15.75	129.75 ± 27.43
Lat pulldown 3RM (kg)	74.41 ± 9.85	74.66 ± 17.26	68.51 ± 9.19	72.60 ± 12.73
Overhead press 3RM (kg)	61.25 ± 10.53	55.19 ± 15.97	54.22 ± 5.18	56.83 ± 11.67

All data presented as means ± standard deviation values.

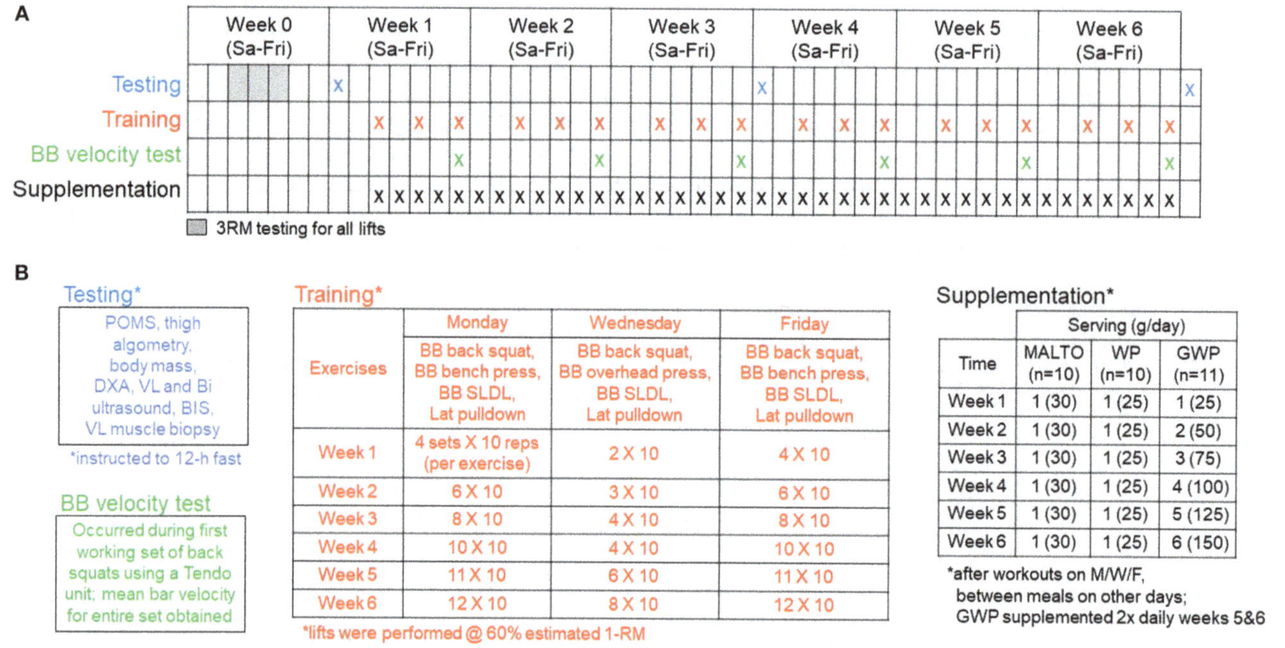

FIGURE 1 | Study design. Panel **(A)** outlines testing, training, and supplementation days. Panel **(B)** (upper left inset) describes the testing battery which included (in order) a profile and mood state questionnaire (POMS), outer thigh pain assessment using algometry, body mass assessment, and whole-body dual x-ray absorptiometry (DXA) scan, a vastus lateralis (VL) and biceps (Bi) ultrasound, total body water assessment using bioelectrical impedance spectroscopy (BIS), and a VL muscle biopsy. Panel **(B)** (lower left inset) describes the BB squat velocity test that occurred during the first set of barbell squats every Friday from weeks 1 to 6 of training. Panel **(B)** (middle inset) outlines the supervised training regimen described in greater detail in the methods. Panel **(B)** (right inset) outlines the supplementation regimen described in greater detail in the methods.

During training sessions, participants provided a repetition in reserve (RIR) rating after each set of each exercise to a researcher, having been instructed to provide a number of repetitions the participant felt he could have completed with good technique beyond the 10 repetitions completed for the set. If the execution of repetitions during a working set was deemed unsafe, or the participant felt unsafe or too fatigued to continue the set or the session, the set or session was terminated. This occurred on only a few occasions, and if repetitions were missed, attempts were made to make these up within the same week of training. The number of repetitions completed for each exercise and the load used for each exercise each week were recorded in Google Sheets (Mountain View, CA, USA), along with the RIR rating provided by the participant for each individual set. RT volume and RIR data are available in the supplementary .csv file (**Supplementary SDC 1**). Based on pilot testing, we elected a systematic approach to load manipulation within each training session; the load was decreased by 5% for each repetition below 10 (e.g., 9 repetitions = −5%, 8 repetitions = −10%, 7 repetitions = −15%, etc.). However, this was only necessary on a few occasions, and the majority of the training was executed according to the planned study design. BB velocity was also measured using a Tendo unit (TENDO Sports Machines, Trencin, Slovak Republic) on Friday of each week as a proxy of fatigue status and recovery on the first set of BB back squats similar to the methods of Zourdos et al. (15). However, due to logistical constraints, BB velocity was only obtained from a subset of participants at all sampling times ($n = 6$–7 per group). Finally, participants were allowed to train from either 07:00 to 09:00 or 15:30 to 18:30 on Monday, Wednesday, and Friday of each week, and were instructed to perform no other vigorous exercise outside of the study.

Supplementation

As illustrated in **Figure 1**, participants were assigned to either MALTO, WP, or GWP groups. All supplements were donated by Dymatize Nutrition® (Dallas, TX, USA). Packaging and delivery was designed to blind participants to the supplement condition; however, investigators of the study were not blinded. The WP (Elite 100% Whey) was comprised of the following nutrition profile per scoop: calories—140, total fat—2 g, cholesterol—70 mg, sodium—70 mg, potassium—150 mg, total carbohydrate—3 g, protein—25 g. Additionally, one WP scoop contained 5.5 g branched chain amino acids (2.7 g L-leucine, 1.4 g L-isoleucine, 1.4 g L-valine), 6.3 g of other essential amino acids, 4.4 g of L-glutamine, 2.4 g of conditionally essential amino acids, and 6.5 g of non-essential amino acids. The MALTO supplement contained 120 calories from 30 g of maltodextrin powder (~30 g of carbohydrates) with <1 g of vanilla flavoring.

Drinks were formulated by research staff for each participant by combining the appropriate serving size with ~500 ml of tap water, and participants consumed drinks after each training session under investigator supervision. The MALTO and WP groups consumed a single scoop each day for the duration of the study; specifically, 1 after training sessions on training days and 1 between meals on non-training days which participants prepared themselves. The GWP group consumed the protein supplement according to the following dosage and timing breakdown:

Week 1: 1 scoop with 500 ml of water post-training on training days, 1 scoop with 500 ml of water between meals on non-training days (1 total scoop each day)
Week 2: 2 scoops with 500 ml of water post-training on training days, 2 scoops with 500 ml of water between meals on non-training days (2 total scoops each day)
Week 3: 3 scoops with 500 ml of water post-training on training days, 3 scoops with 500 ml of water between meals on non-training days (3 total scoops each day)
Week 4: 4 scoops with 500 ml of water post-training on training days, 4 scoops with 500 ml of water between meals on non-training days (4 total scoops each day)
Week 5: 4 scoops with 500 ml of water post-training on training days, 4 scoops with 500 ml of water between meals on non-training days, 1 scoop prior to bed each day (5 total scoops each day)
Week 6: 4 scoops with 500 ml of water post-training on training days, 4 scoops with 500 ml of water between meals on non-training days, 2 scoops prior to bed each day (6 total scoops each day)

Relative supplemental whey intake for the WP group was ~0.30 g/kg/d (i.e., 25 grams of whey/~87 kg body mass). The most the GWP subjects consumed at once post-workout was 100 g. Therefore, the relative intake values for each week post-workout based on the average body mass of the GWP subjects was as follows: 0.30 g/kg/d for week 1, 0.59 g/kg/d for week 2, 0.89 g/kg/d for week 3, and 1.18 g/kg/d for weeks 4–6. As stated above, the remaining GWP doses for weeks 5 and 6 (i.e., 25 additional grams during week 5 and 50 additional grams for week 6) were instructed to be consumed either between meals or before bed. Thus, total supplemental whey values for weeks 5 and 6 were 1.48 g/kg/d and 1.77 g/kg/d, respectively. Beyond post-exercise supplementation which was supervised, participants from all groups verbally reported compliance to the supplementation paradigm on a weekly basis to the research staff. Additionally, participants were asked to refrain from the use of other protein supplements or protein bars throughout the duration of the study.

Nutritional Recommendations and Monitoring Throughout the Protocol

In collaboration with a Registered Dietitian (AK., Ph.D., RD), participants were provided with calorie and macronutrient recommendations along with lists of potential food choices to help meet recommendations for each day during the study. Specifically, recommended values and calculations can be found in the supplementary .csv file (**Supplementary SDC 2**). These recommendations were based on the following: (a) resting metabolic rate estimates from the Harris-Benedict equation, (b) an estimated non-exercise activity expenditure in this age cohort, (c) an estimated energy expenditure from training each week, and (d) the desire for participants to be in a modest calorie surplus [~500 calories above the estimated total daily energy expenditure (TDEE)] throughout the study. Calculations and supplementary formulae can be found in the supplementary .csv file (**Supplementary SDC 2**). Additionally, recommendations were provided directly to participants through Google Sheets. Participants were asked to enter dietary intakes each day throughout the study, and include the consumption of their supplement in their daily tracking using a mobile application (MyFitnessPal, Inc.; Baltimore, MD, USA). This mobile application has been validated against paper-based food records (16). Data were exported on a weekly basis for analysis. A de-identified generic food item was created in the application's database for WP, and participants were instructed to log this food item each time a single scoop of their respective supplement was consumed. Entries by participants in the MALTO group were corrected following the study to account for macronutrient differences between the WP and MALTO supplements.

During week 1, participants in the WP and GWP groups were instructed to consume the same daily amount of dietary protein (1.6 g/kg/day) assuming the consumed supplement contributed 25 g/scoop to this total. Participants in the MALTO group were also instructed to consume 1.6 g/kg/day protein during the entire 6-week protocol. This recommendation was based on the findings of Morton et al. (5) suggesting a maximum effective dose of daily protein around this value in young, resistance-trained men. Following week 1, the WP and GWP participants were recommended to increase protein intakes by 25 g per week. However, the GWP group accomplished this increase through supplemental whey protein, whereas the WP group were recommended to consume more protein-rich food sources. Hence, there was no difference in protein dose recommendations between the WP and GWP groups, but the GWP group was expected to obtain more protein on a weekly basis through supplementation. All participants were instructed to consume ~3 g/kg/day of dietary carbohydrate starting on week 1 of the study. A modest amount of carbohydrates (~30 g) were added to this value on training days each week to account for potential reductions in muscle glycogen from increases in training volume based on the recommendations from Scott et al. (17). Fat recommendations were based on remaining calorie values upon setting targeted protein and carbohydrate values. Participants were instructed to attempt to meet the dietary fat recommendation through primarily monounsaturated and polyunsaturated fatty acid sources, while confining saturated fat intakes to no more than 10% of total calorie intake. Logged nutrition data were stored in Google Drive and are provided in a supplementary file in .csv format (**Supplementary SDC 1**).

Testing Battery Procedures

As outlined in **Figure 1**, the following tests were performed prior to (PRE), during (MID), and following the 6-week protocol (POST). Participants were encouraged to arrive to these testing sessions in an overnight fasted condition approximately 24 h after the third training session during week 3 (for MID) and week 6 (for POST). Participants were told to refrain from physical activity prior to the testing sessions, and participants voided their bladders during urinalysis described below. The following tests were performed during each testing session:

Hydration Status and Profile of Mood State

Participants were instructed to submit a urine sample (~5 mL) to assess normal hydration specific gravity levels (1.005–1.020 ppm) using a handheld refractometer (ATAGO; Bellevue, WA, USA). Participants with a urine specific gravity >1.020 were asked to consume 400 ml tap water and were re-tested ~10 min later. Following urinalysis, profiles of mood state (POMS) were collected on Google Forms using the questionnaire published by Grove and Prappavessis (18). Total mood disturbances (TMD) were calculated by summing negative emotion scores and subtracting positive emotion scores from this summed value.

Algometry

Following the POMS questionnaire, pressure-to-pain threshold (PPT) of the outer aspect of the right upper thigh was measured using a handheld algometer (Force Ten FDX, Wagner Instruments, Greenwich, CT, USA) according to methods described in our previous work (19). Briefly, focal pressure was applied by the algometer to proximal, medial, and distal portions of the right vastus lateralis (VL) which were marked for accurate application of force. Algometry pressure was applied at a rate of approximately 5 Newtons (N) per second at each site until the participant audibly indicated the specific moment at which the applied pressure became painful. At this point, the PPT value in N was recorded. The digital display of the algometer indicating the force value was blinded to participants. The PPT was measured sequentially at proximal, medial, and distal sites, respectively, three times for triplicate measures with ~30 s between cycles of measurement. The average of the triplicate measures at each site was calculated as the respective PPT of the site, and these values were averaged for a total PPT.

Body Composition Assessment

Following algometry, height and body mass were assessed using a digital column scale (Seca 769; Hanover, MD, USA) with weights and heights being collected to the nearest 0.1 kg and 0.5 cm, respectively. After this, participants partook in a full body dual x-ray absorptiometry (DXA) scan (Lunar Prodigy; GE Corporation, Fairfield, CT, USA). All DXA scans were completed by the same investigator (M.A.R.). According to previous data published by our laboratory (20), the same-day reliability of the DXA during a test-calibrate-retest on 10 participants produced an intra-class correlation coefficient (ICC) of 0.998 for total body lean mass.

Ultrasound Muscle Thickness Measurements

Participants also underwent duplicate ultrasound assessments on the right side of the body during each testing session to determine average right leg VL muscle and right bicep brachii thicknesses with a 3–12 MHz multi-frequency linear phase array transducer (Logiq S7 R2 Expert; General Electric, Fairfield, CT, USA). VL measurements were taken at the midway point between the iliac crest and patella of the right femur, which was marked with a cross for probe placement. Participants were instructed to stand and displace bodyweight more to the left leg to ensure the right leg was relaxed. Thereafter, the probe was placed horizontally at the previously marked location and an image was captured. The probe was removed, and the aforementioned steps were repeated for a second subsequent image. Similarly, bicep brachii thickness measurements were taken ~60% distal from the acromial process of the scapula to the lateral epicondyle of the humerus, which was marked with a cross for probe placement. Thereafter, the probe was placed horizontally at the previously marked location and an image was captured. The probe was removed, and the aforementioned steps were repeated for a second subsequent image. All ultrasound assessments were completed by the same investigator (P.W.M.). Reliability of duplicate ultrasound muscle thickness measurements on 33 participants at PRE produced an ICC of 0.994.

Total Body Water Assessment

Total body water (TBW), extracellular water (ECW), and intracellular water (ICW) were measured by bioimpedance spectroscopy (BIS) using the SFB7 device (ImpediMed Limited, Queensland, AU) according to the methods described by Moon et al. (21). The SFB7 device measures whole-body bioelectrical impedance at more than 200 frequencies, and uses complex Cole models to estimate TBW, ICW and ECW. Moreover, the SFB7 device: (a) has excellent agreement with TBW assessed via deuterium oxide (21), (b) has excellent agreement with ECW assessed via sodium bromide dilution (22), and (c) has been posited to be the best non-invasive methodology for the determination of fluid compartmentalization (23). This test involved the participant resting in a supine position for 5–10 min, after which TBW, ICW, and ECW estimates were determined while the participants laid supine on a table with his arms ≥30° away from the torso and legs separated. The average of two readings was used to represent the participants' TBW, ICW, and ECW. All BIS tests were supervised by the same investigator (K.C.Y.). Reliability of duplicate TBW measurements on 24 participants at PRE produced an ICC of 0.999. Notably, while unadjusted whole body DXA LBM raw scores are presented herein, we also calculated changes in DXA LBM from weeks 1–3 and weeks 3–6 (ΔLBM) corrected for changes in ECW at these time points (i.e., ECW-corrected ΔLBM). This correction is illustrated in the equation below:

$$\begin{aligned} ECW - corrected\ \Delta LBM = &\ POST\ (or\ MID)\ DXA\ LBM \\ &- PRE\ DXA\ LBM \\ &- [POST\ (or\ MID)\ BIS\ ECW \\ &- PRE\ BIS\ ECW] \end{aligned}$$

The justification for this correction comes from literature suggesting expansions of ECW being representative of edema or inflammation, and such expansions potentially masking true alterations in functional skeletal muscle mass (24).

Muscle Biopsies and Tissue Processing

After body composition and ultrasound measurements, VL muscle biopsies from the right leg were collected using a 5-gauge needle under local anesthesia as previously described (25). Immediately following sampling, tissue was teased of blood and connective tissue, and ~20-40 mg was embedded in cryomolds containing optimal cutting temperature (OCT) media (Tissue-Tek®, Sakura Finetek Inc.; Torrence, CA, USA). Embedding was performed by positioning the tissue in cryomolds for perpendicular slicing in a non-stretched state prior to rapid freezing. Cryomolds were then frozen using liquid nitrogen-cooled isopentane and subsequently stored at −80°C until immunofluorescent staining for determination of fiber cross sectional area (fCSA). The remaining tissue was wrapped in pre-labeled foils, flash frozen in liquid nitrogen, and subsequently stored at −80°C. All biopsies were obtained by the same investigators (M.D.R. and C.T.H.), and biopsies were obtained ~2 cm apart at the same approximate depth each testing session.

Immunohistochemistry for Fiber Cross Sectional Area Assessment

Similar methods for immunohistochemistry have been employed previously in our laboratory (25). Sections from OCT-preserved samples were cut at a thickness of 8 μm using a cryotome (Leica Biosystems; Buffalo Grove, IL, USA) and were adhered to positively-charged histology slides. Once all samples were sectioned, batch processing occurred for immunohistochemistry. During batch processing sections were air-dried at room temperature for 10 min, permeabilized in a phosphate-buffered saline (PBS) solution containing 0.5% Triton X-100 for 10 min, and blocked with 100% Pierce Super Blocker (Thermo Fisher Scientific) for 10 min. For fiber type staining, sections were subsequently washed for 2 min in PBS. Sections were then incubated for 10 min with a pre-diluted commercially-available rabbit anti-dystrophin IgG antibody solution (catalog #: GTX15277; Genetex Inc.; Irvine, CA, USA) and spiked in mouse anti-myosin I IgG (catalog #: A4.951 supernatant; Hybridoma Bank, Iowa City, IA, USA; 40 μL added per 1 mL of dystrophin antibody solution). Sections were then washed for 2 min in PBS and incubated in the dark for 15 min with a secondary antibody solution containing Texas Red-conjugated anti-rabbit IgG (catalog #: TI-1000; Vector Laboratories, Burlingame, CA, USA), and Alexa Fluor 488-conjugated anti-mouse IgG (catalog #: A-11001; Thermo Fisher Scientific) (~6.6 μL of all secondary antibodies per 1 mL of blocking solution). Sections were washed for 2 min in PBS, air-dried, and mounted with fluorescent media containing 4,6-diamidino- 2-phenylindole (DAPI; catalog #: GTX16206; Genetex Inc.). Following mounting, slides were stored in the dark at 4°C until immunofluorescent images were obtained. After staining was performed on all sections, digital 10x objective images were captured using a fluorescence microscope (Nikon Instruments, Melville, NY, USA). All images were captured by a laboratory technician who was blinded to the group assignment of each participant. Approximate exposure times were 400 ms for TRITC and FITC imaging. Our staining method allowed the identification of cell membranes (detected by the Texas Red filter), type I fiber green cell bodies (detected by the FITC filter), type II fiber black cell bodies (unlabeled), and myonuclei (detected by the DAPI filter). Measurements of type I and II fCSAs were performed using custom-written pipelines in the open-sourced software CellProfiler™ (26) per modified methods previously described whereby the number of pixels counted within the border of each muscle fiber was converted to a total area (μm^2). A calibrator slide containing a 250,000 μm^2 square image was also captured, and pixels per fiber from imaged sections were converted to area using this calibrator image. On average, 113 ± 26 fibers per cross-section were identified for analysis at each sampling time. A *post-hoc* experiment performed in our laboratory to examine potential differences in fCSA measurements between sections on the same slide ($n = 23$ slides) revealed strong reliability using this method (ICC = 0.929).

Statistical Analysis

Statistical tests were performed in RStudio (Version 1.0.143; R Foundation for Statistical Computing, Vienna, AT), SPSS (Version 23; IBM SPSS Statistics Software, Chicago, IL, USA), and Google Sheets. Group [3 levels (WP, GWP, MALTO)] and time [3 levels (PRE, MID, POST), or 6 levels (Week 1–6) for weekly measures] served as independent variables. A mean-centered covariate for each baseline measurement was added as a parameter to models to examine the explained variance in dependent variables relative to values at PRE. Since nutrition-related data were not available at PRE, and only after collection of data during week 1, no covariate was utilized in this model and a repeated-measures ANOVA was performed after assumptions testing. Statistical assumptions tests were completed prior to analysis consisting of: (1) Shapiro-Wilks tests of residual distributions for normality, (2) Levene's test of homogeneity of variance, and (3) Mauchly's test for Sphericity, given that a repeated-measures analysis of covariance (ANCOVA) was performed for the provision of p-values. Violation of these assumptions and appropriate data transformations (i.e., square root or $\log_{10}$ transformations) when residuals were not normally distributed were completed prior to ANCOVA for the avoidance of type 1 or type 2 errors. Data transformation and data removal were avoided with intention to analyze all raw data. For this reason, if the majority of levels of group (2 of 3 groups) at each level of time were normally distributed, ANCOVA proceeded without data transformation. If the assumptions of homogeneity of variance or sphericity were violated, Greenhouse-Geisser corrections to degrees of freedom were made. The alpha level of significance was set at $p < 0.05$. For significant main effects of time and group × time interactions, LSD *post-hoc* tests were performed at each level of time to elucidate specific differences. A priori power analysis in RStudio using general linear model parameters in the "pwr" package (Version 1.2-1) revealed 84.5% power (power = 1 − β) for the discovery of a large effect size when 2 predictors and 31 observations were employed [e.g., $k = 2$ (time, y-intercept), $n = 31$ (31 participants), $f^2 = 0.35$ (large effect), $p = 0.05$ (a-priori level of significance)]. However, a power analysis to detect a significantly large difference of an effect between groups when 3 groups ($k = 3$) included 10 participants each ($n = 10$) revealed 44% power. Therefore, Cohen's d effect sizes and 95% confidence intervals were also calculated for each dependent variable, aside from nutrition data, to examine mean differences between groups from PRE to POST considering the pooled standard deviation of a dependent variable at baseline since population-based inferences were underpowered. **Supplementary Tables 2–11** provide descriptive statistics, effect sizes, and 95% confidence intervals for each dependent variable. Additionally, raw data are provided in

.csv files (**Supplementary SDC 1**, **Supplementary SDC 2**) and supplementary tables including effect size calculations and 95% confidence intervals are provided in a .pdf file (**Supplementary SDC 3**).

RESULTS

Self-Reported Nutrition

Nutritional analyses were performed on participants who logged >90% of days throughout the study. Twelve participants irregularly reported or did not report nutritional intakes each week resulting in 19 complete sets of nutritional data. Hence, **Table 2** contains self-reported dietary intakes from these 19 participants. For these participants, no significant main effect of group, time, or group × time interaction was observed for self-reported absolute or relative energy, protein, or carbohydrate intakes ($p > 0.05$). A significant main effect of time and group, but no interaction, was observed on reported fat intake. Fat intake decreased over time ($p = 0.006$), and WP averaged higher reported intakes than GWP and MALTO ($p = 0.017$). In reference to participant adherence to nutrition recommendations provided by the R.D., GWP reported less protein consumption than recommended during weeks 1 and 6 ($p < 0.05$), and the reported consumption of dietary fat relative to that recommended was significantly different during weeks 1–6 in MALTO, weeks 1–3 in GWP, and weeks 4–6 in WP ($p < 0.05$).

Training Volume, Soreness, BB Velocity, and Total Mood Disturbance

Training volume significantly increased over time on a weekly basis ($p < 0.001$), but no significant group or group × time interaction was observed (**Figure 2A**, **Supplementary Tables 13, 14**). No significant main effects or group × time interaction was observed for BB velocity assessed during set 1 of the back squat exercise at the beginning of each Friday training session (**Figure 2B**). Algometry PPT measures significantly decreased over time ($p < 0.001$), but no significant group or group × time interaction was observed (**Figure 2C**). PPT was significantly lower at MID compared to PRE ($p = 0.002$), and POST compared to PRE ($p < 0.001$), but not at POST compared to MID ($p = 0.122$). POMS TMD significantly increased over time ($p = 0.002$) but no significant effect of group or group × time interaction was observed (**Figure 2D**). TMD was significantly higher at MID compared to PRE ($p = 0.002$), and at POST compared to PRE ($p < 0.001$), but not at POST compared to MID ($p = 0.254$).

TABLE 2 | Self-reported dietary data.

	week	MALTO (*n* = 6)				WP (*n* = 6)				GWP (*n* = 7)				TOTAL (*n* = 19)			
		Abs	SD	Rel	SD	Abs	SD	Rel	SD	Abs	SD	Rel	SD	Abs	SD	Rel	SD
Energy	1	2,870	462	35.2	5.4	2994	462	35.2	5.4	2,625	845	32.2	10.3	2819	595	34.1	7.0
(kcal/d)	2	2,733	583	36.0	6.9	3065	583	36.0	6.9	2,832	582	34.7	7.1	2874	520	34.7	6.1
or	3	2,737	614	34.9	7.3	2959	614	34.9	7.3	2,677	515	32.6	6.3	2785	479	33.5	5.7
(kcal/kg/d)	4	2,827	211	38.6	2.4	3288	211	38.6	2.4	2,744	573	33.3	6.9	2942	442	35.2	5.2
	5	2,912	281	37.5	3.2	3199	281	37.5	3.2	2,558	827	30.9	10.1	2872	586	34.3	7.0
	6	2,209	350	35.8	4.2	3047	350	35.8	4.2	2,319	903	28.0	10.8	2514	828	30.1	10.0
PRO	1	148	38	2.1	0.5	178	38	2.1	0.5	186	61	2.3	0.8	171	45	2.1	0.4
(g/d)	2	151	27	2.1	0.2	181	27	2.1	0.2	184	48	2.3	0.5	173	36	2.1	0.4
or	3	166	52	2.3	0.7	191	52	2.3	0.7	170	53	2.1	0.5	176	46	2.1	0.4
(g/kg/d)	4	183	38	2.4	0.5	205	38	2.4	0.5	187	56	2.3	0.8	191	44	2.3	0.4
	5	190	57	2.5	0.7	214	57	2.5	0.7	184	82	2.2	1.1	195	65	2.3	0.9
	6	172	55	2.4	0.7	204	55	2.4	0.7	168	87	2.0	1.1	181	79	2.2	0.9
CHO	1	278	91	3.1	1.0	261	91	3.1	1.0	251	87	3.1	1.1	263	78	3.2	0.9
(g/d)	2	260	53	3.1	0.7	262	53	3.1	0.7	279	55	3.4	0.8	268	50	3.2	0.4
or	3	254	45	3.1	0.5	267	45	3.1	0.5	267	47	3.3	0.5	263	47	3.2	0.4
(g/kg/d)	4	271	41	3.4	0.5	286	41	3.4	0.5	263	76	3.2	0.8	273	53	3.3	0.4
	5	288	28	3.5	0.2	298	28	3.5	0.2	251	79	3.0	1.1	277	67	3.3	0.9
	6	207	35	3.4	0.5	290	35	3.4	0.5	211	91	2.5	1.1	234	82	2.8	0.9
FAT	1	123	21	1.7	0.2	141	21	1.7	0.2	102	39	1.3	0.5	121	33	1.5	0.4
(g/d)	2	118	27	1.6	0.2	137	27	1.6	0.2	110	28	1.3	0.3	121	27	1.5	0.4
or	3	111	33	1.5	0.5	130	33	1.5	0.5	101	26	1.2	0.3	113	27	1.4	0.4
(g/kg/d)	4	113	12	1.7	0.2	146	12	1.7	0.2	107	29	1.3	0.3	121	27	1.4	0.4
	5	108	15	1.5	0.2	126.7	15	1.5	0.2	91	32	1.1	0.3	108	25	1.3	0.4
	6	82	20	1.5	0.2	129.7	20	1.5	0.2	90	31	1.1	0.3	100	33	1.2	0.4

All data absolute (Abs) or relative (Rel) self-reported dietary intake data are presented as means ± standard deviation (SD) values. Data from only 19 participants were included in the nutritional analyses given that 12 participants irregularly reported (or did not report) nutritional intakes. No significant main effect of group, time, or group × time interaction was observed for reported absolute or relative calories, protein intake, or carbohydrate intake ($p > 0.05$); thus no significance is indicated.

Body Composition Data

TBW significantly increased over time ($p < 0.001$), but no significant group or group × time interaction was observed (**Figure 3A**). Both ICW (**Figure 3B**) and ECW (**Figure 3C**) significantly increased over time, but no significant group or group × time interactions were observed for these metrics.

DXA LBM significantly increased over time ($p < 0.001$; **Figure 3D**). A significant group × time interaction ($p = 0.007$) was observed for LBM, although LSD *post-hoc* tests revealed no significant differences among groups at any sampling time. When corrected for changes in ECW, a significant increase in DXA LBM was observed from PRE to POST ($p < 0.001$). No significant group or group × time interaction was observed (**Figure 3E**). DXA fat mass significantly decreased over time ($p = 0.004$; **Figure 3F**). A significant group × time interaction ($p = 0.012$) was observed and, while LSD *post-hoc* tests revealed no significant differences among groups at any sampling time, the difference between GWP and MALTO at MID and POST approached significance ($p = 0.088$ and $p = 0.064$, respectively).

Segmental DXA Data

DXA dual-arm LBM significantly increased over time ($p = 0.001$; **Figure 4A**). Additionally, DXA dual-leg LBM significantly increased over time ($p < 0.001$; **Figure 4B**), and there was a significant group × time interaction ($p = 0.046$). However, LSD *post-hoc* tests revealed no significant differences among groups at any sampling time.

Muscle Thicknesses and fCSA

A significant effect of time was observed for bicep thickness with a greater thickness at MID compared to PRE ($p = 0.001$) and POST ($p = 0.040$), but there was no significant group × time interaction (**Figure 5A**). A significant effect of time was

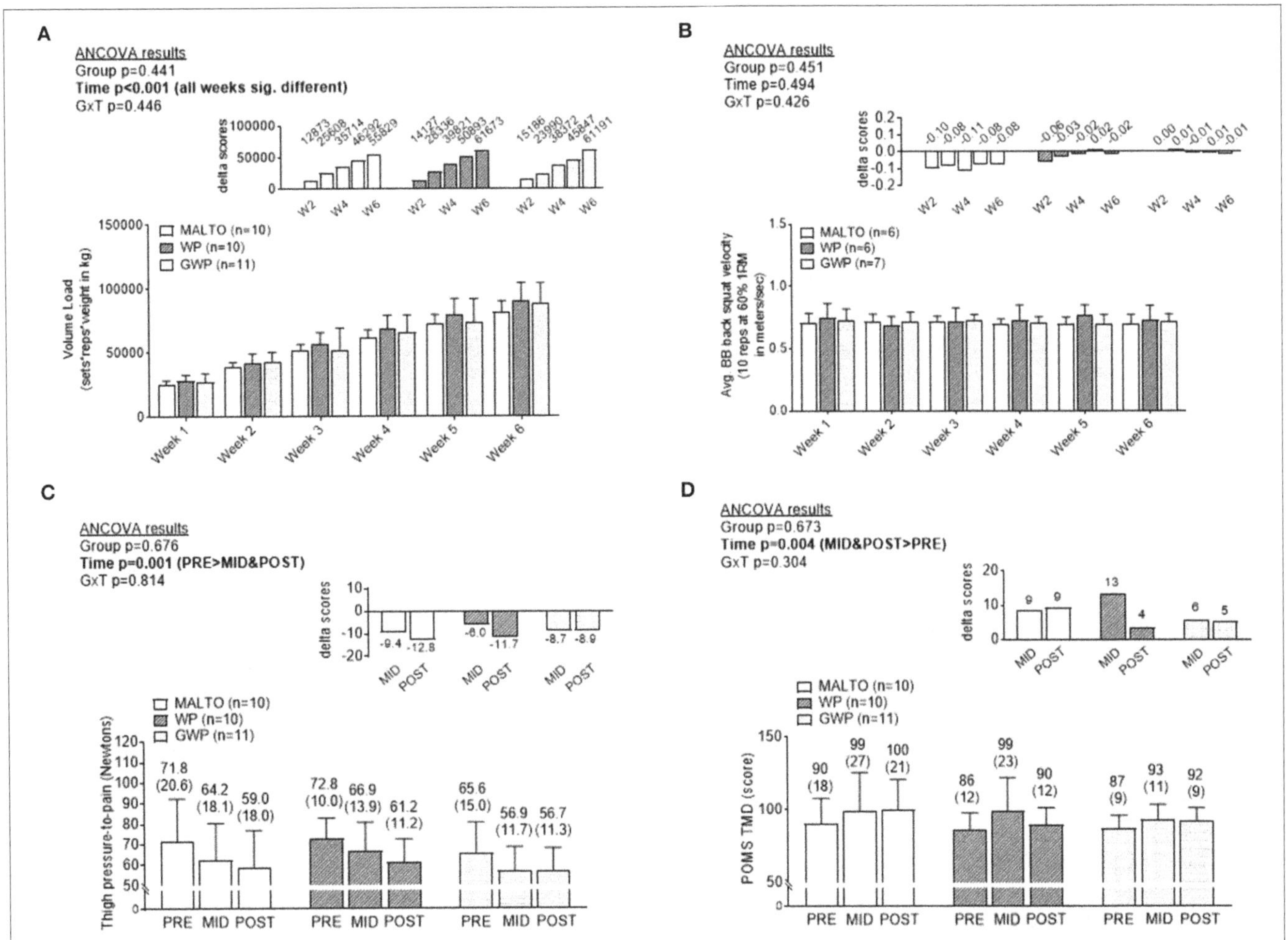

FIGURE 2 | Differences in training volume, back squat lifting velocity, thigh soreness, and total mood disturbance among supplementation groups. Only a significant time effect was observed for training volume with values increasing on a weekly basis **(A)**. No main effects or group×interaction was observed for back squat lifting velocity **(B)**. Only a significant time effect was observed for thigh pressure-to-pain values (lower values indicates greater soreness) **(C)**. Only a significant time effect was observed for profile of mood state (POMS) total mood disturbance (TMD) (greater values indicates more mood disturbance) **(D)**. All data are presented as means ± standard deviation values, and values in **(C,D)** are indicated above each bar; values for panels a and b are not indicated due to space constraints but are provided in the raw data file. Additionally, each data panel has delta values from PRE included as inset data. MALTO, maltodextrin group; WP, standardized whey protein group; GWP, graded whey protein group.

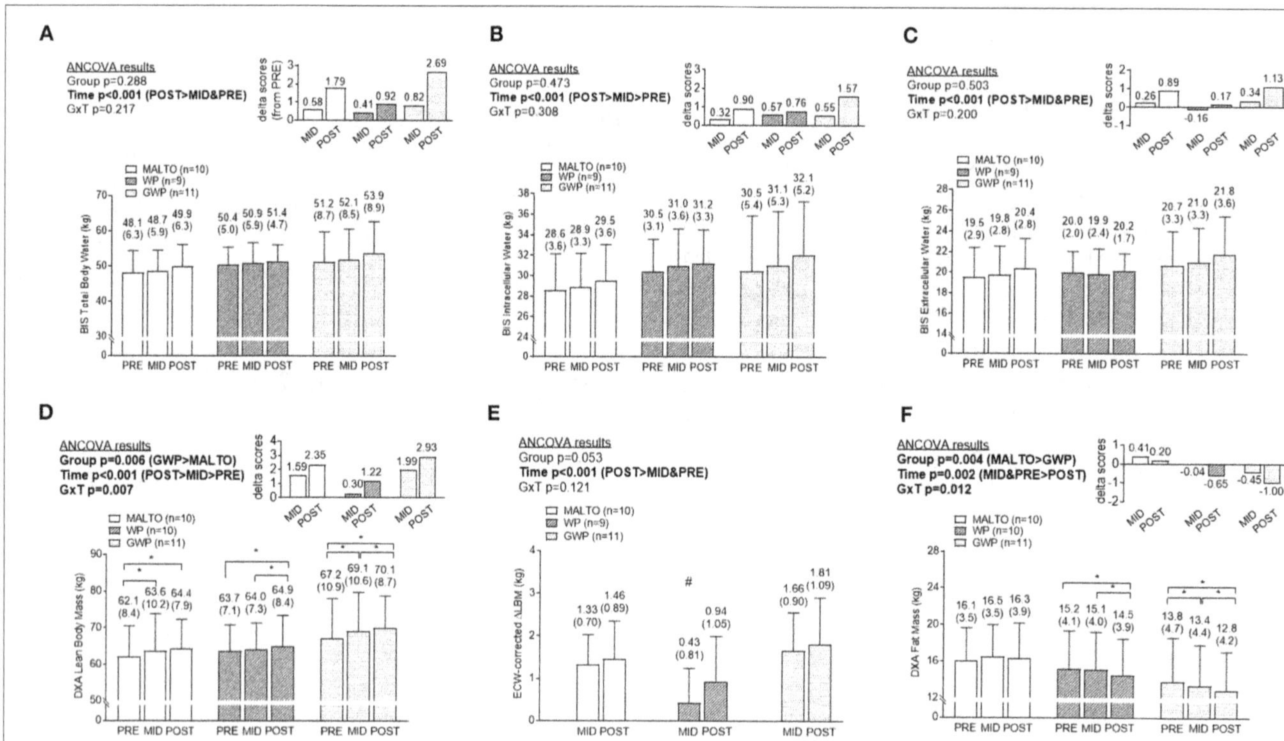

FIGURE 3 | Body composition differences between supplementation groups. Only significant time effects were observed for total body water content **(A)** assessed via bioelectrical impedance spectroscopy (BIS), BIS intracellular water content **(B)**, and BIS extracellular water content **(C)**. For all of these metrics, POST values were significantly greater than PRE and MID values. Significant main group and time effects as well as a group × time interaction were observed for lean body mass **(D)** assessed via dual x-ray absorptiometry (DXA). *Post-hoc* tests indicated lean body mass increased within groups from PRE to MID (MALTO and GWP; $^*p < 0.05$), MID to POST (WP abd GWP; $^*p < 0.05$), and PRE to POST (all groups; $^*p < 0.05$). However, no significant between-group differences existed at each level of time. A significant main time effect as well as a group × time interaction was observed for change scores in DXA lean body mass corrected for change scores in ECW **(E)**. *Post-hoc* tests indicated this metric increased within groups from PRE to MID (MALTO and GWP; $^*p < 0.05$), and PRE to POST (all groups; $^*p < 0.05$). Additionally, MID WP was significantly lower than MID GWP ($\#p = 0.004$). Significant main group and time effects as well as a group × time interaction were observed for fat mass **(F)** assessed via DXA. *Post-hoc* tests indicated fat mass decreased within groups from PRE to MID (GWP; $^*p < 0.05$), MID to POST (WP and GWP; $^*p < 0.05$), and PRE to POST (WP and GWP; $^*p < 0.05$). However, no significant between-group differences existed at any level of time. All data are presented as means ± standard deviation values, and values are indicated above each bar. Additionally, each data panel (except **E**) has delta values from PRE included as inset data. MALTO, maltodextrin group; WP, standardized whey protein group; GWP, graded whey protein group.

also observed for VL thickness ($p = 0.003$) with *post-hoc* tests revealing lower values at MID compared to POST ($p < 0.001$), and lower values at MID compared to PRE approaching significance ($p = 0.053$; significance **Figures 5B,C**). However, a significant group × time interaction was not observed. When summing biceps and VL thicknesses at each level of time, there were no significant differences between groups at each level of time. However, a significant main effect of time revealed that the summed values of thickness measurements were significantly higher at POST compared to PRE ($p = 0.049$). The summed value at POST was 7.16 ± 0.77 cm where the summed value was 6.98 ± 0.81 cm at PRE (data not shown). Significant reductions in VL total fCSA, type I fCSA, and type II fCSA were observed from PRE to MID ($p = 0.045$, $p = 0.009$, and $p = 0.0410$, respectively), followed by a significant increase from MID to POST ($p = 0.004$, $p = 0.004$, and $p = 0.001$, respectively) (**Figures 5D–F, Supplementary Table 12**). However, values in these metrics at POST were not significantly different from values at PRE, and no significant group or group × time interactions were observed.

Training Volume vs. Change in DXA Lean Body Mass

As previously stated, a primary goal was to determine the whole-body hypertrophic response in all participants given that the RT volume is the highest ever attempted in a laboratory-based study over a 6-week period. Interestingly, a significant increase in LBM occurred from PRE to MID ($p < 0.001$) and MID to POST ($p < 0.001$), and these increases were proportional to the significant increase in weekly training volume (**Figure 6**). When considering ECW-corrected ΔLBM, a similar increase was observed from PRE to MID ($p < 0.001$), but a non-significant increase from MID to POST ($p = 0.131$).

DISCUSSION

Large numerical increases in DXA LBM (+2.93 kg on average) and significant reductions in DXA fat mass (−1.00 kg on average) were observed in the GWP group. However, it is also notable that the MALTO group experienced a PRE to POST increase

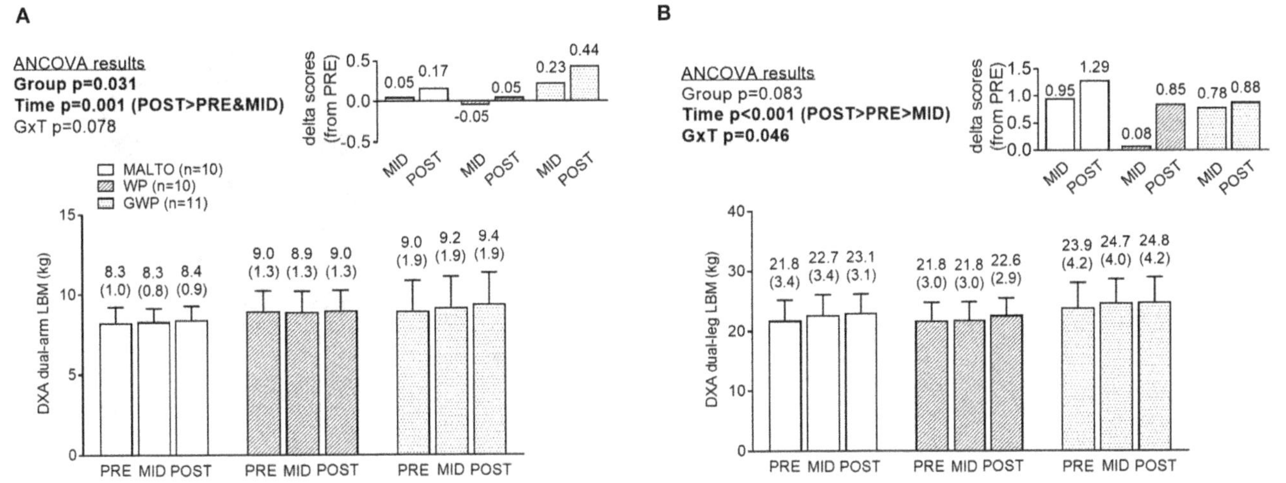

FIGURE 4 | Segmental DXA data differences between supplementation groups. Significant time effects were observed for DXA dual-arm LBM **(A)** and DXA dual-leg LBM **(B)**, with MID, and/or POST values being greater than PRE. While a significant group × time interaction was observed for DXA dual-leg LBM, no significant between-group differences at each time point were observed. All data are presented as means ± standard deviation values, and values are indicated above each bar. Additionally, each data panel has delta values from PRE included as inset data. MALTO, maltodextrin group; WP, standardized whey protein group; GWP, graded whey protein group.

DXA LBM (+2.35 kg, $p < 0.05$), and the GWP and MALTO groups experienced similar PRE to POST increases in type II muscle fiber cross-sectional area (+~300 μm^2). Thus, similar hypertrophic effects observed in the MALTO group preclude us from suggesting that GWP supplementation is clearly superior to MALTO supplementation in facilitating skeletal muscle hypertrophy.

As stated prior, several studies have indicated that single dose ingestion or longer-term supplementation with higher whey protein doses enhances anabolic outcomes. For example, Macnaughton et al. (4) recently reported significantly greater MPS responses to a resistance exercise bout and whey protein ingestion when 40 g were consumed post-exercise compared to 20 g. Additionally, Witard et al. (3) compared myofibrillar protein synthesis responses following the ingestion of 40 g of whey protein to 0, 10, and 20 g in younger resistance-trained males. These authors noted numerically larger, but not significantly different, responses from ingestion of 40 vs. 20 g, while 0 and 10 g resulted in significantly lower responses. Regarding longer-term supplementation data, and as stated previously, four studies in previously-trained subjects have reported that high-dose (80–120 g/d) supplementation with whey protein (or a protein blend containing whey protein) significantly increases LBM following 6–12 weeks of RT (9–12). Additionally, Antonio et al. (27) reported ~2 kg increases in LBM (assessed via air displacement plethysmography) in a group of 20 participants consuming ~4.4 g/kg/day of dietary protein over an 8-week period, much of which was supplemented via whey protein in the diet, compared to ~1.3 kg increases in LBM in another group of participants consuming ~1.8 g/kg/day. Antonio et al. (28) conducted a follow-up investigation wherein a total of 31 participants consumed ≥3 g/kg/d, and 17 participants consumed their normal amount of dietary protein (1.8–2.3 g/kg/d) for 8 weeks while undergoing 5 days of RT per week. These authors reported statistically equivalent LBM gains in both groups (+1.5 kg), although the three highest hypertrophic responders in the study consumed ≥3 g/kg/d. Collectively, our data and these previous reports suggest that high daily whey protein intake appears to promote skeletal muscle hypertrophy. However, given that MALTO supplementation herein also promoted similar anabolic effects and subjects from all groups self-reported consuming >2.0 g/kg/d of dietary protein, it does not appear that high-dose whey protein supplementation during high volume RT in lieu of adequate protein intake (i.e., >1.6 g/kg/d) is clearly superior in promoting hypertrophy.

Our data suggesting GWP promotes the greatest loss in fat mass is intriguing and agrees with prior literature. For instance, Cribb et al. (10) reported that participants supplementing with ~120 g/d of whey protein lost a significant amount of fat mass compared to casein-supplemented participants (−1.4 vs. +0.1 kg). Additionally, Antonio et al. (28) reported that participants consuming high amounts of protein lost significantly more fat mass relative to a lower protein intake group (−1.6 vs. −0.3 kg). There are mechanistic rodent data (29, 30) and longer-term human data (13) suggesting whey protein possesses lipolytic properties. However, this research has mainly indicated that hydrolyzed whey protein could possess lipolytic properties rather than whey protein concentrate; the latter being the source of whey provided to the WP and GWP groups. Given that self-reported caloric intakes were non-significantly but numerically lower on a weekly basis in GWP vs. WP and MALTO participants throughout the study, an alternative explanation of our data could be that the observed loss in fat mass in the GWP group occurred due to a lower calorie intake relative to the other groups. Indeed, these data agree with studies which have mechanistically

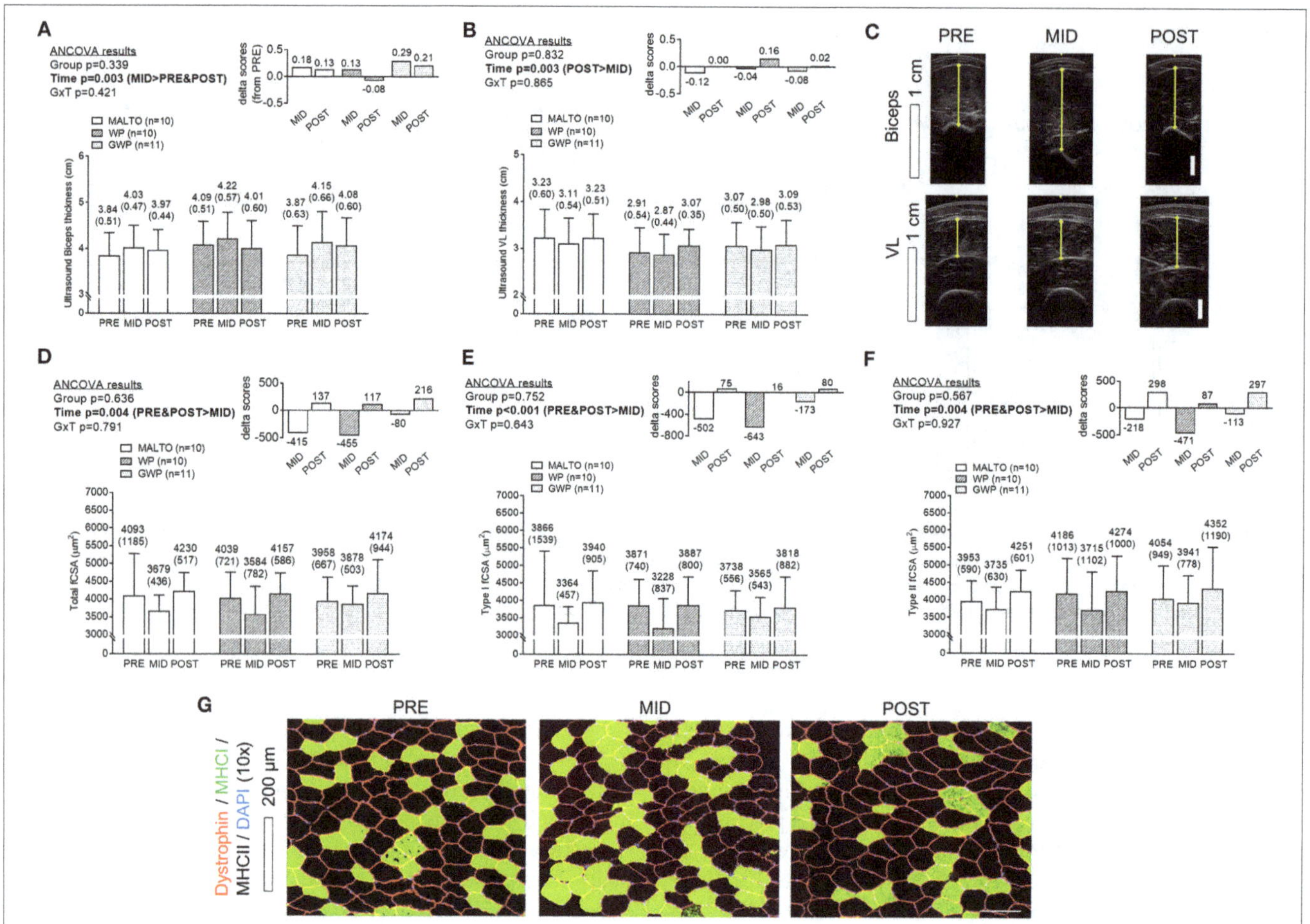

FIGURE 5 | Muscle thickness and VL fiber size differences between supplementation groups. Only a significant time effect was observed for biceps thickness **(A)** assessed via ultrasound with MID values being greater than PRE- and POST values. Only a significant time effect was observed for VL thickness **(B)** assessed via ultrasound with MID values being less than POST values. Panel **(C)** provides representative images of ultrasound scans from the same participants. Only significant time effects were observed for total fiber cross sectional area (fCSA) **(D)**, type I fCSA **(E)**, and type II fCSA **(F)** assessed via histology with MID values being less than PRE and POST values. Panel **(G)** provides representative 10x objective histology images from VL biopsies of the same participant. All data are presented as means ± standard deviation values, and values are indicated above each bar. Additionally, each data panel has delta values from PRE included as inset data. MALTO, maltodextrin group; WP, standardized whey protein group; GWP, graded whey protein group.

demonstrated that whey protein consumption acutely increases circulating levels of satiety-related hormones and reduces food intake [reviewed in (31)].

Beyond the observed supplementation effects, a unique finding of this investigation is the apparent dose-response relationship observed between RT volume and LBM changes corrected for alterations in ECW (**Figure 6**). It has been suggested that a positive relationship exists between RT volume and skeletal muscle hypertrophy up to a certain volume threshold (32). A recent meta-analysis by Schoenfeld et al. (14) demonstrated significantly greater hypertrophic responses after completion of 10 sets per week of a resistance exercise emphasizing specific musculature compared to <5 sets per week. However, others have suggested that a plateau in the hypertrophic response exists beyond select RT doses (33). Our data indicate no clear plateau in RT-induced muscle mass increases when RT volumes are increased from 10 sets of 10 repetitions at 60% 1RM per exercise per week up to 32 sets per week, and this interpretation stems from the significant increases observed in DXA LBM from weeks 1 to 3 and 3 to 6. However, when changes in DXA LBM were corrected for changes in ECW, a different interpretation arises. Notably, subtractions of ECW changes from LBM changes were completed in an attempt to control for transient extracellular fluid retention (e.g., local swelling) related to tissue trauma potentially due to the extreme RT volumes completed by participants. In this regard, Yamada et al. (24) suggest expansions of ECW may be representative of edema or inflammation and can mask true alterations in functional skeletal muscle mass. Further, these authors suggest the measurements of fluid compartmentalization (e.g., ICW, ECW), which are not measured by DXA, are needed if accurate representation of functional changes in LBM are to be inferred. When ECW-corrected ΔLBM changes are considered, week 1–3 increases were similar in magnitude to uncorrected DXA

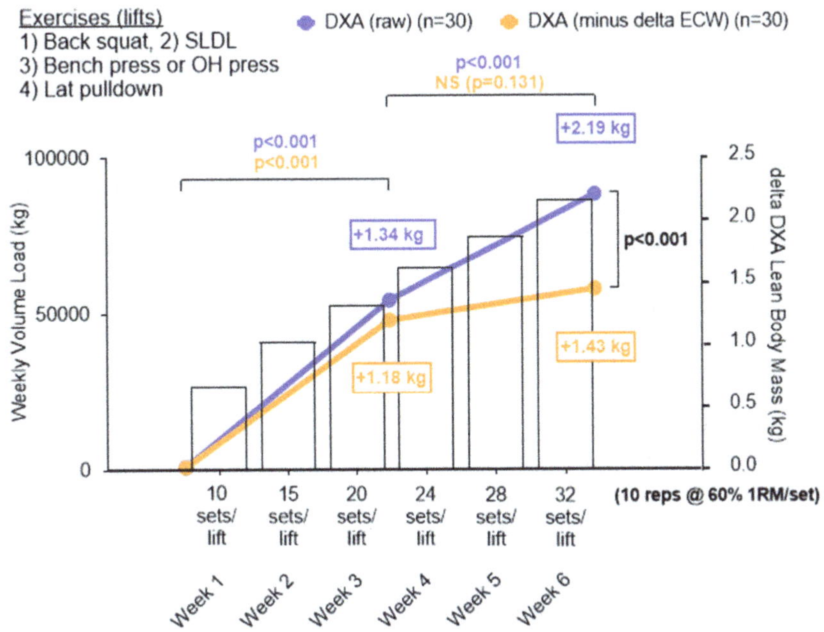

FIGURE 6 | Change in DXA lean body mass plotted against increases in training volume for all participants. Data in this figure include DXA lean body mass changes (blue line graph), changes in LBM by subtracting changes in extracellular water (i.e., ECW-corrected ΔLBM), and training volume (bar data) from all 30 participants who underwent DXA and BIS testing. A significant increase in LBM from PRE to MID ($p < 0.001$) and MID to POST ($p < 0.001$) was observed in DXA LBM and this was proportional to the increase in training volume over time. When considering ECW-corrected ΔLBM changes, a similar increase occurred across groups from PRE to MID ($p < 0.001$), but the increase from MID to POST was not significant ($p = 0.131$). Additionally, POST DXA LBM was significantly higher than POST ECW-corrected ΔLBM. All data is presented as mean changes, and bars depicting standard deviation were left off of these panels in order to simplify the figure.

LBM changes (+1.18 vs. +1.34 kg, respectively). However, ECW-corrected ΔLBM changes from weeks 3–6 were significantly lower than uncorrected DXA LBM changes (+0.85 vs. +0.25 kg, respectively). We speculate the latter observation could be related to local inflammation or edema induced by increasing RT volume above 20 sets per exercise per week. Thus, when considering uncorrected DXA LBM changes, one interpretation of these data is that participants did not experience a hypertrophy threshold to increasing volumes up to 32 sets per week. However, if accounting for ECW changes during RT does indeed better reflect changes in functional muscle mass, then it is apparent participants were approaching a maximal adaptable volume at ~20 sets per exercise per week. First, it is critical to note that more research is needed in order to determine if correcting changes in DXA LBM relative to changes in ECW is a valid method which better reflects changes in functional muscle mass. Second, and in regard to a set volume threshold, we are careful to generalize these findings across populations to avoid promotion of an assumed RT volume ceiling for eliciting hypertrophy since there is likely no "one size fits all" RT dose for eliciting a maximal hypertrophic response (34, 35). Rather, optimally dosing RT for hypertrophic outcomes should depend on the physiological status of an individual and particularly as it pertains to recent historical training (36).

Other interesting effects related to training emerged from the current study. First, divergent adaptive responses in the bicep brachii and VL muscles as assessed via ultrasound were observed. Specifically, increases in biceps thickness and decreases in VL thickness occurred from PRE to MID and the inverse effects occurred from MID to POST. While fiber type data in human biceps brachii muscle are lacking, Dahmane et al. (37) reported ~60% of fibers in the biceps brachii were type II, while ~40% were type I. Herein, we observed the VL consisted of ~50% type II fibers, on average. Type II fibers typically hypertrophy to a greater extent in response to RT relative to type I fibers (38), and the observed divergent responses in the biceps and VL muscle thickness measurements may be related to fiber-type distributions of these muscles. However, this hypothesis is speculative at best and more work is needed to determine how different muscle groups mechanistically adapt to high volume RT. Another striking observation was the PRE to MID decrease in VL thickness and fCSA values followed by the MID to POST increase in these metrics. Damas et al. (36) recently reported significant increases in muscle damage after a single bout of RT, followed by an attenuation of damage measured from a similar bout 3 and 10 weeks later. Additionally, while these authors observed significant elevations in MPS after bouts at weeks 3 and 10, significant increases in fCSA were only observed after 10 weeks. The authors posited that significant increases in muscle damage and MPB from weeks 1–3 outpaced increases in MPS resulting in no significant increase in fCSA until the RT-induced damage response subsided from weeks 3–10. Relating these findings to our data, the initial atrophic VL muscle response during the first 3 weeks of training may have been due to high levels of muscle damage/MPB counteracting increases in MPS. However, during weeks 3–6, MPS levels may have outpaced muscle damage/MPB leading to increases in muscle thickness and fCSA. Again, these findings are speculative at best since we did not assess markers of muscle protein turnover.

Experimental Considerations

Our study is limited in that only 31 participants completed the intervention. As such, we were underpowered to detect small, but significant, effects. Second, an unresolved limitation is that not all participants adhered to the dietary self-reporting protocol. We felt that 2 to 4-day food logs would not entirely reflect what participants consumed throughout the study. For this reason, we sought to implement a convenient and more ecologically valid method of self-reporting dietary data which persuaded our utilization of daily mobile application entries. However, despite consistent verbal encouragement by research staff, only ~60% of participants were adherent. In regard to dietary adherence it is also worth noting that, while our intent was to grade dietary protein intakes on a weekly basis in the WP and GWP groups, all groups (including MALTO) self-reported consuming similar amounts of protein throughout the study (>2.0 g/kg/d). Thus, results observed in the GWP group could be interpreted as physiological effects due to the replacement of dietary protein with whey protein on a weekly basis rather than increases in overall protein intake. We do not propose that this protein replacement strategy should be adopted by recreational lifters or athletes, and future studies should try to resolve if strictly maintaining dietary habits while increasing whey protein dosing promotes physiological benefits. A methodological consideration is our reliance upon DXA assessments reflecting true whole-body muscle mass changes. While numerous forms of body composition assessment exist, the scientific literature supports the utilization of DXA for detecting changes in body composition. Buckinx et al. (39) recently posited DXA as a reference standard (but not gold standard) method for measurement of LBM in research and clinical practice. As mentioned previously, our laboratory has observed excellent same-day reliability of the DXA during a test-calibrate-retest. Notwithstanding, others have suggested a modest overestimation of fat mass using DXA compared to a 4-compartment model of body composition (40). Therefore, we acknowledge that LBM or fat mass assessed via DXA could have been under- or overestimated in an absolute sense. Additionally, PRE to POST increases in DXA dual-arm and DXA dual-leg LBM seemingly did not agree well with the ultrasound data suggesting PRE to POST increases in biceps thickness occurred and only a MID to POST increase in VL thickness occurred. While this finding is difficult to reconcile, it is notable that Franchi et al. (41) have recently reported that change scores in VL ultrasound thickness and VL muscle area assessed via magnetic resonance spectroscopy poorly agree following weeks of RT. Hence, the lack of agreement between DXA and ultrasound could be similarly reflective of between-method comparison limitations reported by Franchi et al. Finally, while a 6-week RT program seems rather abbreviated, we chose to implement this duration due to the concern *a priori* that the implemented volume would lead to injuries past 6 weeks of training. Furthermore, traditional training periodization strategies commonly employed in practical settings organize training phases or "blocks" emphasizing specific adaptations (e.g., hypertrophy, strength) into 3–6 week durations (42). In spite of these limitations, we posit that our findings are novel in the sense that these were the highest RT volumes formally studied in humans to date in a 6-week timeframe.

CONCLUSIONS

GWP participants exhibited robust increases in DXA LBM, and reductions in DXA fat mass. These data imply graded whey protein consumption in conjunction with increases in RT volume (i.e., a proportional supplemental protein hypothesis) is a viable strategy to improve body composition during high volume RT. However, similar PRE to POST effects regarding DXA LBM and VL fCSA changes were observed in the MALTO group and, given that all groups herein consumed >2.0 g/kg/d of dietary protein, this finding suggests that GWP may not provide substantial benefit in promoting hypertrophy when protein intakes are >1.6 g/kg/d as suggested by Morton et al. (5). Additionally, the RT volumes investigated in this study are the highest formally studied in human participants in a 6-week timeframe. Significant increases in LBM corrected for alterations in ECW were observed from weeks 1–3, although this response was dampened from weeks 3–6 suggesting that ~20 sets per exercise per week may approach a maximal adaptable volume in younger resistance-trained men.

AUTHOR CONTRIBUTIONS

CH was primarily responsible for the design, execution, analysis, and writing of the manuscript. CV critically assisted with all aspects of execution and analysis. All other co-authors assisted in multiple aspects of data collection as well as the preparation of the manuscript. MDR is the principal investigator of the laboratory where much of the work for this study was performed, and assisted in all aspects of the study as well as in the preparation of the manuscript.

FUNDING

Funding for participant compensation and assays were provided by a gift donation from Renaissance Periodization (Charlotte, NC, USA) and contract through Impedimed Inc. (Queensland, AU).

ACKNOWLEDGMENTS

We would like to thank the participants for participating in this difficult training study. We would also like to thank Nick Shaw (CEO, Renaissance Periodization) for his generosity.

Additionally, we would like to thank Dr. Rob Wildman from Dymatize Nutrition in coordinating the donation of nutritional supplement products. Finally, we would like to thank Dr. David Pascoe for his assistance with purchasing weight equipment and allowing us to use his laboratory space for testing procedures. We graciously acknowledge Casey Sexton, Jazzylyn Pepper, James Creel, Lauren Mussell, Brooke Anderson, Mclelland-Rae Johnson, Jacobs Brewer, Denico Jackson, and JoAnna Roberts for their helpful assistance throughout the training portion of the study and/or data analysis.

SUPPLEMENTARY MATERIAL

Supplementary SDC 1 | haun_supplementary_data.csv—this file includes all raw data.

Supplementary SDC 2 | haun_supplementary_diet.csv—this file includes dietary recommendations as well as self-reported dietary intakes.

Supplementary SDC 3 | haun_supplementary_tables.pdf—this file includes descriptive tables for each dependent variable.

Supplementary Table 1 | Pre-study body composition and strength descriptive measurements.

Supplementary Table 2 | Body mass.

Supplementary Table 3 | Total lean body mass (DXA).

Supplementary Table 4 | Total body fat mass (DXA).

Supplementary Table 5 | Vastus lateralis thickness (ultrasound).

Supplementary Table 6 | Biceps brachii thickness (ultrasound).

Supplementary Table 7 | Total body water (BIS).

Supplementary Table 8 | Extracellular water (BIS).

Supplementary Table 9 | Intracellular water (BIS).

Supplementary Table 10 | Total mood disturbance scores (POMS Questionnaire).

Supplementary Table 11 | Pressure to pain threshold (Algometry).

Supplementary Table 12 | Fiber count and fiber cross sectional area.

Supplementary Table 13 | Training design.

Supplementary Table 14 | Training volume load and repetitions in reserve.

REFERENCES

1. Burd NA, Holwerda AM, Selby KC, West DW, Staples AW, Cain NE, et al. Resistance exercise volume affects myofibrillar protein synthesis and anabolic signalling molecule phosphorylation in young men. *J Physiol.* (2010) 588:3119–30. doi: 10.1113/jphysiol.2010.192856
2. Atherton PJ, Smith K. Muscle protein synthesis in response to nutrition and exercise. *J Physiol.* (2012) 590:1049–57. doi: 10.1113/jphysiol.2011.225003
3. Witard OC, Jackman SR, Breen L, Smith K, Selby A, Tipton KD. Myofibrillar muscle protein synthesis rates subsequent to a meal in response to increasing doses of whey protein at rest and after resistance exercise. *Am J Clin Nutr.* (2014) 99:86–95. doi: 10.3945/ajcn.112.055517
4. Macnaughton LS, Wardle SL, Witard OC, Mcglory C, Hamilton DL, Jeromson S, et al. The response of muscle protein synthesis following whole-body resistance exercise is greater following 40 g than 20 g of ingested whey protein. *Physiol Rep.* (2016) 4: e12893. doi: 10.14814/phy2.12893
5. Morton RW, Murphy KT, Mckellar SR, Schoenfeld BJ, Henselmans M, Helms E, et al. A systematic review, meta-analysis and meta-regression of the effect of protein supplementation on resistance training-induced gains in muscle mass and strength in healthy adults. *Br J Sports Med.* (2018) 52:376–84. doi: 10.1136/bjsports-2017-097608
6. Moore DR, Churchward-Venne TA, Witard O, Breen L, Burd NA, Tipton KD, et al. Protein ingestion to stimulate myofibrillar protein synthesis requires greater relative protein intakes in healthy older versus younger men. *J Gerontol A Biol Sci Med Sci.* (2015) 70:57–62. doi: 10.1093/gerona/glu103
7. Kumar V, Atherton P, Smith K, Rennie MJ. Human muscle protein synthesis and breakdown during and after exercise. *J Appl Physiol.* (2009) 106:2026–39. doi: 10.1152/japplphysiol.91481.2008
8. Wolfe RR. Skeletal muscle protein metabolism and resistance exercise. *J Nutr.* (2006) 136:525S–8. doi: 10.1093/jn/136.2.525S
9. Burke DG, Chilibeck PD, Davidson KS, Candow DG, Farthing J, Smith-Palmer T. The effect of whey protein supplementation with and without creatine monohydrate combined with resistance training on lean tissue mass and muscle strength. *Int J Sport Nutr Exerc Metab.* (2001) 11:349–64. doi: 10.1123/ijsnem.11.3.349
10. Cribb PJ, Williams AD, Carey MF, Hayes A. The effect of whey isolate and resistance training on strength, body composition, and plasma glutamine. *Int J Sport Nutr Exerc Metab.* (2006) 16:494–509. doi: 10.1123/ijsnem.16.5.494
11. Hoffman JR, Ratamess NA, Kang J, Falvo MJ, Faigenbaum AD. Effects of protein supplementation on muscular performance and resting hormonal changes in college football players. *J Sports Sci Med.* (2007) 6:85–92. Available online at: https://www.jssm.org/hf.php?id=jssm-06-85.xml#
12. Hoffman JR, Ratamess NA, Tranchina CP, Rashti SL, Kang J, Faigenbaum AD. Effect of protein-supplement timing on strength, power, and body-composition changes in resistance-trained men. *Int J Sport Nutr Exerc Metab.* (2009) 19:172–85. doi: 10.1123/ijsnem.19.2.172
13. Lockwood CM, Roberts MD, Dalbo VJ, Smith-Ryan AE, Kendall KL, Moon JR, et al. Effects of hydrolyzed whey versus other whey protein supplements on the physiological response to 8 weeks of resistance exercise in college-aged males. *J Am Coll Nutr.* (2017) 36:16–27. doi: 10.1080/07315724.2016.1140094
14. Schoenfeld BJ, Ogborn D, Krieger JW. Dose-response relationship between weekly resistance training volume and increases in muscle mass: a systematic review and meta-analysis. *J Sports Sci.* (2017) 35:1073–82. doi: 10.1080/02640414.2016.1210197
15. Zourdos MC, Klemp A, Dolan C, Quiles JM, Schau KA, Jo E, et al. Novel resistance training-specific rating of perceived exertion scale measuring repetitions in reserve. *J Strength Cond Res.* (2016) 30:267–75. doi: 10.1519/JSC.0000000000001049
16. Teixeira V, Voci SM, Mendes-Netto RS, Da Silva DG. The relative validity of a food record using the smartphone application MyFitnessPal. *Nutr Diet* (2018) 75:219–25. doi: 10.1111/1747-0080.12401
17. Scott CB, Luchini A, Knausenberger A, Steitz A. Total energy costs - aerobic and anaerobic, exercise and recovery - of five resistance exercises. *Cent Eur J Sport Sci Med.* (2014) 8:53–9. Available online at: https://wnus.edu.pl/cejssm/en/issue/22/article/175/
18. Grove JR, Prapavessis H. Preliminary evidence for the reliability and validity of an abbreviated Profile of Mood States. *Int J Sport Psych.* (1992) 23:93–109.
19. Haun CT, Mumford PW, Roberson PA, Romero MA, Mobley CB, Kephart WC, et al. Molecular, neuromuscular, and recovery responses to light versus heavy resistance exercise in young men. *Physiol Rep.* (2017) 5:e13457. doi: 10.14814/phy2.13457
20. Kephart WC, Wachs TD, Mac Thompson R, Brooks Mobley C, Fox CD, Mcdonald JR, et al. Ten weeks of branched-chain amino acid supplementation improves select performance and immunological variables in trained cyclists. *Amino Acids* (2016) 48:779–89. doi: 10.1007/s00726-015-2125-8
21. Moon JR, Tobkin SE, Roberts MD, Dalbo VJ, Kerksick CM, Bemben MG, et al. Total body water estimations in healthy men and women using bioimpedance spectroscopy: a deuterium oxide comparison. *Nutr Metab.* (2008) 5:7. doi: 10.1186/1743-7075-5-7

22. Birzniece V, Khaw CH, Nelson AE, Meinhardt U, Ho KK. A critical evaluation of bioimpedance spectroscopy analysis in estimating body composition during GH treatment: comparison with bromide dilution and dual X-ray absorptiometry. *Eur J Endocrinol.* (2015) 172:21–8. doi: 10.1530/EJE-14-0660
23. Moon JR. Body composition in athletes and sports nutrition: an examination of the bioimpedance analysis technique. *Eur J Clin Nutr.* (2013) 167(Suppl.):S54–9. doi: 10.1038/ejcn.2012.165
24. Yamada Y, Matsuda K, Bjorkman MP, Kimura M. Application of segmental bioelectrical impedance spectroscopy to the assessment of skeletal muscle cell mass in elderly men. *Geriatr Gerontol Int.* (2014) 1(Suppl. 14):129–34. doi: 10.1111/ggi.12212
25. Mobley CB, Haun CT, Roberson PA, Mumford PW, Romero MA, Kephart WC, et al. Effects of whey, soy or leucine supplementation with 12 weeks of resistance training on strength, body composition, and skeletal muscle and adipose tissue histological attributes in college-aged males. *Nutrients* (2017) 9:E972. doi: 10.3390/nu9090972
26. Carpenter AE, Jones TR, Lamprecht MR, Clarke C, Kang IH, Friman O, et al. CellProfiler: image analysis software for identifying and quantifying cell phenotypes. *Genome Biol.* (2006) 7:R100. doi: 10.1186/gb-2006-7-10-r100
27. Antonio J, Peacock CA, Ellerbroek A, Fromhoff B, Silver T. The effects of consuming a high protein diet (4.4 g/kg/d) on body composition in resistance-trained individuals. *J Int Soc Sports Nutr.* (2014) 11:19. doi: 10.1186/1550-2783-11-19
28. Antonio J, Ellerbroek A, Silver T, Orris S, Scheiner M, Gonzalez A, et al. A high protein diet (3.4 g/kg/d) combined with a heavy resistance training program improves body composition in healthy trained men and women–a follow-up investigation. *J Int Soc Sports Nutr.* (2015) 12:39. doi: 10.1186/s12970-015-0100-0
29. Roberts MD, Cruthirds CL, Lockwood CM, Pappan K, Childs TE, Company JM, et al. Comparing serum responses to acute feedings of an extensively hydrolyzed whey protein concentrate versus a native whey protein concentrate in rats: a metabolomics approach. *Appl Physiol Nutr Metab.* (2014) 39:158–67. doi: 10.1139/apnm-2013-0148
30. Mobley CB, Fox CD, Ferguson BS, Pascoe CA, Healy JC, Mcadam JS, et al. Effects of protein type and composition on postprandial markers of skeletal muscle anabolism, adipose tissue lipolysis, and hypothalamic gene expression. *J Int Soc Sports Nutr.* (2015) 12:14. doi: 10.1186/s12970-015-0076-9
31. Luhovyy BL, Akhavan T, Anderson GH. Whey proteins in the regulation of food intake and satiety. *J Am Coll Nutr.* (2007) 26:704S–12. doi: 10.1080/07315724.2007.10719651
32. Wernbom M, Augustsson J, Thomee R. The influence of frequency, intensity, volume and mode of strength training on whole muscle cross-sectional area in humans. *Sports Med.* (2007) 37:225–64. doi: 10.2165/00007256-200737030-00004
33. La Scala Teixeira CV, Motoyama Y, De Azevedo P, Evangelista AL, Steele J, Bocalini DS. Effect of resistance training set volume on upper body muscle hypertrophy: are more sets really better than less? *Clin Physiol Funct Imaging* (2017) 38:727–32. doi: 10.1111/cpf.12476
34. Bamman MM, Petrella JK, Kim JS, Mayhew DL, Cross JM. Cluster analysis tests the importance of myogenic gene expression during myofiber hypertrophy in humans. *J Appl Physiol.* (2007) 102:2232–9. doi: 10.1152/japplphysiol.00024.2007
35. Mobley CB, Haun CT, Roberson PA, Mumford PW, Kephart WC, Romero MA, et al. Biomarkers associated with low, moderate, and high vastus lateralis muscle hypertrophy following 12 weeks of resistance training. *PLoS ONE* (2018) 13:e0195203. doi: 10.1371/journal.pone.0195203
36. Damas F, Phillips SM, Libardi CA, Vechin FC, Lixandrao ME, Jannig PR, et al. Resistance training-induced changes in integrated myofibrillar protein synthesis are related to hypertrophy only after attenuation of muscle damage. *J Physiol.* (2016) 594:5209–22. doi: 10.1113/JP272472
37. Dahmane R, Djordjevic S, Simunic B, Valencic V. Spatial fiber type distribution in normal human muscle Histochemical and tensiomyographical evaluation. *J Biomech.* (2005) 38:2451–9. doi: 10.1016/j.jbiomech.2004.10.020
38. Fry AC. The role of resistance exercise intensity on muscle fibre adaptations. *Sports Med.* (2004) 34:663–79. doi: 10.2165/00007256-200434100-00004
39. Buckinx F, Landi F, Cesari M, Fielding RA, Visser M, Engelke K, et al. Pitfalls in the measurement of muscle mass: a need for a reference standard. *J Cachexia Sarcopenia Muscle* (2018) 9:269–78. doi: 10.1002/jcsm.12268
40. Santos DA, Silva AM, Matias CN, Fields DA, Heymsfield SB, Sardinha LB. Accuracy of DXA in estimating body composition changes in elite athletes using a four compartment model as the reference method. *Nutr Metab.* (2010) 7:22. doi: 10.1186/1743-7075-7-22
41. Franchi MV, Longo S, Mallinson J, Quinlan JI, Taylor T, Greenhaff PL, et al. Muscle thickness correlates to muscle cross-sectional area in the assessment of strength training-induced hypertrophy. *Scand J Med Sci Sports* (2018) 28:846–53. doi: 10.1111/sms.12961
42. Stone MH, O'bryant H, Garhammer J, Mcmillan J, Rozenek R. A theoretical model of strength training. *Strength Cond J.* (1982) 4:36–39. doi: 10.1519/0199-610X(1982)004<0036:ATMOST>2.3.CO;2

17

Is an Energy Surplus Required to Maximize Skeletal Muscle Hypertrophy Associated with Resistance Training

Gary John Slater[1,2], Brad P. Dieter[3], Damian James Marsh[4], Eric Russell Helms[5], Gregory Shaw[6] and Juma Iraki[7]*

[1] School of Health and Sport Sciences, University of the Sunshine Coast, Maroochydore, QLD, Australia, [2] Australian Institute of Sport, Canberra, ACT, Australia, [3] Department of Pharmaceutical Sciences, Washington State University, WA Spokane, WA, United States, [4] Fiji Rugby Union, Suva, Fiji, [5] Auckland University of Technology, Sports Performance Research Institute New Zealand, Auckland, New Zealand, [6] Swimming Australia, Brisbane, QLD, Australia, [7] Iraki Nutrition AS, Fjerdingby, Norway

***Correspondence:**
Gary John Slater
gslater@usc.edu.au

Resistance training is commonly prescribed to enhance strength/power qualities and is achieved via improved neuromuscular recruitment, fiber type transition, and/ or skeletal muscle hypertrophy. The rate and amount of muscle hypertrophy associated with resistance training is influenced by a wide array of variables including the training program, plus training experience, gender, genetic predisposition, and nutritional status of the individual. Various dietary interventions have been proposed to influence muscle hypertrophy, including manipulation of protein intake, specific supplement prescription, and creation of an energy surplus. While recent research has provided significant insight into optimization of dietary protein intake and application of evidence based supplements, the specific energy surplus required to facilitate muscle hypertrophy is unknown. However, there is clear evidence of an anabolic stimulus possible from an energy surplus, even independent of resistance training. Common textbook recommendations are often based solely on the assumed energy stored within the tissue being assimilated. Unfortunately, such guidance likely fails to account for other energetically expensive processes associated with muscle hypertrophy, the acute metabolic adjustments that occur in response to an energy surplus, or individual nuances like training experience and energy status of the individual. Given the ambiguous nature of these calculations, it is not surprising to see broad ranging guidance on energy needs. These estimates have never been validated in a resistance training population to confirm the "sweet spot" for an energy surplus that facilitates optimal rates of muscle gain relative to fat mass. This review not only addresses the influence of an energy surplus on resistance training outcomes, but also explores other pertinent issues, including "how much should energy intake be increased," "where should this extra energy come from," and "when should this extra energy be consumed." Several gaps in the literature are identified, with the hope this will stimulate further research interest in this area. Having a broader appreciation of these issues will assist practitioners in the establishment of dietary strategies that facilitate resistance training adaptations while also addressing other important nutrition related issues such as optimization of fuelling and recovery goals. Practical issues like the management of satiety when attempting to increase energy intake are also addressed.

Keywords: muscle hypertrophy, sports nutrition, resistance exercise, diet, nutrient timing

INTRODUCTION

Resistance training is commonly prescribed to increase underlying strength and power qualities in an attempt to improve athletic performance. The enhancement of these qualities may be derived from a range of potential adaptations including improved neuromuscular recruitment, fiber type transition, and/ or skeletal muscle hypertrophy. Promoting hypertrophy is especially important in strength sports, given the strong relationship between fat free mass (FFM) and competitive lifting performance (1, 2). Furthermore, in contact sports such as rugby union, larger players have a clear advantage (3) which is highlighted in World Cup data where total mass of forwards is correlated with success (4, 5). Amongst elite youth rugby league players, quadriceps muscle hypertrophy is related to enhancement of running speed (6). However, this may not be appropriate for all athletes with skeletal muscle hypertrophy possibly resulting in adverse adaptations, including a transition away from fast twitch glycolytic fibers and slower contraction velocity characteristics (7) if inappropriately prescribed. Thus, unless the increase in power proportionally exceeds any associated weight gain, performance is unlikely to be enhanced by skeletal muscle hypertrophy. Collectively there is support for the potential of skeletal muscle hypertrophy enhancing athletic performance, but individual athlete nuances must be considered by coaching personnel and training prescribed so as to facilitate adaptations in both muscle hypertrophy and power so that any associated increase in body mass does not negatively affect variables like speed (8).

The manipulation of dietary intake is common among individuals attempting to facilitate resistance training gains in strength and skeletal muscle hypertrophy. Aside from water (75%), skeletal muscle is made up of protein (20%), with the remainder from other materials including fat, glycogen, inorganic salts, and minerals (9). Given the protein content of skeletal muscle, it is perhaps not surprising resistance trained athletes emphasize the importance of dietary protein in their meal plans (10). This is also reflected in the scientific literature with significant attention given to protein focused nutritional interventions to facilitate resistance training induced adaptations (11), including manipulation of total daily dietary protein intake (12), protein dosage per meal (13–15), protein quality (16), and protein distribution (17). While a recent meta-analysis suggested dietary protein supplementation enhances resistance training induced gains in muscle mass and strength, at least when dietary protein intake is suboptimal (<1.6 g·kg^{-1} daily) (18), resistance training alone provides a far greater stimulus than protein supplementation (14). Given this, a number of other dietary strategies have previously been proposed to augment the resistance training response, including the creation of a positive energy balance (19, 20). While facilitating a positive energy balance is not supported by others because of the potential for increments in fat mass (FM) (21), there is clear evidence of a whole body anabolic response to overfeeding, even in the absence of a resistance training stimulus in sedentary populations (22, 23). This raises a question about composition of the lean mass accretion in this scenario i.e., skeletal muscle vs. splanchnic protein (24), especially given the lack of change in mammalian target of rapamycin (mTOR) (25). Furthermore, additional energy does not appear to further modulate the acute muscle protein synthesis (MPS) response to dietary protein ingestion at rest (26), or following resistance exercise (27, 28). Despite this, numerous textbooks used in the training of nutrition professionals advocate the creation of an energy surplus when attempting to facilitate skeletal muscle hypertrophy (29–32).

The exact energy cost of skeletal muscle hypertrophy is not known. Likewise, it is not clear if this energy cost can be met purely from endogenous (i.e., internal fat stores) and/or exogenous sources (i.e., diet). Indeed, there is clear evidence of marked skeletal muscle hypertrophy in response to a novel resistance training stimulus in otherwise healthy, overweight individuals in conjunction with a hypoenergetic, higher protein meal plan (33, 34). While similar concurrent reductions in FM and gains in FFM have been observed in elite and professional athletes following return to sport after an off-season break (35) or injury (36, 37), this response is less evident in highly trained individuals exposed regularly to a resistance training stimulus (38). This raises the possibility that individual nuances may need to be considered, including energy status and training history. Indeed, there is research confirming initial body fat stores influence metabolic response to starvation (39), while individuals with higher FFM and cardiorespiratory fitness gain less FM relative to FFM during isoenergetic, isonitrogenous overfeeding in a sedentary state (40). Preliminary research indicates younger athletes experience more pronounced physique and physical characteristic training adaptations compared to their older peers (41), a trend also even amongst mature professional athletes (38). A better appreciation of these individual nuances may assist with establishing realistic training adaptation aspirations, plus prescription of training and diet interventions to facilitate skeletal muscle hypertrophy.

It is not known if any adjustment in dietary intake to support muscle hypertrophy is required to merely contribute the building blocks of skeletal muscle while also accounting for the metabolic cost of generating new skeletal muscle mass (SMM), or if the physiological response to an energy surplus amplifies the anabolic signal created by resistance training. Addressing these fundamental questions is paramount to future prescription of energy intake guidance associated with dietary strategies to optimize skeletal muscle hypertrophy. Given the dearth of research specifically examining the influence of an energy surplus on resistance training outcomes, an exploration of overfeeding studies independent of resistance exercise has also been included in this review. This needs to be considered, given the impact of resistance training on sensitivity to nutrition support. Indeed, a single resistance training session can serve to potentiate MPS in response to protein feeding (42), an effect which may persist for upwards of 24–48 h after resistance exercise (43, 44).

Overfeeding alone is not sufficient to produce favorable body composition changes such that proportionally more FFM is gained than FM. Indeed, while 100 days of energy surplus (totaling 353 MJ) among young lean males resulted in significant individual variation in body composition change, ~2 kg of FM were accrued for each 1 kg of lean mass (45). In Leaf and Antonio's summary of overfeeding studies, they also note that predominantly more FM is gained with overfeeding in the absence of resistance training (46). However, it seems unlikely that overfeeding alone would produce meaningful increases in contractile tissue as the initiating event which induces skeletal muscle hypertrophy after maturation is the production of sufficient tension (47) and subsequent mechanotransduction at the muscle fiber level (48). In an exercise or strength and conditioning setting, this stimulus is supplied via progressive resistance training. Other related factors such as the resultant muscle damage, metabolic fatigue, and hormonal response to resistance training are speculated to either correlate with, be additive to, or play a permissive role in training-induced hypertrophy, but are not yet fully understood (49). It is plausible that nutrition could influence some of these factors.

This review not only addresses the impact of energy balance on resistance training outcomes, with an emphasis on skeletal muscle hypertrophy, but also explores other important issues, including "how big should the energy surplus be," "where should the extra energy come from," and "when should this extra energy be consumed." Having a broader understanding of these issues will help establish nutrition strategies to optimize resistance training adaptations and at the same time address nutritional issues such as optimizing recovery and fuelling goals. A broader understanding of the physiological implications of an energy surplus not only has clear application to the resistance trained athlete but may also be applicable to clinical populations where retention or promotion of SMM may be advantageous. While it is recognized supplement use is common amongst resistance trained athletes (50), and there is empirical evidence to support the use of supplements like creatine monohydrate in facilitating resistance training adaptations (51), the focus of this review remains with exploring the impact of energy balance on resistance training outcomes.

ENERGY BALANCE

The daily energy cost of protein turnover accounts for ~20% of resting energy needs or 18 kJ·kg^{-1} body mass (52). Skeletal muscle hypertrophy requires the further remodeling of muscle, ensuring it is an energy intensive process. As such, there has been much discussion around the role of energy balance (i.e., energy surpluses, energy deficits, and isocaloric states) in modulating hypertrophy. Currently, there is a paucity of literature that directly addresses the precise role energy deficits, surpluses, and net balance states play in muscle hypertrophy.

Only a few studies have directly assessed the role of energy balance on skeletal muscle hypertrophy in response to resistance training and these focus specifically on the impact of an energy deficit. Indeed, an acute, moderate energy deficit (~80% of estimated energy requirements) that promoted ~1.0 kg weight loss over 10 days amongst young healthy volunteers resulted in a 16% reduction in MPS at rest despite moderate dietary protein intake (1.5 g·kg^{-1}·day^{-1}), with corresponding reductions in signaling pathways involved in the protein translation protein E4-EBP1 (53). Similar findings were observed following 5 days of energy restriction (energy availability of 30 kcal·kg FFM^{-1}·day^{-1}), resulting in ~30% reduction in MPS amongst a group of young resistance trained volunteers, with corresponding reductions in activation of mTOR and P70S6K, protein kinases that regulate protein synthesis (54). However, a single resistance training session was able to restore MPS to levels observed in energy balance and this was further enhanced by protein ingestion (15–30 g) post-exercise, resulting in elevation of MPS ~30% above those observed at rest when in energy balance. Taken together, these acute investigations confirm an energy deficit can impair the molecular machinery involved in protein synthesis, but the overall impact on MPS will depend on other relevant factors such as dietary protein intake and resistance exercise.

The complex interaction between resistance training and diet in an energy deficit has also been explored chronically. In one study, 21 obese women were randomized to either a control arm or a resistance training arm and fed a very low energy liquid formula diet (3,369 kJ·day^{-1} containing 80 g protein, 97 g carbohydrate, 10 g fat) for 90 days. The control group and weight training group lost 16.2 and 16.8% of their body mass, respectively. Changes in body mass, FM, and FFM were similar between groups. However, muscle biopsies revealed an increase in the cross-sectional area of fast twitch muscle fibers (55). In another study on 31 women (69 ± 12 kg, 164 ± 6 cm) who engaged in 24 weeks of combined resistance and endurance training found that the cross-sectional area of thigh muscle, measured by magnetic resonance imaging, increased 7 cm, despite a 2.2% loss in body mass throughout the study (56). Similar gains in lean body mass (LBM) have been observed amongst resistance training naive overweight males in response to regular training (6 days per week, including two resistance training sessions weekly) and a higher protein diet (2.4 g·kg^{-1}·day^{-1}), despite a substantial energy deficit (~60% of estimated energy requirements) (34). Thus, skeletal muscle hypertrophy is possible in an energy deficit, but we propose this response may be more likely among resistance training naive, overweight, or obese individuals. The influence of training status on resistance training response to adjustments in energy balance warrants further investigation.

To our knowledge, there are no rigorously controlled investigations to date that have directly assessed the role of an energy surplus on resistance training outcomes such as skeletal muscle hypertrophy and strength/power traits over an extended period of time. However, there is an array of circumferential evidence to support the idea that an energy surplus does enhance gains in FFM, even independent of the resistance training stimulus. In an early overfeeding study in which 12 pairs of identical male twins were fed a total energy surplus of 353 MJ (with 15% of total daily energy intake from protein) over a span of 100 days (or 4,200 kJ·day^{-1}), the volunteers gained an average of 5.4 kg FM and 2.7 kg FFM (45), despite maintaining a relatively sedentary lifestyle. There was a high level of intra-pair correlation among twins, but significant variance between groups of twins, indicating a significant genetic contribution to the adaptation. Another overfeeding study explored the effect of a similar energy surplus (~40% above estimated daily needs or ~4,000 kJ energy surplus daily) but with varying levels of protein intake (5, 15, or 25% of total energy intake) on body composition over an 8-week period. While all groups increased body fat by similar amounts (~3.5 kg) during this tightly controlled metabolic unit investigation, gains in LBM (~3 kg) were only evident with the two higher protein intakes, suggesting a minimum amount of dietary protein is necessary to facilitate gains in LBM, even in an energy surplus (23).

In a preliminary exploration of the combined effects of an energy surplus and resistance training, it was found that only those individuals who consumed an energy dense liquid supplement twice daily on training days observed significant gains in body mass and FFM, as inferred via hydrodensitometry, over an 8-week training period (57). Furthermore, there was no difference in response whether the extra energy was consumed as carbohydrate or a combination of carbohydrate and protein, suggesting the energy content of the diet had the biggest impact on body composition changes when dietary protein intake is already adequate. This is supported by earlier pilot work on the influence of an energy surplus on resistance training adaptations (58). Interestingly, while both investigations confirmed a favorable influence of an energy surplus on FFM gains, this was not reflected in strength changes, perhaps because of the brief duration of training or due to nuances in the techniques used to assess strength and body composition. A recently published pilot study on male bodybuilders also supports the concept of greater body mass and muscle mass gains with a more aggressive energy intake (282 kJ·kg^{-1}·day^{-1}), although further inferences from this study are difficult due to methodological concerns (59).

While much still needs to be done to understand the precise role an energy surplus has in facilitating skeletal muscle hypertrophy, the following discussion explores what is known about the magnitude of a surplus, macronutrient composition, and the mechanisms surrounding the role an energy surplus has on skeletal muscle hypertrophy. Given the lack of research within this environment, exploration of overfeeding studies, independent of the resistance training stimulus, are included in the discussion on this topic. This needs to be considered given the influence resistance training has on protein metabolism, highlighting the symbiotic influence of training, and diet on resistance training adaptations.

ENERGY SURPLUS... HOW MUCH

Common text book recommendations for the energy surplus required to gain 1 kg of SMM range from ~1,500 to 2,000 kJ·day^{-1} in weight stable athletes to an additional 4,000 kJ·day^{-1} in individuals who struggle with lean mass gains or during heavy training loads (31, 32). Guidance on the energy surplus necessary to facilitate skeletal muscle hypertrophy is often based solely on the foundation that if 1 kg of skeletal muscle is 75% water, 20% protein, and 5% fat, glycogen and other minerals and metabolites, then the energy required to accumulate such tissue must at a minimum equal the sum of its parts. Given the assumed composition of skeletal muscle, the energy stored in 1 kg of muscle is ~5,000–5,200 kJ, with ~3,400 kJ from protein, ~1,400–1,500 kJ from fat, and ~300–450 kJ from muscle glycogen. Furthermore, energy intake should also be sufficient to supply substrate to fuel the protein synthetic machinery stimulated by resistance exercise, a potentially costly process (11, 60). Finally, adequate energy may be needed to account for the increased metabolic cost of accumulated muscle mass and diet induced thermogenesis (DIT), all while minimizing additional energy stored as FM. However, the foundations of these estimates fail to recognize the complicated and energetically expensive process of tissue accretion, an energy value which remains to be systematically quantified. To date, the authors are not aware of any studies that have clearly demonstrated a consistent energy cost of tissue accumulation, specifically that which is associated with skeletal muscle hypertrophy in response to a resistance training stimulus.

Throughout the twentieth century numerous obesity researchers investigated the influence an energy surplus has on body composition. Most studies consistently demonstrate a strong association between body mass gain and the energy surplus (61). However, there is large inter-individual variability in the composition of this mass gain with between 33 and 40% of body mass accretion accounted for by increases in FFM (61). In non-exercising populations some have suggested that the composition of tissue change associated with an energy surplus is a fixed relationship (62), but in athletic populations where exercise and adequate protein intake are the main stimuli for SMM adaptation, this seems unlikely. Of interest from this obesity research is Forbes and colleagues attempt to estimate the energy cost of tissue deposition by using theoretical values of deposition and comparing them to their own findings (22). They reported that by using the values suggested by Spady et al. (63), which were 36.2 kJ·g^{-1} of protein and 50.2 kJ·g^{-1} of fat deposited, in combination with composition ratios of FM:FFM observed in their research, that the energy cost of depositing 1 kg was closely aligned with theoretical values (31,600 and 33,800 kJ·kg^{-1}, respectively). As part of this, Forbes surmised that due to SMM being 20% protein and 75% water, the energy cost of depositing 1 kg of SMM was 7,440 kJ·kg^{-1}. More recently, Joosen and Westerp (61) have suggested a figure of 29.4 kJ·g^{-1}

of protein deposition, potentially reducing the cost of SMM deposition to 6,050 $kJ \cdot kg^{-1}$. Both estimates suggest an additional energy cost to deposit tissue above the energy density of the substrate (i.e., 16.7 $kJ \cdot g^{-1}$ for protein) of between 12.7 and 19.5 $kJ \cdot g^{-1}$ protein after overfeeding in non-exercising individuals.

As previously highlighted, research suggests considerable inter-individual variability in body mass and composition changes associated with an energy surplus, perhaps as a consequence of genetics (40, 45) or metabolic responses such as adaptation to DIT or non-exercise activity thermogenesis (NEAT) (18, 64). Numerous mathematical models have been published to predict changes in body composition associated with changes in dietary intake and energy expenditure (65, 66). However, these equations often standardize estimates of whole-body metabolic energy flux due to the non-exercising population they are focused on (e.g., no change in glycogen state over time, constant relationships between FM and FFM based on population norms). In athletic populations, the nature of training for body composition alterations significantly influences exercise energy expenditure and confounds the ratios of tissue deposition these models rely on. Therefore, if practitioners are to provide guidelines on the energy surplus necessary to synthesize 1 kg of SMM with minimal FM change, it is necessary that a more expansive model of energy cost be explored.

A recent review of studies investigating the combination of a protein focused energy surplus with resistance training have indicated favorable improvements in LBM accretion (46). However, to date few studies have focused on a titrated energy surplus to ascertain the exact energy and nutrient cost of SMM accretion. It seems to the authors that the energy cost of SMM accretion would be accounted for by consideration of several issues. These include the energy stored within muscle tissue, the energy cost of resistance exercise plus any associated post-exercise elevation in metabolism, the energy cost of any subsequent tissue generation, plus it's subsequent metabolic function. The metabolic adjustments that occur in response to an energy surplus also need to be considered. **Figure 1** provides an overview of factors contributing to the energy cost of skeletal muscle hypertrophy. An appreciation of the magnitude of these factors would provide greater insight into appropriate energy intake prescription to facilitate quality weight gain i.e., weight gain characterized primarily by gains in FFM.

Numerous studies have attempted to estimate the energy cost of single (67), multiple set (68), and varying speed and intensity (69) resistance exercise sessions, with the net energy cost of an 8 exercise (2 sets of 8–10 repetitions per exercise) hypertrophy program lasting ~30 min being ~300 and 600 kJ, for females and males, respectively (70, 71). These sex differences in net energy expenditure are not evident when normalized for lean mass (72). Given the potential importance of quantifying energy expenditure, estimates of net resistance training energy expenditure are available i.e., total energy expenditure (TEE) minus resting energy expenditure or the specific energy cost of the resistance training alone. Mookerjee et al. (68) report the energy cost of undertaking 3 sets of 10 reps at 70% of one repetition maximum across five upper body exercises (369.4 ± 174.1 kJ), equating to an energy expenditure of ~0.10–0.12 $kJ \cdot kg^{-1}$ $LBM \cdot min^{-1}$. More recently, a regression equation has been established to estimate resistance training relative energy expenditure based on several variables including stature, age, FM, LBM, and total exercise volume (72), giving practitioners several options to assist with quantifying the energy cost of resistance training. While some of these estimates fail to account for any elevation in energy expenditure post exercise, this effect may only be evident for upwards of 20 min post exercise (72), and thus may be considered negligible, at least following shorter duration resistance training. The metabolic implications of resistance training warrant further exploration.

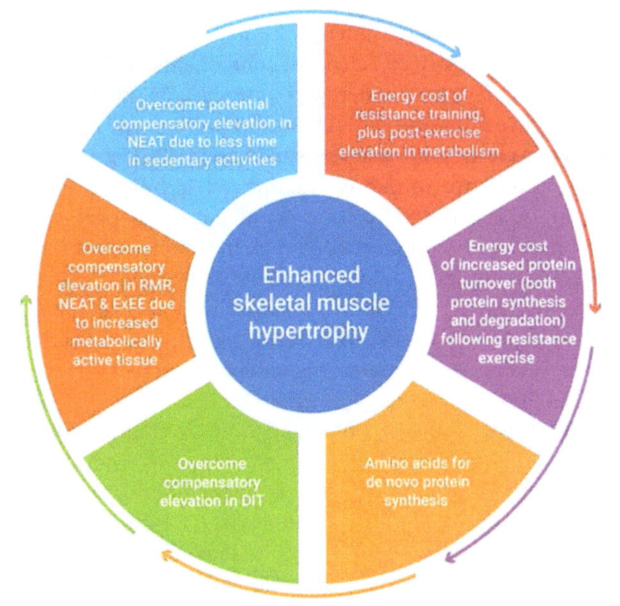
Overcome potential compensatory elevation in NEAT due to less time in sedentary activities
Energy cost of resistance training, plus post-exercise elevation in metabolism
Overcome compensatory elevation in RMR, NEAT & ExEE due to increased metabolically active tissue
Enhanced skeletal muscle hypertrophy
Energy cost of increased protein turnover (both protein synthesis and degradation) following resistance exercise
Overcome compensatory elevation in DIT
Amino acids for de novo protein synthesis

FIGURE 1 | An overview of factors contributing to the energy cost of skeletal muscle hypertrophy.

Given skeletal MPS is elevated for upwards of 24–48 h after resistance exercise, the high metabolic cost of protein synthesis needs to also be accounted for (60, 73, 74). The process of translation elongation is likely to account for a large portion of the synthetic cost with 4 high energy phosphate bonds per peptide bond formed required or 3.6 $kJ \cdot g^{-1}$ of protein synthesized (75). Although significant, translation is one of many energy requiring steps in protein synthesis, with processes such as transcription, folding and movement of proteins within cells all being energy dependent (52). The high energy cost of protein synthesis and the duration over which protein synthetic machinery can be upregulated clearly highlights an underestimated cost of protein synthesis and thus, muscle mass accretion. While any associated increase in protein breakdown has been considered to be negligible, this is unlikely the case (52). Further research is needed to better quantify the energy cost of protein synthesis and degradation, plus the time frame over which this may impact energy needs.

Any increase in LBM will also increase energy expenditure, both at rest and during exercise due to the addition of metabolically active tissue, but the implications of this are likely substantially less than is often presumed. Indeed, estimates of the metabolic activity of individual components of FFM suggest skeletal muscle has an energy cost of just 54 $kJ \cdot kg^{-1} \cdot day^{-1}$ (76, 77). Given this, the elevation in REE in response to a 1–2 kg gain in muscle mass is likely very small (i.e., ~100 kJ), and within the precision error of indirect calorimetry techniques available to quantify REE (78). Less is known about the impact of both training and an energy surplus on high metabolic activity tissues like internal organs. However, just 3 weeks of energy restriction has been shown to significantly decrease liver and kidney mass, with associated reductions in REE (79), confirming manipulation of energy balance may impact high metabolic activity tissue size and thus presumably energy expenditure.

Any adjustment in energy intake away from energy balance results in an adaptive change in energy expenditure, via adjustments in NEAT, DIT, and/or adaptive thermogenesis (AT). Indeed, energy expenditure has been observed to increase after just 24 h in an energy surplus (40% above estimated needs), at least when protein intake is concomitantly increased (25). It has also been proposed that overfeeding induces an increase in heat production from the food consumed as a protective mechanism against obesity, a process termed luxuskonsumption which is claimed to dissipate upwards of 30% of the excess energy consumed (64). This form of AT has more recently been challenged by Muller et al. (80) with their assessment of overfeeding literature suggesting in most studies 60–70% of excess energy was stored and a further 20–30% accounted for by metabolic lean mass accretion and increased cost of movement leaving only about 10% of energy expenditure not explained and likely accounted for by errors of measurement. One component of TEE that increases based on changes to the baseline food consumption is DIT. The DIT associated with a typical western diet accounts for ~8–15% of TEE, depending on the macronutrient breakdown of the diet (81). In a review of 26 studies investigating DIT, Quatela et al. (82) used a mixed model meta-regression process to estimate DIT associated with overfeeding. They suggested for every 100 kJ of additional energy from a mixed diet, DIT increased by 1.1 $kJ \cdot h^{-1}$. Energy surpluses associated with higher protein intakes >3.0 $g \cdot kg^{-1}$ BM are likely to increase this figure further and potentially add an additional energy requirement compared to surpluses with energy coming from carbohydrate and fat. This could require an additional 500 kJ a day for athletes with protein intakes in the rage of 3.0 $g \cdot kg^{-1} \cdot day^{-1}$ compared to intakes of 1.0 $g \cdot kg^{-1} \cdot day^{-1}$. Another significant component of TEE that is highly variable in exercising individuals, and may be influenced by training and eating, is NEAT (83). Levine et al. (84) observed a significant increase in NEAT (1,380 ± 1,080 $kJ \cdot day^{-1}$) among individuals over feed 4,200 $kJ \cdot day^{-1}$ for 56 days. Although there are some arguments against this response (64), it is likely this component of TEE may be highly variable among individuals with different physical activity levels when in an energy surplus.

Finally, the influence dietary energy intake has on the anabolic hormonal environment is becoming better understood. It is now well-established that energy restriction can significantly influence anabolic hormones in exercising individuals, potentially impairing their ability to gain and maintain LBM (85). Although early research by Forbes and colleagues suggested that an energy surplus could improve anabolic hormone levels in women (86), few other studies have demonstrated significant increases in the hormonal environment in response to an energy surplus (87, 88). Irrespective, such acute elevations in circulating anabolic hormones may have little, if any, impact on resistance training adaptations (89, 90). Thus, any benefit of an energy surplus is likely mediated via mechanisms other than acutely influencing the anabolic hormonal environment.

What is clear from the existing literature is that there is yet to be defined a single evidence-based energy estimate for accretion of 1 kg of SMM. This is most likely because of the impact of individual presenting nuances (age, genetics, prior training experience, sex, body composition) as well as adaptation to the energy surplus. **Figure 2** provides a theoretical overview of the energy cost of generating SMM typically reported amongst resistance training individuals (91), the results of which are similar to that estimated previously (22). A better understanding of these variables and their impact on resistance training induced skeletal muscle hypertrophy may afford better individual prescription of the energy surplus. Until then, practitioners are advised to take a conservative approach to creating an energy surplus, within the range of ~1,500–2,000 $kJ \cdot day^{-1}$, to minimize FM gains, with regular review of body composition and functional capacities like strength to further personalize dietary intake.

ENERGY SURPLUS... MACRONUTRIENT CONSIDERATIONS

Within the constraints of an athlete's total daily energy intake, considering appropriate allocation of protein, carbohydrate, and fat may also have a measurable impact on skeletal muscle hypertrophy. Dietary protein has long been identified as a critical macronutrient to consider in skeletal muscle repair and synthesis. Indeed, resistance trained athletes have advocated high protein diets for many years (10). While debate continues on the need for additional protein amongst athletes, general guidelines now recommend that athletes undertaking resistance training ingest approximately twice the current recommendations for protein of their sedentary counterparts or as much as 1.6–2.2 $g \cdot kg^{-1} \cdot day^{-1}$ (92). In a recent meta-regression of 49 studies including 1,863 male and female participants, the protein intake associated with the greatest gains in muscle mass was 1.6 $g \cdot kg^{-1} \cdot day^{-1}$ (18). Exceeding this upper range of protein intake guidelines likely offers no further benefit and simply promotes increased amino acid catabolism and protein oxidation (14). Even extremely high protein intakes, up to double that advocated (18), does not further facilitate skeletal muscle hypertrophy or strength gains (93–95).

Despite a lack of apparent benefits from a high protein diet, athletes who are particularly sensitive to gains in FM may be tempted to source additional energy to facilitate an energy surplus from protein, given it is suggested to be less lipogenic, presumably because of increased DIT (96). However,

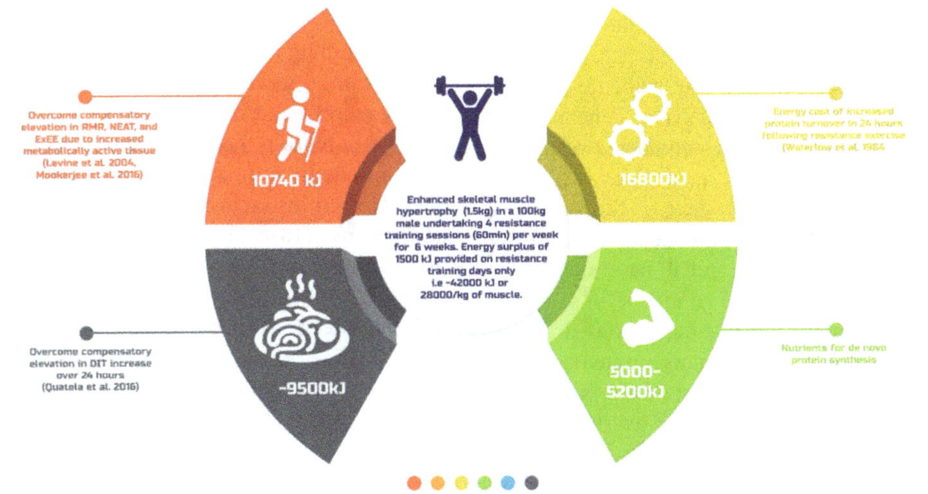
Overcome compensatory elevation in RMR, NEAT, and ExEE due to increased metabolically active tissue (Levine et al. 2004, Mookerjee et al. 2016)
10740 kJ
Enhanced skeletal muscle hypertrophy (1.5kg) in a 100kg male undertaking 4 resistance training sessions (60min) per week for 6 weeks. Energy surplus of 1500 kJ provided on resistance training days only i.e ~42000 kJ or 28000/kg of muscle.
16800kJ
Energy cost of increased protein turnover in 24 hours following resistance exercise (Waterlow et al. 1984
Overcome compensatory elevation in DIT increase over 24 hours (Quatela et al. 2016)
~9500kJ
5000-5200kJ
Nutrients for de novo protein synthesis

FIGURE 2 | A theoretical overview of the energy cost of generating skeletal muscle mass typically reported amongst resistance training individuals.

the impact on DIT is small in absolute terms and thus unlikely to significantly influence the response to an energy surplus (97). While it has been claimed protein, and thus energy intake, can be increased substantially without promoting gains in FM (93–95, 98), it is difficult to understand how this is possible, even after considering the impact on DIT. Indeed, tightly controlled research exploring the impact of variable protein intakes while overfeeding in a metabolic hospital ward confirms protein intake impacts lean mass while the energy surplus alone contributes to increases in FM, at least amongst sedentary individuals (23).

Despite previous concerns that high protein diets may be harmful, healthy adults with protein intakes of 1.8 $g{\cdot}kg^{-1}{\cdot}day^{-1}$ show no adverse effect on renal function (99). Furthermore, very high protein diets (2.5–3.3 $g{\cdot}kg^{-1}{\cdot}day^{-1}$) consumed over a year had no deleterious effects on blood lipids, liver, or renal function (100). However, the health implications of very high protein diets over longer periods is yet to be elucidated. Taken collectively, it is hard to justify the very high protein intakes consumed by some resistance training athletes, given the current lack of supporting research in enhancing resistance training adaptations, nor research confirming such high intakes are without health implications.

In addition to protein requirements, consideration must also be given to appropriate allocation of carbohydrate and fat in a meal plan attempting to facilitate muscle hypertrophy. Short term overfeeding studies in sedentary populations confirm there is no significant difference in body composition changes whether the energy surplus comes predominantly from carbohydrate or fat (101, 102). However, the metabolic implications of exercise must be considered amongst resistance trained individuals. Given the primary substrate used during resistance training is carbohydrate (103), it is logical to explore the provision of additional carbohydrate to help support training demands. This may be especially so for athletes other than weightlifters, powerlifters, and bodybuilders, where resistance training is typically undertaken as an ancillary form of training to complement sport specific training. Resistance training can reduce muscle glycogen stores by 30–40% (104). Therefore, larger volume, hypertrophy focused resistance training may necessitate additional carbohydrate to facilitate resistance training work capacity (105, 106) and restore muscle glycogen (107). While it is difficult to confirm further enhancement in acute training capacity (108) or chronic body composition adaptations (58), when contrasting a moderate vs. high carbohydrate intake, a chronic restrictive carbohydrate intake may impair resistance training adaptations. Indeed, SMM gains have consistently been impaired in studies of resistance trained individuals following high fat, "ketogenic" diets when compared to moderate intakes (109–111). Given this, it seems reasonable to continue to support carbohydrate intakes within the range of 4–7 $g{\cdot}kg^{-1}{\cdot}day^{-1}$ for strength trained athletes (112), with upper ranges advocated for those undertaking resistance exercise as an ancillary form of training to complement sport specific training.

The American College of Sports Medicine advises athletes to keep fat intakes in line with general health guidelines (113), which constitutes 20–35% of energy intake. Athletes should be discouraged from fat intakes below 15–20% of energy intake since such restrictions likely moderate the energy density of a meal plan, making it challenging to facilitate an energy surplus while also reducing intake and absorption of fat-soluble vitamins (114, 115). Furthermore, reducing dietary fat from 33.3 to 13.9% of total energy intake resulted in modest but significant reductions in resting testosterone concentrations (116), a result which has been replicated elsewhere (117, 118). However, the relevance of these small changes in circulating androgens is unknown in the context of chronic resistance training adaptation.

Given the energy density of fat is effectively double that of carbohydrate and protein, it is logical to consider increasing fat intake when attempting to increase the energy density of a meal plan. Indeed, within hypermetabolic clinical conditions such as cystic fibrosis requiring a high energy intake, increasing fat intake is advocated (119). Fat source may also determine the fate of excess energy, with polyunsaturated fat more likely to promote gains in lean mass compared to saturated fat, which is more likely to result in ectopic and general fat accumulation in normal weight volunteers (120). Evolving evidence suggests omega-3 polyunsaturated fatty acid ingestion enhances the anabolic response to nutritional stimuli and increases muscle mass and function in young and middle-aged males (121), plus older adults (122), respectively, independent of the resistance training stimuli. There are also health benefits to consider in the type of fat consumed. Postprandial fat oxidation is higher after monounsaturated (olive oil) compared to saturated (cream) fat meals (123). Simply substituting saturated fat for unsaturated fat, predominantly as monounsaturated fat, was enough to induce favorable improvements in lipid profile and reductions in fat mass in a small sample of overweight and obese males (124). Whilst interesting, further research is required to determine whether the potential benefits in the type of fat ingested are maintained in an athletic population undergoing resistance training in an energy surplus and whether this influences the quality of weight gain. Until then, international recommendations indicate that active individuals may consume up to 35% of their daily energy intake from dietary fat, with saturated fatty acids not exceeding 10% of total energy intake (114).

The type of foods from which macronutrients are sourced may also have implications on lean mass gains. Protein type is important as high biological value protein sources rich in leucine are recommended to maximize protein synthetic rates (125). Consumption of protein in its natural whole-food matrix may also differentially stimulate muscle anabolic properties compared to isolated proteins particularly post resistance training (126). This has been observed with whole milk compared to skim milk (127), and whole eggs compared to egg whites (126). Thus, additional nutrients found in whole foods may offer advantages beyond their amino acid profile to maximize protein synthesis (128), although more research is required to ascertain how this occurs and if benefits remain when total dietary protein and energy is matched.

In conclusion, insufficient data exists to promote an energy surplus that comes primarily from any specific macronutrient. Thus, without further research we can only emphasize that the minimum intakes of macronutrients advised in this section be achieved while ensuring an appropriate energy surplus. Preliminary evidence suggests extra protein may be less lipogenic, perhaps because of an increase in energy expenditure associated with DIT, although this needs to be confirmed with better controlled studies on resistance training populations and may need to merely be corrected by further increasing energy intake if the same energy surplus is desired. Furthermore, the health implications of sustained protein intakes above $\sim$2.5 g·kg^{-1}·day^{-1} remain to be validated. As such, other factors such as individual preference, allocation of extra energy over the day relative to resistance training, existing energy density of the meal plan and potential for increasing the volume of existing food/ fluid intake may be a higher priority when considering the source of any prescribed energy surplus.

ENERGY SURPLUS... NUTRIENT TIMING

Nutrient timing has received significant attention in recent years (129), with interventions aiming to optimize work capacity during exercise and/or facilitate training adaptations. Specifically, primary attention has been given to the timing of protein and carbohydrate intake to support acute fuelling and recovery goals (130), plus facilitate chronic skeletal muscle hypertrophy adaptations (18). However, whenever daily macronutrient distribution is adjusted, so too potentially is energy intake. Thus, the influence of daily energy distribution, including the number of eating occasions, also warrants consideration.

Athletes are encouraged to pay attention to dietary intake pre, during and post exercise, under the assumption that nutritional strategies can influence both acute resistance exercise capacity and/ or training induced adaptations. Indeed, evidence is present for a beneficial role of acute carbohydrate ingestion before and/ or during strength training (105, 131). However, not all investigations show a benefit of acute carbohydrate ingestion (132–134), suggesting the ergogenic potential for carbohydrate ingestion is most likely to be observed when athletes are undertaking longer-duration, high-volume resistance training in isolation, or when resistance training is incorporated into a higher volume total training load that also includes sports specific training. Currently, specific recommendations for an optimum rate or timing of carbohydrate ingestion for resistance trained athletes before and during a resistance training session cannot be made within broader guidance of 4–7 g·kg^{-1} body mass daily (112). However, this warrants investigation given the potential for enhanced substrate availability, plus better alignment of energy intake to expenditure.

The consumption of high biological value protein containing meals/snacks in close proximity to training is widely applied as a strategy to augment the skeletal muscle adaptive response to resistance exercise (135). Less is known about the impact of protein distribution in the meal plan outside of the acute period before and/or after exercise ($<$3 h). There is some evidence to suggest that skeletal MPS may be enhanced with a wider distribution of daily protein intake compared with an acute bolus of protein (17). Indeed, spacing protein-containing meals ($\sim$0.3 g·kg^{-1} of high biological value protein) every 3–5 h throughout the waking period of the day has been advocated when attempting to maximizes MPS (92), although this remains to be validated amongst resistance trained individuals when ingesting protein as part of mixed macronutrient meals while in energy balance or surplus. Indeed, increasing daily distribution of high biological value protein from four to six meals per day had no influence of pre-season gains in lean body mass amongst a group of rugby athletes (91), suggesting a threshold of daily protein containing meals, above which there is likely no further enhancement in skeletal muscle hypertrophy when in energy balance/surplus, perhaps due to the hypothesized refractory period that follows acute protein ingestion (136).

While skeletal MPS is unlikely to be further enhanced by more frequent eating occasions, smaller more frequent eating occasions (5–6+) are advocated when attempting to increase muscle mass, presumably because gastrointestinal tract tolerance is higher with more frequent eating occasions compared to merely increasing the size of existing eating occasions (31). Indeed, smaller, more frequent meals are advocated clinically in the management of early satiety, anorexia and gastrointestinal symptoms (137). Emerging evidence supports this notion, with significantly stronger hunger and desire to eat when following a smaller, more frequent eating pattern (138). This is corroborated by preliminary data in elite athletes, with a moderate association between meal frequency and total energy intake (139). Given that snacks accounted for approximately one-quarter of total energy intake in this athletic population, it seems pertinent to advocate the inclusion of snacks in the meal pattern of athletes attempting to increase overall energy intake. Current evidence suggests athletes ingest food daily typically over ~5 eating occasions, including the three main meals, plus snacks (139, 140). The impact of eating occasion frequency on overall nutrient intake and subsequent resistance training outcomes warrants investigation in athletic populations. Until then, athletes are encouraged to consume a minimum of 3 main meals, with the use of strategic snacks to support fuelling and recovery goals, plus facilitate skeletal MPS.

Similar to the general population (141), athletes allocate more of their daily energy intake to the later part of the day (140, 142). The impact of better alignment of daily energy intake to expenditure, or within day energy balance, is an emerging area of research interest focused on the physiological implications of real-time changes in energy intake and expenditure. Preliminary research suggests unfavorable metabolic and endocrine perturbations with large acute or extended energy deficits amongst athletes focused on leanness (143–145). The implications of manipulating within day energy balance amongst resistance training athletes attempting to promote quality weight gain has not been investigated but warrants consideration.

There is some preliminary evidence to suggest better alignment of energy intake to expenditure may have application in facilitating resistance training outcomes. Ingestion of a creatine monohydrate containing carbohydrate-protein supplement immediately before and after resistance training results in more favorable resistance training adaptations than when the same supplement is ingested away from training (146), although this is not always evident, at least when a lower energy, protein only supplement is ingested according to a similar time frame (147). While it is impossible to ascribe this effect to the timing of macronutrient or energy intake, this approach toward optimizing nutrition support before and after a resistance training session also supports general fuelling and recovery goals. It also better aligns acute energy intake to expenditure, given daily energy expenditure is likely highest during exercise.

For athletes focused on facilitating quality weight gain, consideration of temporal energy patterns may also be warranted given preliminary research suggesting an association between eating more of the day's total energy intake at night and obesity (148, 149). This may be due to the metabolic dysfunction induced by delayed eating, even amongst normal weight individuals (150), or it may merely reflect behavioral mechanisms that influence appetite control (151). Indeed, intake in the late night also appears to lack satiating value, resulting in greater overall daily intake (152). While tempting to advocate athletes to "front end" more of the daily energy intake, especially amongst individuals aiming to minimize fat mass gains, moderating energy intake as the day progresses may be inappropriate for those with high energy needs and/ or those with significant training commitments in the evening. Indeed, there is evidence of enhanced strength and muscle mass gains from resistance training undertaken in the evening when two protein containing meals are ingested prior to bed compared to one (153). As such, manipulation of daily energy distribution should merely be a variable practitioners consider when providing advice to athletes, adjusting according to the individual athlete and their unique circumstances, including specific energy needs, timing of training, and nutrition goals. The influence of daily energy distribution warrants investigation amongst resistance trained athletes attempting to facilitate quality weight gain.

While it is logical to encourage energy intake to vary over a training week to reflect exercise energy expenditure, athletes do not always adjust intake to reflect expenditure (154), perhaps in part because of the variable impact exercise has on appetite (155). If the creation of a positive energy balance is desired to facilitate resistance training adaptations, one variable to consider is whether that energy surplus should be applied throughout the week or just on resistance training days. Supplemental energy has typically only been provided on resistance training days in the limited research in which a positive energy balance has been achieved in conjunction with resistance training (57). While this better mirrors energy intake to expenditure, it could be argued given that skeletal MPS is elevated for upwards of 48 h following a single resistance training session (43), that a positive energy balance is also warranted for upwards of 24–48 h post training. Presumably the creation of a positive energy balance on both resistance training and non-training days may help to optimize the potential for enhanced skeletal muscle hypertrophy. This issue warrants further investigation in resistance trained populations, especially amongst those individuals aiming to facilitate quality weight gain. The concept of intermittent energy restriction shows preliminary potential for facilitating more effective quality weight loss by moderating any associated metabolic adjustments (156). It would be interesting to explore if the reverse was also true with the intermittent application of a positive energy balance for facilitating quality weight gain. Indeed, there is preliminary evidence to suggest an acute energy surplus (facilitated via an increase in all macronutrients) results in preferential gains in fat free mass (157).

MANAGING SATIETY

Attempts to increase total energy intake by merely increasing the total volume of food ingested may result in early satiety, limiting the potential for creation of an energy surplus. Thus, consideration may need to be given to increasing the energy density of the meal plan. While increasing dietary fat intake is a logical option, other novel strategies to better manage early satiety include changing the food form. For example, regardless of the predominant energy source, drinks have lower satiety than solid foods and thus, provide greater potential for facilitating a positive energy balance (158, 159). Furthermore, nutritious drinks can be particularly practical following exercise when the appetite may be suppressed, while also supporting nutritional recovery goals. A high intake of low energy density vegetables may also moderate total energy intake at a meal (160). However, given the health benefits of individuals achieving public health guidance on vegetable intake (161), practitioners are advised to balance the pursuit of enhancing energy density with overall health benefits of the meal plan. Advocating the ingestion of only moderate servings of protein rich foods at meals may also be appropriate, given the satiating effect of protein (162), although the implications of higher protein meals on satiety when in a positive energy balance remain to be confirmed. However, given moderate protein servings will also help optimize the skeletal muscle protein synthetic response (92), guidance on moderated protein servings appears logical.

FUTURE DIRECTIONS

Further research into this area is clearly warranted, but challenged by individual responsiveness, including the potential for rapid metabolic adjustment to the energy surplus and the need to consider not only the energy surplus, but potentially where that energy comes from and how it is allocated in the meal plan over the day relative to the resistance training stimulus. Methodological issues associated with the quantification of key outcome measures such as energy intake, energy expenditure and body composition are also very relevant when attempting to interpret the literature. For example, an increase in dietary carbohydrate intake to facilitate a positive energy balance will acutely increase muscle metabolites and associated water content, significantly influencing estimates of body composition via dual energy x-ray absorptiometry (163), and other commonly used techniques, including air displacement plethysmography and bioimpedance analysis (164), while acute resistance exercise induced water retention can influence magnetic resonance imaging estimates of muscle cross-sectional area for at least 52 h (165). Given such physique assessment nuances, concurrent review of associated functional capacity adaptations would appear pertinent for future investigations.

Several gaps in the literature have been identified in this review, which warrant further exploration. Some of these are expanded upon here in the hope of facilitating research interest in this area. A broader understanding of these issues has the potential to not only impact on dietary guidance for athletic populations, but also clinical populations where retention or promotion of SMM is advocated.

Should the Prescribed Energy Surplus Be Adjusted Based on the Anticipated Muscle Hypertrophy Potential of the Athlete?

Younger, less experienced athletes have a greater potential for skeletal muscle hypertrophy in response to resistance training than their more experienced counterparts (38). It could be argued that if the energy surplus is merely required to contribute the building blocks of newly generated tissue, then the prescribed energy surplus should be adjusted based on muscle hypertrophy potential. Preliminary research in a small group of elite Norwegian athletes supports this hypothesis (166). However, if the energy surplus facilitates a physiological response that amplifies the anabolic signal created by resistance training, then perhaps the energy surplus should be maintained in experienced athletes, at least in these where muscle hypertrophy and strength gains are prioritized over short term FM increments.

What Factors Influence Whether Endogenous and/or Exogenous Energy Sources Can Support the Energy Cost of Muscle Hypertrophy?

The presence of muscle hypertrophy in response to resistance training while in an energy deficit clearly confirms the energy cost of hypertrophy can be obtained endogenously (34, 55, 56), but is more likely evident amongst resistance training naïve, overweight individuals. Thus, individual nuances such as presenting energy status and training history may need to be considered when prescribing energy intake.

Does Better Temporal Alignment of Daily Energy Intake to Expenditure (Within Day and Between Day) Result in More Favorable Gains in FFM Relative to FM When in an Energy Surplus?

While preliminary research suggests unfavorable metabolic and endocrine perturbations with large acute, within day energy deficits amongst athletes (144, 145), less is known about the potential benefit of better aligning daily energy intake to expenditure when in an energy surplus. Encouraging preliminary research indicates a more favorable response to resistance training when more of the daily energy intake is allocated immediately before and after exercise (146). The influence of better aligning daily energy intake to expenditure across a training week also warrants investigation, the results of which would help to identify if any energy surplus should be applied on raining days only or throughout the training week.

CONCLUSIONS

The creation of an energy surplus is commonly advocated by sports nutrition practitioners when attempting to optimize resistance training induced skeletal muscle hypertrophy. Such guidance is often based solely on the assumed energy stored within the tissue being assimilated. Unfortunately, this fails to account for other energetically expensive processes, including the energy cost of tissue generation, plus the metabolic adjustments that occur in response to an energy surplus. An appreciation of the magnitude of these factors would provide greater insight into appropriate energy prescription to facilitate optimal rates of muscle hypertrophy while minimizing fat mass gain. Until that time, practitioners are advised to start conservatively with an energy surplus within the range of ~1,500–2,000 kJ·day^{-1} and closely monitor response to the intervention, using changes in body composition and functional capacity to further personalize dietary interventions. So long as minimum guidelines for macronutrients advocated for resistance training individuals are achieved, there does not appear to be any metabolic or functional benefit to the source of the energy surplus, affording the practitioner an opportunity to adjust intake based on other variables such as existing energy density of the meal plan, eating occasions and distribution of energy, and macronutrient intake relative to training, plus potential for further increasing food intake.

AUTHOR CONTRIBUTIONS

BD, DM, EH, GS, GJS, and JI drafted, critically reviewed, and revised the manuscript for important intellectual content, contributed to manuscript revision, read, and approved the submitted version.

REFERENCES

1. Brechue WF, Abe T. The role of FFM accumulation and skeletal muscle architecture in powerlifting performance. *Eur J Appl Physiol.* (2002) 86:327–36. doi: 10.1007/s00421-001-0543-7
2. Siahkouhian M, Hedayatneja M. Correlations of anthropometric and body composition variables with the performance of young elite weightlifters. *J Hum Kinet.* (2010) 25:125–31. doi: 10.2478/v10078-010-0040-3
3. Bell W, Evans WD, Cobner DM, Eston RG. Regional placement of bone mineral mass, fat mass, and lean soft tissue mass in young adult rugby union players. *Ergonomics.* (2005) 48:1462–72. doi: 10.1080/00140130500101007
4. Olds T. The evolution of physique in male rugby union players in the twentieth century. *J Sports Sci.* (2001) 19:253–62. doi: 10.1080/026404101750158312
5. Barr MJ, Newton RU, Sheppard JM. Were height and mass related to performance at the 2007 and 2011 rugby world cups? *Int J Sports Sci Coach.* (2014) 9:671–80. doi: 10.1260/1747-9541.9.4.671
6. Waldron M, Worsfold P, Twist C, Lamb K. Changes in anthropometry and performance, and their interrelationships, across three seasons in elite youth rugby league players. *J Strength Cond Res.* (2014) 28:3128–36. doi: 10.1519/JSC.0000000000000445
7. Alway SE, MacDougall JD, Sale DG, Sutton JR, McComas AJ. Functional and structural adaptations in skeletal muscle of trained athletes. *J Appl Physiol.* (1988) 64:1114–20. doi: 10.1152/jappl.1988.64.3.1114
8. Barr MJ, Sheppard JM, Gabbett TJ, Newton RU. Long-term training-induced changes in sprinting speed and sprint momentum in elite rugby union players. *J Strength Cond Res.* (2014) 28:2724–31. doi: 10.1519/JSC.0000000000000364
9. Frontera WR, Ochala J. Skeletal muscle: a brief review of structure and function. *Calcif Tissue Int.* (2015) 96:183–95. doi: 10.1007/s00223-014-9915-y
10. Mitchell L, Hackett D, Gifford J, Estermann F, O'Connor H. Do bodybuilders use evidence-based nutrition strategies to manipulate physique? *Sports.* (2017) 5:E76. doi: 10.3390/sports5040076
11. Morton RW, McGlory C, Phillips SM. Nutritional interventions to augment resistance training-induced skeletal muscle hypertrophy. *Front Physiol.* (2015) 6:245. doi: 10.3389/fphys.2015.00245
12. Tarnopolsky MA, Atkinson SA, MacDougall JD, Chesley A, Phillips S, Schwarcz HP. Evaluation of protein requirements for trained strength athletes. *J Appl Physiol.* (1992) 73:1986–95. doi: 10.1152/jappl.1992.73.5.1986
13. Moore DR, Robinson MJ, Fry JL, Tang JE, Glover EI, Wilkinson SB, et al. Ingested protein dose response of muscle and albumin protein synthesis after resistance exercise in young men. *Am J Clin Nutr.* (2009) 89:161–8. doi: 10.3945/ajcn.2008.26401
14. Witard OC, Jackman SR, Breen L, Smith K, Selby A, Tipton KD. Myofibrillar muscle protein synthesis rates subsequent to a meal in response to increasing doses of whey protein at rest and after resistance exercise. *Am J Clin Nutr.* (2014) 99:86–95. doi: 10.3945/ajcn.112.055517
15. Macnaughton LS, Wardle SL, Witard OC, McGlory C, Hamilton DL, Jeromson S, et al. The response of muscle protein synthesis following whole-body resistance exercise is greater following 40 g than 20 g of ingested whey protein. *Physiol Rep.* (2016) 4:e12893. doi: 10.14814/phy2.12893
16. Devries MC, Phillips SM. Supplemental protein in support of muscle mass and health: advantage whey. *J Food Sci.* (2015) 80(Suppl. 1):A8–15. doi: 10.1111/1750-3841.12802
17. Areta JL, Burke LM, Ross ML, Camera DM, West DW, Broad EM, et al. Timing and distribution of protein ingestion during prolonged recovery from resistance exercise alters myofibrillar protein synthesis. *J Physiol.* (2013) 591:2319–31. doi: 10.1113/jphysiol.2012.244897
18. Morton RW, Murphy KT, McKellar SR, Schoenfeld BJ, Henselmans M, Helms E, et al. A systematic review, meta-analysis and meta-regression of the effect of protein supplementation on resistance training-induced gains in muscle mass and strength in healthy adults. *Br J Sports Med.* (2018) 52:376–84. doi: 10.1136/bjsports-2017-097608
19. Grandjean A. Nutritional requirements to increase lean mass. *Clin Sports Med.* (1999) 18:623–32. doi: 10.1016/S0278-5919(05)70172-1
20. Houston ME. Gaining weight: the scientific basis of increasing skeletal muscle mass. *Can J Appl Physiol.* (1999) 24:305–16. doi: 10.1139/h99-024
21. Kreider RB. Dietary supplements and the promotion of muscle growth with resistance exercise. *Sports Med.* (1999) 27:97–110. doi: 10.2165/00007256-199927020-00003
22. Forbes GB, Brown MR, Welle SL, Lipinski BA. Deliberate overfeeding in women and men: energy cost and composition of the weight gain. *Br J Nutr.* (1986) 56:1–9. doi: 10.1079/BJN19860080
23. Bray GA, Smith SR, de Jonge L, Xie H, Rood J, Martin CK, et al. Effect of dietary protein content on weight gain, energy expenditure, and body composition during overeating: a randomized controlled trial. *JAMA.* (2012) 307:47–55. doi: 10.1001/jama.2011.1918
24. Churchward-Venne TA, Murphy CH, Longland TM, Phillips SM. Role of protein and amino acids in promoting lean mass accretion with resistance exercise and attenuating lean mass loss during energy deficit in humans. *Amino Acids.* (2013) 45:231–40. doi: 10.1007/s00726-013-1506-0
25. Bray GA, Redman LM, de Jonge L, Covington J, Rood J, Brock C, et al. Effect of protein overfeeding on energy expenditure measured in a metabolic chamber. *Am J Clin Nutr.* (2015) 101:496–505. doi: 10.3945/ajcn.114.091769
26. Gorissen SH, Burd NA, Hamer HM, Gijsen AP, Groen BB, van Loon LJ. Carbohydrate coingestion delays dietary protein digestion and absorption but does not modulate postprandial muscle protein accretion. *J Clin Endocrinol Metab.* (2014) 99:2250–8. doi: 10.1210/jc.2013-3970
27. Koopman R, Beelen M, Stellingwerff T, Pennings B, Saris WH, Kies AK, et al. Coingestion of carbohydrate with protein does not further augment postexercise muscle protein synthesis. *Am J Physiol Endocrinol Metab.* (2007) 293:E833–42. doi: 10.1152/ajpendo.00135.2007
28. Glynn EL, Fry CS, Timmerman KL, Drummond MJ, Volpi E, Rasmussen BB. Addition of carbohydrate or alanine to an essential amino acid mixture does not enhance human skeletal muscle protein anabolism. *J Nutr.* (2013) 143:307–14. doi: 10.3945/jn.112.168203
29. Manore M, Meyer N, Thompson J. Achieving healthy body weight. In: *Sport Nutiriton for Health and Performance.* 2nd ed. Champaogn, IL: Human Kinetics (2009). p. 167–204.
30. Williams MH, Anderson DE, Rawson ES. Weight gaining through proper nutrition and exercise. In: *Nutrition for Health, Fitness and Sport.* 10th ed. New York, NY: McGraw Hill (2013). p. 517–44.
31. Moore D, Phillips S, Slater G. Protein. In: Burke L, Deakin V, editors. *Clinical Sports Nutrition.* 5th ed. North Ryde, NSW: McGRaw Hill (2015). p. 94–113.

32. Dunford M, Macedonio MA. Weight management. In: Karpinski C, Rosenbloom CA, editors. *Sports Nutrition. A Handbook for Professionals.* Chicago, IL: Academy of Nutrition and Dietetics (2018). p. 218–37.
33. Josse AR, Tang JE, Tarnopolsky MA, Phillips SM. Body composition and strength changes in women with milk and resistance exercise. *Med Sci Sports Exerc.* (2010) 42:1122–30. doi: 10.1249/MSS.0b013e3181c854f6
34. Longland TM, Oikawa SY, Mitchell CJ, Devries MC, Phillips SM. Higher compared with lower dietary protein during an energy deficit combined with intense exercise promotes greater lean mass gain and fat mass loss: a randomized trial. *Am J Clin Nutr.* (2016) 103:738–46. doi: 10.3945/ajcn.115.119339
35. Zemski AJ, Keating SE, Broad EM, Marsh DJ, Hind K, Slater GJ. Preseason body composition adaptations in elite white and polynesian rugby union athletes. *Int J Sport Nutr Exerc Metab.* (2018) 29, 9–17. doi: 10.1123/ijsnem.2018-0059
36. Haakonssen EC, Martin DT, Burke LM, Jenkins DG. Increased lean mass with reduced fat mass in an elite female cyclist returning to competition: case study. *Int J Sports Physiol Perform.* (2013) 8:699–701. doi: 10.1123/ijspp.8.6.699
37. Milsom J, Barreira P, Burgess DJ, Iqbal Z, Morton JP. Case study: muscle atrophy and hypertrophy in a premier league soccer player during rehabilitation from ACL injury. *Int J Sport Nutr Exerc Metab.* (2014) 24:543–52. doi: 10.1123/ijsnem.2013-0209
38. Jones B, Till K, Roe G, O'Hara J, Lees M, Barlow MJ, et al. Six-year body composition change in male elite senior rugby league players. *J Sports Sci.* (2018) 36:266–71. doi: 10.1080/02640414.2017.1300313
39. Elia M, Stubbs RJ, Henry CJ. Differences in fat, carbohydrate, and protein metabolism between lean and obese subjects undergoing total starvation. *Obes Res.* (1999) 7:597–604. doi: 10.1002/j.1550-8528.1999.tb00720.x
40. Bouchard C, Tchernof A, Tremblay A. Predictors of body composition and body energy changes in response to chronic overfeeding. *Int J Obes.* (2014) 38:236–42. doi: 10.1038/ijo.2013.77
41. Till K, Jones B, Darrall-Jones J, Emmonds S, Cooke C. Longitudinal development of anthropometric and physical characteristics within academy rugby league players. *J Strength Cond Res.* (2015) 29:1713–22. doi: 10.1519/JSC.0000000000000792
42. Biolo G, Tipton KD, Klein S, Wolfe RR. An abundant supply of amino acids enhances the metabolic effect of exercise on muscle protein. *Am J Physiol.* (1997) 273:E122–9. doi: 10.1152/ajpendo.1997.273.1.E122
43. Phillips SM, Tipton KD, Aarsland A, Wolf SE, Wolfe RR. Mixed muscle protein synthesis and breakdown after resistance exercise in humans. *Am J Physiol.* (1997) 273:E99–107. doi: 10.1152/ajpendo.1997.273.1.E99
44. Burd NA, West DW, Moore DR, Atherton PJ, Staples AW, Prior T, et al. Enhanced amino acid sensitivity of myofibrillar protein synthesis persists for up to 24 h after resistance exercise in young men. *J Nutr.* (2011) 141:568–73. doi: 10.3945/jn.110.135038
45. Bouchard C, Tremblay A, Despres JP, Nadeau A, Lupien PJ, Theriault G, et al. The response to long-term overfeeding in identical twins. *N Engl J Med.* (1990) 322:1477–82. doi: 10.1056/NEJM199005243222101
46. Leaf A, Antonio J. The effects of overfeeding on body composition: the role of macronutrient composition - a narrative review. *Int J Exerc Sci.* (2017) 10:1275–96.
47. Goldberg AL, Etlinger JD, Goldspink DF, Jablecki C. Mechanism of work-induced hypertrophy of skeletal muscle. *Med Sci Sports.* (1975) 7:185–98. doi: 10.1249/00005768-197500730-00016
48. Gonzalez AM, Hoffman JR, Stout JR, Fukuda DH, Willoughby DS. Intramuscular anabolic signaling and endocrine response following resistance exercise: implications for muscle hypertrophy. *Sports Med.* (2016) 46:671–85. doi: 10.1007/s40279-015-0450-4
49. Wackerhage H, Schoenfeld BJ, Hamilton DL, Lehti M, Hulmi JJ. Stimuli and sensors that initiate skeletal muscle hypertrophy following resistance exercise. *J Appl Physiol.* (2019) 126:30–43. doi: 10.1152/japplphysiol.00685.2018
50. Hackett DA, Johnson NA, Chow CM. Training practices and ergogenic aids used by male bodybuilders. *J Strength Cond Res.* (2013) 27:1609–17. doi: 10.1519/JSC.0b013e318271272a
51. Kreider RB, Kalman DS, Antonio J, Ziegenfuss TN, Wildman R, Collins R, et al. International Society of Sports Nutrition position stand: safety and efficacy of creatine supplementation in exercise, sport, and medicine. *J Int Soc Sports Nutr.* (2017) 14:18. doi: 10.1186/s12970-017-0173-z
52. Bier DM. The energy costs of protein metabolism: lean and mean on uncle Sam's team. In: Poos MI, Costello R, Carlson-Newberry SJ, editors. *The Role of Protein and Amino Acids in Sustaining and Enhancing Performance.* Washington, DC: National Acadamies Press (1999). p. 109–19.
53. Pasiakos SM, Vislocky LM, Carbone JW, Altieri N, Konopelski K, Freake HC, et al. Acute energy deprivation affects skeletal muscle protein synthesis and associated intracellular signaling proteins in physically active adults. *J Nutr.* (2010) 140:745–51. doi: 10.3945/jn.109.118372
54. Areta JL, Burke LM, Camera DM, West DW, Crawshay S, Moore DR, et al. Reduced resting skeletal muscle protein synthesis is rescued by resistance exercise and protein ingestion following short-term energy deficit. *Am J Physiol Endocrinol Metab.* (2014) 306:E989–97. doi: 10.1152/ajpendo.00590.2013
55. Donnelly JE, Sharp T, Houmard J, Carlson MG, Hill JO, Whatley JE, et al. Muscle hypertrophy with large-scale weight loss and resistance training. *Am J Clin Nutr.* (1993) 58:561–5. doi: 10.1093/ajcn/58.4.561
56. Nindl BC, Harman EA, Marx JO, Gotshalk LA, Frykman PN, Lammi E, et al. Regional body composition changes in women after 6 months of periodized physical training. *J Appl Physiol.* (2000) 88:2251–9. doi: 10.1152/jappl.2000.88.6.2251
57. Rozenek R, Ward P, Long S, Garhammer J. Effects of high-calorie supplements on body composition and muscular strength following resistance training. *J Sports Med Phys Fitness.* (2002) 42:340–7.
58. Rinehardt KF. Effects of diet on muscle and strength gains during resistive training. In: Garrett WE, Malone TR, editors. *Ross Symposium on Muscle Development: Nutritional Alternatives to Anabolic Steroids.* Columbus, OH: Ross (1988). p. 78–83.
59. Ribeiro AS, Nunes JP, Schoenfeld BJ, Aguiar AF, Cyrino ES. Effects of different dietary energy intake following resistance training on muscle mass and body fat in bodybuilders: a pilot study. *J Hum Kinet.* (2019). [Epub ahead of print].
60. Hamilton DL, Philp A. Can AMPK mediated suppression of mTORC1 explain the concurrent training effect? *Cell Mol Exerc Physiol.* (2013) 2:e4. doi: 10.7457/cmep.v2i1.e4
61. Joosen AM, Westerterp KR. Energy expenditure during overfeeding. *Nutr Metab.* (2006) 3:25. doi: 10.1186/1743-7075-3-25
62. Forbes Dagger GB. Some adventures in body composition, with special reference to nutrition. *Acta Diabetol.* (2003) 40(suppl 1):S238–41. doi: 10.1007/s00592-003-0075-1
63. Spady DW, Payne PR, Picou D, Waterlow JC. Energy balance during recovery from malnutrition. *Am J Clin Nutr.* (1976) 29:1073–88. doi: 10.1093/ajcn/29.10.1073
64. Stock MJ. Gluttony and thermogenesis revisited. *Int J Obes Relat Metab Disord.* (1999) 23:1105–17. doi: 10.1038/sj.ijo.0801108
65. Chow CC, Hall KD. The dynamics of human body weight change. *PLoS Comput Biol.* (2008) 4:e1000045. doi: 10.1371/journal.pcbi.1000045
66. Thomas DM, Martin CK, Heymsfield S, Redman LM, Schoeller DA, Levine JA. A simple model predicting individual weight change in humans. *J Biol Dyn.* (2011) 5:579–99. doi: 10.1080/17513758.2010.508541
67. Scott CB, Leighton BH, Ahearn KJ, McManus JJ. Aerobic, anaerobic, and excess postexercise oxygen consumption energy expenditure of muscular endurance and strength: 1-set of bench press to muscular fatigue. *J Strength Cond Res.* (2011) 25:903–8. doi: 10.1519/JSC.0b013e3181c6a128
68. Mookerjee S, Welikonich MJ, Ratamess NA. Comparison of energy expenditure during single-set vs. multiple-set resistance exercise. *J Strength Cond Res.* (2016) 30:1447–52. doi: 10.1519/JSC.00000000000001230
69. Roberson KB, Jacobs KA, White MJ, Signorile JF. Loads and movement speed affect energy expenditure during circuit resistance exercise. *Appl Physiol Nutr Metab.* (2017) 42:637–46. doi: 10.1139/apnm-2016-0552
70. Rawson ES, Walsh TM. Estimation of resistance exercise energy expenditure using accelerometry. *Med Sci Sports Exerc.* (2010) 42:622–8. doi: 10.1249/MSS.0b013e3181b64ef3
71. Stec MJ, Rawson ES. Estimation of resistance exercise energy expenditure using triaxial accelerometry. *J Strength Cond Res.* (2012) 26:1413–22. doi: 10.1519/JSC.0b013e318248d7b4

72. Lytle JR, Kravits DM, Martin SE, Green JS, Crouse SF, Lambert BS. Predicting energy expenditure of an acute resistance exercise. *Med Sci Sports Exerc.* (2019) 51:1532–7. doi: 10.1249/MSS.0000000000001925
73. Proud CG. Regulation of mammalian translation factors by nutrients. *Eur J Biochem.* (2002) 269:5338–49. doi: 10.1046/j.1432-1033.2002.03292.x
74. Browne GJ, Proud CG. Regulation of peptide-chain elongation in mammalian cells. *Eur J Biochem.* (2002) 269:5360–8. doi: 10.1046/j.1432-1033.2002.03290.x
75. Waterlow JC. Protein turnover with special reference to man. *Q J Exp Physiol.* (1984) 69:409–38. doi: 10.1113/expphysiol.1984.sp002829
76. Elia M. Organ and tissue contribution to metabolic rate. In: Kinney JM, Tucker HN, editors. *Energy Metabolism: Tissue Determinants and Cellular Corollaries.* New York, NY: Raven (1992). p. 61–80.
77. Illner K, Brinkmann G, Heller M, Bosy-Westphal A, Muller MJ. Metabolically active components of fat free mass and resting energy expenditure in nonobese adults. *Am J Physiol Endocrinol Metab.* (2000) 278:E308–15. doi: 10.1152/ajpendo.2000.278.2.E308
78. MacKenzie-Shalders KL, Byrne NM, King NA, Slater GJ. Are increases in skeletal muscle mass accompanied by changes to resting metabolic rate in rugby athletes over a pre-season training period? *Eur J Sport Sci.* (2019) 19:885–92. doi: 10.1080/17461391.2018.1561951
79. Muller MJ, Enderle J, Pourhassan M, Braun W, Eggeling B, Lagerpusch M, et al. Metabolic adaptation to caloric restriction and subsequent refeeding: the Minnesota Starvation Experiment revisited. *Am J Clin Nutr.* (2015) 102:807–19. doi: 10.3945/ajcn.115.109173
80. Muller MJ, Enderle J, Bosy-Westphal A. Changes in energy expenditure with weight gain and weight loss in humans. *Curr Obes Rep.* (2016) 5:413–23. doi: 10.1007/s13679-016-0237-4
81. Raben A, Agerholm-Larsen L, Flint A, Holst JJ, Astrup A. Meals with similar energy densities but rich in protein, fat, carbohydrate, or alcohol have different effects on energy expenditure and substrate metabolism but not on appetite and energy intake. *Am J Clin Nutr.* (2003) 77:91–100. doi: 10.1093/ajcn/77.1.91
82. Quatela A, Callister R, Patterson A, MacDonald-Wicks L. The energy content and composition of meals consumed after an overnight fast and their effects on diet induced thermogenesis: a systematic review, meta-analyses and meta-regressions. *Nutrients.* (2016) 8:E670. doi: 10.3390/nu8110670
83. Levine JA. Nonexercise activity thermogenesis (NEAT): environment and biology. *Am J Physiol Endocrinol Metab.* (2004) 286:E675–85. doi: 10.1152/ajpendo.00562.2003
84. Levine JA, Eberhardt NL, Jensen MD. Role of nonexercise activity thermogenesis in resistance to fat gain in humans. *Science.* (1999) 283:212–4. doi: 10.1126/science.283.5399.212
85. Mountjoy M, Sundgot-Borgen J, Burke L, Carter S, Constantini N, Lebrun C, et al. The IOC consensus statement: beyond the Female Athlete Triad–Relative Energy Deficiency in Sport (RED-S). *Br J Sports Med.* (2014) 48:491–7. doi: 10.1136/bjsports-2014-093502
86. Forbes GB, Brown MR, Welle SL, Underwood LE. Hormonal response to overfeeding. *Am J Clin Nutr.* (1989) 49:608–11. doi: 10.1093/ajcn/49.4.608
87. Pritchard J, Despres JP, Gagnon J, Tchernof A, Nadeau A, Tremblay A, et al. Plasma adrenal, gonadal, and conjugated steroids before and after long-term overfeeding in identical twins. *J Clin Endocrinol Metab.* (1998) 83:3277–84. doi: 10.1210/jc.83.9.3277
88. Sato K, Samocha-Bonet D, Handelsman DJ, Fujita S, Wittert GA, Heilbronn LK. Serum sex steroids and steroidogenesis-related enzyme expression in skeletal muscle during experimental weight gain in men. *Diabetes Metab.* (2014) 40:439–44. doi: 10.1016/j.diabet.2014.03.006
89. West DW, Phillips SM. Associations of exercise-induced hormone profiles and gains in strength and hypertrophy in a large cohort after weight training. *Eur J Appl Physiol.* (2012) 112:2693–702. doi: 10.1007/s00421-011-2246-z
90. Morton RW, Sato K, Gallaugher MPB, Oikawa SY, McNicholas PD, Fujita S, et al. Muscle androgen receptor content but not systemic hormones is associated with resistance training-induced skeletal muscle hypertrophy in healthy, young men. *Front Physiol.* (2018) 9:1373. doi: 10.3389/fphys.2018.01373
91. MacKenzie-Shalders KL, King NA, Byrne NM, Slater GJ. Increasing protein distribution has no effect on changes in lean mass during a rugby preseason. *Int J Sport Nutr Exerc Metab.* (2016) 26:1–7. doi: 10.1123/ijsnem.2015-0040
92. Stokes T, Hector AJ, Morton RW, McGlory C, Phillips SM. Recent perspectives regarding the role of dietary protein for the promotion of muscle hypertrophy with resistance exercise training. *Nutrients.* (2018) 10:E180. doi: 10.3390/nu10020180
93. Antonio J, Peacock CA, Ellerbroek A, Fromhoff B, Silver T. The effects of consuming a high protein diet (4.4 g/kg/d) on body composition in resistance-trained individuals. *J Int Soc Sports Nutr.* (2014) 11:19. doi: 10.1186/1550-2783-11-19
94. Antonio J, Ellerbroek A, Silver T, Orris S, Scheiner M, Gonzalez A, et al. A high protein diet (3.4 g/kg/d) combined with a heavy resistance training program improves body composition in healthy trained men and women–a follow-up investigation. *J Int Soc Sports Nutr.* (2015) 12:39. doi: 10.1186/s12970-015-0100-0
95. Antonio J, Ellerbroek A, Silver T, Vargas L, Peacock C. The effects of a high protein diet on indices of health and body composition–a crossover trial in resistance-trained men. *J Int Soc Sports Nutr.* (2016) 13:3. doi: 10.1186/s12970-016-0114-2
96. Halton TL, Hu FB. The effects of high protein diets on thermogenesis, satiety and weight loss: a critical review. *J Am Coll Nutr.* (2004) 23:373–85. doi: 10.1080/07315724.2004.10719381
97. Eisenstein J, Roberts SB, Dallal G, Saltzman E. High-protein weight-loss diets: are they safe and do they work? A review of the experimental and epidemiologic data. *Nutr Rev.* (2002) 60:189–200. doi: 10.1301/00296640260184264
98. Campbell BI, Aguilar D, Conlin L, Vargas A, Schoenfeld BJ, Corson A, et al. Effects of high versus low protein intake on body composition and maximal strength in aspiring female physique athletes engaging in an 8-week resistance training program. *Int J Sport Nutr Exerc Metab.* (2018) 28:580–5. doi: 10.1123/ijsnem.2017-0389
99. Devries MC, Sithamparapillai A, Brimble KS, Banfield L, Morton RW, Phillips SM. Changes in kidney function do not differ between healthy adults consuming higher- compared with lower- or normal-protein diets: a systematic review and meta-analysis. *J Nutr.* (2018) 148:1760–75. doi: 10.1093/jn/nxy197
100. Antonio J, Ellerbroek A, Silver T, Vargas L, Tamayo A, Buehn R, et al. A high protein diet has no harmful effects: a one-year crossover study in resistance-trained males. *J Nutr Metab.* (2016) 2016:9104792. doi: 10.1155/2016/9104792
101. Horton TJ, Drougas H, Brachey A, Reed GW, Peters JC, Hill JO. Fat and carbohydrate overfeeding in humans: different effects on energy storage. *Am J Clin Nutr.* (1995) 62:19–29. doi: 10.1093/ajcn/62.1.19
102. Lammert O, Grunnet N, Faber P, Bjornsbo KS, Dich J, Larsen LO, et al. Effects of isoenergetic overfeeding of either carbohydrate or fat in young men. *Br J Nutr.* (2000) 84:233–45. doi: 10.1017/S0007114500001471
103. Tesch PA, Colliander EB, Kaiser P. Muscle metabolism during intense, heavy-resistance exercise. *Eur J Appl Physiol Occup Physiol.* (1986) 55:362–6. doi: 10.1007/BF00422734
104. Koopman R, Manders RJ, Jonkers RA, Hul GB, Kuipers H, van Loon LJ. Intramyocellular lipid and glycogen content are reduced following resistance exercise in untrained healthy males. *Eur J Appl Physiol.* (2006) 96:525–34. doi: 10.1007/s00421-005-0118-0
105. Lambert CP, Flynn MG, Boone JBJ, Michaud TJ, Rodriguez-Zayas J. Effects of carbohydrate feeding on multiple-bout resistance exercise. *J Strength Cond Res.* (1991) 5:192–7. doi: 10.1519/00124278-199111000-00004
106. Haff GG, Schroeder CA, Koch AJ, Kuphal KE, Comeau MJ, Potteiger JA. The effects of supplemental carbohydrate ingestion on intermittent isokinetic leg exercise. *J Sports Med Phys Fitness.* (2001) 41:216–22.
107. Tesch PA, Ploutz-Snyder LL, Ystrom L, Castro MJ, Dudley GA. Skeletal muscle glycogen loss evoked by resistance exercise. *J Strength Cond Res.* (1998) 12:67–73. doi: 10.1519/00124278-199805000-00001
108. Mitchell JB, DiLauro PC, Pizza FX, Cavender DL. The effect of preexercise carbohydrate status on resistance exercise performance. *Int J Sport Nutr.* (1997) 7:185–96. doi: 10.1123/ijsn.7.3.185
109. Greene DA, Varley BJ, Hartwig TB, Chapman P, Rigney M. A low-carbohydrate ketogenic diet reduces body mass without compromising performance in powerlifting and olympic weightlifting athletes. *J Strength Cond Res.* (2018) 32:3373–82. doi: 10.1519/JSC.0000000000002904

110. Kephart WC, Pledge CD, Roberson PA, Mumford PW, Romero MA, Mobley CB, et al. The three-month effects of a ketogenic diet on body composition, blood parameters, and performance metrics in crossfit trainees: a pilot study. *Sports.* (2018) 6:1. doi: 10.3390/sports6010001
111. Vargas S, Romance R, Petro JL, Bonilla DA, Galancho I, Espinar S, et al. Efficacy of ketogenic diet on body composition during resistance training in trained men: a randomized controlled trial. *J Int Soc Sports Nutr.* (2018) 15:31. doi: 10.1186/s12970-018-0236-9
112. Slater G, Phillips SM. Nutrition guidelines for strength sports: sprinting, weightlifting, throwing events, and bodybuilding. *J Sports Sci.* (2011) 29 (suppl 1):S67–77. doi: 10.1080/02640414.2011.574722
113. Thomas DT, Erdman KA, Burke LM. American college of sports medicine joint position statement. Nutrition and athletic performance. *Med Sci Sports Exerc.* (2016) 48:543–68. doi: 10.1249/MSS.0000000000000852
114. Jequier E. Response to and range of acceptable fat intake in adults. *Eur J Clin Nutr.* (1999) 53(suppl 1):S84–8. doi: 10.1038/sj.ejcn.1600747
115. Trumbo P, Schlicker S, Yates AA, Poos M. Dietary reference intakes for energy, carbohydrate, fiber, fat, fatty acids, cholesterol, protein and amino acids. *J Am Diet Assoc.* (2002) 102:1621–30. doi: 10.1016/S0002-8223(02)90346-9
116. Wang C, Catlin DH, Starcevic B, Heber D, Ambler C, Berman N, et al. Low-fat high-fiber diet decreased serum and urine androgens in men. *J Clin Endocrinol Metab.* (2005) 90:3550–9. doi: 10.1210/jc.2004-1530
117. Hamalainen E, Adlercreutz H, Puska P, Pietinen P. Diet and serum sex hormones in healthy men. *J Steroid Biochem.* (1984) 20:459–64. doi: 10.1016/0022-4731(84)90254-1
118. Dorgan JF, Judd JT, Longcope C, Brown C, Schatzkin A, Clevidence BA, et al. Effects of dietary fat and fiber on plasma and urine androgens and estrogens in men: a controlled feeding study. *Am J Clin Nutr.* (1996) 64:850–5. doi: 10.1093/ajcn/64.6.850
119. Collins CE, O'Loughlin EV, Henry RL. Fat gram target to achieve high energy intake in cystic fibrosis. *J Paediatr Child Health.* (1997) 33:142–7. doi: 10.1111/j.1440-1754.1997.tb01017.x
120. Rosqvist F, Iggman D, Kullberg J, Cedernaes J, Johansson HE, Larsson A, et al. Overfeeding polyunsaturated and saturated fat causes distinct effects on liver and visceral fat accumulation in humans. *Diabetes.* (2014) 63:2356–68. doi: 10.2337/db13-1622
121. Smith GI, Atherton P, Reeds DN, Mohammed BS, Rankin D, Rennie MJ, et al. Omega-3 polyunsaturated fatty acids augment the muscle protein anabolic response to hyperinsulinaemia-hyperaminoacidaemia in healthy young and middle-aged men and women. *Clin Sci.* (2011) 121:267–78. doi: 10.1042/CS20100597
122. Smith GI, Julliand S, Reeds DN, Sinacore DR, Klein S, Mittendorfer B. Fish oil-derived n-3 PUFA therapy increases muscle mass and function in healthy older adults. *Am J Clin Nutr.* (2015) 102:115–22. doi: 10.3945/ajcn.114.105833
123. Piers LS, Walker KZ, Stoney RM, Soares MJ, O'Dea K. The influence of the type of dietary fat on postprandial fat oxidation rates: monounsaturated (olive oil) vs saturated fat (cream). *Int J Obes Relat Metab Disord.* (2002) 26:814–21. doi: 10.1038/sj.ijo.0801993
124. Piers LS, Walker KZ, Stoney RM, Soares MJ, O'Dea K. Substitution of saturated with monounsaturated fat in a 4-week diet affects body weight and composition of overweight and obese men. *Br J Nutr.* (2003) 90:717–27. doi: 10.1079/BJN2003948
125. Tang JE, Moore DR, Kujbida GW, Tarnopolsky MA, Phillips SM. Ingestion of whey hydrolysate, casein, or soy protein isolate: effects on mixed muscle protein synthesis at rest and following resistance exercise in young men. *J Appl Physiol.* (2009) 107:987–92. doi: 10.1152/japplphysiol.00076.2009
126. van Vliet S, Shy EL, Abou Sawan S, Beals JW, West DW, Skinner SK, et al. Consumption of whole eggs promotes greater stimulation of postexercise muscle protein synthesis than consumption of isonitrogenous amounts of egg whites in young men. *Am J Clin Nutr.* (2017) 106:1401–12. doi: 10.3945/ajcn.117.159855
127. Elliot TA, Cree MG, Sanford AP, Wolfe RR, Tipton KD. Milk ingestion stimulates net muscle protein synthesis following resistance exercise. *Med Sci Sports Exerc.* (2006) 38:667–74. doi: 10.1249/01.mss.0000210190.64458.25
128. Burd NA, Beals JW, Martinez IG, Salvador AF, Skinner SK. Food-first approach to enhance the regulation of post-exercise skeletal muscle protein synthesis and remodeling. *Sports Med.* (2019) 49:59–68. doi: 10.1007/s40279-018-1009-y
129. Kerksick CM, Arent S, Schoenfeld BJ, Stout JR, Campbell B, Wilborn CD, et al. International society of sports nutrition position stand: nutrient timing. *J Int Soc Sports Nutr.* (2017) 14:33. doi: 10.1186/s12970-017-0189-4
130. Alghannam AF, Gonzalez JT, Betts JA. Restoration of muscle glycogen and functional capacity: role of post-exercise carbohydrate and protein co-ingestion. *Nutrients.* (2018) 10:E253. doi: 10.3390/nu10020253
131. Krings BM, Rountree JA, McAllister MJ, Cummings PM, Peterson TJ, Fountain BJ, et al. Effects of acute carbohydrate ingestion on anaerobic exercise performance. *J Int Soc Sports Nutr.* (2016) 13:40. doi: 10.1186/s12970-016-0152-9
132. Kulik JR, Touchberry CD, Kawamori N, Blumert PA, Crum AJ, Haff GG. Supplemental carbohydrate ingestion does not improve performance of high-intensity resistance exercise. *J Strength Cond Res.* (2008) 22:1101–7. doi: 10.1519/JSC.0b013e31816d679b
133. Escobar KA, Morales J, Vandusseldorp TA. The effect of a moderately low and high carbohydrate intake on crossfit performance. *Int J Exerc Sci.* (2016) 9:460–70.
134. Rountree JA, Krings BM, Peterson TJ, Thigpen AG, McAllister MJ, Holmes ME, et al. Efficacy of carbohydrate ingestion on crossfit exercise performance. *Sports.* (2017) 5:61. doi: 10.3390/sports5030061
135. Phillips SM, Van Loon LJ. Dietary protein for athletes: from requirements to optimum adaptation. *J Sports Sci.* (2011) 29(suppl 1):S29–38. doi: 10.1080/02640414.2011.619204
136. Atherton PJ, Smith K. Muscle protein synthesis in response to nutrition and exercise. *J Physiol.* (2012) 590:1049–57. doi: 10.1113/jphysiol.2011.225003
137. Dashti HS, Mogensen KM. Recommending small, frequent meals in the clinical care of adults: a review of the evidence and important considerations. *Nutr Clin Pract.* (2017) 32:365–77. doi: 10.1177/0884533616662995
138. Perrigue MM, Drewnowski A, Wang CY, Neuhouser ML. Higher eating frequency does not decrease appetite in healthy adults. *J Nutr.* (2016) 146:59–64. doi: 10.3945/jn.115.216978
139. Burke LM, Slater G, Broad EM, Haukka J, Modulon S, Hopkins WG. Eating patterns and meal frequency of elite Australian athletes. *Int J Sport Nutr Exerc Metab.* (2003) 13:521–38. doi: 10.1123/ijsnem.13.4.521
140. Erdman KA, Tunnicliffe J, Lun VM, Reimer RA. Eating patterns and composition of meals and snacks in elite Canadian athletes. *Int J Sport Nutr Exerc Metab.* (2013) 23:210–9. doi: 10.1123/ijsnem.23.3.210
141. de Castro JM, Bellisle F, Feunekes GIJ, Dalix A-M, De Graaf C. Culture and meal patterns: a comparison of the food intake of free-living American, Dutch, and French students. *Nutr Res.* (1997) 17:807–29. doi: 10.1016/S0271-5317(97)00050-X
142. Anderson L, Naughton RJ, Close GL, Di Michele R, Morgans R, Drust B, et al. Daily distribution of macronutrient intakes of professional soccer players from the english premier league. *Int J Sport Nutr Exerc Metab.* (2017) 27:491–8. doi: 10.1123/ijsnem.2016-0265
143. Deutz RC, Benardot D, Martin DE, Cody MM. Relationship between energy deficits and body composition in elite female gymnasts and runners. *Med Sci Sports Exerc.* (2000) 32:659–68. doi: 10.1097/00005768-200003000-00017
144. Fahrenholtz IL, Sjodin A, Benardot D, Tornberg AB, Skouby S, Faber J, et al. Within-day energy deficiency and reproductive function in female endurance athletes. *Scand J Med Sci Sports.* (2018) 28:1139–46. doi: 10.1111/sms.13030
145. Torstveit MK, Fahrenholtz I, Stenqvist TB, Sylta O, Melin A. Within-day energy deficiency and metabolic perturbation in male endurance athletes. *Int J Sport Nutr Exerc Metab.* (2018) 28:419–27. doi: 10.1123/ijsnem.2017-0337
146. Cribb PJ, Hayes A. Effects of supplement timing and resistance exercise on skeletal muscle hypertrophy. *Med Sci Sports Exerc.* (2006) 38:1918–25. doi: 10.1249/01.mss.0000233790.08788.3e
147. Hoffman JR, Ratamess NA, Tranchina CP, Rashti SL, Kang J, Faigenbaum AD. Effect of protein-supplement timing on strength, power, and body-composition changes in resistance-trained men. *Int J Sport Nutr Exerc Metab.* (2009) 19:172–85. doi: 10.1123/ijsnem.19.2.172
148. Bo S, Musso G, Beccuti G, Fadda M, Fedele D, Gambino R, et al. Consuming more of daily caloric intake at dinner predisposes to obesity. A 6-year population-based prospective cohort study. *PLoS ONE.* (2014) 9:e108467. doi: 10.1371/journal.pone.0108467

149. Wang JB, Patterson RE, Ang A, Emond JA, Shetty N, Arab L. Timing of energy intake during the day is associated with the risk of obesity in adults. *J Hum Nutr Diet.* (2014) 27(suppl 2):255–62. doi: 10.1111/jhn.12141
150. Allison KC, Goel N. Timing of eating in adults across the weight spectrum: metabolic factors and potential circadian mechanisms. *Physiol Behav.* (2018) 192:158–66. doi: 10.1016/j.physbeh.2018.02.047
151. Timlin MT, Pereira MA. Breakfast frequency and quality in the etiology of adult obesity and chronic diseases. *Nutr Rev.* (2007) 65:268–81. doi: 10.1111/j.1753-4887.2007.tb00304.x
152. de Castro JM. The time of day of food intake influences overall intake in humans. *J Nutr.* (2004) 134:104–11. doi: 10.1093/jn/134.1.104
153. Snijders T, Res PT, Smeets JS, van Vliet S, van Kranenburg J, Maase K, et al. Protein ingestion before sleep increases muscle mass and strength gains during prolonged resistance-type exercise training in healthy young men. *J Nutr.* (2015) 145:1178–84. doi: 10.3945/jn.114.208371
154. Bradley WJ, Cavanagh B, Douglas W, Donovan TF, Twist C, Morton JP, et al. Energy intake and expenditure assessed 'in-season' in an elite European rugby union squad. *Eur J Sport Sci.* (2015) 15:469–79. doi: 10.1080/17461391.2015.1042528
155. King NA, Caudwell PP, Hopkins M, Stubbs JR, Naslund E, Blundell JE. Dual-process action of exercise on appetite control: increase in orexigenic drive but improvement in meal-induced satiety. *Am J Clin Nutr.* (2009) 90:921–7. doi: 10.3945/ajcn.2009.27706
156. Peos JJ, Norton LE, Helms ER, Galpin AJ, Fournier P. Intermittent dieting: theoretical considerations for the athlete. *Sports.* (2019) 7:E22. doi: 10.3390/sports7010022
157. Sagayama H, Jikumaru Y, Hirata A, Yamada Y, Yoshimura E, Ichikawa M, et al. Measurement of body composition in response to a short period of overfeeding. *J Physiol Anthropol.* (2014) 33:29. doi: 10.1186/1880-6805-33-29
158. DellaValle DM, Roe LS, Rolls BJ. Does the consumption of caloric and non-caloric beverages with a meal affect energy intake? *Appetite.* (2005) 44:187–93. doi: 10.1016/j.appet.2004.11.003
159. Mourao DM, Bressan J, Campbell WW, Mattes RD. Effects of food form on appetite and energy intake in lean and obese young adults. *Int J Obes.* (2007) 31:1688–95. doi: 10.1038/sj.ijo.0803667
160. Rolls BJ, Roe LS, Meengs JS. Salad and satiety: energy density and portion size of a first-course salad affect energy intake at lunch. *J Am Diet Assoc.* (2004) 104:1570–6. doi: 10.1016/j.jada.2004.07.001
161. Aune D, Giovannucci E, Boffetta P, Fadnes LT, Keum N, Norat T, et al. Fruit and vegetable intake and the risk of cardiovascular disease, total cancer and all-cause mortality-a systematic review and dose-response meta-analysis of prospective studies. *Int J Epidemiol.* (2017) 46:1029–56. doi: 10.1093/ije/dyw319
162. Westerterp-Plantenga MS, Lemmens SG, Westerterp KR. Dietary protein - its role in satiety, energetics, weight loss and health. *Br J Nutr.* (2012) 108(suppl 2):S105–12. doi: 10.1017/S0007114512002589
163. Bone JL, Ross ML, Tomcik KA, Jeacocke NA, Hopkins WG, Burke LM. Manipulation of muscle creatine and glycogen changes dual X-ray absorptiometry estimates of body composition. *Med Sci Sports Exerc.* (2017) 49:1029–35. doi: 10.1249/MSS.0000000000001174
164. Shiose K, Yamada Y, Motonaga K, Sagayama H, Higaki Y, Tanaka H, et al. Segmental extracellular and intracellular water distribution and muscle glycogen after 72-h carbohydrate loading using spectroscopic techniques. *J Appl Physiol.* (2016) 121:205–11. doi: 10.1152/japplphysiol.00126.2016
165. Kristiansen MS, Uhrbrand A, Hansen M, Shiguetomi-Medina JM, Vissing K, Stodkilde-Jorgensen H, et al. Concomitant changes in cross-sectional area and water content in skeletal muscle after resistance exercise. *Scand J Med Sci Sports.* (2014) 24:e260–8. doi: 10.1111/sms.12160
166. Garthe I, Raastad T, Refsnes PE, Sundgot-Borgen J. Effect of nutritional intervention on body composition and performance in elite athletes. *Eur J Sport Sci.* (2013) 13:295–303. doi: 10.1080/17461391.2011.643923

18

The Impact of Step Reduction on Muscle Health in Aging: Protein and Exercise as Countermeasures

*Sara Y. Oikawa, Tanya M. Holloway and Stuart M. Phillips**

Exercise Metabolism Research Group, Department of Kinesiology, McMaster University, Hamilton, ON, Canada

***Correspondence:**
Stuart M. Phillips
phillis@mcmaster.ca

Declines in strength and muscle function with age—sarcopenia—contribute to a variety of negative outcomes including an increased risk of: falls, fractures, hospitalization, and reduced mobility in older persons. Population-based estimates of the loss of muscle after age 60 show a loss of ~1% per year while strength loss is more rapid at ~3% per year. These rates are not, however, linear as periodic bouts of reduced physical activity and muscle disuse transiently accelerate loss of muscle and declines in muscle strength and power. Episodic complete muscle disuse can be due to sickness-related bed rest or local muscle disuse as a result of limb immobilization/surgery. Alternatively, relative muscle disuse occurs during inactivity due to illness and the associated convalescence resulting in marked reductions in daily steps, often referred to as step reduction (SR). While it is a "milder" form of disuse, it can have a similar adverse impact on skeletal muscle health. The physiological consequences of even short-term inactivity, modeled by SR, show losses in muscle mass and strength, as well as impaired insulin sensitivity and an increase in systemic inflammation. Though seemingly benign in comparison to bed rest, periodic inactivity likely occurs, we posit, more frequently with advancing age due to illness, declining mental health and declining mobility. Given that recovery from inactivity in older adults is slow or possibly incomplete we hypothesize that accumulated periods of inactivity contribute to sarcopenia. Periodic activity, even in small quantities, and protein supplementation may serve as effective strategies to offset the loss of muscle mass with aging, specifically during periods of inactivity. The aim of this review is to examine the recent literature encompassing SR, as a model of inactivity, and to explore the capacity of nutrition and exercise interventions to mitigate adverse physiological changes as a result of SR.

Keywords: step reduction, physical inactivity, protein, muscle, older adults

PHYSICAL ACTIVITY AND AGING

In Canada, ~85% of individuals are not meeting physical activity guidelines (1). This highlights the potential for improvement that could be achieved given the potential for increased physical activity to reduce risk for a number of diseases and for all-cause mortality (2, 3). Older adults tend to engage in less physical activity in comparison to younger adults (4) with a notable decline in levels of leisure time physical activity in older adults (5–7). Interestingly, social isolation in older persons may be result from numerous factors: inability to leave the house due to poor mobility, lack of transportation, or adverse weather conditions, illness of the individual or in their social circles, all of which highlight the complexity for the capacity of intervention in aging adults.

Exacerbating low levels of habitual physical activity in older adults are abrupt and acute reductions in activity resulting in lower levels of mechanical loading of muscle. Acute bouts of inactivity that result in unloading of muscles manifest due to a variety of circumstances (illness, injury, poor weather conditions) and are distinctly different from habitual sedentary behavior. Though these acute disruptions in activity may be seemingly benign, we hypothesize that accumulated bouts of marked inactivity superimposed on a physically inactive population is a major risk for negative physiological health outcomes and may accelerate sarcopenia and the development of chronic cardiometabolic conditions associated with aging.

Sarcopenia and Physical Inactivity

Cyclical bouts of pronounced inactivity, even in relatively healthy persons, can have significant detrimental physiological effects on health particularly with advancing age (8). Specifically, acute periods of physical inactivity (9–14) lead to reductions in skeletal muscle size and strength that transiently expedite the usual declines resulting from sarcopenia (15). Population-based estimates of sarcopenia show muscle loss occurring at a rate of ~1% per year with losses in muscle strength and power, more rapid at rates of ~3% and ~8% per year, respectively, (16, 17). Though the progression of sarcopenia is seen as a normal consequence of aging it can be accelerated due to inactivity, which transiently accelerates muscle loss (15). Indeed, numerous factors can affect the progression of sarcopenic muscle loss with inactivity events further accelerating muscle loss as shown in **Figure 1**. Lifestyle factors such as exercise and nutrition may moderate the progression of normal muscle loss with increasing age. In particular, declines in physical activity, insufficient or excess energy intake, and protein malnutrition may act to synergistically accelerate sarcopenic declines and thus increase the risk for subsequent hospitalization or disuse resulting in accelerated muscle loss (18). Importantly with each disuse event, muscle mass loss decreases and muscle cross sectional area is drastically reduced with an increase in intramuscular fat content (19). Physical activity is a potent regulator of factors associated with aging and skeletal muscle health [inactivity and inflammation (14), reactive oxygen species, glycemic control (20), loss of motor neurons (21)] and when combined with proper nutrition (adequate protein intake) may serve to attenuate the rate of muscle decline.

STEP REDUCTION AS A MODEL OF PERIODIC INACTIVITY

Previous studies have employed various models to study physical inactivity in humans ranging from a brief reduction in habitual physical activity (90% reduction in daily steps for 1 day) (22) to spaceflight and microgravity (23). As shown in **Figure 2**, each reduced activity model results in differences in daily activity level, which are notably reduced from habitual physical activity levels in older adults. Inactivity during bed rest has provided researchers with a characteristic change in muscle phenotype in order to better understand the physiological consequences of disuse (29). Given that bed rest requires inactivity of the whole body, it provides an excellent model to understand the systemic effect of disuse on multiple physiological systems and is clinically relevant (30). Conversely, single limb immobilization studies in older (11, 12) and younger (11, 31, 32) adults have emphasized the significant physiological consequences occurring with local muscle-level disuse. Immobilization-induced muscle loss is largely applicable to clinical scenarios of single-limb immobilization or elective orthopedic surgery, during which the recovery of the affected limb may be without loading for several weeks (11, 12, 20). More recently, the investigation of SR as a form of abrupt physical inactivity has been employed, to investigate the effects of abrupt reductions in activity but not complete disuse. During SR, participants are asked to reduce their daily steps (usually externally monitored by a pedometer or similar device) to a low maximal daily step count (750–5,000 steps/d) (14, 27, 33). The lower end of daily step count (~750 steps/d) used in studies is in line with steps performed by patients in acute hospital stays (34). Alarmingly, the daily steps of patients in hospital (out of 708 days examined) exceeded 300 steps per day only 50% of the time; however, on average daily steps per patient were ~740 (34). Reductions of physical activity with SR to these low levels would not obviously constitute complete muscle disuse, but do have profound physiological consequences. Importantly, SR has similar whole body systemic effects, but obviously to a lesser degree, as bed rest, in comparison to unilateral limb immobilization which largely targets peripheral tissues (**Figure 3**). Additionally, episodes of bed rest (typically due to hospital admittance) arguably occur less frequently than episodes of inactivity that occur periodically throughout due to weather or illness such as influenza and likely affect a greater proportion of the population than is affected by complete bed rest. Thus, the purpose of this review is to highlight the physiological consequences resulting from purposeful reduced daily steps in younger and older adults with insight on recent studies using SR and the potential for exercise and nutrition to combat disuse atrophy in this model.

Physiological Consequences of SR in Young Adults

The first study establishing the physiological consequences of SR was by Olsen et al. who elegantly demonstrated that reducing daily steps for as little as 3-wks had marked negative impacts on skeletal muscle (35). Participants (young healthy adults) reduced their step count by simply taking the elevator instead of stairs and utilizing cars instead of walking or bicycling resulting in daily average steps totalling ~1,300 steps/d (reduced from a habitual step count of ~10000 steps/d). Following 21 days of SR, participants had decreased insulin sensitivity, attenuation of postprandial lipid metabolism, and increased intra-abdominal fat mass (35). The negative alterations in glycemic control and impaired lipid metabolism (35) highlight the rapidity of how healthy and mobile individuals move to metabolic dysfunction simply through a period of SR as well as how easily, through

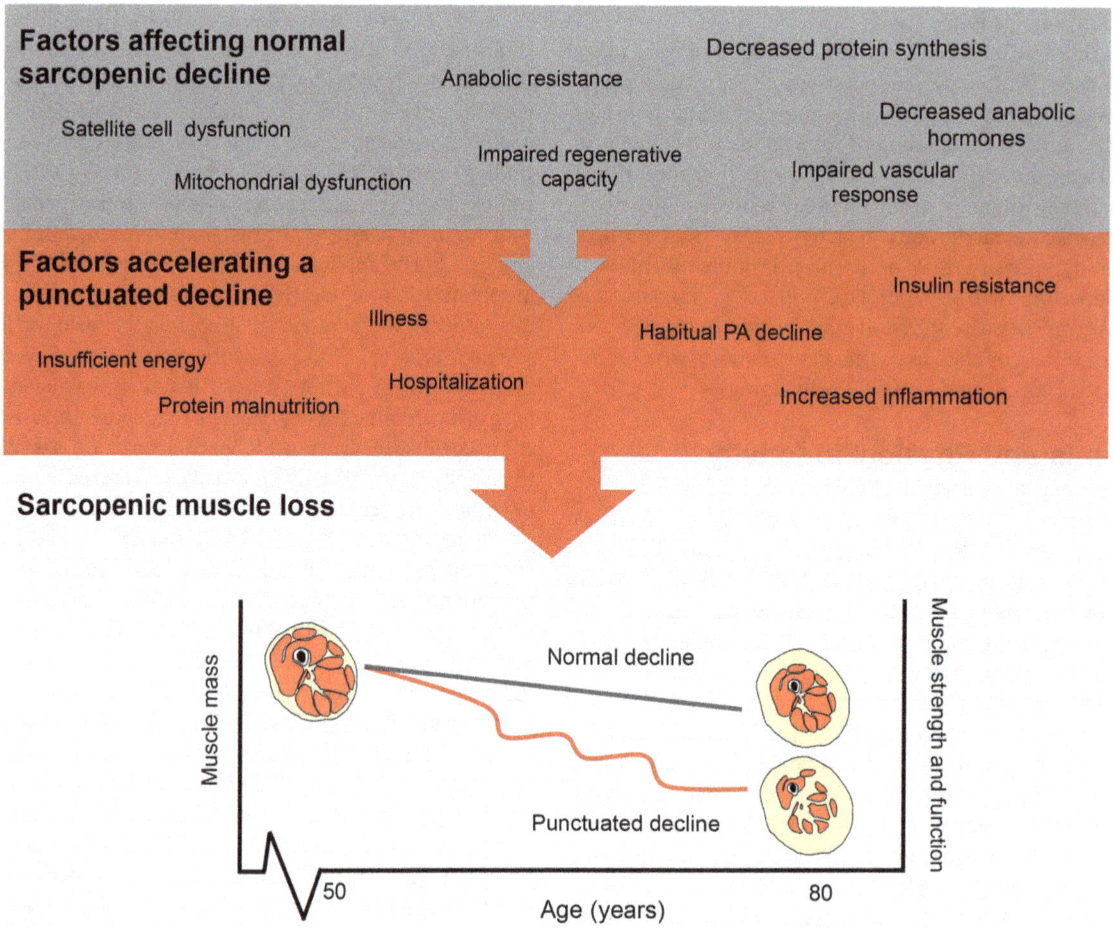

FIGURE 1 | Factors influencing the progression of sarcopenia. Representations of normal sarcopenic muscle loss and accelerated muscle loss as shown by a punctuated decline.

alterations in use of personal and publication transportation that adults can reduce daily step count.

Knudsen et al. also demonstrated that reducing daily steps from 10,000 to 1500, in combination with over-feeding, increased visceral adiposity by 49% and decreased insulin sensitivity by 44% in healthy, active, young adults (36). Likewise, Krogh-Madsen et al. showed that reducing daily physical activity to levels similar to the previously described intervention but maintaining energy balance (36), resulted in a reduced insulin sensitivity, a reduction in VO_2 max of 7 mL/kg/min and a 0.5 kg decrease in leg lean mass (LLM) in healthy young men (27). Taken together, data from Knudsen et al. (36), and Krogh-Madsen et al. (27), demonstrate the potency of a SR model and the susceptibility of healthy young adult populations to significant negative metabolic health outcomes following even brief periods of inactivity.

Interestingly, Stephens et al. (22) showed that even 1 day of limited physical activity (~260 steps) was a sufficient stimulus to induce a impairments in insulin action, as measured by whole body rate of glucose disappearance, in physically active, young men and women by ~39%. Though the steps per day in that investigation (22) were low for a healthy adult, when viewed in the context of severe illness or hospital stay, the daily step counts are on par with those of hospitalized patients (34). Further, given that the impairments to reduced steps in young healthy adults are notably adverse, then it is not unreasonable to hypothesize that the effects would be of greater magnitude in a compromised aging population (18). Nevertheless, measures to mitigate rapid declines in physical activity even in young adults should be further explored in order to offset the negative physiological adaptations to SR.

Physiological Consequences of SR in Older Adults

Older adults, compared to their younger counterparts, may be at a greater risk for periods of inactivity in addition to a declines in habitual physical activity (4). In addition to the frequency of periodic SR, the adverse consequences of such periods of inactivity in older persons are also likely much greater than

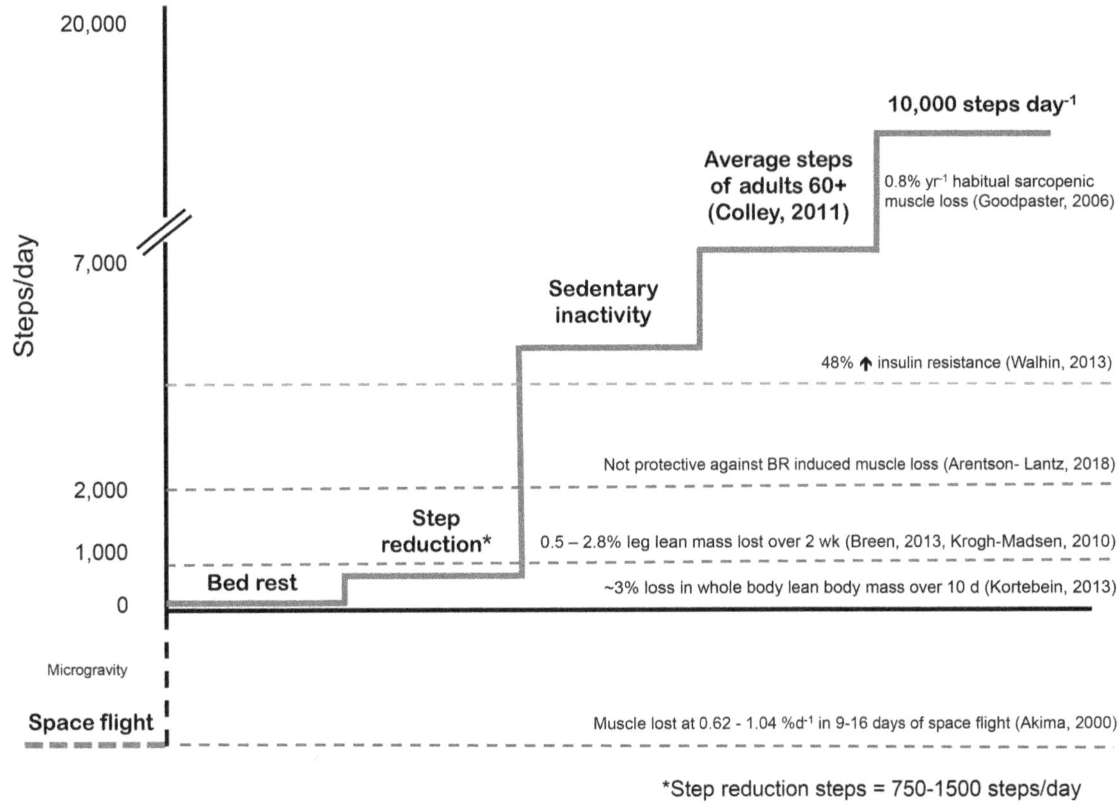

FIGURE 2 | Physical inactivity models used in human skeletal muscle metabolism. Typical sarcopenic muscle loss based on population estimates (24). Sedentary behavior as categorized by Walhin et al. as < 4000 steps per day induced significant insulin resistance in healthy young adults (25). Interestingly, during one week of bed rest, participants walked for ~22 minutes per day (~2000 steps) in an effort to offset bed rest induced muscle atrophy however exercise was not able to mediate this effect and muscle loss was similar to controls (26). Step reduction, or abruptly reducing habitual daily steps to 750-1500 steps per day results in leg lean mass loss over two weeks in healthy young and older adults (13, 14, 27). Bed rest induces rapid muscle atrophy in healthy older adults (9) however the rate of muscle loss per day as a result of space flight or exposure to microgravity are staggering (28).

they are in younger persons. For example, in a seminal study by Suetta et al. (11), the authors found that following 2-weeks of unilateral leg casting and subsequent intensive resistance training that older adults were not able to fully recover losses of skeletal muscle in comparison to a cohort of young adults who demonstrated full recovery of quadriceps cross sectional area (CSA) (11). Similarly, healthy older adults have shown marked susceptibility to acute reductions in daily stepping impacting glycemic control, markers of inflammation, and skeletal muscle, the recovery from which is incomplete following SR, underlining an obvious impaired regenerative capacity in aging skeletal muscle (20).

Glucose Handling and Inflammation With SR in Older Adults

Similar to healthy young adults, healthy older adults also demonstrate negative effects on glucoregulation with SR. McGlory et al. (20), examined how pre-diabetic older adults responded metabolically to 2 weeks of SR and importantly whether participants were able to recover to pre-SR levels. In this study (20), participants reduced their daily steps to <1000 steps/d followed by a two-week recovery period in which they returned to habitual levels of activity while maintaining energy balance. Fasted plasma glucose and insulin levels were significantly elevated following SR by 8 and 31%, respectively and these values did not return to pre-SR levels following a two-week recovery (20). Comparably, Breen et al. had participants reduce their daily step count by ~75% or to ~1500 steps/day for 2 weeks and monitored changes in glycemic control. Though the authors found no significant elevation in fasted blood glucose following SR, they noted a significant elevation in fasted plasma insulin as well as an increase in glucose and insulin area under the curve by 9 and 12%, respectively confirming an impaired glycemic handling in response to SR (13). It is notable that in both studies (13, 20), that SR resulted in small but significant increases in systemic inflammatory cytokines. Breen et al. observed elevated levels of TNF- α and CRP in response to inactivity in normoglycemic participants while McGlory et al. observed an increase in levels of TNF-α, IL-6 and CRP following SR in overweight and obese pre-diabetic participants. The concentrations of inflammatory markers were partially recovered following return to habitual activity in pre diabetic participants (20). Interestingly, older

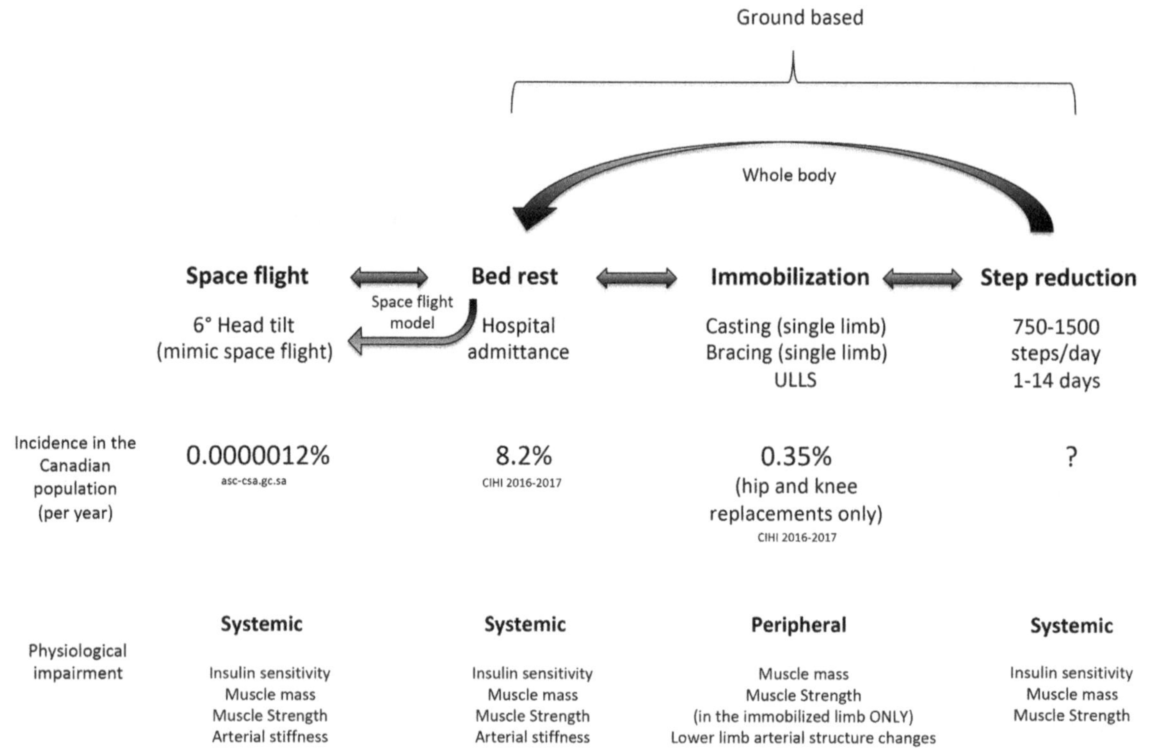

FIGURE 3 | Comparison of disuse models used to study inactivity highlighting the whole body systemic nature of bed rest and step reduction compared to limb immobilization. Data regarding the prevalence of events with induced step reduction is currently unknown.

adults showed a rise in inflammatory cytokines (13, 20), which is something that was not seen in younger adults in response to SR (27, 36). While we acknowledge that this is an observation, we posit that this may be of some significance in explaining why younger persons do and older persons do not recover from SR (37); however, this would require specific examination.

Changes in Muscle Protein Turnover and Muscle With SR

Previous work from our group (13, 20, 38) and others (39, 40), have attributed the loss of muscle mass with muscle disuse, for the most part, to a reduction in both fasted- and fed-state muscle protein synthesis (MPS) (41). Indeed, alterations in skeletal muscle protein synthesis are highly sensitive to modifications in physical activity and mechanical loading to similar extent in both younger and older adults (9, 31). To date, no studies have examined the impact of SR on modifications in MPS in younger adults in response to SR. Nonetheless, Krogh-Madsen et al. (27) did observe a loss of leg lean mass of 2.8% following 2 weeks of reduced daily stepping (<1500 steps per day), an observation that emphasizes the impact of SR in healthy young adults. Several studies have investigated the effects of SR on losses in lean body mass (LBM) and modifications in rates of MPS in older adults (13, 14, 20, 38). Consistent with the concept of muscle disuse-induced "anabolic resistance" (12, 31) work from our laboratory has shown consistent reductions in MPS in response to 2 weeks of SR of varying degrees (750–1500 steps per day) (13, 14, 20) with rates reduced 13–26% from baseline. Importantly, in healthy older adults McGlory et al. demonstrated that in the absence of rehabilitative measures (i.e., additional physical activity/loading above baseline levels, nutritional intervention) the reduced rates of MPS seen during inactivity were not recovered following 2 weeks of return to habitual activity (17).

Given that MPS is a strong regulator of skeletal muscle mass in healthy populations (42), strategies to improve MPS in response to SR may prove to be promising in the maintenance of skeletal muscle during and in recovery from acute inactivity due to illness. Importantly, older adults typically have less muscle mass in comparison to younger adults (43) when they become inactive. While the absolute loss of skeletal muscle in older adults in response to reduced activity models may be less (11) the relative loss is significantly greater than losses in younger adults in bed rest protocols (44). Nonetheless, the lack of recovery seen in older as opposed to younger adults is a troubling observation (11, 20).

Changes in Muscle Function and Physical Capacity With SR

The association of skeletal muscle mass and skeletal muscle strength has been well-established, where reductions in muscle mass/area are roughly correlated with reductions in muscle strength and power (24, 45). Low skeletal muscle strength (but not mass) is an independent risk factor for mortality (46). Thus, determining the impact of seemingly benign periods of reduced daily activity, via models such as SR, on skeletal muscle functional outcomes is imperative, specifically for older adults for whom losses in strength have a substantial effect on quality of life (47).

As mentioned previously, young adults exhibit notable decrements in maximal aerobic capacity [3–7% (27, 36)] following SR (<1500 steps per day) lasting only 14 days. Evidence substantiating alterations in maximum voluntary strength of the lower limbs in response to SR in older adults have been varied (14, 17, 38). Reidy et al. found that knee extensor maximum voluntary contraction (MVC) was significantly reduced by ~8% in older adults during moderate SR (<3,000 steps per day, 2 weeks) (48) while we observed a reduction in MVC of 9% and 6% in men and women, respectively, following SR (<750 steps per day, 2 weeks) (49). Further in the investigation by Reidy et al. strength losses were not recovered (48) after 14 days of return to normal activity and were only recovered in men in work by Oikawa et al. (49). Conversely, reductions in knee extensor MVC were not observed in previous investigations of SR despite marked metabolic and physiological perturbations in glucose regulation, inflammation and reductions in MPS (13, 20, 38); however, we speculate that differences in familiarization procedures might underpin this heterogeneity of response. Substantial familiarization is required in order to obtain a true baseline strength measurement especially in older persons (50), along with the small changes in strength expected with SR (compared to complete disuse) may be responsible for the observed heterogeneity in MVC as measured by dynamometry following SR. To date, no study has examined the impact of SR on strength or clinical functional parameters in healthy young adults though these outcomes appear to be preserved in older adults following SR, unlike the decrements observed in models of complete unloading (bed rest) (9, 51). Though the decrements in muscle strength reported by Reidy and Oikawa are small, it should be acknowledged that a lack of strength recovery poses a significant threat in the progression of healthy aging. Without recovery of lost strength, each future perturbation in physical activity will reduce an individual's maximal strength output increasing risk for disability and mobility impairments (47). Thus, strategies to restore muscle strength and function following SR are imperative in order for maintenance of independence and quality of life throughout aging.

MITIGATING THE PHYSIOLOGICAL CONSEQUENCES OF DISUSE AND SR WITH EXERCISE

Muscular contraction is a potent stimulus to attenuate the negative effects of muscle disuse on skeletal muscle loss (38, 52). Resistance training (RT) has been shown to increase skeletal muscle mass (53, 54), capillary density (55), and satellite cell activation in older adults (56) making it an obvious countermeasure to combat skeletal muscle atrophy.

Previous literature employing resistance exercise to offset declines in LBM during bed rest have been successful (52, 57–59). Bamman et al. found significant decreases in Type I and II fiber CSA while myofibre CSA was maintained in the exercise and bed rest group of young men (57) while Kawakami et al. found that exercise attenuated the decline in muscle CSA as measured by magnetic resonance imaging (MRI) in young men (58). Similarly, Alkner et al. showed that following 90 days of bed rest that a RT group showed no decrease in total quadriceps muscle volume while the non-exercise control group showed a decrease decreased of ~18% (52). Trappe et al. showed that whole quadriceps muscle volume as measured by MRI decreased by ~17% while there was no decline in muscle volume in the RT group after 84 days of bed rest (59). Oates et al. also showed that even a very low volume of RT performed every other day was sufficient to mitigate declines in muscle CSA of the triceps surae and knee extensors (60).

To date, only one study has been conducted in which periodic low-level resistance exercise has been used to offset SR-induced muscle atrophy (38). Devries et al. utilized a unilateral model of resistance training during SR in which older participants were asked to reduce their daily step count to <1500 steps per day for 2 weeks (38) and performed unilateral low-load resistance exercise at 30% of their maximal strength (~20-25 repetitions) three times per week. Low load RT has significant promise to induce skeletal muscle hypertrophy and even strength (61, 62) and could possibly be useful in situations where high load exercises are not possible such as hospitalization or when home bound due to illness. Following 2-weeks of SR, the leg that performed RT was protected against the SR-induced reduction in postabsorptive and postprandial MPS seen in the non-exercised SR leg (38). Data from the same group of participants was analyzed for alterations in satellite cell activation in both the SR and SR plus RT limbs and found that RT was effective at preserving Type I and II fiber cross sectional area, similar to findings during bed rest (57), and in the preservation of Pax7$^+$ positive cells (satellite cells) in type I and II fibers (63), which were lower in the SR leg. Given the robust impact of resistance exercise on skeletal muscle anabolism in younger and older adults (56, 61) it is not wholly surprising that RT was able to preserve aged skeletal muscle during SR to levels similar to healthy controls. Though the applicability of these data (38) is debatable since we recognize that older adults who are taking <1500 steps per day may not be able to perform RT if the nature of the inactivity is caused by illness or injury. Nonetheless, we propose that the potentially favorable effects that even infrequent low load muscular contractions may have on the preservation of skeletal muscle health should be considered in an effort to reduce muscle mass and strength loss with disuse. Interestingly, a study by Arentson-Lantz et al. (26), aimed to determine whether taking 2000 steps/d (~22 min of walking per day) during 1 week of bed rest would be a sufficient stimulus to offset losses in skeletal muscle mass and physical function. Following 1 week, participants lost ~1 kg of LLM with no effect of the added daily stepping, findings that were confirmed by immunohistochemistry determining fiber CSA. Further, increased daily stepping did not attenuate the reduction in leg MVC, with participants exhibiting strength losses of ~12% (26). This study provides compelling data, highlighting the powerful effects that complete bed rest can have. Indeed, strategies to reduce the impact of bed rest and disuse are imperative to the conservation of skeletal muscle and functional outcomes in older adults.

The Role for Nutrition in Attenuating LBM Losses With Disuse

The term anabolic resistance describes the reduction in MPS in response to a given protein dose (64) (and subsequent hyperaminoacidemia) and to a bout of resistance exercise with age (65, 66) and is a negative consequence induced by disuse (31). The role of nutrition to mitigate the negative physiological consequences of inactivity has been examined largely in the context of bed rest (40, 51, 67–69) and single leg immobilization (12, 70) with a majority of studies examining protein or amino acid based supplements (40, 69, 71, 72). Supplementation with amino acids may represent an effective strategy to combat both anabolic resistance with age and anabolic resistance as a result of disuse, particularly if the supplemental protein or amino acids are used to create a more even meal-to-meal pattern with protein intake at each meal (73, 74). This is largely because adults tend to consume the largest amounts of protein; amounts sufficient to induce maximal rates of MPS only at the later meals of the day (75) as shown in **Figure 4** and thus the addition of a protein supplement at meals throughout the day may serve to facilitate a better stimulation of MPS and positive net protein accretion (74).

The essential amino acid leucine is a potent stimulator of mTOR and in turn, MPS (76) and therefore, supplements high in leucine content are typically used for their anabolic potential and potential muscle sparing effect during disuse atrophy. To date however, results have been incongruent in bed rest models. Ferrando et al. found that supplementation with 15 g of essential amino acids (5.3 g of leucine) thrice daily, during 10 days of bed rest did not alleviate LBM loss in healthy older adults in comparison to a control group (51). Similarly, English et al. found that meal time supplementation with doses of 4.5 g of leucine only partially protected LBM loss after 7 days of bed rest but did not significantly protect LBM at 14 days of bed rest with supplementation in younger adults (40). Paddon-Jones et al. showed a protective effect of 16.5 g of EAA (3.1 g of leucine) provided three times daily, during 28 days of bed rest on total LBM in young adults (72). Given that the lack of agreement on the efficacy of amino acid supplementation on the sparing of LBM is in both young and older adults during bed rest, much more research is needed in order to definitively determine whether there is indeed a benefit of EAA and leucine supplementation during bed rest.

Interestingly, energy balance appears to play a significant role on LBM loss during bed rest. As might be expected, consumption of a hypocaloric diet results in an accelerated rate of LBM loss during bed rest, largely through suppression of MPS (42). Indeed, Biolo et al. showed that 14 days of bed rest in combination with a 20% caloric deficit led to the greater wasting of LBM compared to the same participants consuming a eucaloric diet in a cross-over study design (68). However, in a subsequent study, Biolo et al. also examined the effects of positive energy balance during bed rest in comparison to negative energy balance. These authors found that during 35 days of bed rest, participants in positive energy balance, lost 1.5 kg more LBM than participants in negative energy balance, a finding that the authors attributed to an activation of inflammatory pathways associated with the increase in fat mass accompanying the positive energy balanced state. Thus, in addition to nutrient supplementation, a consideration should be made to encourage maintenance of energy balance during periods of disuse for optimal nutrition to attenuate skeletal muscle loss.

Fewer studies have examined the effects of nutritional interventions during single limb immobilization in humans. Two studies have examined the effects of creatine supplementation with mixed results. Hespel et al. examined the effects of daily supplementation with 20 g of creatine monohydrate or placebo control for 2 weeks of unilateral lower limb (knee) immobilization in young adults. These authors found a significant loss in quadriceps muscle CSA with no difference between supplemental groups (77). Conversely, Johnston et al. provided young adult participants with both a placebo control and subsequently 20 g of creatine during 7 days of upper limb (elbow joint) immobilization in a cross-over design study and creatine better maintained lean tissue mass compared to the placebo while also maintaining a variety of functional parameters (78). Though there are many differences between the two aforementioned studies (immobilization time, measurement of muscle mass), the difference in immobilized limb (weight bearing vs. non-weight bearing) makes it difficult for comparison between the two studies and thus the effect of creatine supplementation on LBM retention with immobilization requires further investigation.

Protein and amino acid supplementation has not been widely examined in the literature to offset muscle loss during immobilization. Dirks et al. showed that following 5 days of cast immobilization, quadriceps CSA was reduced by 1.5% in controls and by 2% in healthy older men consuming a placebo or twice daily 20.7 g protein supplement, respectively, (12). Interestingly participants in this study were provided with a protein supplement that may have been below optimal thresholds [0.4 g/kg/dose (79)] as based on average mass a protein dose closer to 30 g may have been more effective to attenuate the loss of LBM with cast immobilization of the knee (79).

Recently, McGlory et al. examined the effect of fish oil supplementation on the retention of LBM during unilateral knee bracing for two weeks in young healthy women. Participants were provided with a daily dose of 5 g of n-3 fatty acids or a control oil (sunflower oil) for 28 days prior to 14 days of unilateral knee immobilization. Following immobilization, supplementation with n-3 fatty acids attenuated the decline in quadriceps muscle volume by 6% (14 vs. 8% in the control vs. supplement group, respectively) and also promoted an elevation of MPS above rates of the control group at all measured time points (70). Thus, the addition of n-3 fatty acid supplementation in addition to an adequate protein dose and energy balance may serve to attenuate the decline in LBM during unilateral limb immobilization and bed rest.

To date no study has examined the effect of dietary manipulations on SR through supplementation or changes in energy intake. Given that protein, specifically, high quality protein (high in EAA) in large quantities has a potent anabolic

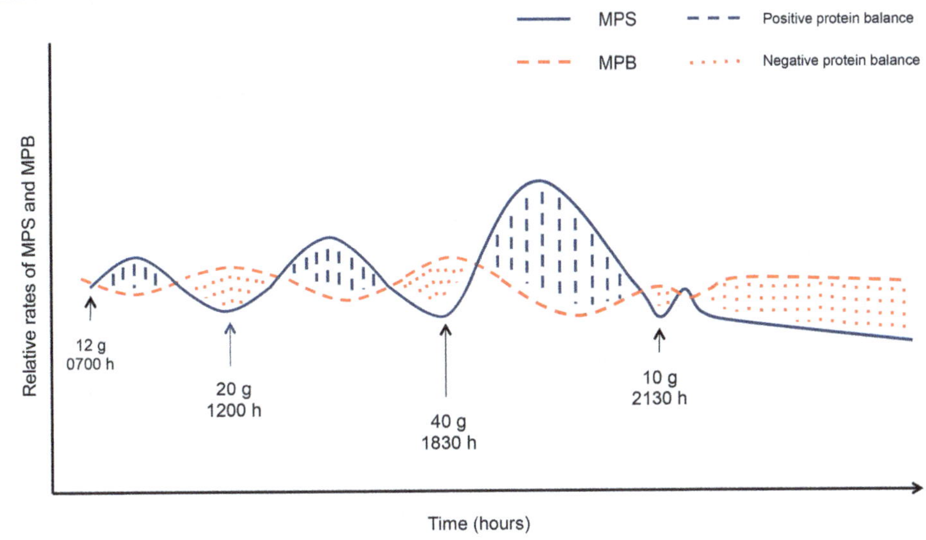

FIGURE 4 | Muscle protein synthesis (MPS) and muscle protein breakdown (MPB) in responses to grams of protein per meal. Solid lines indicate MPS, dashed lines indicate MPB. Blue hashed areas indicate positive protein balance while the red dotted areas indicate negative protein balance. Blue hashed areas and red dotted areas equate to the same area under the curve indicating net protein balance.

effect on older skeletal muscle, we recently aimed to examine the effects of a high protein diet to mitigate skeletal muscle loss and reductions in MPS in healthy older adults during SR. To recapitulate circumstances associated with a period of SR in older adults (i.e., hospitalization), participants were provided with a high protein (1.6 g/kg/day) by supplementation with either a 60 g daily dose of whey protein or collagen peptides, and an energy restricted diet (−500 kcal, in addition to the reduction in energy intake accounted for by the SR) during a 2-week SR period. Supplementation with whey protein or an isonitrogenous quantity of hydrolyzed collagen peptide supplement allowed for the comparison of supplementation with high and low quality, high protein on LBM changes with SR (14). Following 1 week of energy restriction alone, there were no significant losses in LBM, however there was a marked reduction in MPS of ~16% in both groups [findings similar to previous investigations in SR (20)]. Interestingly, with energy restriction and SR, there were no further reductions in MPS, indicating a potential protective mechanism by which healthy older adults are able to mitigate additive catabolic stimuli. However, following a 1 week recovery which featured a return to normal daily steps, during which participants maintained supplementation, whey protein proved to be superior in stimulating rates of MPS above the SR period with no effect of collagen peptide supplementation (14). The lack of recovery of rates of MPS in the collagen supplemented group following return to normal activity is similar to previous findings from our laboratory in which participants resumed consumption of their habitual diets after SR (20). These data highlight the promising observation that high quality protein supplementation may serve to improve skeletal muscle health in conjunction with an increase in physical activity in older adults following convalescence, results that could be possibly further enhanced when combined with structured resistance exercise training.

CONCLUSION

Though it would be considered a significantly less catabolic stimulus than bed rest, SR as a model of reduced activity results in marked negative alterations in skeletal muscle health in younger and older adults. Periods of SR may occur at increased frequencies in comparison to complete unloading and with, we speculate, underappreciated consequences. In younger persons such periods may not be as deleterious as in older persons since, even given the small number of observations, it appears that older persons have difficulty fully recovering from SR or disuse. We propose that the periodic effects of muscle disuse and SR and the cumulative negative consequences that should be considered in addressing the longer-term health of aging individuals. These periods accelerate muscle loss and induce metabolic dysfunction from which for older persons would have deleterious consequences. Resistance exercise, even low load and sporadically performed, may serve as an effective strategy to offset disuse induced losses in skeletal muscle with SR. Importantly, resistive exercise combined with nutritional stimuli (high quality protein, creatine, and n-3 fatty acids, energy balance) may aid in attenuating the decline in LBM with disuse and aid in the rehabilitation of muscle mass. Given, that nutritional modification or RT is not always feasible during disuse, future research should aim to examine how to improve the recovery period from SR using exercise, rehabilitation, or supplementation to improve the physiological decline with disuse.

AUTHOR CONTRIBUTIONS

SO prepared the original draft of the manuscript. SO, TH, and SP contributed to the editing and preparation of the final manuscript.

ACKNOWLEDGMENTS

SO was supported by the Ontario Graduate Scholarship. SP is supported by grants from The Canadian Institutes for Health Research, The National Science and Engineering Research Council, The McMaster Institute for Research on Aging, and the Canada Research Chairs program and gratefully acknowledges these sources of funding.

REFERENCES

1. Colley RC, Garriguet D, Janssen I, Craig CL, Clarke J, Tremblay MS. Physical activity of Canadian adults: Accelerometer results from the 2007 to 2009 Canadian Health Measures Survey. *Health Rep.* (2011) 22:7–14. doi: 10.1016/j.yspm.2011.03.006
2. Samitz G, Egger M, Zwahlen M. Domains of physical activity and all-cause mortality: systematic review and dose-response meta-analysis of cohort studies. *Int J Epidemiol.* (2011) 40:1382–400. doi: 10.1093/ije/dyr112
3. Lollgen H, Bockenhoff A, Knapp G. Physical activity and all-cause mortality: an updated meta-analysis with different intensity categories. *Int J Sports Med.* (2009) 30:213–24. doi: 10.1055/s-0028-1128150
4. Trost SG, Owen N, Bauman AE, Sallis JF, Brown W. Correlates of adults' participation in physical activity: review and update. *Med Sci Sports Exerc.* (2002) 34:1996–2001. doi: 10.1097/00005768-200212000-00020
5. King AC, Castro C, Wilcox S, Eyler AA, Sallis JF, Brownson RC. Personal and environmental factors associated with physical inactivity among different racial–ethnic groups of U.S. middle-aged and older-aged women. *Health Psychol.* (2000) 19:354–64. doi: 10.1037//0278-6133.19.4.354
6. Sasidharan V, Payne L, Orsega-Smith E, Godbey G. Older adults' physical activity participation and perceptions of wellbeing: examining the role of social support for leisure. *Manag Leisure.* (2007) 11:164–85. doi: 10.1080/13606710600715242
7. Willey JZ, Paik MC, Sacco R, Elkind MS, Boden-Albala B. Social determinants of physical inactivity in the Northern Manhattan Study (NOMAS). *J Commun Health.* (2010) 35:602–8. doi: 10.1007/s10900-010-9249-2
8. Hartley P, Costello P, Fenner R, Gibbins N, Quinn E, Kuhn I, et al. Change in skeletal muscle associated with unplanned hospital admissions in adult patients: a systematic review and meta-analysis. *PLoS ONE.* (2019) 14:e0210186. doi: 10.1371/journal.pone.0210186
9. Kortebein P, Ferrando AA, Lombeida J, Wolfe RR, Evans WJ. Effect of 10 days of bed rest on skeletal muscle in healthy older adults. *J Am Med Assoc.* (2007) 297:1769–74. doi: 10.1001/jama.297.16.1772-b
10. Coker RH, Hays NP, Williams RH, Wolfe RR, Evans WJ. Bed rest promotes reductions in walking speed, functional parameters, and aerobic fitness in older, healthy adults. *J Gerontol Series A. Biol Sci Med Sci.* (2015) 70:91–6. doi: 10.1093/gerona/glu123
11. Suetta C, Hvid LG, Justesen L, Christensen U, Neergaard K, Simonsen L, et al. Effects of aging on human skeletal muscle after immobilization and retraining. *J Appl Physiol.* (2009) 107:1172–80. doi: 10.1152/japplphysiol.00290.2009
12. Dirks ML, Wall BT, Nilwik R, Weerts DH, Verdijk LB, van Loon LJ. Skeletal muscle disuse atrophy is not attenuated by dietary protein supplementation in healthy older men. *J Nutr.* (2014) 144:1196–203. doi: 10.3945/jn.114.194217
13. Breen L, Stokes KA, Churchward-Venne TA, Moore DR, Baker SK, Smith K, et al. Two weeks of reduced activity decreases leg lean mass and induces "anabolic resistance" of myofibrillar protein synthesis in healthy elderly. *J Clin Endocrinol Metab.* (2013) 98:2604–12. doi: 10.1210/jc.2013-1502
14. Oikawa SY, McGlory C, D'Souza LK, Morgan AK, Saddler NI, Baker SK, et al. A randomized controlled trial of the impact of protein supplementation on leg lean mass and integrated muscle protein synthesis during inactivity and energy restriction in older persons. *Am J Clin Nutr.* (2018) 108:1060–8. doi: 10.1093/ajcn/nqy193
15. Bell KE, von Allmen MT, Devries MC, Phillips SM. Muscle disuse as a pivotal problem in sarcopenia-related muscle loss and dysfunction. *J Frailty Aging.* (2016) 5:33–41. doi: 10.14283/jfa.2016.78
16. English KL, Paddon-Jones D. Protecting muscle mass and function in older adults during bed rest. *Curr Opin Clin Nutr Metab Care.* (2010) 13:34–9. doi: 10.1097/MCO.0b013e328333aa66
17. Reid KF, Pasha E, Doros G, Clark DJ, Patten C, Phillips EM, et al. Longitudinal decline of lower extremity muscle power in healthy and mobility-limited older adults: influence of muscle mass, strength, composition, neuromuscular activation and single fiber contractile properties. *Eur J Appl Physiol.* (2014) 114:29–39. doi: 10.1007/s00421-013-2728-2
18. Welch C, Hassan-Smith ZK, Greig, CA, Lord, JM, Jackson, TA. Acute sarcopenia secondary to hospitalisation - an emerging condition affecting older adults. *Aging Dis.* (2018) 9:151–64. doi: 10.14336/AD.2017.0315
19. Atherton PJ, Greenhaff PL, Phillips SM, Bodine SC, Adams CM, Lang CH. Control of skeletal muscle atrophy in response to disuse: clinical/preclinical contentions and fallacies of evidence. *Am J Physiol Endocrinol Metab.* (2016) 311:E594–604. doi: 10.1152/ajpendo.00257.2016
20. McGlory C, von Allmen MT, Stokes T, Morton RG, Hector AJ, Lago BA, et al. Failed recovery of glycemic control and myofibrillar protein synthesis with two weeks of physical inactivity in overweight, pre-diabetic older adults. *J Gerontol A Biol Sci Med Sci.* (2017) 73:1070–7. doi: 10.1093/gerona/glx203
21. Aagaard P, Suetta C, Caserotti P, Magnusson SP, Kjaer M. Role of the nervous system in sarcopenia and muscle atrophy with aging: strength training as a countermeasure. *Scand J Med Sci Sports.* (2010) 20:49–64. doi: 10.1111/j.1600-0838.2009.01084.x
22. Stephens BR, Granados K, Zderic TW, Hamilton MT, Braun B. Effects of 1 day of inactivity on insulin action in healthy men and women: interaction with energy intake. *Metabolism.* (2011) 60:941–9. doi: 10.1016/j.metabol.2010.08.014
23. Fitts RH, Trappe SW, Costill DL, Gallagher PM, Creer AC, Colloton PA, et al. Prolonged space flight-induced alterations in the structure and function of human skeletal muscle fibres. *J Physiol.* (2010) 588(Pt, 18):3567–92. doi: 10.1113/jphysiol.2010.188508
24. Goodpaster BH, Park SW, Harris TB, Kritchevsky SB, Nevitt M, Schwartz AV, et al. The loss of skeletal muscle strength, mass, and quality in older adults: the health, aging and body composition study. *J Gerontol. Med. Sci.* (2006) 61A:1059–64. doi: 10.1093/gerona/61.10.1059
25. Walhin JP, Richardson JD, Betts JA, Thompson D. Exercise counteracts the effects of short-term overfeeding and reduced physical activity independent of energy imbalance in healthy young men. *J Physiol.* (2013) 591:6231–43. doi: 10.1113/jphysiol.2013.262709
26. Arentson-Lantz E, Galvan E, Wacher A, Fry CS, Paddon-Jones D. 2000 Steps/day does not fully protect skeletal muscle health in older adults during bed rest. *J Aging Phys Act.* (2018) 27:1–25. doi: 10.1123/japa.2018-0093.
27. Krogh-Madsen R, Thyfault JP, Broholm C, Mortensen OH, Olsen RH, Mounier R, et al. A 2-wk reduction of ambulatory activity attenuates peripheral insulin sensitivity. *J Appl Physiol.* (2010) 108:1034–40. doi: 10.1152/japplphysiol.00977.2009
28. Akima H, Kawakami Y, Kubo K, Sekiguchi C, Ohshima H, Miyamoto A, et al. Effect of short-duration spaceflight on thigh and leg muscle volume. *Med Sci Sports Exerc.* (2000) 32:1743–7. doi: 10.1097/00005768-200010000-00013
29. Narici MV, de Boer MD. Disuse of the musculo-skeletal system in space and on earth. *Eur J Appl Physiol.* (2011) 111:403–20. doi: 10.1007/s00421-010-1556-x
30. Hughson RL, Robertson AD, Arbeille P, Shoemaker JK, Rush JW, Fraser KS, et al. Increased postflight carotid artery stiffness and inflight insulin resistance resulting from 6-mo spaceflight in male and female astronauts. *Am J Physiol Heart Circ Physiol.* (2016) 310:H628–38. doi: 10.1152/ajpheart.00802.2015
31. Glover EI, Phillips SM, Oates BR, Tang JE, Tarnopolsky MA, Selby A, et al. Immobilization induces anabolic resistance in human myofibrillar protein synthesis with low and high dose amino acid infusion. *J Physiol.* (2008) 586(Pt. 24):6049–61. doi: 10.1113/jphysiol.2008.160333
32. D'Antona G, Pellegrino MA, Adami R, Rossi R, Carlizzi CN, Canepari M, et al. The effect of ageing and immobilization on structure and function of human skeletal muscle fibres. *J Physiol.* (2003) 552(Pt. 2):499–511. doi: 10.1113/jphysiol.2003.046276
33. Mikus CR, Oberlin DJ, Libla JL, Taylor AM, Booth FW, Thyfault JP. Lowering physical activity impairs glycemic control in healthy volunteers.

Med Sci Sports Exerc. (2012) 44:225–31. doi: 10.1249/MSS.0b013e31822acOc0
34. Fisher SR, Goodwin JS, Protas EJ, Kuo YF, Graham JE, Ottenbacher KJ, et al. Ambulatory activity of older adults hospitalized with acute medical illness. *J Am Geriatr Soc.* (2011) 59:91–5. doi: 10.1111/j.1532-5415.2010.03202.x
35. Olsen RH, Krogh-Madsen R, Thomsen C, Booth FW, Pedersen BK. Metabolic responses to reduced daily steps in healthy nonexercising men. *J Am Med Assoc.* (2008) 299:1261–3. doi: 10.1001/jama.299.11.1259
36. Knudsen SH, Hansen LS, Pedersen M, Dejgaard T, Hansen J, Hall GV, et al. Changes in insulin sensitivity precede changes in body composition during 14 days of step reduction combined with overfeeding in healthy young men. *J Appl Physiol (1985).* (2012) 113:7–15. doi: 10.1152/japplphysiol.00189.2011
37. Cesari M, Penninx BWJH, Pahor M, Lauretani F, Corsi A, Williams GR, et al. Inflammatory markers and physical performance in older persons: The InCHIANTI study. *J Gerontol. Med. Sci.* (2004) 59A:242–8. doi: 10.1093/gerona/59.3.M242
38. Devries MC, Breen L, Von Allmen M, MacDonald MJ, Moore DR, Offord EA, et al. Low-load resistance training during step-reduction attenuates declines in muscle mass and strength and enhances anabolic sensitivity in older men. *Physiol Rep.* (2015) 3:e12493. doi: 10.14814/phy2.12493
39. Wall BT, Dirks ML, Snijders T, van Dijk JW, Fritsch M, Verdijk LB, et al. Short-term muscle disuse lowers myofibrillar protein synthesis rates and induces anabolic resistance to protein ingestion. *Am J Physiol Endocrinol Metab.* (2016) 310:E137–47. doi: 10.1152/ajpendo.00227.2015
40. English KL, Mettler JA, Ellison JB, Mamerow MM, Arentson-Lantz E, Pattarini JM, et al. Leucine partially protects muscle mass and function during bed rest in middle-aged adults. *Am J Clin Nutr.* (2015) 103:465–73 doi: 10.3945/ajcn.115.112359
41. Phillips SM, McGlory C. CrossTalk proposal: The dominant mechanism causing disuse muscle atrophy is decreased protein synthesis. *J Physiol.* (2014) 592:5341–3. doi: 10.1113/jphysiol.2014.273615
42. Hector AJ, McGlory C, Damas F, Mazara N, Baker SK, Phillips SM. Pronounced energy restriction with elevated protein intake results in no change in proteolysis and reductions in skeletal muscle protein synthesis that are mitigated by resistance exercise. *FASEB J.* (2017) 32:265–75. doi: 10.1096/fj.201700158RR
43. Baumgartner RN, Koehler KM, Gallagher D, Romero L, Heymsfield SB, Ross RR, et al. Epidemiology of sarcopenia among the elderly in New Mexico. *Am J Epidemiol.* (1998) 147:755–63. doi: 10.1093/oxfordjournals.aje.a009520
44. Pisot R, Marusic U, Biolo G, Mazzucco S, Lazzer S, Grassi B, et al. Greater loss in muscle mass and function but smaller metabolic alterations in older compared with younger men following 2 wk of bed rest and recovery. *J Appl Physiol.* (2016) 120:922–9. doi: 10.1152/japplphysiol.00858.2015
45. Trombetti A, Reid KF, Hars M, Herrmann FR, Pasha E, Phillips EM, et al. Age-associated declines in muscle mass, strength, power, and physical performance: impact on fear of falling and quality of life. *Osteoporos Int.* (2016) 27:463–71. doi: 10.1007/s00198-015-3236-5
46. Newman A, Kupelian V, Visser M, Simonsick E, Goodpaster BH, Kritchevsky SB, et al. Strength, but not muscle mass, is associated with mortality in the health, aging and body composition study cohort. *J Gerontol Series.* (2006) 61:72–7. doi: 10.1093/gerona/61.1.72
47. Clark BC, Manini TM. Functional consequences of sarcopenia and dynapenia in the elderly. *Curr Opin Clin Nutr Metab Care.* (2010) 13:271–6. doi: 10.1097/MCO.0b013e328337819e
48. Reidy PT, McKenzie AI, Mahmassani Z, Morrow VR, Yonemura NM, Hopkins PN, et al. Skeletal muscle ceramides and relationship with insulin sensitivity after 2 weeks of simulated sedentary behaviour and recovery in healthy older adults. *J Physiol.* (2018) 596:5217–36. doi: 10.1113/JP276798
49. Oikawa SY, Callahan DM, McGlory C, Toth MJ, Phillips SM. Maintenance of skeletal muscle function following reduced daily physical activity in healthy older adults: a pilot trial. *Appl Physiol Nutr Metab.* (2019). doi: 10.1139/apnm-2018-0631. [Epub ahead of print].
50. Wallerstein LF, Barroso R, Tricoli V, Mello MT, Urgrinowitsch C. The influence of familiarization sessions on the stability of ramp and ballistic isometric torque in older adults. *J Aging Phys Activit.* (2010) 18:390–400. doi: 10.1123/japa.18.4.390
51. Ferrando AA, Paddon-Jones D, Hays NP, Kortebein P, Ronsen O, Williams RH, et al. EAA supplementation to increase nitrogen intake improves muscle function during bed rest in the elderly. *Clin Nutr.* (2010) 29:18–23. doi: 10.1016/j.clnu.2009.03.009
52. Alkner BA, Tesch PA. Knee extensor and plantar flexor muscle size and function following 90 days of bed rest with or without resistance exercise. *Eur J Appl Physiol.* (2004) 93:294–305. doi: 10.1007/s00421-004-1172-8
53. Nicholson VP, McKean MR, Burkett BJ. Low-load high-repetition resistance training improves strength and gait speed in middle-aged and older adults. *J Sci Med Sport.* (2015) 18:596–600. doi: 10.4324/9781315776422
54. Reid KF, Martin KI, Doros G, Clark DJ, Hau C, Patten C, et al. Comparative effects of light or heavy resistance power training for improving lower extremity power and physical performance in mobility-limited older adults. *J Gerontol A Biol Sci Med Sci.* (2015) 70:374–80. doi: 10.1093/gerona/glu156
55. Holloway TM, Snijders T, Vank J, Vanl LJC, Verdijk LB. Temporal response of angiogenesis and hypertrophy to resistance training in young men. *Med Sci Sports Exerc.* (2018) 50:36–45. doi: 10.1249/MSS.0000000000001409
56. Verdijk LB, Gleeson BG, Jonkers RA, Meijer K, Savelberg HH, Dendale P, et al. Skeletal muscle hypertrophy following resistance training is accompanied by a fiber type-specific increase in satellite cell content in elderly men. *J Gerontol A Biol Sci Med Sci.* (2009) 64:332–9. doi: 10.1093/gerona/gln050
57. Bamman MM, Clarke MS, Feedback DL, Talmadge RJ, Stevens BR, Leiberman SA, et al. Impact of resistance exercise during bed rest on skeletal muscle sarcopenia and myosin isoform distribution. *J Appl Physiol.* (1998) 84:157–63. doi: 10.1152/jappl.1998.84.1.157
58. Kawakami Y, Muraoka Y, Kubo K, Suzuki Y, Fukunaga T. Changes in muscle size and architecture following 20 days of bed rest. *J Gravitat Physiol.* (2000) 7:53–9. doi: 10.1007/s004210000330
59. Trappe S, Trappe T, Gallagher P, Harber M, Alkner B, Tesch P. Human single muscle fibre function with 84 day bed-rest and resistance exercise. *J Physiol.* (2004) 557(Pt 2):501–13. doi: 10.1113/jphysiol.2004.062166
60. Oates BR, Glover EI, West DW, Fry JL, Tarnopolsky MA, Phillips SM. Low-volume resistance exercise attenuates the decline in strength and muscle mass associated with immobilization. *Muscle Nerve.* (2010) 42:539–46. doi: 10.1002/mus.21721
61. Morton RW, Oikawa SY, Wavell CG, Mazara N, McGlory C, Quadrilatero J, et al. Neither load nor systemic hormones determine resistance training-mediated hypertrophy or strength gains in resistance-trained young men. *J Appl Physiol.* (2016):jap 00154 2016. doi: 10.1152/japplphysiol.00154.2016
62. Mitchell CJ, Churchward-Venne TA, West DW, Burd NA, Breen L, Baker SK, et al. Resistance exercise load does not determine training-mediated hypertrophic gains in young men. *J Appl Physiol.* (2012) 113:71–7. doi: 10.1152/japplphysiol.00307.2012
63. Moore DR, Kelly RP, Devries MC, Churchward-Venne TA, Phillips SM, Parise G, et al. Low-load resistance exercise during inactivity is associated with greater fibre area and satellite cell expression in older skeletal muscle. *J Cachexia Sarcopenia Muscle.* (2018) 9:747–54. doi: 10.1002/jcsm.12306
64. Breen L, Phillips SM. Skeletal muscle protein metabolism in the elderly: Interventions to counteract the 'anabolic resistance' of ageing. *Nutr Metab.* (2011) 8:68. doi: 10.1186/1743-7075-8-68
65. Cuthbertson D, Smith K, Babraj J, Leese G, Waddell T, Atherton P, et al. Anabolic signaling deficits underlie amino acid resistance of wasting, aging muscle. *FASEB J.* (2005) 19:422–4. doi: 10.1096/fj.04-2640fje
66. Yang Y, Churchward-Venne TA, Burd NA, Breen L, Tarnopolsky MA, Phillips SM. Myofibrillar protein synthesis following ingestion of soy protein isolate at rest and after resistance exercise in elderly men. *Nutr Metab.* (2012) 9:57. doi: 10.1186/1743-7075-9-57
67. Biolo G, Agostini F, Simunic B, Sturma M, Torelli L, Preiser JC, et al. Positive energy balance is associated with accelerated muscle atrophy and increased erythrocyte glutathione turnover during 5 wk of bed rest. *Am J Clin Nutr.* (2008) 88:950–8. doi: 10.1093/ajcn/88.4.950
68. Biolo G, Ciocchi B, Stuelle M, Bosutti A, Barazzoni R, Zanetti M, et al. Calorie restriction accelerates the catabolism of lean body mass during 2 wk of bed rest. *Am J Clin Nutr.* (2007) 86:366-72. doi: 10.1093/ajcn/86.2.366
69. Deutz NE, Pereira SL, Hays NP, Oliver JS, Edens NK, Evans CM, et al. Effect of beta-hydroxy-beta-methylbutyrate (HMB) on lean body mass during 10 days of bed rest in older adults. *Clin Nutr.* (2013) 32:704–12. doi: 10.1016/j.clnu.2013.02.011
70. McGlory C, Gorissen SHM, Kamal M, Bahniwal R, Hector AJ, Baker SK, et al. Omega-3 fatty acid supplementation attenuates skeletal muscle disuse atrophy

during two weeks of unilateral leg immobilization in healthy young women. *FASEB J.* (2019) 33:4586–97. doi: 10.1096/fj.201801857RRR

71. Kortebein P, Symons TB, Ferrando A, Paddon-Jones D, Ronsen O, Protas E. Functional impact of 10 days of bed rest in healthy older adults. *J Gerontol A Biol Sci Med Sci.* (2008) 63:1076–81. doi: 10.1093/gerona/63.10.1076
72. Paddon-Jones D, Sheffield-Moore M, Urban RJ, Sanford AP, Aarsland A, Wolfe RR, et al. Essential amino acid and carbohydrate supplementation ameliorates muscle protein loss in humans during 28 days bedrest. *J Clin Endocrinol Metab.* (2004) 89:4351–8. doi: 10.1210/jc.2003-032159
73. Murphy CH, Churchward-Venne TA, Mitchell CJ, Kolar NM, Kassis A, Karagounis LG, et al. Hypoenergetic diet-induced reductions in myofibrillar protein synthesis are restored with resistance training and balanced daily protein ingestion in older men. *Am J Physiol Endocrinol Metab.* (2015) 308:E734–43. doi: 10.1152/ajpendo.00550.2014
74. Murphy CH, Oikawa SY, Phillips SM. Dietary protein to maintain muscle mass in aging: a case for per-meal protein recommendations. *J Frailty Aging.* (2016) 5:49–58. doi: 10.14283/jfa.2016.80
75. ARS. *Nutrient Intakes from Food and Beverages: Mean Amounts Consumed per Individual, by Gender and Age, In the United States, What We Eat in America.* Agriculture USDo, editor. NHANES 2015-2016. Available oline at: https://www.ars.usda.gov/ARSUserFiles/80400530/pdf/1516/tables_1-36_2015-2016.pdf (accessed May 10, 2019).
76. Churchward-Venne TA, Burd NA, Mitchell CJ, West DW, Philp A, Marcotte GR, et al. Supplementation of a suboptimal protein dose with leucine or essential amino acids: effects on myofibrillar protein synthesis at rest and following resistance exercise in men. *J Physiol.* (2012) 590(Pt 11):2751–65. doi: 10.1113/jphysiol.2012.228833
77. Hespel P, Op't Eijnde B, Van Leemputte M, Ursøt B, Greenhaff P, Labarque V, et al. Oral creatine supplemenation facilitates the rehabilitation of disuse atrophy and alters the expression of muscle myogenic factors in humans. *J Physiol.* (2001) 536:625–33. doi: 10.1111/j.1469-7793.2001.0625c.xd
78. Johnston AP, Burke DG, MacNeil LG, Candow DG. Effect of creatine supplementation during cast-induced immobilization on the preservation of muscle mass, strength, and endurance. *J Strength Condit Res.* (2009) 23:116–20. doi: 10.1519/JSC.0b013e31818efbcc
79. Moore DR, Churchward-Venne TA, Witard O, Breen L, Burd NA, Tipton KD, et al. Protein ingestion to stimulate myofibrillar protein synthesis requires greater relative protein intakes in healthy older versus younger men. *J Gerontol A Biol Sci Med Sci.* (2015) 70:57–62. doi: 10.1093/gerona/glu103

19

Integrated Myofibrillar Protein Synthesis in Recovery from Unaccustomed and Accustomed Resistance Exercise with and without Multi-Ingredient Supplementation in Overweight Older Men

*Kirsten E. Bell[1], Matthew S. Brook[2], Tim Snijders[3], Dinesh Kumbhare[4], Gianni Parise[5], Ken Smith[6], Philip J. Atherton[6] and Stuart M. Phillips[5]**

[1] *Department of Kinesiology, University of Waterloo, Waterloo, ON, Canada,* [2] *School of Life Sciences, University of Nottingham, Nottingham, United Kingdom,* [3] *Department of Human Biology, NUTRIM School of Nutrition and Translational Research in Metabolism, Maastricht University, Maastricht, Netherlands,* [4] *Department of Medicine, University of Toronto, Toronto, ON, Canada,* [5] *Exercise Metabolism Research Group, Department of Kinesiology, McMaster University, Hamilton, ON, Canada,* [6] *School of Graduate Entry Medicine and Health, University of Nottingham, Derby, United Kingdom*

Correspondence:
Stuart M. Phillips
phillis@mcmaster.ca

Background: We previously showed that daily consumption of a multi-ingredient nutritional supplement increased lean mass in older men, but did not enhance lean tissue gains during a high-intensity interval training (HIIT) plus resistance exercise training (RET) program. Here, we aimed to determine whether these divergent observations aligned with the myofibrillar protein synthesis (MyoPS) response to acute unaccustomed and accustomed resistance exercise.

Methods: A sub-sample of our participants were randomly allocated ($n = 15$; age: 72 $\pm$ 7 years; BMI: 26.9 $\pm$ 3.1 kg/m^2 [mean $\pm$ SD]) to ingest an experimental supplement (SUPP, $n = 8$: containing whey protein, creatine, vitamin D, and n-3 PUFA) or control beverage (CON, $n = 7$: 22 g maltodextrin) twice per day for 21 weeks. After 7 weeks of consuming the beverage alone (Phase 1: SUPP/CON only), subjects completed 12 weeks of RET (twice per week) + HIIT (once per week) (Phase 2: SUPP/CON + EX). Orally administered deuterated water was used to measure integrated rates of MyoPS over 48 h following a single session of resistance exercise pre- (unaccustomed) and post-training (accustomed).

Results: Following an acute bout of accustomed resistance exercise, 0–24 h MyoPS was 30% higher than rest in the SUPP group (effect size: 0.86); however, in the CON group, 0–24 h MyoPS was 0% higher than rest (effect size: 0.04). Nonetheless, no within or between group changes in MyoPS were statistically significant. When collapsed across group, rates of MyoPS in recovery from acute unaccustomed resistance exercise were positively correlated with training-induced gains in whole body lean mass ($r = 0.63$, $p = 0.01$).

Conclusion: There were no significant between-group differences in MyoPS pre- or post-training. Integrated rates of MyoPS post-acute exercise in the untrained state were positively correlated with training-induced gains in whole body lean mass. Our finding that supplementation did not alter 0–48 h MyoPS following 12 weeks of training suggests a possible adaptive response to longer-term increased protein intake and warrants further investigation. This study was registered at ClinicalTrials.gov.

Clinical Trial Registration: www.ClinicalTrials.gov, identifier: NCT02281331

Keywords: fractional synthesis rate, deuterated water, resistance exercise training, high-intensity interval training, whey protein, creatine, vitamin D, n-3 PUFA

INTRODUCTION

Reduced muscularity, a component of sarcopenia (1), appears to be driven to a large extent by the relative resistance of older skeletal muscle to the anabolic effects of loading (i.e., resistance exercise) (2) and protein ingestion (3). Relatively large bolus doses (compared to younger persons) of at least 0.4–0.5 g/kg/meal of protein are required to optimally stimulate myofibrillar protein synthesis (MyoPS) following resistance exercise in older muscle (3). To combat sarcopenic muscle loss, recommendations often suggest combining daily protein supplementation with resistance exercise training (RET). Although this combined strategy has yet to be proven with protein alone (4), multi-nutrient supplementation combined with RET may be effective in preventing and treating sarcopenia (5). We (6) and others (7–9) have shown that RET plus aerobic exercise or high-intensity interval training (HIIT) combined with multi-ingredient supplementation supports lean mass and strength gains in various groups of older adults (overweight, sarcopenic, healthy). Furthermore, the regular practice of both exercise modalities along with multi-ingredient supplementation induces other physiological changes important for healthy aging, such as increased cardiovascular fitness, heightened insulin sensitivity, and reduced inflammation (6, 10).

We previously reported that 6 weeks of ingesting a whey protein-based multi-ingredient supplement increased both appendicular and trunk lean body mass [measured by dual-energy X-ray absorptiometry (DXA)] and strength in a group of older men (6). Yet the subsequent completion of 12 weeks of combined RET + HIIT did not further increase regional or whole body lean mass (6). Although DXA does not measure skeletal muscle directly, increases in lean tissue mass generally align with hypertrophy (11). As such, it is possible that augmented rates of MyoPS underpinned the initial gains in whole body lean mass; however, the specific response of MyoPS to several weeks of multi-ingredient supplementation (with and without exercise training) is unknown. Importantly, we previously reported a high degree of concordance between integrated MyoPS and hypertrophy (12).

The main objective of this study was to determine whether daily integrated rates of MyoPS in response to acute resistance exercise would be altered following regular consumption of a multi-ingredient nutritional supplement alone and in combination with multimodal exercise training. A secondary objective was to examine the association between integrated rates of MyoPS and indicators of muscle hypertrophy during exercise training. We hypothesized that supplementation would stimulate MyoPS to a greater extent than a control beverage independently but not when combined with multimodal exercise training. We further hypothesized that integrated rates of MyoPS would correlate positively with training-related changes in DXA measurements of lean mass and muscle fiber cross-sectional area (CSA).

METHODS

Participants

The present study was a distinct sub-analysis of participants from our original trial (6), which was approved by the Hamilton Integrated Research Ethics Board and registered at ClinicalTrials.gov as NCT02281331. From the 49 participants in the original trial, we screened and recruited 15 healthy non-smoking men, all ≥65 years, each of whom gave their written and informed consent to participate. During a 75 g oral glucose tolerance test, fasting plasma glucose was normal (<5.6 mM; $n = 7$ and $n = 4$ in the supplemented and control groups, respectively) or elevated (5.6–6.0 mM; $n = 1$ and $n = 3$ in the supplemented and control groups, respectively). Two-hour plasma glucose (2hPG) concentrations were normal (<7.8 mM) in all participants (13). No participants were diabetic or prediabetic. Resting blood pressure was <140/90 mmHg in all subjects. Exclusion criteria included regular use of non-steroidal anti-inflammatory drugs, use of simvastatin, and injury or chronic illness that would prevent safe participation in the study. Additionally, subjects were excluded if they regularly consumed any of the following dietary supplements: whey protein, creatine, calcium, vitamin D, or n-3 PUFA.

Study Overview

Following baseline strength, aerobic fitness, and body composition assessments, eligible and consenting participants were randomly assigned to consume an experimental nutritional supplement (SUPP $n = 8$; 30 g whey protein, 2.5 g creatine, 500 IU vitamin D; 400 mg calcium; 1,500 mg n-3 PUFA) or a carbohydrate-based control drink (CON $n = 7$; 22 g maltodextrin). Participants consumed their designated study beverages twice per day for 21 weeks (see **Figure 1A**). Strength and body composition were reassessed at weeks 7 (Phase 1: SUPP/CON only) and 20 (Phase 2: SUPP/CON + EX). From weeks 8 to 19 inclusive, participants completed a 12 weeks progressive exercise training program, which consisted of whole body RET twice weekly (Mondays and Fridays) and HIIT on a cycle ergometer once per week (Wednesdays).

The 0–24 h and 0–48 h integrated MyoPS response to acute resistance exercise was assessed during participants' initial RET session (UT, untrained; week 8; see **Figure 1B**), and 10 days following their final RET session (TR, trained; week 21). Participants continued to take the study beverages twice daily throughout weeks 8 and 21, including during the 48 h post-exercise recovery period.

Training Outcomes

Whole body lean soft tissue mass (i.e., fat- and bone-free mass) and % body fat were measured by DXA (GE-LUNAR iDXA; Mississauga, ON). One-repetition maximum (1RM) strength tests were conducted for leg press, chest press, horizontal row, shoulder press, lateral pulldown, and leg extension. We assessed aerobic fitness using a peak oxygen uptake (VO_2peak) test on a cycle ergometer. Particulars of these procedures can be found in our original trial (6). Type I and type II muscle fiber CSA were measured at weeks 0, 7, and 20 using immunohistochemistry. Muscle fiber CSA measurements were made on resting muscle samples only [i.e., −8 weeks (baseline), and Day 2 (0 h) during the UT and TR acute MyoPS assessments]. For details, please refer to our previous publications (14, 15).

Tracer Protocol

Following collection of a baseline saliva sample (Day 0; **Figure 1B**) for the measurement of background deuterium (^2H) enrichment of body water, participants consumed a single bolus dose of 150 mL 70% deuterated water (D_2O). Serial saliva samples were obtained on Days 1–4 to capture the change in ^2H enrichment of body water in response to D_2O ingestion (**Figure S1**). Participants reported to the laboratory after an overnight fast the mornings of Days 2, 3, and 4 for a muscle biopsy (~30–50 mg) from the *vastus lateralis* muscle using a custom-modified 5 mm Bergstrom biopsy needle as described elsewhere (16). Biopsies were taken alternately from the left and right legs at least 5 cm apart beginning distally and moving proximally with successive biopsies. Directly following their biopsy on Day 2, participants completed a single session of resistance exercise.

A baseline muscle biopsy for the measurement of background ^2H enrichment in skeletal muscle was obtained at the beginning of the study (8 weeks prior to the UT acute MyoPS response). Due to the already high number of biopsies per participant, we elected not to obtain a second "baseline" muscle biopsy immediately prior to the TR acute MyoPS response. As such, the measurement of resting (pre-acute RE) MyoPS was possible only in the UT state in this study.

Acute Resistance Exercise

Each session began with a 5 min warm-up at 25 W on a cycle ergometer (ISO1000 Upright Bike; SCIFIT, Tulsa, OK). Participants then completed three sets of four exercises at 65% 1RM in the following order: leg press, chest press, horizontal row, and leg extension (HUR; Northbrook IL). The first two sets of each exercise consisted of 10–12 repetitions. The last set was performed to volitional fatigue, which we defined as the inability to smoothly move the weight through a full range of motion. Sets were separated by 1–2 min, and the workout was concluded with a 5 min cool-down on the cycle ergometer. In both the UT and TR states, 1RM was assessed 5–7 days prior to the acute resistance exercise session.

Muscle Protein Synthesis

Body water ^2H enrichment was measured as previously described (17). Briefly, 100 μL of saliva was placed in an inverted autosampler vial for 4 h at 100°C to extract body water. Vials were then immediately placed on ice in an upright position, and condensed body water was transferred to a clean autosampler vial. We then injected 0.1 μL body water into a high-temperature conversion elemental analyzer (Thermo Finnigan, Thermo Scientific, Hemel Hempstead, UK) connected to an isotope ratio mass spectrometer (Delta V Advantage, Thermo Scientific).

To measure ^2H incorporation into myofibrillar proteins, we homogenized muscle samples (~30–50 mg) on ice and centrifuged them for 10 min at 2,300 g and 4°C to separate the myofibrillar and sarcoplasmic sub-fractions. The myofibrillar sub-fraction was purified, the protein-bound amino acids released by acid hydrolysis, and the sample eluted from an ion exchange resin as outlined elsewhere (16). Dried samples were then converted to their *n*-methoxycarbonyl methyl ester derivatives (18) for analysis by gas chromatography-*pyrolysis*-isotope ratio mass spectrometry (GC-*pyrolysis*-IRMS; Delta V Advantage, Thermo Scientific).

Calculations

The fractional synthesis rate (FSR) of myofibrillar proteins was calculated using the standard precursor-product method (17):

$$\text{FSR}\ (\%\text{d}^{-1}) = \left[\frac{E_{Ala2} - E_{Ala1}}{E_{BW} \times t}\right] \times 3.7 \times 100$$

Where E_{AlaX} is the protein-bound enrichment (in atom percent excess) from muscle samples at time *X*. Therefore, the difference between time points is the change in protein-bound alanine enrichment between two time points with appropriate correction for ^2H incorporation into alanine (17, 19). E_{BW} is the mean ^2H enrichment (in atom percent excess) in total body water between time points. Two-day resting FSR was calculated using the difference in muscle protein ^2H enrichments between Day 2 and baseline (collected at *-8 weeks*; **Figure 1B**); FSR at 0–24 h and 0–48 h post-resistance exercise were calculated using the difference between Days 2–3 and Days 2–4, respectively. Lastly, *t* is the tracer incorporation time in days. Multiplication by 3.7 adjusts for the average number of ^2H atoms that are incorporated into alanine (17, 19), and multiplication by 100 converts the values to percentages.

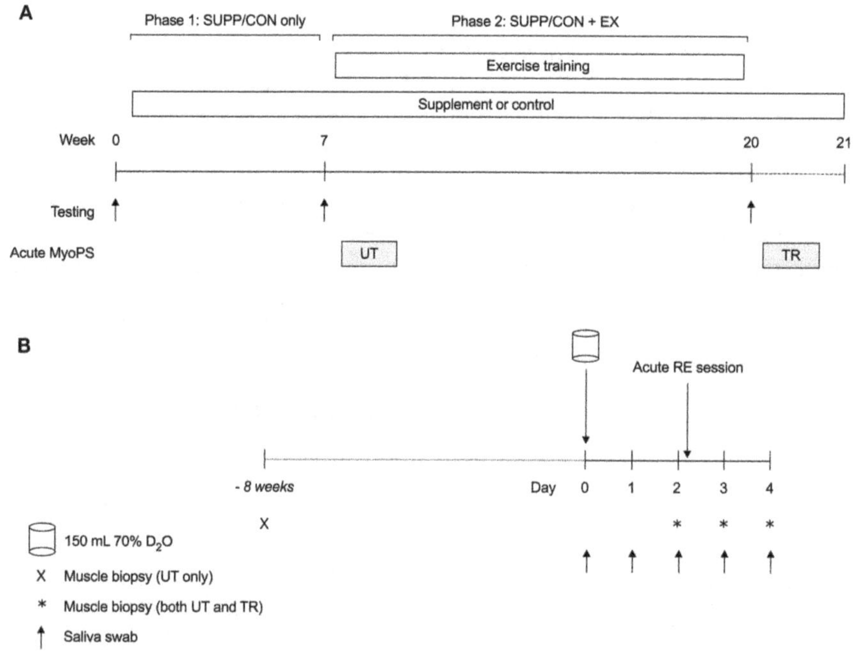

FIGURE 1 | Overall study schematic **(A)** and acute MyoPS response protocol **(B)**. **(A)** Participants were randomly assigned to consume a multi-ingredient supplement (SUPP, $n = 8$) or control (CON, $n = 7$) beverage twice per day for 21 weeks. Between weeks 8 and 19, inclusive, participants completed a 12 weeks combined RET (twice per week) + HIIT (once per week) exercise training program. Lean tissue mass (DXA) and strength (1RM) were assessed at baseline (week 0), as well as pre- (week 7; Phase 1: SUPP/CON) and post-training (week 20; Phase 2: SUPP/CON + EX). The integrated MyoPS response to acute resistance exercise was assessed during participants' initial RET session (UT, untrained; week 8) and 10 days following their last RET session (TR, trained; week 21). **(B)** Following a baseline saliva sample, participants consumed 150 mL 70% deuterated water (D_2O; Day 0). On Days 2–4, we obtained a fasting muscle sample from the *vastus lateralis*. Immediately after their muscle biopsy on Day 2, participants completed a session of resistance exercise at 65% 1RM. Saliva samples were collected regularly throughout each acute response period to assess deuterium (^2H) enrichment of total body water. Eight weeks prior to the untrained acute response (*–8 weeks*), we obtained an unenriched, fasted muscle sample for the measurement of resting FSR. SUPP, supplement; CON, control; RET, resistance exercise training; HIIT, high-intensity interval training; DXA, dual-energy x-ray absorptiometry; 1RM, one repetition maximum; MyoPS, myofibrillar protein synthesis; ^2H, deuterium; D_2O, deuterated water; UT, untrained; TR, trained; FSR, fractional synthesis rate.

Statistical Analysis

Baseline physical characteristics between the two groups were compared using two-tailed Student's *t*-tests. The following outcomes were evaluated using two-way repeated measures ANOVA with group (SUPP or CON) and time as between- and within-subject factors, respectively, body composition and strength (0, 7, and 20 weeks); and FSR (rest, 0–24 h UT, 24–48 h UT 0–48 h UT, 0–24 h TR,24–48 h TR and 0–48 h TR). Muscle fiber CSA was evaluated using two-way repeated measures ANOVA with group (SUPP or CON) as a between-subjects factor, and time (0, 7, and 20 weeks) and fiber type (type I or type II) as within-subject factors. Notably, DXA, strength, and fiber size data for these subjects have been reported elsewhere (6, 14, 15) (albeit from different participant cohorts containing individuals not included in the tracer analysis), and are also presented in this study for the reader's convenience. Any significant *F* ratios were further scrutinized using Tukey's *post hoc* test. We examined the effect sizes of the changes in FSR using Cohen's D. Associations between FSR and changes in whole body and leg lean mass over training were examined using two-tailed Pearson correlations. For all analyses, statistical significance was accepted as $p < 0.05$. Data are presented in text and tables as mean ± SD.

TABLE 1 | Baseline characteristics of participants.

	SUPP ($n = 8$)	CON ($n = 7$)	*p*-value
Age (years)	71 ± 7	73 ± 7	0.78
Weight (kg)	78.9 ± 11.2	83.0 ± 13.4	0.53
Height (m)	1.71 ± 0.06	1.75 ± 0.09	0.31
BMI (kg/m^2)	26.9 ± 3.0	27.0 ± 3.4	0.96
% body fat	29.6 ± 6.5	30.6 ± 5.8	0.76
Whole body lean mass (kg)	53.1 ± 5.5	55.0 ± 7.2	0.57
Leg lean mass (kg)	18.4 ± 2.3	19.2 ± 3.3	0.61
VO_2peak (mL/kg/min)	25.6 ± 4.3	25.7 ± 5.9	0.99
Leg extension 1RM (kg)	27 ± 6	28 ± 6	0.61
Leg press 1RM (kg)	80 ± 13	73 ± 27	0.54

Values are means ± SD.

RESULTS

Participants and Compliance

At baseline, participants were 72 ± 7 years of age and overweight according to BMI (**Table 1**). No significant differences in age or baseline measures of lean tissue mass (whole body or

TABLE 2 | Body composition and strength changes over training.

	SUPP ($n = 8$)			CON ($n = 7$)		
	Baseline (week 0)	**Pre-training (week 7)**	**Post-training (week 20)**	**Baseline (week 0)**	**Pre-training (week 7)**	**Post-training (week 20)**
Whole body lean mass (kg)[1]	53.1 ± 5.6^{a}	53.9 ± 6.4^{a}	54.5 ± 6.3^{b}	55.0 ± 7.2^{a}	55.0 ± 7.2^{a}	55.5 ± 6.5^{b}
Leg lean mass (kg)[2]	18.4 ± 2.3^{a}	18.6 ± 2.7^{a}	18.9 ± 2.6^{b}	19.2 ± 3.3^{a}	19.2 ± 3.4^{a}	19.5 ± 3.0^{b}
Appendicular lean mass (kg)[1]	24.6 ± 2.9^{a}	25.0 ± 3.4^{a}	25.3 ± 3.2^{b}	25.5 ± 4.1^{a}	25.7 ± 4.4^{a}	26.0 ± 3.8^{b}
Trunk lean mass (kg)[3]	24.8 ± 2.8^{a}	25.3 ± 3.2^{b}	25.5 ± 3.2^{b}	25.7 ± 3.1^{a}	25.4 ± 2.8^{a}	25.6 ± 2.7^{a}
% body fat[2]	29.6 ± 6.5^{a}	28.8 ± 6.7^{a}	28.0 ± 6.3^{b}	30.6 ± 5.8^{a}	31.3 ± 5.8^{a}	30.3 ± 6.2^{b}
Σ upper body 1RM (kg)[1]	104 ± 14^{a}	112 ± 12^{b}	127 ± 12^{c}	96 ± 20^{a}	95 ± 20^{b}	107 ± 22^{c}
Σ lower body 1RM (kg)[1]	107 ± 16^{a}	113 ± 17^{b}	144 ± 19^{c}	102 ± 31^{a}	105 ± 29^{b}	127 ± 35^{c}

Values are mean ± SD.
[1] Main effect of time, $p < 0.01$.
[2] Main effect of time, $p < 0.05$.
[3] Group by time interaction, $p = 0.015$.
Dissimilar letters indicate differences over time within each treatment group.

TABLE 3 | Muscle fiber cross-sectional area.

	SUPP ($n = 8$)			CON ($n = 7$)		
	Baseline (week 0)	**Pre-training (week 7)**	**Post-training (week 20)**	**Baseline (week 0)**	**Pre-training (week 7)**	**Post-training (week 20)**
MUSCLE FIBER SIZE (μm^2)						
Type I	6,907 ± 2,110	6,880 ± 1,090	6,883 ± 1,252	8,630 ± 1,737	6,765 ± 1,324	7,626 ± 1,565
Type II	6,409 ± 2,268	6,449 ± 1,214	6,676 ± 601	5,327 ± 1,349	4,924 ± 1,078	5,281 ± 1,003

Values are mean ± SD.
No significant differences.

regional), strength, or aerobic fitness were observed between groups. Compliance (assessed by questionnaire and returned drink sachets) with the nutritional supplements was 95 ± 4% (SUPP) and 95 ± 7% (CON). Participants attended 97 ± 3% (SUPP) and 94 ± 5% (CON) of their training sessions, and no participant missed more than two HIIT or RET sessions.

Exercise Training Adaptations

We observed a main effect of time for whole body lean mass ($p < 0.01$; **Table 2**), leg lean mass ($p = 0.01$), appendicular lean mass ($p < 0.01$), and % body fat ($p = 0.02$). No changes were observed during Phase 1, however over Phase 2 participants gained an average of 0.6 kg whole body (SUPP: +0.6 kg; CON: +0.5 kg), 0.3 kg leg (SUPP: +0.3 kg; CON: +0.3 kg), and 0.4 kg appendicular (SUPP: +0.3 kg; CON: +0.3 kg) lean mass, with no significant difference between groups. Percent body fat did not change during Phase 1, but decreased 0.9% after Phase 2 (SUPP: −0.8%; CON: −1.0%) with no difference between groups. We observed a group by time interaction for trunk lean mass ($p = 0.015$), such that the SUPP group gained 0.5 kg over Phase 1 with no further gains during exercise training in Phase 2. Trunk lean mass did not change over the course of the study in the CON group.

Muscle fiber CSA was not different between groups, and did not change over the course of the study (**Table 3**).

We observed a main effect of time for the sum of upper and lower body 1RM (both $p < 0.001$). Upper body strength increased 4% during Phase 1 (SUPP: +8%; CON: 0%), and a further 13% following Phase 2 (SUPP: +13%; CON: +11%), with no differences between groups. Lower body strength increased 5% during Phase 1 (SUPP: +6%; CON: +3%), and a further 27% following Phase 2 (SUPP: +27%; CON: +22%), with no differences between groups.

Acute Resistance Exercise Session

The volume lifted (weight [in kg] x repetitions/set x number of sets) during the acute resistance exercise session was greater after vs. before the 12 weeks training program ($p < 0.01$), but was not different between groups either pre- (SUPP: 3093 ± 484 kg; CON: 3370 ± 1521 kg) and post-training (SUPP: 4107 ± 938 kg; CON: 3911 ± 2136 kg).

Myofibrillar Protein Synthesis

Resting FSR was similar in the SUPP (1.36 ± 0.24 $\%d^{-1}$; **Figure 2**) and CON (1.44 ± 0.23$\%d^{-1}$) groups. Although we observed trends for main effects of time for day-to-day (i.e., temporal; $p = 0.08$, **Figure 2A**) and cumulative FSR ($p = 0.09$, **Figure 2B**), these changes were not statistically significant.

Following a bout of acute exercise in the untrained state, 0–24 h FSR was ~30% above resting rates (SUPP: 1.74 ± 0.44%d^{-1}; CON: 1.91 ± 0.64%d^{-1}) but 24–48 h FSR was slightly below rest (SUPP: 1.18 ± 0.41%d^{-1}; CON: 1.11 ± 0.75%d^{-1}; **Figure 2A**). However, when integrated over the entire 2-day post-exercise period (0–48 h), FSR was ~10% above resting rates (SUPP: 1.48 ± 0.16%d^{-1}; CON: 1.53 ± 0.26%d^{-1}; **Figure 2B**).

In the SUPP group post-training, 0–24 h FSR was ~30% above resting rates (1.76 ± 0.46%d^{-1}, effect size: 0.86), and 24–48 h FSR was ~7% above resting rates (1.46 ± 0.96%d^{-1}; **Figure 2A**); cumulative FSR over 0–48 h was ~20% above resting rates (1.61 ± 0.51%d^{-1}; **Figure 2B**). In the CON group post-training, 0–24 h FSR was similar to resting rates (1.42 ± 0.71%d^{-1}, effect size: 0.04), and 24–48 h FSR was ~20% above resting rates (1.75 ± 1.23%d^{-1}; **Figure 2A**); cumulative FSR over 0–48 h was ~10% above resting rates (1.63 ± 0.67%d^{-1}; **Figure 2B**). Again, whether expressed as day-to-day ($p = 0.08$) or cumulative ($p = 0.09$) values, FSR did not change significantly over time. We did not observe any between-group differences in FSR.

Correlation Analysis

When collapsed across group, we observed a significant positive correlation between 0 and 24 h UT FSR and the amount of whole body and leg fat- and bone-free (i.e., lean) mass (**Figure 3**) gained over the course of exercise training. No other FSR time points were associated with changes in DXA measurements of lean body mass or muscle fiber CSA.

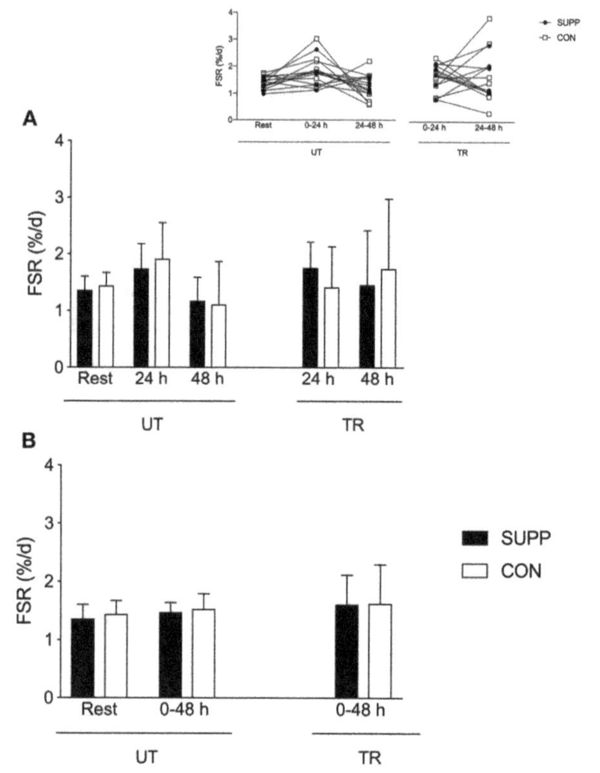

FIGURE 2 | Integrated day-to-day **(A)** and cumulative **(B)** myofibrillar protein synthesis in response to acute resistance exercise pre- and post-training. Individual day-to-day (i.e., temporal) data are presented on the inset line graph in **(A)**. The SUPP group is presented in black; the CON group is presented in white. SUPP, supplement; CON, control; UT, untrained; TR, trained; FSR, fractional synthetic rate.

DISCUSSION

To our knowledge, this is the first study to examine the influence of a comprehensive multimodal exercise training program combined with a multi-ingredient nutrition intervention on integrated rates of MyoPS in previously inactive but healthy older men. We observed that 7 weeks of whey protein-based multi-ingredient supplementation did not augment the MyoPS response to an acute bout of RE. Furthermore, we were unable to detect a statistically significant increase in MyoPS to acute resistance exercise following the completion of a 12 weeks RET + HIIT program, despite sustained supplementation. We did, however, show a significant association between FSR 0 and 24 h following unaccustomed resistance exercise and lean tissue mass gains made over the course of the exercise training program, which is in contrast to our previous work showing no correlation between integrated post-exercise FSR assessed at the outset of a resistance training program and skeletal muscle hypertrophy (12).

The ingestion of whey protein independently stimulates MyoPS for 3–4 h (3, 20) as well as amplifies the rise in MyoPS immediately following resistance exercise in older men (3). Emerging evidence suggests that other ingredients such as vitamin D and n-3 PUFA may contribute to further increases in muscle protein synthesis (MPS) during hyperaminoacidemia (21–23). In middle-aged (24) and older (25) overweight and obese adults, 2–3 weeks of energy restriction has been shown to reduce both postabsorptive and postprandial rates of MyoPS, even when protein intake is maintained at 1.3 g/kg/d (i.e., above the recommended daily allowance [RDA] of 0.8 g/kg/d). In younger adults, 3 weeks of energy restriction depressed postprandial rates of mixed MPS despite protein intakes of 2–3 times the RDA (26). However, the impact of prolonged higher protein diets on resting postabsorptive and postprandial MyoPS in the absence of energy restriction is not well-described. To our knowledge, only two studies (27, 28) to date have measured resting MPS after *several weeks* of dietary intervention where weight loss was not an intended outcome. Hursel et al. (28) observed no difference in postabsorptive mixed MPS between young adults who underwent 12 weeks of a deficient (0.4 g/kg/d) or very high (2.4 g/kg/d) protein diet. Similarly, Gorissen et al. (27) observed no difference in postabsorptive or postprandial MyoPS between older men who completed 2 weeks of a lower (0.7 g/kg/d) or higher (1.5 g/kd/d) protein diet. The lack of change in postabsorptive and postprandial MPS following 2–12 weeks of increased protein intake in these two studies supports our observation in the present study that resting integrated rates of MyoPS (which incorporate both fasted and fed periods, as well as habitual physical activity) were unaffected by 7 weeks of whey protein-based multi-ingredient supplementation [which

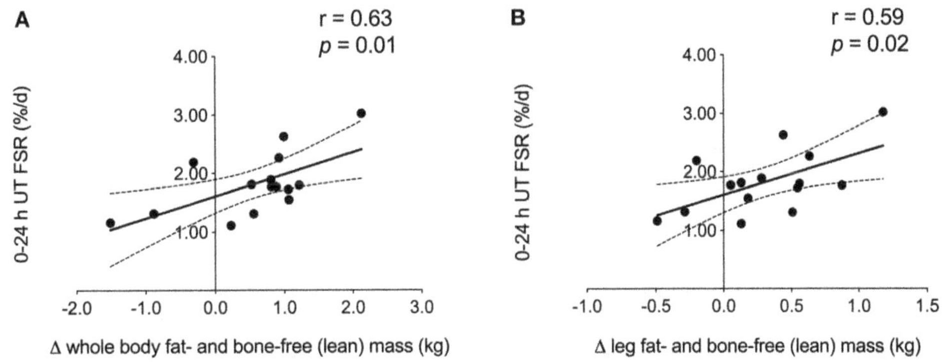

FIGURE 3 | Correlation analysis. FSR 0–24 h after unaccustomed acute resistance exercise was positively associated with the change in **(A)** whole body and **(B)** leg fat- and bone-free (i.e., lean) mass during 12 weeks of multimodal (RET + HIIT) exercise training (Phase 2). Linear regression lines of best fit are shown in black. Dotted lines indicate 95% confidence intervals. UT, untrained; TR, trained; FSR, fractional synthesis rate; RET, resistance exercise training; HIIT, high-intensity interval training.

raised protein intake from 1.1 to 1.6 g/kg/d in the SUPP group (6)]. Considering the well-described anabolic effects of protein (3, 23), these findings are somewhat unexpected but may represent an adaptive response to longer-term increased protein intake.

Given that resistance exercise is a more potent anabolic stimulus compared to dietary protein (3, 29, 30), it is surprising that we did not observe an increase in integrated MyoPS 0–24 h or 0–48 h after acute resistance exercise in this previously sedentary group of older men. In the untrained state, rates of MyoPS were 38% (SUPP group) and 33% (CON group) higher than resting rates at 24 h post-resistance exercise, and had subsequently decreased in both groups by 48 h post-resistance exercise; yet, this trend for a change over time did not achieve statistical significance ($p = 0.08$ and $p = 0.09$ for temporal and cumulative FSR data, respectively). This is in contrast to our previous work showing substantial (~20–90%) increases in MyoPS 24 h post-resistance exercise in younger (12) and older adults (31); as well as more conservative (~15%), yet significant, increases in the 3-day integrated MyoPS response to acute resistance exercise in older adults (32). A key comparison can be made between the present study and Bell et al. (31), since both studies assessed integrated MyoPS 0–24 and 24–48 h following a similar bout of unaccustomed resistance exercise in older men. In Bell et al. (31) we reported a nearly 2-fold increase in MyoPS 0–24 h post-resistance exercise, which was slightly dampened (although still above resting rates) after 24–48 h. In contrast, we observed no significant increase in MyoPS at any timepoint following acute resistance exercise in the current study. A notable difference between the two studies is that resting (1.59 ± 0.03 vs. $1.40 \pm 0.23\%d^{-1}$) and 0–24 h post-exercise (3.10 ± 0.25 vs. $1.82 \pm 0.53\%d^{-1}$) FSR values were higher in Bell et al. (31) compared to this study, possibly due to differences in the D_2O dosing protocol and/or time-frame over which the resting FSR measurements were made. In Bell et al. (31), participants ingested 120–180 mL D_2O daily throughout the experiment, and resting measurements were made over the 24 h immediately prior to the resistance exercise bout. In the present study, participants ingested a single bolus 150 mL dose of D_2O pre- and post-training, and resting measurements integrated the 8 weeks of the study prior to exercise training (Phase 1). In addition, the standard deviations of the FSR measurements appeared larger in the current study, suggesting that this pool of participants was more heterogeneous compared to Bell et al. (31), reducing our ability to detect changes over time or between groups. Other factors that may have contributed to the disparate findings between these two studies include the higher age (72 ± 7 vs. 67 ± 4 years), greater adiposity (% body fat: 30.0 ± 6.0 vs. 24.4 ± 4.9), and lower muscularity (whole body lean mass: 54.0 ± 6.3 vs. 61.4 ± 5.9 kg) at baseline of participants in the current study, relative to the subjects in Bell et al. (31). In fact, when appendicular lean mass is included as covariate in the two-way repeated measures ANOVA for FSR, we observe a main effect of time ($p = 0.04$) whereby—prior to exercise training—MyoPS 0–24 h post-resistance exercise is significantly elevated above both resting and 24–48 h rates, with no difference between groups. Clearly, additional work in carefully controlled studies is required to fully understand the integrated MyoPS response to unaccustomed resistance exercise in overweight older men.

The null findings in the present study are in line with a number of other studies that were unable to detect a significant increase in MPS in older adults despite subjects performing relatively strenuous exercise (3-12 sets of 8–12 repetitions at ≥ 65% 1RM) (33-35). Older individuals demonstrate a blunted rise in the MyoPS response to acute resistance exercise compared to their younger counterparts (2). This anabolic resistance to exercise combined with our use of integrated MyoPS measurements may have "diluted" the rise in MyoPS immediately following an acute bout of unaccustomed resistance exercise. Our participants were overweight, which is another factor that may have blunted the post-exercise rise in MyoPS. Recent work in young adults has shown that obesity may attenuate the ability of acute resistance exercise to increase fed-state MyoPS (36). Notably, however, the overweight status of the older adults in our previously published studies

(31, 32) did not prevent us from detecting acute exercise-induced increases in integrated MyoPS. Moving forwards, researchers should be mindful that the evidence supporting the stimulatory effect of unaccustomed resistance exercise on MyoPS is equivocal in older adults, and future studies should endeavor to elucidate the underlying reasons for the discrepancy between studies.

Work using stable isotope infusions has shown that, in both younger and older untrained adults, the degree to which unaccustomed resistance exercise increases acute MyoPS over 4 h is not related to training-induced gains in muscle volume (37) or lean tissue mass (33). A novel finding of the current study is that *integrated* rates of MyoPS 0–24 h in response to unaccustomed resistance exercise were positively associated with the magnitude of lean mass gained during 12 weeks of RET + HIIT in older men, as measured by DXA. The association we observed herein at the outset of training is not as robust as the correlation between FSR and direct measures (e.g., muscle fiber CSA and ultrasound measures of *vastus lateralis* CSA) of skeletal muscle hypertrophy that we previously reported in younger men after 3–10 weeks of habituation to training and attenuation of the initial damage response to resistance exercise (12). Possible explanations for the discrepancy between our findings and those of Damas et al. (12) include the distinct study populations (overweight older men vs. normal weight young men), as well as the difference in baseline myofiber size. The relatively large pre-training fiber CSA in the present study [~6,000–7,000 μm^2 vs. ~4,500 μm^2 in Damas et al. (12)] may have inhibited our ability to detect hypertrophy following exercise training. The 0.6 kg increase in whole body lean tissue mass that we observed following exercise training is modest compared to other data (38); however, when examined individually most subjects (11 out of 15) demonstrated a change in lean mass of at least +0.5 kg. The magnitude of change in these subjects exceeds the error threshold for DXA-derived lean mass measurements of roughly ±0.5 kg (39), suggesting there was accretion of lean mass. Importantly, although the increase in lean tissue mass over Phase 1 in the SUPP group was restricted to the trunk (+0.5 kg), the majority of lean tissue gained in both groups over exercise training was in the limbs (+0.4 kg). These observations are consistent with recent work by Mitchell et al. (40) demonstrating a significant increase in whole body and trunk lean mass by DXA (both roughly +1.5 kg), but no change in appendicular lean mass, in older men who consumed a higher protein diet (1.6 g/kg/d) for 10 weeks. The gains in trunk lean mass observed in the present study and in Mitchell et al. (40) are likely due to hypertrophy of visceral non-muscle lean tissue (e.g., organs), which has been demonstrated following increased protein intake in animal studies (41, 42). Following the addition of 12 weeks RET + HIIT, we did not detect further increases in trunk lean mass, despite sustained protein-based supplementation in the SUPP group. Appendicular lean mass significantly increased across all subjects during exercise training, which is supportive of muscle growth because skeletal muscle comprises the majority of soft lean tissue in the limbs. Further, we have previously shown in a sample of CON subjects (which included $n = 7$ subjects from the current study) that muscle fiber CSA tended to increase over exercise training ($p = 0.066$) (15). We do not report a change in fiber size in the present study, despite the increase in lean tissue mass, likely due to the large variability inherent to studies with small samples sizes. Although the training-induced gains in whole body (SUPP: +0.6 kg; CON: +0.5 kg, see **Table 2**) and appendicular (SUPP: +0.3 kg; CON: +0.3 kg) lean mass were similar between groups, a single bout of accustomed resistance exercise (i.e., post-training) resulted in a 30% increase in MyoPS in the SUPP group relative to resting measurements of MyoPS made prior to training (effect size: 0.86; **Figure 2**). In contrast, in the CON group, a bout of accustomed resistance exercise did not appear to elevate MyoPS relative to rest (effect size: 0.04). Therefore, despite the fact that we report no significant changes in FSR in this study, we propose that multi-ingredient supplementation, together with RET + HIIT, has the potential to enhance exercise-induced increases in MyoPS but that we lacked the statistical power to detect such differences.

There are several limitations to the present study. Our relatively small sample size may have limited our statistical power and contributed to the null findings. Additionally, the subset of participants included in this study demonstrated divergent body composition changes compared to what we report in the main clinical trial. In the main study, lean tissue mass increased during Phase 1 for subjects in the SUPP group, with no further increase during Phase 2; whereas no changes in lean tissue mass were detected in the CON group. As such, we cannot generalize the findings of the present study to the rest of the subjects in the clinical trial. Lastly, although we report an association between gains in lean tissue mass over training and rates of post-exercise MyoPS prior to training, it is difficult to use DXA-derived lean mass as a surrogate for myofibrillar protein. As we have previously acknowledged, DXA measures fat-free mass (using hydration) rather than skeletal muscle directly. Further, factors that affect hydration, such as plasma volume and muscle water content, may change with protein supplementation and exercise training. Therefore, caution should be used when interpreting these data.

In conclusion, several weeks of whey protein-based multi-ingredient nutrition supplementation did not appear to enhance integrated MyoPS at rest or in recovery from acute RE in this group of healthy older men. However, integrated MyoPS measurements made 24 h post-resistance exercise in the untrained state were positively associated with hypertrophic gains made during a 12 weeks RET + HIIT program.

AUTHOR CONTRIBUTIONS

GP and SP acquired funding for this trial. KB, TS, GP, and SP conceived of and designed the study. KB, TS, and DK collected the data. KB, MB, KS, PA, and SP conducted the biochemical and statistical analysis. KB wrote the original draft, and all authors read and approved the final version of the manuscript.

FUNDING

This work was supported by funding from the Labarge Optimal Aging Initiative from McMaster University (to GP) and a Canadian Institutes of Health Research (CIHR) grant (MOP-123296) to SP. KB was supported by a CIHR Canada Graduate Scholarship (CGS-D). The funders had no role in study design, data collection and analysis, decision to publish, or preparation of the manuscript.

ACKNOWLEDGMENTS

The authors would like to acknowledge the participants for their time and effort, as well as all the undergraduate students who volunteered their time to help with the trial.

SUPPLEMENTARY MATERIAL

Figure S1 | Body water ^{2}H enrichment in the untrained **(A)** and trained **(B)** state. Data were analyzed using a two-way repeated measures ANOVA with group (SUPP or CON) and time (Days 1–4) as factors. Dissimilar letters indicate significant differences over time. Both pre- and post-training, body water APE increased to approximately 0.20% and decreased significantly in a linear fashion each day thereafter ($p < 0.0001$). No differences between groups were observed. ^{2}H, deuterium; APE, atom percent excess; SUPP, supplement; CON, control.

REFERENCES

1. Marzetti E, Calvani R, Tosato M, Cesari M, Di Bari M, Cherubini A, et al. Sarcopenia: an overview. *Aging Clin Exp Res.* (2017). 29:11–7. doi: 10.1007/s40520-016-0704-5
2. Kumar V, Selby A, Rankin D, Patel R, Atherton P, Hildebrandt W, et al. Age-related differences in the dose-response relationship of muscle protein synthesis to resistance exercise in young and old men. *J Physiol.* (2009) 587:211–7. doi: 10.1113/jphysiol.2008.164483
3. Yang Y, Breen L, Burd NA, Hector AJ, Churchward-Venne TA, Josse AR, et al. Resistance exercise enhances myofibrillar protein synthesis with graded intakes of whey protein in older men. *Br J Nutr.* (2012) 108:1780–8. doi: 10.1017/S0007114511007422
4. Morton RW, Murphy KT, McKellar SR, Schoenfeld BJ, Henselmans M, Helms E, et al. A systematic review, meta-analysis and meta-regression of the effect of protein supplementation on resistance training-induced gains in muscle mass and strength in healthy adults. *Br J Sports Med.* (2018) 52:376–84. doi: 10.1136/bjsports-2017-097608
5. O'Bryan KR, Doering TM, Morton RW, Coffey VG, Phillips SM, Cox GR. Do multi-ingredient protein supplements augment resistance training-induced gains in skeletal muscle mass and strength? A systematic review and meta-analysis of 35 trials. *Br J Sports Med.* (2019). doi: 10.1136/bjsports-2018-099889. [Epub ahead of print].
6. Bell KE, Snijders T, Zulyniak M, Kumbhare D, Parise G, Chabowski A, et al. A whey protein-based multi-ingredient nutritional supplement stimulates gains in lean body mass and strength in healthy older men: a randomized controlled trial. *PLoS ONE.* (2017) 12:e0181387. doi: 10.1371/journal.pone.0181387
7. Rondanelli M, Klersy C, Terracol G, Talluri J, Maugeri R, Guido D, et al. Whey protein, amino acids, and vitamin D supplementation with physical activity increases fat-free mass and strength, functionality, and quality of life and decreases inflammation in sarcopenic elderly. *Am J Clin Nutr.* (2016) 103:830–40. doi: 10.3945/ajcn.115.113357
8. Verreijen AM, Verlaan S, Engberink MF, Swinkels S, de Vogel-van den Bosch J, Weijs PJ. A high whey protein-, leucine-, and vitamin D-enriched supplement preserves muscle mass during intentional weight loss in obese older adults: a double-blind randomized controlled trial. *Am J Clin Nutr.* (2015) 101:279–86. doi: 10.3945/ajcn.114.090290
9. Candow DG, Little JP, Chilibeck PD, Abeysekara S, Zello GA, Kazachkov M, et al. Low-dose creatine combined with protein during resistance training in older men. *Med Sci Sports Exerc.* (2008) 40:1645–52. doi: 10.1249/MSS.0b013e318176b310
10. Bell KE, Snijders T, Zulyniak MA, Kumbhare D, Parise G, Chabowski A, et al. A multi-ingredient nutritional supplement enhances exercise training-related reductions in markers of systemic inflammation in healthy older men. *Appl Physiol Nutr Metab.* (2018) 43:299–302. doi: 10.1139/apnm-2017-0533
11. West DW, Phillips SM. Associations of exercise-induced hormone profiles and gains in strength and hypertrophy in a large cohort after weight training. *Eur J Appl Physiol.* (2012) 112:2693–702. doi: 10.1007/s00421-011-2246-z
12. Damas F, Phillips SM, Libardi CA, Vechin FC, Lixandrao ME, Jannig PR, et al. Resistance training-induced changes in integrated myofibrillar protein synthesis are related to hypertrophy only after attenuation of muscle damage. *J Physiol.* (2016) 594:5209–22. doi: 10.1113/JP272472
13. Diabetes Canada Clinical Practice Guidelines Expert Committee. Diabetes Canada 2018 clinical practice guidelines for the prevention and management of diabetes in Canada. *Can J Diabetes.* (2018) 42(Suppl. 1):S1–S325. Available online at: https://www.diabetes.ca/health-care-providers/clinical-practice-guidelines?Categories=&SearchText=&Page=1
14. Snijders T, Bell KE, Nederveen JP, Saddler NI, Mazara N, Kumbhare DA, et al. Ingestion of a multi-ingredient supplement does not alter exercise-induced satellite cell responses in older men. *J Nutr.* (2018) 148:891–9. doi: 10.1093/jn/nxy063
15. Snijders T, Nederveen JP, Bell KE, Lau SW, Mazara N, Kumbhare DA, et al. Prolonged exercise training improves the acute type II muscle fibre satellite cell response in healthy older men. *J Physiol.* (2019) 597:105–19. doi: 10.1113/JP276260
16. Burd NA, West DW, Staples AW, Atherton PJ, Baker JM, Moore DR, et al. Low-load high volume resistance exercise stimulates muscle protein synthesis more than high-load low volume resistance exercise in young men. *PLoS ONE.* (2010) 5:e12033. doi: 10.1371/journal.pone.0012033
17. Wilkinson DJ, Franchi MV, Brook MS, Narici MV, Williams JP, Mitchell WK, et al. A validation of the application of D(2)O stable isotope tracer techniques for monitoring day-to-day changes in muscle protein subfraction synthesis in humans. *Am J Physiol Endocrinol Metab.* (2014) 306:E571–9. doi: 10.1152/ajpendo.00650.2013
18. Brook MS, Wilkinson DJ, Mitchell WK, Lund JN, Phillips BE, Szewczyk NJ, et al. Synchronous deficits in cumulative muscle protein synthesis and ribosomal biogenesis underlie age-related anabolic resistance to exercise in humans. *J Physiol.* (2016) 594:7399–417. doi: 10.1113/JP272857
19. MacDonald AJ, Small AC, Greig CA, Husi H, Ross JA, Stephens NA, et al. A novel oral tracer procedure for measurement of habitual myofibrillar protein synthesis. *Rapid Commun Mass Spectrom.* (2013) 27:1769–77. doi: 10.1002/rcm.6622
20. Burd NA, Yang Y, Moore DR, Tang JE, Tarnopolsky MA, Phillips SM. Greater stimulation of myofibrillar protein synthesis with ingestion of whey protein isolate v. micellar casein at rest and after resistance exercise in elderly men. *Br J Nutr.* (2012) 108:958–62. doi: 10.1017/S0007114511006271

21. Smith GI, Atherton P, Reeds DN, Mohammed BS, Rankin D, Rennie MJ, et al. Dietary omega-3 fatty acid supplementation increases the rate of muscle protein synthesis in older adults: a randomized controlled trial. *Am J Clin Nutr.* (2011) 93:402–12. doi: 10.3945/ajcn.110.005611
22. Smith GI, Atherton P, Reeds DN, Mohammed BS, Rankin D, Rennie MJ, et al. Omega-3 polyunsaturated fatty acids augment the muscle protein anabolic response to hyperinsulinaemia-hyperaminoacidaemia in healthy young and middle-aged men and women. *Clin Sci.* (2011) 121:267–78. doi: 10.1042/CS20100597
23. Chanet A, Verlaan S, Salles J, Giraudet C, Patrac V, Pidou V, et al. Supplementing breakfast with a vitamin D and leucine-enriched whey protein medical nutrition drink enhances postprandial muscle protein synthesis and muscle mass in healthy older men. *J Nutr.* (2017) 147:2262–71. doi: 10.3945/jn.117.252510
24. Hector AJ, Marcotte GR, Churchward-Venne TA, Murphy CH, Breen L, von Allmen M, et al. Whey protein supplementation preserves postprandial myofibrillar protein synthesis during short-term energy restriction in overweight and obese adults. *J Nutr.* (2015) 145:246–52. doi: 10.3945/jn.114.200832
25. Murphy CH, Churchward-Venne TA, Mitchell CJ, Kolar NM, Kassis A, Karagounis LG, et al. Hypoenergetic diet-induced reductions in myofibrillar protein synthesis are restored with resistance training and balanced daily protein ingestion in older men. *Am J Physiol Endocrinol Metab.* (2015) 308:E734–43. doi: 10.1152/ajpendo.00550.2014
26. Pasiakos SM, Cao JJ, Margolis LM, Sauter ER, Whigham LD, McClung JP, et al. Effects of high-protein diets on fat-free mass and muscle protein synthesis following weight loss: a randomized controlled trial. *FASEB J.* (2013) 27:3837–47. doi: 10.1096/fj.13-230227
27. Gorissen SH, Horstman AM, Franssen R, Kouw IW, Wall BT, Burd NA, et al. Habituation to low or high protein intake does not modulate basal or postprandial muscle protein synthesis rates: a randomized trial. *Am J Clin Nutr.* (2017) 105:332–42. doi: 10.3945/ajcn.115.129924
28. Hursel R, Martens EA, Gonnissen HK, Hamer HM, Senden JM, van Loon LJ, et al. Prolonged adaptation to a low or high protein diet does not modulate basal muscle protein synthesis rates - a substudy. *PLoS ONE.* (2015) 10:e0137183. doi: 10.1371/journal.pone.0137183
29. Pennings B, Boirie Y, Senden JM, Gijsen AP, Kuipers H, van Loon LJ. Whey protein stimulates postprandial muscle protein accretion more effectively than do casein and casein hydrolysate in older men. *Am J Clin Nutr.* (2011) 93:997–1005. doi: 10.3945/ajcn.110.008102
30. Churchward-Venne TA, Murphy CH, Longland TM, Phillips SM. Role of protein and amino acids in promoting lean mass accretion with resistance exercise and attenuating lean mass loss during energy deficit in humans. *Amino Acids.* (2013) 45:231–40. doi: 10.1007/s00726-013-1506-0
31. Bell KE, Seguin C, Parise G, Baker SK, Phillips SM. Day-to-day changes in muscle protein synthesis in recovery from resistance, aerobic, and high-intensity interval exercise in older men. *J Gerontol A Biol Sci Med Sci.* (2015) 70:1024–9. doi: 10.1093/gerona/glu313
32. Murphy CH, Saddler NI, Devries MC, McGlory C, Baker SK, Phillips SM. Leucine supplementation enhances integrative myofibrillar protein synthesis in free-living older men consuming lower- and higher-protein diets: a parallel-group crossover study. *Am J Clin Nutr.* (2016) 104:1594–606. doi: 10.3945/ajcn.116.136424
33. Mayhew DL, Kim JS, Cross JM, Ferrando AA, Bamman MM. Translational signaling responses preceding resistance training-mediated myofiber hypertrophy in young and old humans. *J Appl Physiol (1985).* (2009) 107:1655–62. doi: 10.1152/japplphysiol.91234.2008
34. Dickinson JM, Gundermann DM, Walker DK, Reidy PT, Borack MS, Drummond MJ, et al. Leucine-enriched amino acid ingestion after resistance exercise prolongs myofibrillar protein synthesis and amino acid transporter expression in older men. *J Nutr.* (2014) 144:1694–702. doi: 10.3945/jn.114.198671
35. Sheffield-Moore M, Paddon-Jones D, Sanford AP, Rosenblatt JI, Matlock AG, Cree MG, et al. Mixed muscle and hepatic derived plasma protein metabolism is differentially regulated in older and younger men following resistance exercise. *Am J Physiol Endocrinol Metab.* (2005) 288:E922–9. doi: 10.1152/ajpendo.00358.2004
36. Beals JW, Skinner SK, McKenna CF, Poozhikunnel EG, Farooqi SA, van Vliet S, et al. Altered anabolic signalling and reduced stimulation of myofibrillar protein synthesis after feeding and resistance exercise in people with obesity. *J Physiol.* (2018) 596:5119–33. doi: 10.1113/JP276210
37. Mitchell CJ, Churchward-Venne TA, Parise G, Bellamy L, Baker SK, Smith K, et al. Acute post-exercise myofibrillar protein synthesis is not correlated with resistance training-induced muscle hypertrophy in young men. *PLoS ONE.* (2014) 9:e89431. doi: 10.1371/journal.pone.0089431
38. Peterson MD, Sen A, Gordon PM. Influence of resistance exercise on lean body mass in aging adults: a meta-analysis. *Med Sci Sports Exerc.* (2011) 43:249–58. doi: 10.1249/MSS.0b013e3181eb6265
39. Nana A, Slater GJ, Stewart AD, Burke LM. Methodology review: using dual-energy X-ray absorptiometry (DXA) for the assessment of body composition in athletes and active people. *Int J Sport Nutr Exerc Metab.* (2015) 25:198–215. doi: 10.1123/ijsnem.2013-0228
40. Mitchell CJ, Milan AM, Mitchell SM, Zeng N, Ramzan F, Sharma P, et al. The effects of dietary protein intake on appendicular lean mass and muscle function in elderly men: a 10-wk randomized controlled trial. *Am J Clin Nutr.* (2017) 106:1375–83. doi: 10.3945/ajcn.117.160325
41. Fluharty FL, McClure KE. Effects of dietary energy intake and protein concentration on performance and visceral organ mass in lambs. *J Amin Sci.* (1997) 75:604–10. doi: 10.2527/1997.753604x
42. Hammond KA, Janes DN. The effects of increased protein intake on kidney size and function. *J Exp Biol.* (1998) 201:2081–90.

20

Amount, Source and Pattern of Dietary Protein Intake Across the Adult Lifespan

Benoit Smeuninx [1,2], *Carolyn A. Greig* [1,2,3] *and Leigh Breen* [1,2,3*]

[1] *School of Sport, Exercise and Rehabilitation Sciences, University of Birmingham, Birmingham, United Kingdom,* [2] *MRC-Arthritis Research UK Centre for Musculoskeletal Ageing, Birmingham, United Kingdom,* [3] *NIHR Birmingham Biomedical Research Centre, Birmingham, United Kingdom*

Correspondence:
Leigh Breen
l.breen@bham.ac.uk

Objectives: Sub-optimal dietary protein consumption may partially underlie the age-related loss of muscle mass and function (sarcopenia). Specifically, dose, timing, source and distribution of dietary protein across the day might influence muscle anabolism in individuals from across the lifespan.

Design: The present study aimed to assess daily and meal-specific protein intake, protein source and protein intake pattern in 40 young (23.8 ± 4.3 years), 40 middle-aged (51.6 ± 4.1 years), and 40 old (77.4 ± 7.4 years) individuals using 3-day weighed food diaries.

Results: Old individuals consumed on average 83.4 ± 24.6 g of daily protein, which was significantly lower compared with young but not middle-aged individuals who consumed, respectively, 105.1 ± 43.0 g and 97.0 ± 31.1 g of daily protein ($P = 0.013$). No significant difference in daily protein intake was found with middle-aged individuals. Dietary protein intake pattern was uneven across meals for all groups ($P < 0.001$ for all). Sources of protein consumption were similar between groups except at lunch where old individuals ingested lower quality proteins compared with middle aged and young individuals.

Conclusion: Although total daily protein intake was sufficient in the majority of participants, per-meal protein intake and protein distribution contend the current knowledge regarding optimal protein intakes. Increasing protein intake, especially at breakfast and lunch, could mitigate age-related muscle loss.

Keywords: sarcopenia, nutrition, aging, skeletal muscle, protein

INTRODUCTION

The progressive decline in skeletal muscle mass and function observed with advancing age, termed sarcopenia, can lead to an increased risk of falls, frailty and mortality (1). Skeletal muscle maintenance is therefore a cornerstone for healthy aging. Changes in muscle mass are ultimately the product of the complex interplay between muscle protein synthesis (MPS) and muscle protein breakdown (MPB) (2). Dietary protein provision robustly stimulates MPS and, to a lesser extent, decreases MPB, resulting in net muscle protein accretion (3). However, an impaired muscle anabolic response to the ingestion of lower protein doses in old individuals (termed "anabolic resistance"), is thought to be a pivotal factor in sarcopenia (4, 5). Less well documented is the role of dietary protein on muscle mass regulation during middle-age, a potential transition period between normal and impaired muscle anabolic sensitivity. As muscle mass begins to noticeably decline from ~45 years of age (6), it is therefore important to understand dietary protein intakes/requirements at this stage of life, in order to identify an appropriate time at which to introduce dietary strategies to delay the consequences of sarcopenia.

The Recommended Dietary Allowance (RDA) for protein of 0.8 $g{\cdot}kg^{-1}{\cdot}day^{-1}$ is deemed adequate and meets the metabolic demands of this nutrient, irrespective of age and gender. However, the dietary protein RDA is thought to be insufficient for repeated, robust stimulation of MPS and, hence, maintenance of muscle mass in old adults. Indeed, higher protein intakes of 1.0–1.5 $g{\cdot}kg^{-1}{\cdot}day^{-1}$ are associated with increased muscle mass and strength in old individuals (7–9). The proposal that dietary protein requirements are higher in older age are reinforced by recent data demonstrating that older individuals require considerably more protein on a per-meal-basis to maximally stimulate MPS compared with their younger counterparts (0.4 vs. 0.24 $g{\cdot}kg^{-1}$) (10). This is problematic for many older individuals, who typically consume dietary protein unevenly across meals, with the majority of protein intake being consumed during one meal (11). This uneven pattern of daily protein intake likely results in a failure to meet the threshold for maximal MPS stimulation during most meals. Developing dietary protein strategies that enable maximal MPS stimulation with every meal may be essential for attenuating the progression of sarcopenia.

The source of dietary protein is an important determinant of postprandial MPS stimulation. Specifically, the AA profile and absorption/digestive properties of ingested protein may determine the extent of MPS stimulation. Proteins that elicit a rapid increase in blood aminoacidemia/leucinemia, generally stimulate MPS to a greater extent than proteins with slower digestive properties or an inferior AA/leucine profile (12). In a typical Western diet, protein consumption primarily originates from meat and dairy products. The majority of animal-derived proteins have an AA profile that closely matches the bodily requirements and, as such, are able to evoke greater MPS stimulation compared with plant-derived proteins (13). However, reductions in appetite brought on by physiological (impaired sensory perception, poor chewing capability) and psychosocial factors (loneliness, cost), make it challenging for many older individuals to consume sufficient protein with each meal (14, 15), particularly from animal sources (16). Therefore, more pragmatic approaches are required in order to develop feasible protein intake guidelines for older individuals, formulated on a meal-to-meal basis.

The dearth of evidence on dietary protein habits across the adult lifespan hampers the development of tailored dietary interventions to support skeletal muscle health in older age. Therefore, the purpose of the present study was to assess the habitual dietary intakes of healthy young, middle-aged and community-dwelling old individuals living in the UK, with a focus on the amount, source and pattern of intake.

TABLE 1 | Participant characteristics.

	Young	Middle	Old
Sample size (N)	40	40	40
Male/Female (N/N)	26/14	12/28	21/19
Age (y)	23.8 ± 4.3	51.6 ± 4.1*	77.4 ± 7.4*†
Weight (kg)	70.9 ± 11.9	74.1 ± 15.1	72.0 ± 12.7
Height (cm)	173.6 ± 8.3	168.2 ± 13.4	170.8 ± 8.6
BMI ($kg{\cdot}m^{-1}$)	23.5 ± 2.6	26.6 ± 6.2*	24.5 ± 3.0

indicates a significant difference from young ($P < 0.05$), †indicates a significant difference from middle ($P < 0.05$). Values are presented as means ± SD.

METHODS

Participants

Young ($n = 40$; 23 ± 4.3 years), middle-aged ($n = 40$; 51.6 ± 4.1 years), and old ($n = 40$; 77.4 ± 7.4 years) adults were recruited from the Birmingham area (West Midlands, UK). Participants were eligible if deemed healthy based on a general health questionnaire and ambulatory. Institutionalized or dependent living individuals were excluded from study participation. Group characteristics are presented in **Table 1**. All participants were informed of the study procedures and provided written consent to participate. Ethical approval was obtained through the University of Birmingham Research Ethics Committee (#13-1475A). The study conformed to the latest guidelines set by the Declaration of Helsinki (7th edition).

Dietary Intake Recording

Participants' height and body mass were assessed in light clothing to the nearest 0.1 cm and 0.1 kg, respectively, using a stadiometer and digital scales. Participants were given a 3-day weighed food diary to be completed over 2 week-days and 1 weekend-day. The food diary required participants to provide the time, preparation method, brand and weight of all food ingredients and drinks consumed. Participants were given written and verbal instructions on how to accurately complete the food diary. Kitchen scales (Wuwangni, WeiHeng, Hong Kong) were provided to accurately determine the weight of foods and drinks ingested.

Nutritional Data Analyses

Weighed food diaries were analyzed using Dietplan 7 software (Forestfield Ltd, West Sussex, UK, V7.00.46). Daily total energy intake (TEI), macronutrient and micronutrient composition data were generated. Dietary macronutrient values were calculated relative to participants' body mass ($g{\cdot}kg^{-1}$), and as a relative percentage of total daily energy intake. Relative protein intakes were compared with the current RDA for protein consumption (0.8 $g{\cdot}kg^{-1}{\cdot}day^{-1}$), and with an alternative recommendation for higher protein in older individuals (1.0 $g{\cdot}kg^{-1}{\cdot}day^{-1}$) (8). Daily dietary intake was divided into 4 time points; T1, T2, T3, and T4, respectively corresponding to breakfast (6.00–10.00 h), lunch (11.30–14.30 h), dinner (17.30–22.00 h), and snacks (remainder of the day outside T1, T2, and T3). Relative protein intake at each meal was compared against the 0.24 and 0.40 g·kg^{-1} thresholds for maximal MPS stimulation for young and old individuals, respectively (10), and used to assess the proportion of meals that reached these respective thresholds. Furthermore, participants' daily protein intake pattern for T1, T2, and T3 was determined. The meal with the highest relative protein content was given a score of 3 and used as a reference value. Meal protein intake differed from the reference meal if a 10–20% (score 2) or >20% (score 1) decrease was observed in relative protein intake. This resulted in 18 distinct protein intake patterns. Finally, the protein source contributing the highest absolute amount of protein at each meal time-point was determined for all participants, and presented as a percentage of individuals consuming the respective protein source. Most commonly identified protein sources included: bread, red meat, poultry/eggs, milk, cheese, yogurt, protein supplements, fish, nuts, soya, vegetarian meat substitutes and oats/muesli.

Statistical Analysis

Sample size was determined using point estimate calculations for protein intake, with a population mean based on a study by Cardon-Thomas et al. (11), to allow a margin for random error of 0.05 g·kg^{-1}·day^{-1}. Data were analyzed using Graphpad Prism V7.0 (Graphpad Software, CA, USA). Between-group differences for total nutrient intakes and participant characteristics were assessed using an ordinary 1-way ANOVA. Within and between-group differences for meal-specific protein intakes were identified using an ordinary 2-way ANOVA. Tukey *post-hoc* analyses were used. *F*-values represent the ratio of systematic to unsystematic variation, with a value greater than one indicating an effect beyond extraneous factors. Spearman's correlations were used to determine all associations between protein intake (absolute and relative) and daily total energy intake (TEI), with the exception of the correlation between absolute protein intake and TEI in the old group where a Pearson correlation was used. A binomial test was used to determine whether differences within groups for protein intake pattern (even or uneven intake) existed. A Fisher's exact test was used to determine whether protein intake pattern (even or uneven) differed between groups. Significance was set at $P < 0.05$. All values are expressed as mean ± SD unless stated otherwise.

RESULTS

Dietary Energy and Macronutrient Intake

Average daily energy and macronutrient intakes are presented in **Table 2**. No differences between groups were found for TEI, or absolute and relative CHO, fat and alcohol consumption. Absolute ($P = 0.013$) and relative ($P = 0.005$) daily protein intakes were 26% higher in young compared with old individuals. Expressed as a percentage of TEI, old individuals consumed less protein and alcohol compared with young ($P = 0.01$ for both) and middle-aged individuals ($P = 0.034$ and $P < 0.001$, respectively), but more CHO compared with middle-aged individuals ($P = 0.001$). Absolute and relative daily protein intake in young and old individuals was positively associated with TEI, whereas only absolute protein intake showed a positive correlation with TEI in middle-aged individuals (**Table 3**). Over the entire 3-day measurement period, 95, 100, and 98% of young, middle-aged and old individuals, respectively, met the current RDA for protein intake of 0.8 g·kg^{-1}·day^{-1} (**Figure 1**). However, only 70, 62, and 65% of, respectively, young, middle-aged and old individuals met this threshold on all 3 individual measurement days. When compared to the alternative protein recommendation of 1.0 g·kg^{-1}·day^{-1}, a significantly greater proportion of young individuals (60%) reached this protein intake on all 3 individual measurement days as opposed to middle-aged and old individuals (both 35%) ($P = 0.034$).

TABLE 2 | Average daily energy and macronutrient intakes in young, middle and old.

	Young	Middle	Old
Total energy intake (kcal)	2,257 ± 576.5	2,181 ± 606.9	2,169 ± 496.6
Total protein intake (g)	105.1 ± 43.0	97.0 ± 31.1	83.4 ± 24.6*
Protein intake (g·kg^{-1})	1.5 ± 0.5	1.3 ± 0.4	1.2 ± 0.4*
Protein (% TEI)	18.6 ± 6.4	18.1 ± 4.4	15.4 ± 3.0*†
Total CHO intake (g)	236.4 ± 73.6	211.1 ± 64.2	231.5 ± 64.6
CHO intake (g·kg^{-1})	3.4 ± 1.1	2.9 ± 0.9	3.3 ± 1.1
CHO (% TEI)	43.8 ± 6.4	41.4 ± 8.4	47.3 ± 6.3†
Total fat intake (g)	85.7 ± 23.4	86.7 ± 34.6	88.8 ± 25.0
Fat intake (g·kg^{-1})	1.2 ± 0.3	1.2 ± 0.5	1.3 ± 0.4
Fat (% TEI)	34.2 ± 5.8	35.1 ± 6.6	36.9 ± 6.4
Total alcohol intake (g)	11.6 ± 17.6	17.3 ± 21.7	9.3 ± 8.9
Alcohol (g·kg^{-1})	0.2 ± 0.2	0.2 ± 0.3	0.1 ± 0.1
Alcohol (% TEI)	3.5 ± 5.0	5.4 ± 6.4	0.4 ± 0.4*†

** indicates a significant difference from young (P < 0.05), † indicates a significant difference from middle (P < 0.05). Values are presented as means ± SD.*

TABLE 3 | Correlations between protein intake (absolute and relative) and total energy intake (TEI), and between protein intake (absolute and relative) and age.

	r	*r*^{2}	*P*
Young TEI – Protein Intake (g·kg^{-1})	0.636	0.404	<0.001
Young TEI – Protein Intake (g)	0.505	0.255	<0.001
Middle TEI – Protein Intake (g·kg^{-1})	0.515	0.265	0.001
Middle TEI – Protein Intake (g)	0.290	0.084	0.069
Old TEI – Protein Intake (g·kg^{-1})	0.765	0.585	<0.001
Old TEI – Protein Intake (g)	0.643	0.413	<0.001
Age – Protein Intake (g·kg^{-1})	−0.288	0.082	0.001
Age – Protein Intake (g)	−0.349	0.122	<0.001

Dietary Protein Distribution

Meal-specific relative protein intakes are presented in **Figure 2**. Daily dietary protein intake was distributed unevenly across meals with ~16, 30, 39, and 15% of protein in young, ~14, 31, 44, and 11% of protein in middle-aged and ~8, 12, 75, and 5% of protein in old individuals being consumed at T1, T2, T3, and T4, respectively. A significant main effect for time and group was found for relative [$F_{(3, 468)} = 115.53$ and $F_{(2, 468)} = 5.72$, respectively] and absolute [$F_{(3, 468)} = 107.31$ and $F_{(2, 468)}$

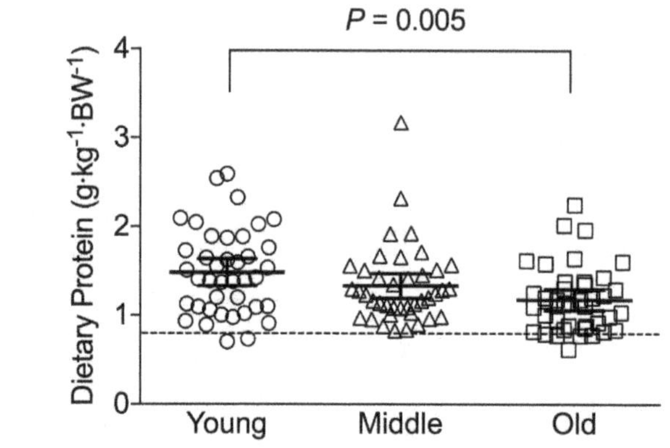

FIGURE 1 | Average relative daily protein intake in young, middle-aged and older individuals. Scatter plots display mean with 95% confidence intervals. Dashed line indicates current recommended daily allowance for dietary protein allowance of 0.8 $g{\cdot}kg^{-1}{\cdot}day^{-1}$.

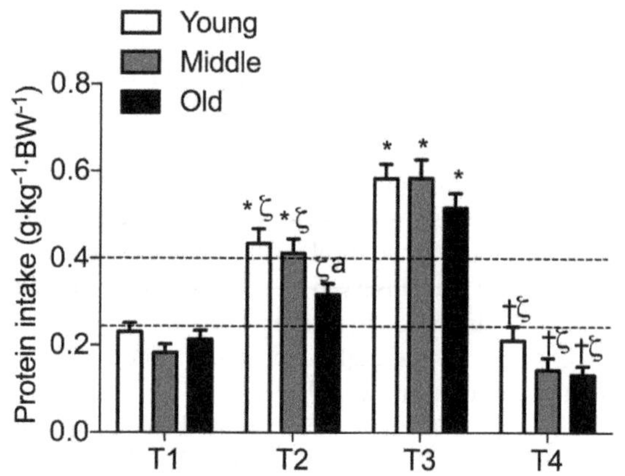

FIGURE 2 | Meal-specific average protein intakes in young, middle-aged and older individuals. Dashed lines represent threshold protein intakes of 0.24 and 0.4 $g{\cdot}kg^{-1}$, suggested for maximal stimulation of MPS in young and older individuals, respectively. *indicates significantly different from T1, ς indicates significantly different from T3, †indicates significantly different from T2, [a]indicates significantly different from young at same time-point. Significance was set at $P < 0.05$.

= 5.91, respectively] protein intake. No significant interaction effects were found for both relative [$F_{(6, 468)} = 1.13$] and absolute protein intake [$F_{(6, 468)} = 1.31$]. Relative and absolute protein intake was higher at T3 (dinner) compared with all other time-points for all groups ($P < 0.01$ for all). Greater relative and absolute protein intakes were observed at T2 compared with T1 in young and middle-aged individuals ($P < 0.001$ for both). Absolute and relative protein intakes were similar at T1 and T4 for all groups. Between-group differences in relative and absolute protein intake were found at T2 (lunch) only, where absolute protein intake was lower in old compared with young ($P = 0.01$) and middle-aged individuals ($P = 0.03$), and relative protein intake was lower in old compared with young ($P = 0.01$). On a meal-to-meal basis, the proposed dietary protein threshold for maximal MPS (0.24 $g{\cdot}kg^{-1}$ in young and 0.40 $g{\cdot}kg^{-1}$ in old) was met on all 3 measurement occasions by 28, 50, and 75% of young and 7.5, 7.5, and 30% of old individuals at T1, T2, and T3, respectively (**Figures 3A,B**). Snacks were often not consumed as a single-meal; therefore, it was not possible/appropriate to determine whether dietary protein MPS thresholds were met at T4 for young, middle-aged and old.

Dietary Intake Protein Patterns

A significantly greater proportion of young, middle-aged and old individuals displayed an uneven protein intake pattern ($P < 0.001$ for all) with no differences between groups ($P = 0.617$). The uneven protein distribution across the day, resulted in 18 observed protein intake patterns (**Figure 4**). Approximately 67, 63, and 53% of, respectively, young, middle-aged and old individuals distributed their daily protein intake according to one of three most frequently observed intake patterns. In young and middle-aged individuals, 72% of the meals highest in protein were consumed at T3, whereas 76% of the meals highest in protein were consumed at T3 in old individuals.

Sources of Dietary Protein Intake

At T1 and T4, milk was the most common source of protein intake for all three groups. At T2, young and middle-aged individuals primarily consumed animal-derived proteins in the form of poultry, fish and red meat, whereas plant-based proteins (bread) were the main source of protein in old individuals. At T3, animal-based proteins were most commonly consumed by all three groups. **Table 4** represents the 5 most commonly consumed protein sources for each meal in young, middle-aged and old individuals.

DISCUSSION

The present study is, to our knowledge, the first to directly compare dietary habits in young, middle-aged and old individuals with a focus on the amount, pattern and source of dietary protein intake. Absolute and relative protein intake was lower in old compared with young individuals. The RDA for protein (0.8 $g{\cdot}kg^{-1}{\cdot}day^{-1}$) was met by a majority of young, middle-aged and old individuals, whereas the number of old and middle-aged individuals (35%) meeting the proposed alternative higher protein RDA (1.0 $g{\cdot}kg^{-1}{\cdot}day^{-1}$) on all 3 measurement days was lower than young individuals (60%). Further to this, an uneven pattern of dietary protein intake was observed across meals for all groups, which was likely insufficient to reach the proposed threshold for maximal MPS stimulation at each meal in old, and potentially middle-aged individuals. Sources of protein consumption were similar between groups, except at T2 (lunch) where old individuals ingested mainly plant-based proteins compared with animal-based proteins in young and middle-aged individuals. These findings support increasing total daily protein intake on a per-meal basis in older individuals, to ensure a maximal muscle anabolic benefit is achieved.

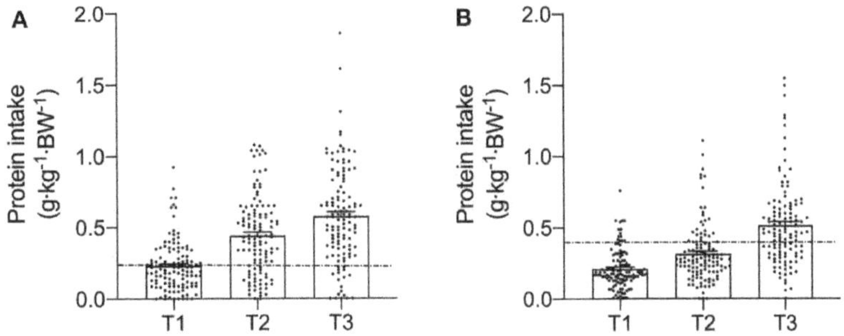

FIGURE 3 | Meal-specific relative protein intakes for each meal consumed at breakfast (T1), lunch (T2), and dinner (T3) in young **(A)** and old **(B)**. Dashed lines represent threshold protein intakes of 0.24 and 0.4 g·kg^{-1}, suggested for maximal stimulation of MPS in young and older individuals, respectively.

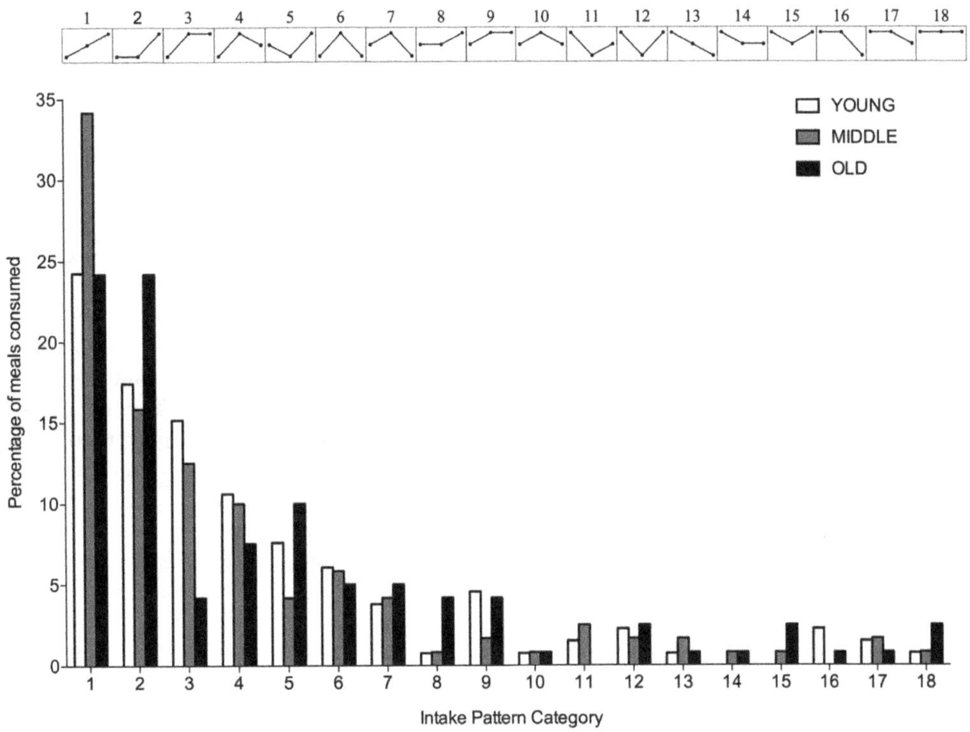

FIGURE 4 | Percentage of young, middle-aged and older individuals for each observed protein intake pattern. Intake patterns are depicted above each bar and represent the relationship between protein intake at T1, T2, and T3, respectively.

The current RDA for dietary protein to prevent deficiencies in this macronutrient is 0.8 g·kg^{-1}·day^{-1}. However, despite strong evidence to suggest a benefit/need for higher protein intakes to support muscle mass and strength in old individuals (17, 18), no guidelines exist for RDA requirements in this population. Indeed, the cumulative caloric intake when consuming the RDA for the three macronutrients (protein, carbohydrates and fat) would only result in 50% of the TEI observed in the present study, with the remaining 50% of energy intake classified as *flexible* calories. Therefore, it is little surprise that the majority of young, middle-aged and old individuals in the current study achieved the protein RDA. Alternative guidelines for dietary protein intakes of 1.0-1.2 g·kg^{-1}·day^{-1} have been proposed for older individuals (8). Herein, we report that 40% of young and 65% middle-aged and old individuals, respectively, did not reach a protein intake of 1.0 g·kg^{-1}·day^{-1} on all 3 measurement days, clearly emphasizing the need for novel strategies to increase daily protein intake. The positive association between TEI and dietary protein intake in old individuals reported here and elsewhere (19), lends to the idea that increasing TEI would increase protein intake. Important to note here, is that we did not observe any difference in TEI between groups. Thus, whilst increasing TEI may increase dietary protein delivery for old individuals, this may come at the expense of an increase in body fat mass. Furthermore, increasing TEI is likely difficult to achieve for many old individuals, due to the well-described anorexia of aging

TABLE 4 | Top 5 most commonly consumed protein sources during breakfast (T1), lunch (T2), dinner (T3), and snacks (T4) in young, middle-aged and old.

Young				Middle				Old			
T1	**T2**	**T3**	**T4**	**T1**	**T2**	**T3**	**T4**	**T1**	**T2**	**T3**	**T4**
Milk (25%)	Poultry (35%)	Meat (red) (37.5%)	Milk (32.5%)	Milk (47.5%)	Poultry (30%)	Poultry (42.5%)	Milk (50%)	Milk (67.5%)	Bread (32.5%)	Meat (red) (32.5%)	Milk (65%)
Bread (17.5%)	Fish (22.5%)	Poultry (37.5%)	Protein supplement (17.5%)	Poultry (25%)	Fish (27.5%)	Meat (red) (32.5%)	Yogurt (10%)	Bread (12%)	Fish (22.5%)	Poultry (30%)	Bread (5%)
Poultry (15%)	Meat (red) (20%)	Fish (7.5%)	Cake (12.5%)	Yogurt (10%)	Meat (red) (17.5%)	Fish (17.5%)	Bread (7.5%)	Yogurt (7.5%)	Poultry 15%)	Fish (27.5%)	Cake (5%)
Oats (12.5%)	Bread (15%)	Pizza (7.5%)	Poultry (7.5%)	Bread (5%)	Bread (10%)	Yogurt (2.5%)	Cake (7.5%)	Oats (5%)	Meat (red) 10%	Vegetarian substitute (2.5%)	Chocolate (5%)
Yogurt (12.5%)	Milk (2.5%)	Vegetarian substitute (5%)	Meat (red) (5%)	Oats (5%)	Cheese (7.5%)	Vegetarian substitute (2.5%)	Nuts (7.5%)	Poultry (5%)	Milk (7.5%)	Bread (2.5%)	Yogurt (2.5%)

Percentages represent the fraction of individuals consuming the respective protein source.

(20). Instead, altering the composition of the *flexible* calories in favor of protein consumption might be a prosperous strategy to maintain muscle mass in old age.

The distribution pattern of daily protein intake has been proposed to distinctly stimulate MPS, with an evenly spread protein intake thought to enhance daily net postprandial muscle anabolism compared with an uneven intake pattern (21). However, others have challenged this idea (22, 23), proposing that the quantity of per-meal protein, rather than intake pattern *per se*, is key for maximizing muscle anabolism in old individuals (21, 24). The concept of an age-related impairment in the muscle anabolic response to protein provision was demonstrated by Moore et al. (10), who showed that maximal MPS stimulation occurs with the ingestion of 0.24 $g{\cdot}kg^{-1}$ in young and 0.40 $g{\cdot}kg^{-1}$ in old individuals. Comparing present study results against the threshold values for maximal MPS stimulation revealed that a majority of young individuals did not reach their threshold at T1 and T2 on all three measurement days, whilst most old individuals failed to reach their threshold at all eating occasions. Therefore, it is plausible that the dietary protein habits of our old cohort are insufficient to support skeletal muscle mass due to a failure to maximally stimulate MPS with every meal, as opposed to the uneven pattern of intake *per se*. These data are consistent with observations in British (11), Dutch (19), and US (25) cohorts of older individuals of varying health status. Taken together, these findings support calls for future studies to investigate whether increasing per-meal protein intakes in older individuals, particularly at breakfast and lunch, could maintain skeletal muscle health. Whether this is best achieved through protein supplementation, fortifying commonly consumed foods with protein/leucine, or altering meal macronutrient composition in favor of protein, remains to be elucidated.

A paucity of studies of muscle protein metabolism in middle-aged individuals, and absence of any direct comparisons of MPS against young or old individuals, make it difficult to formulate a specific MPS stimulatory threshold for this population. However, evidence shows that the postprandial MPS response to lower-dose protein ingestion does not increase above postabsorptive rates in middle-aged individuals (26, 27), similar to reported values in old individuals. Indeed, we recently reported that muscle anabolic resistance is an inevitable part of chronological aging, exacerbated by aspects of biological aging [i.e., inactivity, obesity (28)]. Thus, one might expect the MPS stimulatory threshold to fall somewhere between values for young and old individuals (0.24–0.4 $g{\cdot}kg^{-1}$) (10). Therefore, if we apply a hypothetical mid-point value of 0.32 $g{\cdot}kg^{-1}$ of dietary protein for maximal postprandial MPS stimulation in our middle-aged cohort, the proportion of individuals reaching this threshold is 5, 15, and 50% at T1, T2, and T3, respectively. However, this conjecture requires clarification through direct comparison of postprandial dose-response MPS rates between young, middle-aged and old individuals. Notwithstanding, an increase in dietary protein at breakfast and lunch in middle-aged individuals, might likely assist in the maintenance of muscle mass with advancing age.

Considering the purported threshold for maximal MPS stimulation is based on studies feeding isolated proteins, it is likely that a higher threshold for MPS saturation exists in the context of a mixed meal containing additional macronutrients. Indeed, it has been suggested that that there is no maximal anabolic response to increasing intakes of dietary protein. Specifically, increasing levels of protein intake have been shown to result in greater suppression of MPB, even when MPS is saturated (29). The suppressive effect of dietary protein on MPB is thought to be mediated by insulin secretion, with a lesser contribution of postprandial insulin directed toward MPS (30). Given that postprandial insulin-mediated regulation of muscle protein turnover may be impaired with aging (31, 32), it is possible that increasing protein consumption beyond the point of MPS saturation in older individuals might facilitate greater net muscle protein accretion through attenuating MPB. This suppressive effect of EAA on MPB is even observed beyond the suppressive effects of insulin. By further increasing intracellular EAA concentrations through protein ingestion, the additional support of MPB in regards to providing EAA precursors becomes more and more obsolete (33). However, it remains to be seen whether very high per-meal dietary protein intake ($\geq$0.4 g·kg^{-1}) leads to greater muscle mass retention in the long-term in middle-aged and old individuals.

The consumption of high-quality protein sources within the diet is essential for a robust increase in MPS (34). High-quality proteins, reflected by superior digestible indispensable amino acid scores, have a greater EAA-to-NEAA ratio, and a favorable EAA profile which closely matches the bodily needs (34). Furthermore, proteins that exhibit fast absorption and digestion kinetics, allow for a more rapid rise in circulating AAs (12). Finally, high-quality proteins have a greater protein density. Based on these characteristics, animal, rather than plant-based proteins are generally considered to be higher quality (19). In the present study, no differences were observed between groups in protein sources consumed at each meal, with the exception of lunch, where old individuals consumed mainly plant-based proteins. Lower quality proteins often exhibit an AA profile which is deficient or lacking in one or more EAA, making it crucial to combine different protein sources to provide a full complement of EAA to facilitate MPS stimulation (35). Noteworthy, is that no two plant-based proteins will be truly complementary as most plant proteins lack lysine (35). Failing to achieve a well-balanced AA profile will render the deficient protein rate-limiting in the muscle building process, as all AA are required to synthesize skeletal muscle (36). Substituting lower- for higher-quality proteins, particularly at lunch, may therefore help to support skeletal muscle maintenance in older age.

It is important to acknowledge several limitations of our study. It has been suggested that there may be potential sex-specific differences in the amount and pattern of dietary protein intake, with reports of lower protein intakes in old compared with younger men, and an opposing trend in women (37). In contrast, our data revealed no discernible difference in the amount, pattern, or source of dietary protein between men and women across age-ranges, hence why data were pooled for analysis. However, given the inherent degree of variability in all dietary protein parameters, we acknowledge that we may have been underpowered to detect significant differences between sexes. Secondly, we did not assess the physical activity status of our participants. This is important to highlight as physical activity status may be an important determinant of muscle anabolic responsiveness, particularly in older individuals (28). Specifically, physical activity/exercise acts in synergy with dietary protein ingestion to further enhance MPS (38, 39), and can therefore improve muscle anabolic responsiveness in older, and mainly frail older, individuals regularly failing to consume adequate daily protein amounts (40). Indeed, it is widely accepted that combining dietary protein strategies with regular physical activity, particularly in the form of structured resistance training, offers the most potent non-pharmacological means of maintaining or improving muscle mass, strength and function in older age (41, 42). Thirdly, our findings are only generalizable for healthy, community-dwelling older individuals, and provide little insight into the dietary protein requirements for sub-populations of older individuals with compromised muscle mass/function (for example, in frail, institutionalized, or hospitalized). Nevertheless, a recent study exploring habitual dietary protein intakes in 1051 free-living Irish individuals aged 18–90 years found comparable protein intakes and patterns to our study (43). These similarities are a likely consequence of investigating a similar study population, i.e., healthy and free-living. When comparing our results against the U.K. National Diet and Nutrition Survey (NDNS), we found that adults aged over 65 y included in the NDNS had a lower total energy intake (1,633 vs. 2,169 kcal) and absolute daily protein intake (67.4 vs. 83.4 g) (44). Whilst relative protein intakes are not presented in the NDNS, it is safe to assume that they would be lower based on the average body mass as measured by the NHS Health Survey for England 2018 (86.1 and 81.1 kg in males and 73.1 and 67.5 kg in females aged 66–74 years and over 75 years, respectively) (45). These discrepancies between the present results and those from national surveys could be due to study population differences. Indeed, studies have shown that protein intakes are similar between community-dwelling and frail older, but lower in institutionalized and hospitalized older individuals (46, 47), with a similar uneven pattern of intake in all groups. Given the rapid muscle atrophy that can occur with inactivity (47, 48), strategies to increase dietary protein delivery in institutionalized and hospitalized older individuals are of paramount importance. However, increasing dietary protein intake in hospitalized and/or malnourished older individuals is not always feasible. In this particular instance, a pattern whereby protein is pulse-fed might be preferred over an equally spread protein intake (49). By providing the majority of protein within one meal (>30 g of protein), MPS will be maximally stimulated and MPB potentially attenuated, contributing to an overall improved NPB. It is hence recommended to, first and foremost, ensure an adequate amount of protein during one meal rather than evenly spreading a suboptimal amount of protein over three main meals. Finally, it is important to acknowledge that the thresholds for maximal MPS used herein are based on a retrospective analysis and, hence, not originally intended for comparing the maximal MPS between young and old participants.

In summary, the majority of young, middle-aged and old individuals in our study met or exceeded current protein intake recommendations, even though relative and absolute protein intakes were lower in old compared with young individuals. Whilst TEI did not differ between groups, this was positively correlated with relative protein intake across age-ranges. Protein distribution throughout the day was uneven and inadequate to reach the proposed threshold for maximal MPS stimulation in old, and potentially in middle-aged individuals. Protein sources ingested at each main meal were similar across age-ranges, except for lunch where old individuals mainly consumed lower-quality plant-based proteins. Increasing protein intake, particularly at breakfast and lunch, in combination with regular physical activity/exercise in middle-aged and older individuals could potentially mitigate age-related muscle loss.

AUTHOR CONTRIBUTIONS

BS, CG, and LB designed the study and wrote the manuscript together and are the guarantors of this work who will take responsibility for the integrity and accuracy of the data analysis. BS and LB carried out data collection and analysis. All authors gave their final approval of the version of the article to be published.

FUNDING

BS was a Biotechnology and Biological Sciences Research Council (BBSRC) funded postdoctoral research fellow (BB/N018214/1). Funding for study consumables was provided internally through the College of Life and Environmental Sciences, University of Birmingham.

ACKNOWLEDGMENTS

The authors would like to thank the research participants for their time and effort. We extend our appreciation to Ms. Leisha Mulvey and Ms. Megan Bailey for their assistance with data collection in the middle-aged cohort. The authors would also like to thank Dr. Danielle Cardon-Thomas for her insights into the protein intake patterns and help regarding the obtainment of ethical approvals.

REFERENCES

1. Goodpaster BH, Park SW, Harris TB, Kritchevsky SB, Nevitt M, Schwartz AV, et al. The loss of skeletal muscle strength, mass, and quality in older adults: the health, aging and body composition study. *J Gerontol A Biol Sci Med Sci.* (2006) 61:1059–64. doi: 10.1093/gerona/61.10.1059
2. Biolo G, Fleming RY, Maggi SP, Wolfe RR. Transmembrane transport and intracellular kinetics of amino acids in human skeletal muscle. *Am J Physiol.* (1995) 268:E75–84.
3. Wolfe RR. Regulation of muscle protein by amino acids (2002). *J Nutr.* 132:3219s–24s. doi: 10.1093/jn/131.10.3219S
4. Cuthbertson D, Smith K, Babraj J, Leese G, Waddell T, Atherton P, et al. Anabolic signaling deficits underlie amino acid resistance of wasting, aging muscle. *FASEB J.* (2005) 19:422–4. doi: 10.1096/fj.04-2640fje
5. Shad BJ, Thompson JL, Breen L. Does the muscle protein synthetic response to exercise and amino acid-based nutrition diminish with advancing age? A systematic review. *Am J Physiol Endocrinol Metab.* (2016) 311:E803–E817. doi: 10.1152/ajpendo.00213.2016
6. Janssen I, Heymsfield SB, Wang ZM, Ross R. Skeletal muscle mass and distribution in 468 men and women aged 18-88 yr. *J Appl Physiol.* (2000) 89:81–8. doi: 10.1152/jappl.2000.89.1.81
7. Morley JE, Argiles JM, Evans WJ, Bhasin S, Cella D, Deutz NEP, et al. Nutritional recommendations for the management of sarcopenia. *J Am Med Direct Assoc.* (2010) 11:391–6. doi: 10.1016/j.jamda.2010.04.014
8. Bauer J, Biolo G, Cederholm T, Cesari M, Cruz-Jentoft AJ, Morley JE, et al. Evidence-based recommendations for optimal dietary protein intake in older people: a position paper from the PROT-AGE study group. *J Am Med Direct Assoc.* (2013) 14:542–59. doi: 10.1016/j.jamda.2013.05.021
9. Traylor DA, Gorissen SHM, Phillips SM. Perspective: protein requirements and optimal intakes in aging: are we ready to recommend more than the recommended daily allowance? *Adv Nutr.* (2018) 9:171–82. doi: 10.1093/advances/nmy003
10. Moore DR, Churchward-Venne TA, Witard O, Breen L, Burd NA, Tipton KD, et al. Protein ingestion to stimulate myofibrillar protein synthesis requires greater relative protein intakes in healthy older versus younger men. *J Gerontol A Biol Sci Med Sci.* (2015) 70:57–62. doi: 10.1093/gerona/glu103
11. Cardon-Thomas DK, Riviere T, Tieges Z, Greig CA. Dietary protein in older adults: adequate daily intake but potential for improved distribution. *Nutrients.* (2017) 9:E184. doi: 10.3390/nu9030184
12. Boirie Y, Dangin M, Gachon P, Vasson MP, Maubois JL, Beaufrere B. Slow and fast dietary proteins differently modulate postprandial protein accretion. *Proc Natl Acad Sci USA.* (1997) 94:14930–5. doi: 10.1073/pnas.94.26.14930
13. van Vliet S, Burd NA, van Loon LJ. The skeletal muscle anabolic response to plant- versus animal-based protein consumption. *J Nutr.* (2015) 145:1981–91. doi: 10.3945/jn.114.204305
14. Pilgrim A, Robinson S, Sayer AA, Roberts H. An overview of appetite decline in older people. *Nurs Older People.* (2015) 27:29–35. doi: 10.7748/nop.27.5.29.e697
15. Giezenaar C, Chapman I, Luscombe-Marsh N, Feinle-Bisset C, Horowitz M, Soenen S. Ageing is associated with decreases in appetite and energy intake–a meta-analysis in healthy adults. *Nutrients.* (2016) 8:E28. doi: 10.3390/nu8010028
16. Gorissen SHM, Witard OC. Characterising the muscle anabolic potential of dairy, meat and plant-based protein sources in older adults. *Proc Nutr Soc.* (2018) 77:20–31. doi: 10.1017/s0029665117 00194x
17. Houston DK, Nicklas BJ, Ding J, Harris TB, Tylavsky FA, Newman AB, et al. Dietary protein intake is associated with lean mass change in older, community-dwelling adults: the Health, Aging, and Body Composition (Health ABC) Study. *Am J Clin Nutr.* (2008) 87:150–5. doi: 10.1093/ajcn/87.1.150
18. Celis-Morales CA, Petermann F, Steell L, Anderson J, Welsh P, Mackay DF, et al. Associations of dietary protein intake with fat free mass and grip strength: cross-sectional study in 146,816 UK Biobank participants. *Am J Epidemiol.* (2018) 187:2405–14. doi: 10.1093/aje/kwy134
19. Tieland M, Borgonjen-Van den Berg KJ, Van Loon LJ, de Groot LC. Dietary protein intake in dutch elderly people: a focus on protein sources. *Nutrients.* (2015) 7:9697–706. doi: 10.3390/nu7125496
20. Landi F, Calvani R, Tosato M, Martone AM, Ortolani E, Savera G, et al. Anorexia of aging: risk factors, consequences, and potential treatments. *Nutrients.* (2016) 8:69. doi: 10.3390/nu8020069
21. Mamerow MM, Mettler JA, English KL, Casperson SL, Arentson-Lantz E, Sheffield-Moore M, et al. Dietary protein distribution positively influences 24-h muscle protein synthesis in healthy adults. *J Nutr.* (2014) 144:876–80. doi: 10.3945/jn.113.185280
22. Kim IY, Schutzler S, Schrader A, Spencer H, Kortebein P, Deutz NE, et al. Quantity of dietary protein intake, but not pattern of intake, affects net protein balance primarily through differences in protein synthesis in older adults. *Am J Physiol Endocrinol Metab.* (2014) 308:E21–8. doi: 10.1152/ajpendo.00382.2014
23. Kim IY, Schutzler S, Schrader AM, Spencer HJ, Azhar G, Wolfe RR, et al. Protein intake distribution pattern does not affect anabolic response, lean body mass, muscle strength or function over 8 weeks in

older adults: a randomized-controlled trial. *Clin Nutr.* (2018) 37:488–93. doi: 10.1016/j.clnu.2017.02.020

24. Loenneke JP, Loprinzi PD, Murphy CH, Phillips SM. Per meal dose and frequency of protein consumption is associated with lean mass and muscle performance. *Clin Nutr.* (2016) 35:1506–11. doi: 10.1016/j.clnu.2016.04.002
25. Paddon-Jones D, Campbell WW, Jacques PF, Kritchevsky SB, Moore LL, Rodriguez NR, et al. Protein and healthy aging. *Am J Clin Nutr.* (2015) 101:1339S–45S. doi: 10.3945/ajcn.114.084061
26. Robinson MJ, Burd NA, Breen L, Rerecich T, Yang Y, Hector AJ, et al. Dose-dependent responses of myofibrillar protein synthesis with beef ingestion are enhanced with resistance exercise in middle-aged men. *Appl Physiol Nutr Metab.* (2013) 38:120–5. doi: 10.1139/apnm-2012-0092
27. Mitchell CJ, D'Souza R, Zeng N, McGregor RA, Fanning AC, Poppitt S, et al. Understanding the sensitivity of muscle protein synthesis to dairy protein in middle-aged men. *Int Dairy J.* (2016) 63:35–41. doi: 10.1016/j.idairyj.2016.07.008
28. Smeuninx B, McKendry J, Wilson D, Martin U, Breen L. Age-related anabolic resistance of myofibrillar protein synthesis is exacerbated in obese inactive individuals. *J Clin Endocrinol Metab.* (2017) 102:3535–45. doi: 10.1210/jc.2017-00869
29. Kim IY, Schutzler S, Schrader A, Spencer HJ, Azhar G, Ferrando AA, et al. The anabolic response to a meal containing different amounts of protein is not limited by the maximal stimulation of protein synthesis in healthy young adults. *Am J Physiol Endocrinol Metab.* (2016) 310:E73–80. doi: 10.1152/ajpendo.00365.2015
30. Greenhaff PL, Karagounis LG, Peirce N, Simpson EJ, Hazell M, Layfield R, et al. Disassociation between the effects of amino acids and insulin on signaling, ubiquitin ligases, and protein turnover in human muscle. *Am J Physiol Endocrinol Metab.* (2008) 295:E595–604. doi: 10.1152/ajpendo.90411.2008
31. Fujita S, Glynn EL, Timmerman KL, Rasmussen BB, Volpi E. Supraphysiological hyperinsulinaemia is necessary to stimulate skeletal muscle protein anabolism in older adults: evidence of a true age-related insulin resistance of muscle protein metabolism. *Diabetologia.* (2009) 52:1889–98. doi: 10.1007/s00125-009-1430-8
32. Wilkes EA, Selby AL, Atherton PJ, Patel R, Rankin D, Smith K, et al. Blunting of insulin inhibition of proteolysis in legs of older subjects may contribute to age-related sarcopenia. *Am J Clin Nutr.* (2009) 90:1343–50. doi: 10.3945/ajcn.2009.27543
33. Kim IY, Shin YA, Schutzler SE, Azhar G, Wolfe RR, Ferrando AA. Quality of meal protein determines anabolic response in older adults. *Clin Nutr.* (2018) 37:2076–83. doi: 10.1016/j.clnu.2017.09.025
34. Phillips SM. The impact of protein quality on the promotion of resistance exercise-induced changes in muscle mass. *Nutr Metab (Lond).* (2016) 13:64. doi: 10.1186/s12986-016-0124-8
35. Young VR, Pellett PL. Plant proteins in relation to human protein and amino acid nutrition. *Am J Clin Nutr.* (1994) 59:1203s–12s. doi: 10.1093/ajcn/59.5.1203S
36. Wolfe RR. Branched-chain amino acids and muscle protein synthesis in humans: myth or reality? *J Int Soc Sports Nutr.* (2017) 14:30. doi: 10.1186/s12970-017-0184-9
37. Rousset S, Patureau Mirand P, Brandolini M, Martin JF, Boirie Y. Daily protein intakes and eating patterns in young and elderly French. *Br J Nutr.* (2003) 90:1107–15. doi: 10.1079/bjn20031004
38. Pennings B, Koopman R, Beelen M, Senden JM, Saris WH, van Loon LJ. Exercising before protein intake allows for greater use of dietary protein-derived amino acids for de novo muscle protein synthesis in both young and elderly men. *Am J Clin Nutr.* (2011) 93:322–31. doi: 10.3945/ajcn.2010.29649
39. Tieland M, Dirks ML, van der Zwaluw N, Verdijk LB, van de Rest O, de Groot LCPGM, et al. Protein supplementation increases muscle mass gain during prolonged resistance-type exercise training in frail elderly people: a randomized, double-blind, placebo-controlled trial. *J Am Med Direct Assoc.* (2012) 13:713–9. doi: 10.1016/j.jamda.2012.05.020
40. Thomas DK, Quinn MA, Saunders DH, Greig CA. Protein supplementation does not significantly augment the effects of resistance exercise training in older adults: a systematic review. *J Am Med Dir Assoc.* (2016) 17:959.e951–959. doi: 10.1016/j.jamda.2016.07.002
41. Cermak NM, de Groot LC, van Loon LJ. Perspective: protein supplementation during prolonged resistance type exercise training augments skeletal muscle mass and strength gains. *J Am Med Direct Assoc.* (2013) 14:71–2. doi: 10.1016/j.jamda.2012.10.003
42. Morton RW, Murphy KT, McKellar SR, Schoenfeld BJ, Henselmans M, Helms E, et al. A systematic review, meta-analysis and meta-regression of the effect of protein supplementation on resistance training-induced gains in muscle mass and strength in healthy adults. *Br J Sports Med.* (2018) 52:376–84. doi: 10.1136/bjsports-2017-097608
43. Hone M, Nugent AP, Walton J, McNulty BA, Egan B. Habitual protein intake, protein distribution patterns and dietary sources in Irish adults with stratification by sex and age. *J Hum Nutr Diet.* (2020). p. 12. doi: 10.1111/jhn.12736
44. Roberts C, Steer T, Maplethorpe N, Cox L, Meadows S, Nicholson S, et al. *National Diet and Nutrition Survey. Results From Years 7-8 (Combined) of the Rolling Programme (2014/15 to 2015/16).* London (2018).
45. Lifestyles Team ND. *Health Survey for England 2018". 03/12/2019 ed.: NHS Digital, Part of the Government Statistical Service* (2019).
46. Tieland M, Borgonjen-Van den Berg KJ, van Loon LJ, de Groot LC. Dietary protein intake in community-dwelling, frail, and institutionalized elderly people: scope for improvement. *Eur J Nutr.* (2011) 51:173–9. doi: 10.1007/s00394-011-0203-6
47. Kouw IWK, Groen BBL, Smeets JSJ, Kramer IF, van Kranenburg JMX, Nilwik R, et al. One week of hospitalization following elective hip surgery induces substantial muscle atrophy in older patients. *J Am Med Dir Assoc.* (2018) 20:35–42. doi: 10.1016/j.jamda.2018.06.018
48. Breen L, Stokes KA, Churchward-Venne TA, Moore DR, Baker SK, Smith K, et al. Two weeks of reduced activity decreases leg lean mass and induces 'anabolic resistance' of myofibrillar protein synthesis in healthy elderly. *J Clin Endocrinol Metab.* (2013) 98:2604–12. doi: 10.1210/jc.2013-1502
49. Bouillanne O, Curis E, Hamon-Vilcot B, Nicolis I, Chretien P, Schauer N, et al. Impact of protein pulse feeding on lean mass in malnourished and at-risk hospitalized elderly patients: a randomized controlled trial. *Clin Nutr.* (2013) 32:186–92. doi: 10.1016/j.clnu.2012.08.015

21

Ingestion of a Pre-Bedtime Protein Containing Beverage Prevents Overnight Induced Negative Whole Body Protein Balance in Healthy Middle-Aged Men

Leonidas G. Karagounis[1,2,3], Maurice Beaumont[1], Laurence Donato-Capel[1], Jean-Philippe Godin[1], Anne-France Kapp[1], Dimitrios Draganidis[1], Stéphane Pinaud[1], Jacques Vuichoud[1], Maya Shevlyakova[1], Koraljka Rade-Kukic[1] and Denis Breuillé[1]*

[1] Nestlé Research, Lausanne, Switzerland, [2] Institute of Social and Preventive Medicine, University of Bern, Bern, Switzerland, [3] Translation Research, Nestlé Health Science, Lausanne, Switzerland

***Correspondence:**
Leonidas G. Karagounis
leonidas.karagounis@nestle.com

Age related muscle wasting leads to overall reductions of lean body mass, reduced muscle strength, and muscle function resulting in compromised quality of life. Utilizing novel nutritional strategies to attenuate such losses is of great importance in elderly individuals. We aimed to test if a complete dietary supplement containing 25 g of milk proteins and ingested in the evening before bed would improve protein metabolism in terms of whole body protein balance over a 10 h overnight period following ingestion of the test drink in healthy middle-aged male subjects. In addition we also assessed the rates of muscle protein synthesis during the second half of the night in order to see if previously reported extended amino acidemia during sleep results in increased rates of muscle protein synthesis. Seventeen healthy middle-aged male subjects (59.4 $\pm$ 3.2 year) consumed a dietary supplement drink at 21:00 containing either 25 g milk protein concentrate, 25 g maltodextrin, 7.75 g canola oil (treatment group), or an isocaloric protein void drink (placebo group). Muscle protein synthesis was assessed from a muscle biopsy following the continuous intravenous infusion of ^{13}C-phenylalanine for 5 h (from 03:00 to 08:00). Whole body protein balance was greater in the treatment group (-0.13 ± 11.30 g prot/10 h) compared to placebo (-12.22 ± 6.91 g prot/10 h) ($P \leq 0.01$). In contrast, no changes were observed on rates of muscle protein synthesis during the second half of the night. Ingestion of a dietary supplement containing 25 g of milk proteins significantly reduced the negative protein balance observed during the night. Therefore, pre-bedtime protein ingestion may attenuate overnight losses of lean tissue in healthy elderly men. Despite increases in aminoacidemia during the second part of the night, no changes were observed in the rates of muscle protein synthesis during this time.

Clinical Trial Registration: www.ClinicalTrials.gov, identifier: NCT02041143.

Keywords: milk protein, aging, sleep, muscle, protein balance

INTRODUCTION

Skeletal muscle is the most abundant tissue in the human body and plays a key role in both locomotion and metabolic health and it is therefore important to maintain healthy muscle mass and function as we age (1). Two triggers known to stimulate adaptations in skeletal muscle include nutrition (macro- and micro-nutrients) (2–5) and contractile activity (weight loading and unloading) (1, 6–9). Repeated exposure to such stimuli over time initiate changes at the molecular level allowing skeletal muscle to adapt and alter its profile to meet the demands of its new environment (10). This regulation of skeletal muscle protein turnover is primarily coordinated by changes in the rates of both muscle protein synthesis (MPS) and muscle protein breakdown (MPB). However, with the progression of age, the rate of muscle protein turnover and especially the lower postprandial MPS response may contribute to a reduction in muscle mass and function (11). Specifically, at a population level it has been demonstrated that after the fifth decade of life muscle mass is reduced by ~1% per year (12). This accumulated loss of muscle mass over time may lead to mobility limitations in older individuals (13).

Fasting, such as that observed during overnight sleep, results in negative muscle protein balance as a result of both, reduced rates of muscle protein synthesis and increased rates of muscle protein breakdown (9, 14–16). Nutritional strategies aimed at maintaining and improving lean tissue body composition may be beneficial for elderly populations who are at risk of muscle atrophy and accelerated muscle loss as observed under sarcopenic conditions. Therefore, attenuating the overnight losses of lean tissue mass (including muscle) would potentially be beneficial in helping maintain lean tissue/muscle mass in the elderly. Several bodies of work have addressed this proof of concept in young, healthy, physically active subjects which have been reviewed in recent work by Trommelen and Van Loon (17). Specifically, Res et al., reported that 25 g post-exercise (21:30) whey protein ingestion followed by a second 40 g bolus ingestion of casein at 23:30 (before bed time) resulted in increased muscle protein balance over an 8-h period in young healthy male subjects (18). In addition, the authors reported that plasma amino acid concentrations remained elevated throughout the sleep duration highlighting a potential extension in the nutrient driven anabolic state. More recently, Kouw et al. (19) showed that the ingestion of 40 g protein before sleep increased myofibrillar protein synthesis during overnight sleep. This effect was not observed after ingestion of 20 g protein. However, what is not clear is whether or not the increased whole body protein balance observed in the morning was due to an extension in the postprandial anabolic window beyond that normally observed (within 3–5 h postprandialy). Moreover, it is not known if such a benefit would be observed in older individuals following the ingestion of a complete oral nutritional supplement containing 25 g of dairy protein together with carbohydrate and fat.

Therefore, the aim of the present study was to investigate if whole body nitrogen balance would be improved after ingestion of a complete oral nutritional supplement (25 g milk protein, 25 g maltodextrin, and 7.5 g canola oil) in healthy elderly individuals. In addition we aimed to identify if there is an extension to the anabolic window of opportunity for muscle protein synthesis beyond the commonly reported 3–5 h postprandial window due to increased amino acid availability.

SUBJECTS AND METHODS

Subject Characteristics

A total of 17 healthy recreationally active men aged 59.4 ± 3.2 year (range: 55–66 year) were selected to participate in this study (**Figure 1**). Subjects were recruited locally, through a recruitment agency (TrialReach, Nyon, Switzerland). Inclusion criteria were healthy males aged 50–70, with a BMI between 19.0 and 27.0 kg/m^2. Main exclusion criteria were any cardiovascular disease including arterial hypertension, any clotting disorders or any chronic intake of medications jeopardizing clotting, participation in any special diet (vegan, vegetarian, high protein intake) or weight loss program, food allergies, medication for chronic disease or any people following a strict exercise regime in order to either lose weight, gain muscle or reach competition standards for a chosen sport. The study was approved by the Commission Cantonale d'Ethique (VD) pour la Recherche sur l'Etre Humain, Switzerland, under the reference 423/13.

Subjects were randomly assigned to either the protein containing supplement (PRO: $n = 9$) or an isocaloric protein void placebo supplement (PLA: $n = 8$) experimental group. One individual in the PLA experiment group had to be excluded because it was not possible to obtain the muscle biopsy. Subject characteristics are presented in **Table 1**. All subjects were fully informed on the nature and possible risks of the experimental procedures before their written informed consent was obtained. Before taking part, all subjects underwent routine medical screening and eligible participants all gave their informed signed consent to take part in the study and were aware that they were free to withdraw from the experiment at any point.

Experimental Design

A detailed schema outlining the study procedure is described in **Figure 2**.

Eligible subjects reported to the Nestlé Metabolic Unit in the morning of the experimental day at 07:30 having fasted from 22:00 the preceding evening. A fasted blood sample was obtained in order to measure blood clotting parameters (prothrombin time, activated partial thromboplastin time, and fibrinogen). Each subject was provided with a standardized breakfast which was consumed on site. Subsequently, each subject was provided with a standardized lunch and advised to consume it at 12:00. All subjects reported back to the Nestlé Metabolic Unit at 17:30 and were provided with a standardized dinner which was consumed at 18:00. Subjects were not controlled for snacks out of the laboratory but they were asked to refrain from consuming protein supplements in the 15 days preceding the testing session. The total amount of protein in each of the standardized meals was defined as 1.2 g protein per kg of body weight. For practical reasons, 1 meal portion was designed to contain 61.15 g of protein (chicken breast) and subjects were given 1, 1.25, 1.5, or 1.75 portions as a function of their body weight. Following

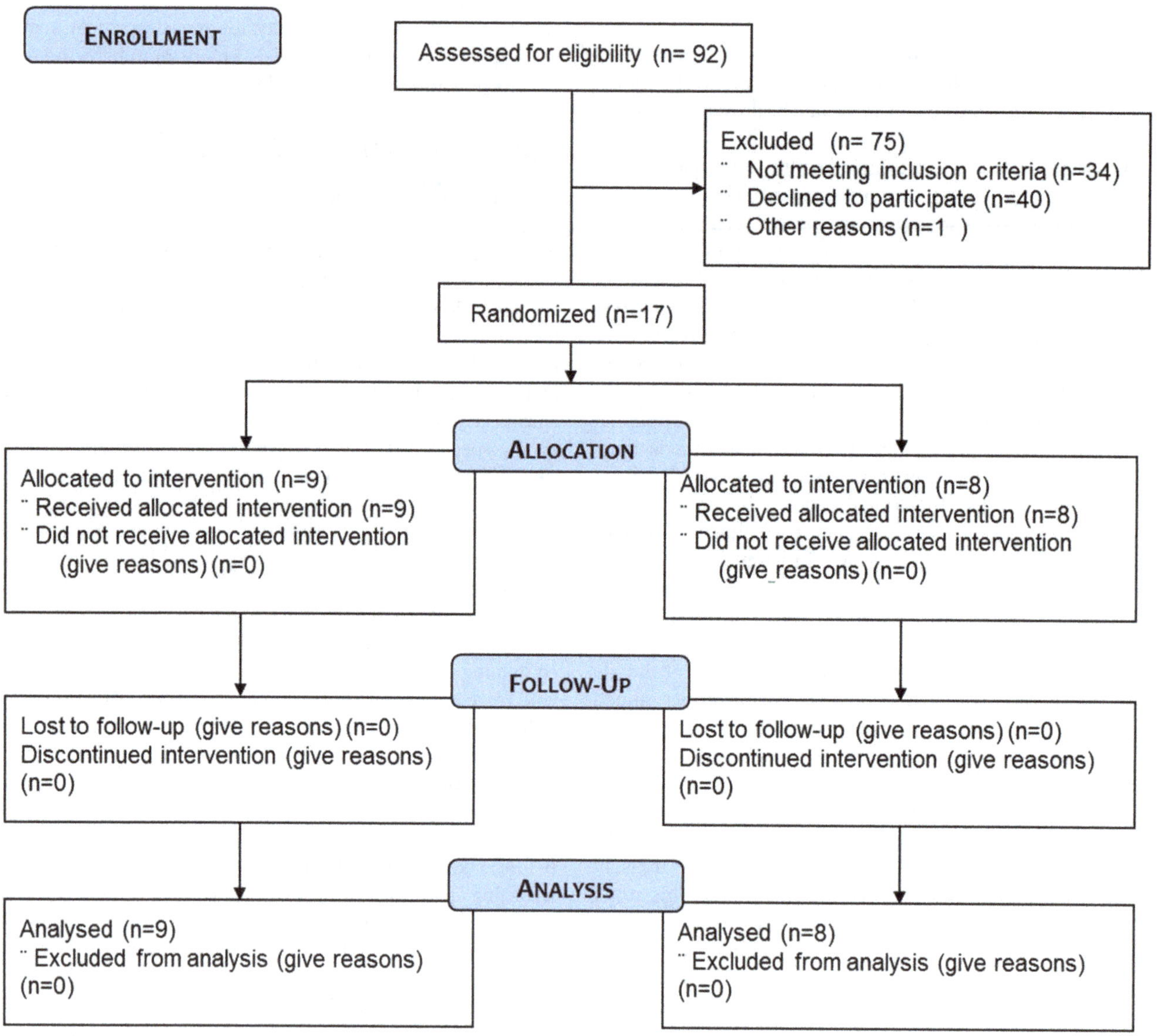

FIGURE 1 | CONSORT flow diagram of the study.

completion of the dinner meal, two catheters were inserted into an antecubital vein.

Prior to the ingestion of the tracer at 21:00 subjects voided their bladder. Subsequently, a blood sample was obtained and used for baseline measurements of plasma amino acids, glucose and insulin. Following this and 15 min before the commencement of the experimental trial, each subject ingested the intervention supplement (at 21:00) containing 200 mg of [^{15}N]glycine stable isotope tracer (Euriso-top, St. Aubin, France). The intervention product contained either 3.1% canola oil, 10% maltodextrin DE21, and 10% milk protein concentrate (test product) or 3.1% canola oil, and 20% maltodextrin DE21 (placebo). Both products were isocaloric with a total calorie content of 270 kcal per drink (test product). Each subject in each group was required to consume 250 g of either the study test product or placebo. Each subject remained in a resting condition for 2 h before going to bed (23:00 h) for an 8-h sleep period.

At 03:00 the plasma phenylalanine pools were primed with a single intravenous dose of [$^{13}C_6$]phenylalanine (2.0 μmol/kg). Thereafter, a continuous stable isotope infusion of [$^{13}C_6$]phenylalanine (Euriso-top, St. Aubin, France) was initiated at an infusion rate of 0.050 μmol kg^{-1} min^{-1} for 300 min. At the end of the infusion (t = 8.00 h) a muscle biopsy was obtained from the vastus lateralis muscle under local anesthesia (see **Figure 2**). During the infusion of the [$^{13}C_6$]phenylalanine, arterialized blood samples were obtained to confirm steady state conditions.

Blood samples were obtained at specific time points throughout the night (−15 min before drink ingestion and 1, 3, 6, 7, 10, and 11 h following drink ingestion) without waking the subjects. Urine was collected once the subjects had woken or during toilet breaks during the night. Subjects woke up at 07:00. Following the muscle biopsy procedure, each subject was provided with a standard breakfast.

Muscle Biopsy

Muscle biopsies were performed according to the Bergstrom methodology. Briefly, local anesthesia [2–3 ml of 1% xylocain (rapidocain®)] was administered to the skin, subcutaneous tissue and fascia of the vastus lateralis in preparation for muscle sampling. A muscle biopsy sample (100–150 mg) of the Vastus lateralis was obtained using a 5 mm Bergstrom needle with manual suction by an experienced practitioner. The muscle sample was then washed and immediately frozen in liquid nitrogen and stored at −80°C for further analysis.

Whole Body Protein Balance

Whole body protein turnover was calculated using the end-product method as described previously (20). The ^{15}N isotopic enrichments of urinary ammonia and urea samples were determined in duplicate after isolation of both components by cation exchange resin (Bio-Rad AG, Reinach, Switzerland) and measured by isotope ratio mass spectrometry (Delta V coupled to an elemental analyzer, Thermo Fischer, Bremen, Germany). Concentrations of urinary urea and creatinine, the major nitrogen containing metabolites in urine, were measured by an automated analyzer (Cobas, Hoffmann- La Roche, Switzerland). Isotopic enrichments were expressed as TTR (tracer to tracee ratio) corrected from baseline isotopic enrichment. Whole body nitrogen turnover (Q) was calculated as Q (mg N/kg/h) = d/Ei/BW/time; where d is the dose of oral [^{15}N]glycine in g, Ei is the isotopic enrichment of ^{15}N ammonia, t is the time of urine collection (i.e., 10 h) and BW is the body weight expressed in kg (21). Whole body protein synthesis (S) and whole body protein breakdown B were then calculated from the expression Q = S + E = B + I; where E is the excretion of nitrogen estimated as the sum of urea and creatinine excretion plus other losses (i.e., fecal and miscellaneous). Protein synthesis and protein breakdown were normalized by body weight (BW) and finally expressed as mg protein/kg BW/h (using 6.25 as coefficient to transform nitrogen to protein fluxes).

TABLE 1 | Baseline characteristics of participants.

	Placebo ($n = 8$)	Treatment ($n = 9$)	p (t-test)
Age (years)	60.4 ± 3.02	57.9 ± 2.93	0.11
Height (cm)	181 ± 7.33	178 ± 7.38	0.55
Weight (kg)	79.6 ± 9.59	76.1 ± 9.85	0.46
BMI (kg/m^2)	24.4 ± 1.47	23.8 ± 1.64	0.48
Diastolic blood pressure (mmHg)	82.6 ± 5.10	80 ± 8.40	0.44
Systolic blood pressure (mmHg)	135 ± 5.98	125 ± 8.82	0.03*

Values are means ± SD. For comparison of numerical values, statistics were obtained with the use of Student's t-test.
**Different from controls (P < 0.05).*

Muscle Protein Synthesis

Mixed muscle fractional synthesis rate (FSR) were based on the single biopsy approach (22, 23). FSR (expressed in %/h) was calculated using the standard precursor-product equation (validated for a single muscle biopsy approach) as described by Burd et al. (23).

$$FSR(\%/h) = (E_{p2} - E_{p1})/E_{ic}/t \times 100;$$

Where, E_{p2} and E_{p1} are the ^{13}C isotopic enrichment of Phe from protein bound in muscle (from the muscle biopsy) and Phe from plasma protein, respectively. E_{ic} is the mean intracellular phenylalanine enrichment from the biopsy and t is the tracer incorporation time.

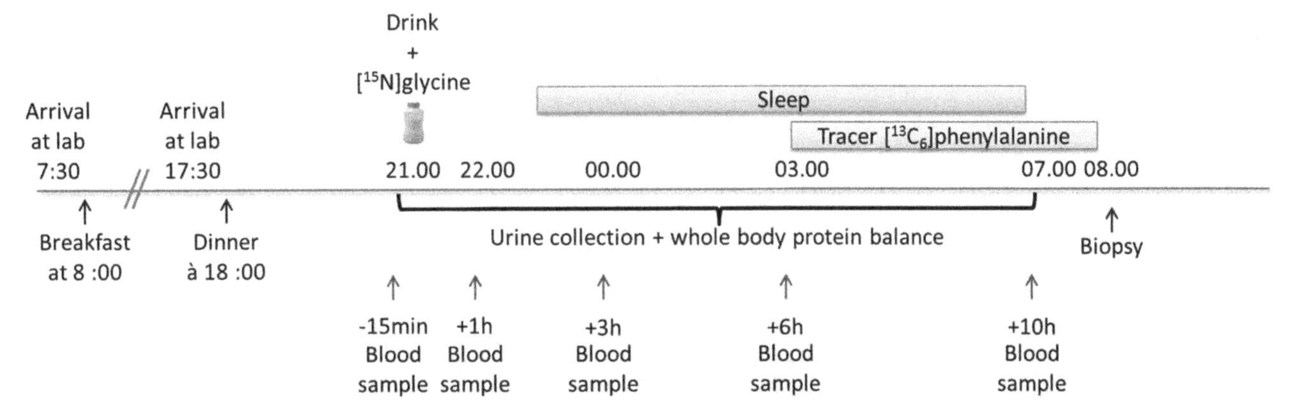

FIGURE 2 | Study overview for the measurement of the effect of pre-bedtime dietary protein intake and its effect on whole body protein balance and rates of muscle protein synthesis. A drink containing 25 g of milk protein concentrate was ingested at 21:00 h. For the measurement of muscle protein synthesis a tracer ([$^{13}C_6$]phenylalanine) infusion was commenced at 03:00 h and a single muscle biopsy was obtained 5 h later at 08:00 h.

Sample Collection, Processing, and Analysis for FSR Determination

Blood samples were collected in pre-chilled tubes containing EDTA. Plasma was separated by centrifugation and then stored at −80°C until analysis. Muscle samples were rinsed in ice-cold saline solution immediately after collection, then cleared from fat tissues and finally frozen in liquid nitrogen.

To determine plasma ^{13}C Phe isotopic enrichment expressed as tracer-to-tracee ratio (TTR), plasma was precipitated with acetonitrile and free amino acids were derivatized by preparing propyl-chloroformate derivatives and analyzed using Phenomenex ZB-AAA column (15 m × 0.25 mm, 0.1 μm I.D film thickness column, from Brechbuller, Switzerland). Plasma Phe TTR were monitored by gas chromatography/mass spectrometry (GC-MS, MSD 5973 System, Hewlett Packard).

^{13}C isotopic enrichment of Phe from plasma protein and muscle protein (biopsy samples) were determined using a gas chromatography-combustion-isotope ratio mass spectrometry (Delta V Hyphenated to GC system from Thermo Fischer, Bremen, Germany). Isotopic data (^{13}C/^{12}C ratio) were expressed in delta per mil value (δ^{13}C, ‰). The pellets containing muscle and plasma proteins was washed and then hydrolyzed with 6 N HCL at 110°C for 24 h. Amino acids obtained were then purified on cation exchange chromatography (Dowex 50W-X8-200, Bio-Rad Laboratories), then derivatized to get N-acetyl-n-propyl ester derivative (NAP) amino acid and analyzed on DB5-MS column (30 m × 0.25 mm; 0.25 μm I.D film thickness column, from Agilent, Germany).

For FSR calculation, in this study, background ^{13}C-Phe enrichment of mixed plasma proteins for the initial isotopic enrichment as described by Burd et al. and intracellular ^{13}C-Phe (as precursor pool) were used. We found that the plasma protein measured before administration of the tracer was $\delta^{13}C = -32.49 \pm 0.52$ ‰ ($n = 17$, expressed as mean ± SD) showing a good repeatability between subjects. Like in most of the studies with ^{13}C-Phe as tracer, we used muscle intracellular free ^{13}C-Phe as precursor (24). Internal validation of this single biopsy approach showed an analytical intra-day repeatability ($n = 6$ days) of FSR of 6%.

Plasma Amino Acid Analysis

Within 30 min following blood sampling, the samples were centrifuged at 1,800 g for 20 min at +4°C (3,200 rpm). About 500 μl of the supernatant were transferred into a fresh 1.5 mL Eppendorf tube and frozen at −80°C.

Samples were thawed and then work on ice at ~4°C. The samples were centrifuged for 1 min at 8,000 rpm at 4°C. The 200 μl aliquot was then transferred to a fresh Eppendorf tube. While vortexing, 20 μl of ice cold (2–8°C) sulfosalycilic acid 40% solution were added to the plasma aliquot. This was then vortexed for 1 min at 1,800 rpm. The samples were then kept between 2 and 8°C for 15 min before centrifuging for 3 min at 13,000 g at 4°C.

Individual amino acid concentrations were measured by ion exchange chromatography with spectrophotometer detection after ninhydrine derivatization using and Amino Acid Analyser (Biochrom 30, Onken, Germany). The sum of all individual AA measured provided the total of plasma amino acids concentration. The sum of all individual essential AA's measured, provided the essential plasma AA concentration.

Western Analysis of AKT/p70S6k Signaling Proteins

Western blot analysis was performed using the NuPage System precast gels as described by the manufacturer (Novex, Life Technologies). About 40 mg of frozen muscle tissue was homogenized in ice cold lysis buffer A (50 mmol/L Tris-HCL, pH 7.5, 1 mmol EDTA/L, 1 mmol EGTA/L, 10%glycerol, 1%triton-X, 50 mmol NaF/L, 5 mmolNa4P2O7/L, 1 mmol dithiothreitol/L, 10 mg trypsin inhibitor/mL, 2 mg aprotinin/mL,1 mmol benzamidine/L, and 1 mmol phenylmethylsulfonylfluoride/L) using a TissueLyser (Qiagen). The lysate was centrifuged (12,000 × g, for 20 min at 4°C) and the supernatant was transferred to fresh Eppendorf tubes for subsequent quantification of protein content. The protein concentration for each muscle extract was determined using the Pierce BCA Protein Assay Kit (Thermo Scientific). Equal amounts (5 μg) of protein samples were denatured by boiling for 5 min. Subsequently, samples were loaded onto 4–12% Bis-Tris midi gels before being transferred onto nitrocellulose membranes (iBlot gel Transfer Stacks, Life Technologies) and blocked for 1 h with Odyssey Blocking Buffer at room temperature. Each membrane was then incubated overnight at 4°C with a primary antibody [Anti-AKT1 phospho (1:2,000) ab66138; Anti-rpS6 (1:1,000) ab40820; Anti-AKT1 (1:1,000) ab91505 were purchased from Abcam; Phospho-p70S6K (1:500) #9205; Phospho-rpS6 (1:1,000) #2211; Phospho mTOR (1:500) #2971; mTOR (1:1,000) #2972; α-Tubulin (1:1,000) #3873 were purchased from Cell Signaling Technology], diluted in 0.1% Tween Odyssey Blocking Buffer PBS (LI-QOR Biosciences). The following morning each membrane was washed with PBS containing 0.1% Tween 20 (PBST). The membranes were then incubated for 1 h at room temperature in a black box with IRDye800CW-conjugated goat anti-rabbit or anti-mouse secondary antibodies (LI-COR Biosciences) diluted in Odyssey Blocking Buffer. The blots were then washed four times with PBST and rinsed with PBS. Proteins were visualized by scanning the membrane on an Odyssey Infrared Imaging System (LI-COR Biosciences) with 800-nm channels.

Insulin and Glucose Analysis

Insulin

Plasma insulin concentrations was measured using the commercially available IBL Insulin Enzyme Immunoassay Kit (IBL International) according to manufacturer's directions.

Glucose

Plasma glucose concentrations were assessed using the Siemens dimension EXL 200 clinical chemistry system (Siemens Healthcare Diagnostics AG, Zurich, Switzerland).

Statistical Analysis

No sample size calculation have been performed due to absence of data on mean difference and variations of endpoints in this study.

Endpoints with a single measure (changes in whole body protein, FSR, signaling pathways and other variables) -were analyzed using a paired t-test or a Wilcoxon rank-sum test, depending on the presence of outliers (outliers were defined as value exceeding the distance from the mean by more than two standard deviations). For parameters with longitudinal measurements, a two-way ANOVA with repeated measurements was employed to test the treatment effect over time and its interaction with time. Pairwise comparisons at different time points were only evaluated in the case when the overall treatment effect was statistically significant. These rules were agreed upon in the statistical analysis plan prior to unblinding of the study. In addition, for data with 5 time points, mean profile of insulin, glucose and amino acids was estimated using spline and summarized by an AUC. Estimates of tmax (time where concentration is maximum), Cmax (value of the maximum concentration), AUC (area under the curve), and AUCc (area under the curve, corrected for baseline value) were based on 1,000 replicates of the mean smoothing curves in each treatment group. No multiplicity adjustments were performed. Data are expressed as means ± SDs. Significance was set at $\alpha = 0.05$. The analyses were performed in R software (version 3.0.1, R Foundation for Statistical Computing).

RESULTS

Baseline Characteristics

All participants in both supplementation groups in the present study had similar baseline values for age and body mass index (**Table 1**).

Plasma Amino Acid Concentrations

No treatment effect was observed for either total amino acids, essential amino acids, branched chain amino acids or leucine plasma concentrations between groups at baseline. However, total amino acid plasma concentrations were significantly greater in the treatment group compared to the placebo group at 1 and 3 h ($P < 0.001$; **Figure 3A**). Essential amino acid plasma concentrations were significantly higher in the treatment group compared to placebo at 1 h ($P < 0.001$), 3 h ($P < 0.001$), 6 h ($P < 0.001$), and 10 h ($P = 0.01$) (**Figure 3B**). Furthermore, branched chain amino acid plasma concentrations were significantly higher in the treatment group compared to placebo at 1 h ($P < 0.001$), 3 h ($P < 0.001$), 6 h ($P < 0.01$), and 10 h ($P = 0.01$) (**Figure 3C**). Finally, leucine plasma concentrations were significantly greater in the treatment group compared to placebo at 1 h ($P < 0.001$), 3 h ($P < 0.001$), 6 h ($P = 0.01$), and 10 h ($P = 0.05$) (**Figure 3D**).

Plasma Insulin and Glucose Concentrations

Plasma insulin and glucose concentrations are presented in **Figures 4A,B**, respectively. A treatment effect was observed at time 1 h for insulin showing a Cmax significantly higher ($P < 0.05$) in the placebo group compared to treatment (**Figure 4B**). A significant difference was observed in the glucose concentrations between treatments at 1 h (placebo group higher) and 10 h (treatment group higher) ($P < 0.001$ and $P < 0.05$, respectively; **Figure 4B**).

Rates of Muscle Protein Synthesis

Plasma free phenylalanine enrichment was significantly different between pre-administration of the tracer and 1 h after (7 h post-drink, data not reported). When plotting the average TTR of free ^{13}C-Ph in plasma over time (7, 10, and 11 h), the slope was not significantly different from 0 ($P = 0.17$). TTR ranged from 0.0702 ± 0.006 at 7 h to 0.0673 ± 0.0082 ($n = 17$). These data suggest that plasma free ^{13}C-Ph reached a plateau and subjects were in isotopic steady state condition throughout the duration of the tracer infusion. The rates of muscle protein synthesis were measured between 03:00 and 08:00. No significant changes were observed in the rate of muscle protein synthesis, over time or between treatments (**Figure 5**).

Whole Body Protein Balance

The ingestion of the placebo drink resulted in negative whole body protein balance across the entire 10 h overnight sleep period (−12.22 g prot/10 h). In contrast, the ingestion of the protein containing drink resulted in a near zero protein balance across the entire 10-h overnight sleep period (−0.13 g prot/10 h) and this difference was significantly different compared to the placebo group ($P < 0.01$) (**Figure 6**). One individual in the placebo group had to be excluded because it was not possible to obtain a muscle sample. No significant differences were observed in either whole body protein synthesis or breakdown (**Figure 6**).

Western Analysis of Muscle Signaling Proteins

Western analysis was carried out on the muscle biopsy obtained at 08:00. No significant changes were observed between treatments for any of the signaling proteins examined (**Figure 7**).

DISCUSSION

To date, only a few studies have investigated the impact of pre-bedtime dietary protein ingestion on either whole body or muscle specific protein turnover and most of this work has been carried out as part of a resistance exercise training program in young and elderly healthy physically active individuals (17, 18, 25–28).

In light of the accelerated loss of lean tissue mass observed in the elderly (including muscle), nutritional strategies aimed at preventing such losses are of key importance in such populations. A recent paper showed that the ingestion of a 40 g protein bolus before sleep increased muscle protein synthesis during overnight sleep (19). In our present study, we report that providing a complete protein containing drink (containing 25 g of dietary protein together with

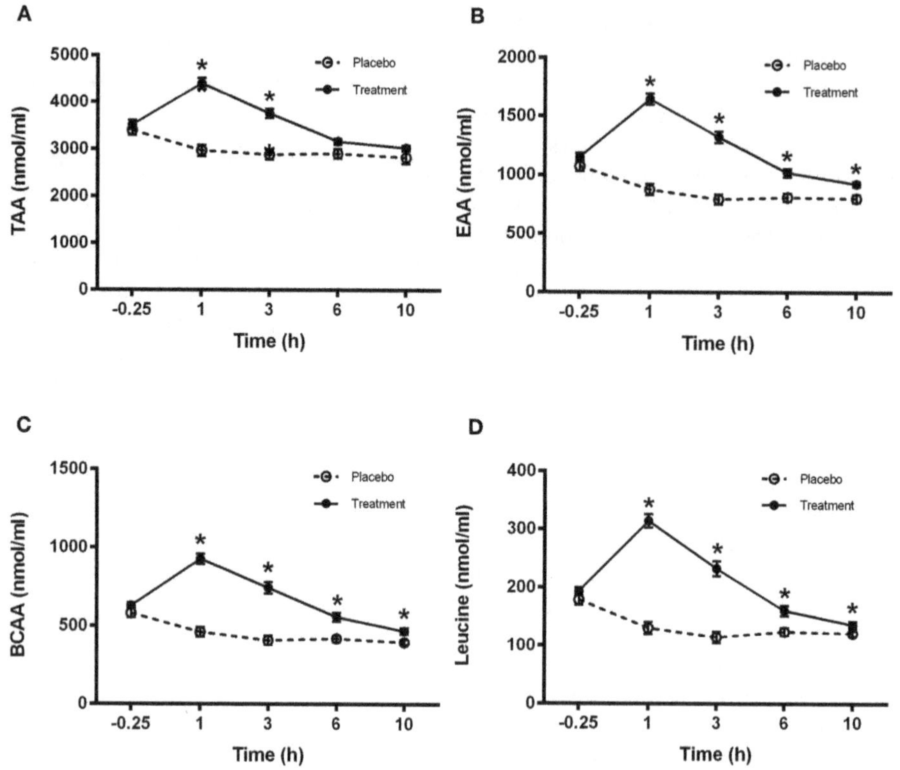

FIGURE 3 | Plasma amino acid concentrations for **(A)** total (TAA), **(B)** essential (EAA), **(C)** branched chain (BCAA), and **(D)** leucine for control (light bars) and treatment (dark bars) groups observed over 10 h post supplement ingestion. Supplement was ingested immediately after the first blood sample was obtained. Values are means ± SD. *Significantly different at corresponding time point between groups ($P < 0.05$).

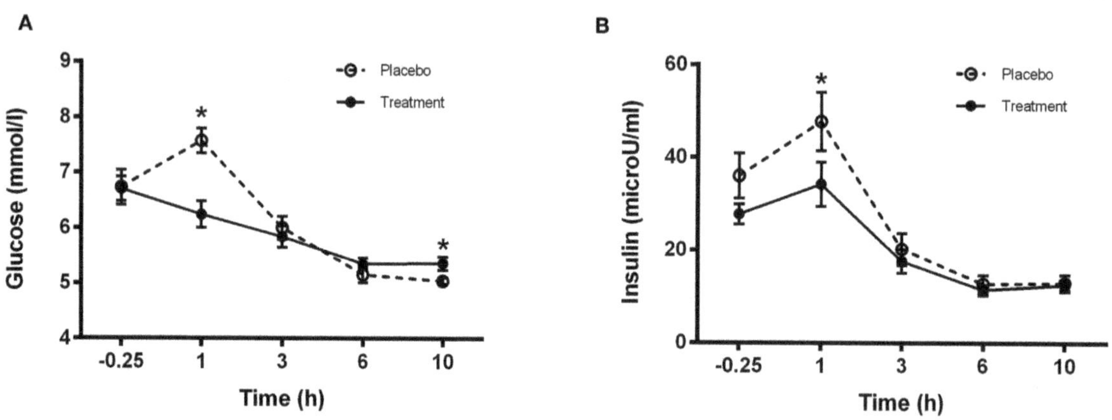

FIGURE 4 | Plasma **(A)** Glucose and **(B)** Insulin concentrations for control (light bars) and treatment (dark bars) groups observed over 10 h post supplement ingestion. Supplement was ingested immediately after the first blood sample was obtained. Values are means ± SD. *Significantly different at corresponding time point between groups ($P < 0.05$).

25 g carbohydrate and 7.5 g oil) to healthy middle-aged individuals before sleep, prevented the negative whole body protein balance and that muscle protein synthesis specifically, is not augmented in the later part of the night despite elevated aminoacidemia.

Interestingly Res et al., previously reported that a total of 60 g of casein resulted in greater whole body protein balance and increased muscle protein synthesis in young exercising participants (18) while Groen et al. showed that nasogastric feeding of 40 g casein commencing at 02:00 in elderly resulted

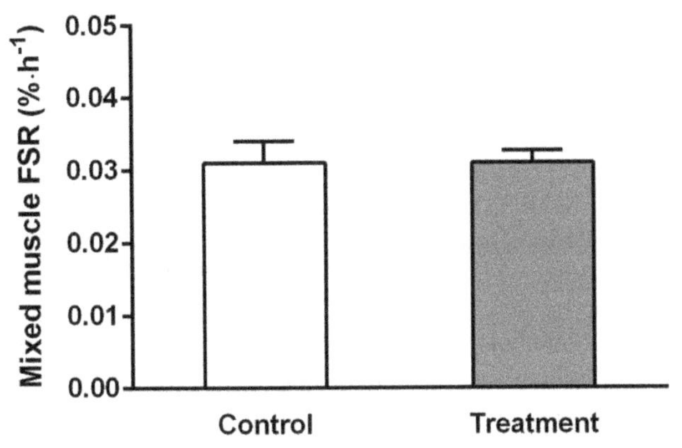

FIGURE 5 | Mixed muscle rates of protein synthesis measured between 03:00 and 08:00 h in control (light bars) and treatment (dark bars) groups. Values are means ± SD. No significant difference was observed between treatments.

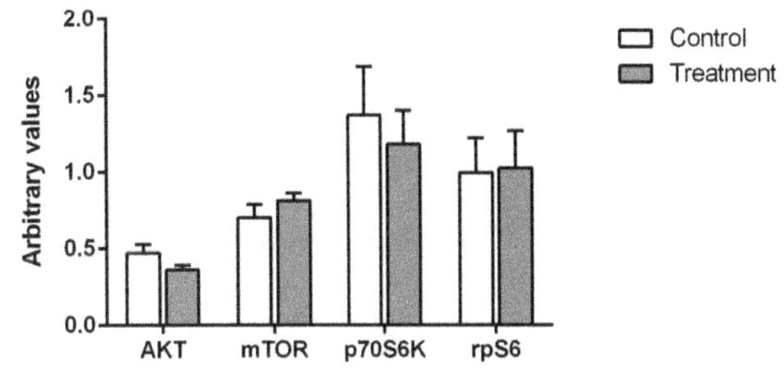

FIGURE 7 | Relative phosphorylation status of proteins involved in skeletal muscle protein synthesis for AKT, mTOR, p70S6K, and rpS6. Values are expressed as means ± SD and are expressed as the ratio between phosphorylated forms to total protein and corrected for a house keeper. No significant differences were observed for any of the proteins between treatments.

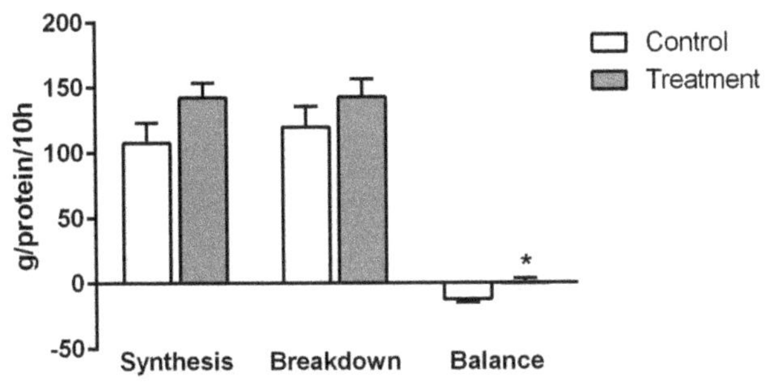

FIGURE 6 | Rates of whole body protein synthesis, breakdown and balance in control (light bars) and treatment groups (dark bars) observed across the 10 h overnight sleep duration. Values are expressed as means ± SD. To test the treatment effect over time, a two-way ANOVA with repeated measurements was employed. Pairwise comparisons at different time points were only evaluated in case when overall treatment effect was statistically significant, *Significantly different from control ($P < 0.05$).

in normal digestion and absorption kinetics, stimulating muscle protein synthesis and improved overnight whole body protein balance (29). In these studies, muscle protein synthesis was measured over the whole night and thus it is unknown if the effect observed was related to a stimulation of protein synthesis occurring all along the night in response to the sustained amino acid availability or only during the first hours after protein ingestion (as usually described when a meal effect is studied).

In our study we still observed amino acid digestion kinetics similar to those previously reported in individuals throughout the night. Specifically, we observed substantial elevations in plasma amino acid concentrations (TAA, BCAA, EAA, Leucine) throughout the night when compared to the isocaloric, protein void control drink which is even more extended than previously reported by Kouw et al. (19) who reported a return to baseline values about 6 h following the ingestion of 20 g whey protein. In our study, we still observed higher aminoacidemia values in the treatment group after 10 h which may in part be due to either a slower digestion rate related to the presence of carbohydrate and fat in our treatment drink, the additional 5 g of protein provided in our treatment drink or a combination of both. Moreover, given that muscle protein synthesis is only stimulated for several hours following an increase in plasma amino acid concentrations (5, 30, 31) it is not clear if the observed benefits in whole body protein balance in our study as well as the increased rates of muscle protein synthesis and whole body net protein balance observed previously by others were driven at specific time points (0–4 h following protein ingestion) or across the whole duration of the night (extended amino acid availability).

Accordingly, Kouw et al. concluded that the greater plasma amino acid availability they observed following 40 g of protein ingestion compared to 20 g during the longer overnight period may have been required in order to allow a measurable increase in muscle protein synthesis rates. To address this question we assessed muscle protein synthesis at the later part of the night between the hours of 03:00–08:00. Despite the extended increases in plasma amino acid concentrations observed in our study (**Figure 3**) we found that rates of muscle protein synthesis at the later part of the night did not differ between groups. In addition we also quantified the activation of the canonical signaling cascade implicated in skeletal muscle protein synthesis and found no significant differences between treatment groups for either AKT, mTOR, rpS6, or p70S6K (**Figure 7**). In light of these observations, it seems therefore that the observed increase in whole body protein balance in our study was most likely driven by the immediate postprandial response to the beverage ingestion (first 4 h post-ingestion).

What is not clear however, is why the extended and elevated amino acid plasma concentrations did not stimulate muscle protein synthesis. One possibility is that the threshold plasma levels of circulating amino acids required to stimulate muscle protein synthesis was not reached. Indeed, when we compared the activation of the mTOR signaling pathway in the morning at waking we did not observe any changes between treatments in relative phosphorylation of either mTOR, rpS6, or p70S6K which are known to be activated by amino acid availability (9). In the absence of changes in the rates of muscle protein synthesis at the later part of the sleep period as well as the lack of observed changes in the anabolic signaling pathway, we propose that any observed change in whole body protein balance was likely due to the postprandial effect of protein ingestion (<4 h following ingestion) or that the improved whole body protein balance was primarily driven by other organs other than muscle. The former is partly supported by a recent study in elderly individuals in which the authors investigated the effect of a bolus vs. a pulse feeding pattern of amino acids on muscle protein synthesis. They reported extended elevated essential aminoacidemia in the absence of increased muscle protein synthesis (32) which the authors attributed to the "muscle full" state (a state describing the point at which stimulation of muscle protein synthesis becomes refractory to the ongoing availability of EAA).

The insulin response to the treatment and placebo beverages displayed significantly different values at the 1 h time point whereby the placebo ingestion resulted in a greater insulin peak compared to the treatment group (**Figure 4B**). This is not surprising given the increased maltodextrin content of the placebo beverage (in order to provide isocaloric properties between treatment and placebo groups). Furthermore, ingestion of the placebo beverage also resulted in a higher glucose peak compared to the protein group 1 h post ingestion. However, despite the lower levels of maltodextrin in the treatment group, plasma glucose levels in the treatment group failed to return to basal levels in the morning (08:00) and therefore, fasting plasma glucose remained higher relative to the control group but no significant effect was observed for insulin. The exact physiological significance of this response however is not clear. Several studies have reported mixed observations on measures of glucose handling in the morning following either pre-bedtime or overnight nutrient provisions (27, 29, 33–35). In a study investigating the effect of providing a pre-bed time protein or carbohydrate snack to overweight sedentary women, the authors reported that plasma insulin concentrations were negatively affected resulting in an increased homeostatic model assessment of insulin resistance score indicating an insulin resistant phenotype (33). In contrast, introducing physical activity to the daily routine prevented the negative responses in insulin (34). It seems therefore that beyond the caloric content, the habitual physical activity status of an individual is an important determinant regulating the metabolic milieu following a pre-bedtime nutrient containing snack. In addition, the overall body composition of an individual may also further impact the results, as lean tissue percentage may impact insulin sensitivity and/or glucose uptake, something we were not able to control for in the present work. However, one limitation in the current study which prohibits us to conclude on the impact of pre-bed protein ingestion on the subsequent morning glycemic control is the absence of a fasting baseline glucose measure. This would have enabled us to better compare fasting glycemia pre and post-intervention.

Moreover, it is important that the circadian rhythm and an integrative physiology approach should be considered when planning pre-bedtime nutritional strategies aimed at promoting specific health outcomes (36–39). For instance controlling for sleep time as well as meal compositions 2–3d prior to an intervention seems ever more important in order to account for circadian rhythm disturbances which may in turn impact the results. Whether these short term benefits are translated into long term functional outcomes remains to be seen. Nonetheless, in a recent study it was shown that long-term pre-bedtime protein supplementation in healthy young men resulted in greater gains in both, strength and muscle mass following a 12 week progressive resistance training program (27). However, what is not clear is whether or not this effect was due to the timing of the protein ingestion *per se* (before bed) or simply due to the extra 25 g of protein ingested above that of the control group in a 24 h period.

In conclusion we show that the ingestion of a complete drink containing 25 g of milk protein before sleep promotes whole body protein balance in the morning compared to the ingestion of an isocaloric, protein void pre-bed supplement in middle-aged healthy men. Moreover, this effect was not related to a stimulation in the rates of skeletal muscle protein synthesis in the second part of the night, suggesting the observed anabolic effect was likely a typical postprandial response observed in the first half of the sleep period. Such nutritional strategies may be implemented in order to attenuate age related losses of lean tissue mass but other metabolic outcomes such as glucose handling need to be incorporated and assessed to prevent any disturbances to the metabolic milieu. Better understanding of the role of chronobiology and how it is impacted by nutrition is of critical significance in promoting long-term benefits of nutrient timing interventions for the promotion and maintenance of health and well-being.

AUTHOR CONTRIBUTIONS

LK conceptualized the research. LK, DB, MB, J-PG, and MS designed the research. LD-C and KR-K were responsible for product development. DD, SP, A-FK, and JV performed the analysis. MS was responsible for the statistical analysis and reporting. LK and DB were responsible for data interpretation. LK wrote the paper and had primary responsibility for final content. All authors read and approved the final manuscript.

FUNDING

The authors declare that this study received full funding from Nestlé Research. The funder had the following involvement with the study: planning of the clinical trial, preparation and development of test products (placebo and active treatment product), clinical trial execution, sample analysis, data analysis, and interpretation.

ACKNOWLEDGMENTS

The authors would like to thank Frederik Delodder, Karine Groulx, Laurence Guignard, Corine Nielsen Moennoz, Sylviane Oguey-Araymon, and Fabienne Praplan for their help in performing the clinical trial.

REFERENCES

1. Karagounis LG, Hawley JA. Skeletal muscle: increasing the size of the locomotor cell. *Int J Biochem Cell Biol.* (2010) 42:1376–9. doi: 10.1016/j.biocel.2010.05.013
2. Bauer JM, Verlaan S, Bautmans I, Brandt K, Donini LM, Maggio M, et al. Effects of a vitamin d and leucine-enriched whey protein nutritional supplement on measures of sarcopenia in older adults, the provide study: a randomized, double-blind, placebo-controlled trial. *J Am Med Dir Assoc.* (2015) 16:740–7. doi: 10.1016/j.jamda.2015.05.021
3. Smith GI, Atherton P, Reeds DN, Mohammed BS, Rankin D, Rennie MJ, et al. Dietary omega-3 fatty acid supplementation increases the rate of muscle protein synthesis in older adults: a randomized controlled trial. *Am J Clin Nutr.* (2011) 93:402–12. doi: 10.3945/ajcn.110.005611
4. Phillips SM, Tang JE, Moore DR. The role of milk- and soy-based protein in support of muscle protein synthesis and muscle protein accretion in young and elderly persons. *J Am Coll Nutr.* (2009) 28:343–54. doi: 10.1080/07315724.2009.10718096
5. Witard OC, Jackman SR, Breen L, Smith K, Selby A, Tipton KD. Myofibrillar muscle protein synthesis rates subsequent to a meal in response to increasing doses of whey protein at rest and after resistance exercise. *Am J Clin Nutr.* (2014) 99:86–95. doi: 10.3945/ajcn.112.055517
6. Tipton KD. Muscle protein metabolism in the elderly: influence of exercise and nutrition. *Can J Appl Physiol.* (2001) 26:588–606. doi: 10.1139/h01-033
7. Collino S, Martin FP, Karagounis LG, Horcajada MN, Moco S, Franceschi C, et al. Musculoskeletal system in the old age and the demand for healthy ageing biomarkers. *Mech Ageing Dev.* (2013) 134:541–7. doi: 10.1016/j.mad.2013.11.003
8. Andersen LL, Tufekovic G, Zebis MK, Crameri RM, Verlaan G, Kjaer M, et al. The effect of resistance training combined with timed ingestion of protein on muscle fiber size and muscle strength. *Metab Clin Exp.* (2005) 54:151–6. doi: 10.1016/j.metabol.2004.07.012
9. Greenhaff PL, Karagounis LG, Peirce N, Simpson EJ, Hazell M, Layfield R, et al. Disassociation between the effects of amino acids and insulin on signaling, ubiquitin ligases, and protein turnover in human muscle. *Am J Physiol Endocrinol Metab.* (2008) 295, E595–604. doi: 10.1152/ajpendo.90411.2008
10. Murphy CH, Shankaran M, Churchward-Venne TA, Mitchell CJ, Kolar NM, Burke LM, et al. Effect of resistance training and protein intake pattern on myofibrillar protein synthesis and proteome kinetics in older men in energy restriction. *J Physiol.* (2018) 596:2091–120. doi: 10.1113/JP275246
11. Cuthbertson D, Smith K, Babraj J, Leese G, Waddell T, Atherton P, et al. Anabolic signaling deficits underlie amino acid resistance of wasting, aging muscle. *FASEB J.* (2005) 19:422–4. doi: 10.1096/fj.04-2640fje
12. Janssen I. Evolution of sarcopenia research. *Appl Physiol Nutr Metab.* (2010) 35:707–12. doi: 10.1139/H10-067
13. Morley JE, Abbatecola AM, Argiles JM, Baracos V, Bauer J, Bhasin S, et al. Sarcopenia with limited mobility: an international consensus. *J Am Med Dir Assoc.* (2011) 12:403–9. doi: 10.1016/j.jamda.2011.04.014
14. Meek SE, Persson M, Ford GC, Nair KS. Differential regulation of amino acid exchange and protein dynamics across splanchnic and skeletal muscle beds by insulin in healthy human subjects. *Diabetes.* (1998) 47:1824–35. doi: 10.2337/diabetes.47.12.1824
15. Baillie AG, Garlick PJ. Responses of protein synthesis in different skeletal muscles to fasting and insulin in rats. *Am J Physiol.* (1991) 260:E891–6. doi: 10.1152/ajpendo.1991.260.6.E891
16. Millward DJ, Garlick PJ. The pattern of protein turnover in the whole animal and the effect of dietary variations. *Proc Nutr Soc.* (1972) 31:257–63. doi: 10.1079/PNS19720049
17. Trommelen J, van Loon LJ. Pre-sleep protein ingestion to improve the skeletal muscle adaptive response to exercise training. *Nutrients.* (2016) 8:E763. doi: 10.3390/nu8120763
18. Res PT, Groen B, Pennings B, Beelen M, Wallis GA, Gijsen AP, et al. Protein ingestion before sleep improves postexercise overnight recovery. *Med Sci Sports Exerc.* (2012) 44:1560–9. doi: 10.1249/MSS.0b013e31824cc363
19. Kouw IWK, Holwerda AM, Trommelen J, Kramer IF, Bastiaanse J, Halson SL, et al. Protein ingestion before sleep increases overnight muscle protein synthesis rates in healthy older men: a randomized controlled trial. *J Nutr.* (2017) 147:2252–61. doi: 10.3945/jn.117.254532
20. Moore DR, Areta J, Coffey VG, Stellingwerff T, Phillips SM, Burke LM, et al. Daytime pattern of post-exercise protein intake affects whole-body protein turnover in resistance-trained males. *Nutr Metab.* (2012) 9:91. doi: 10.1186/1743-7075-9-91
21. Waterlow JC, Golden MH, Garlick PJ. Protein turnover in man measured with 15n: comparison of end products and dose regimes. *Am J Physiol Endocrinol Metab.* (1978) 235:E165. doi: 10.1152/ajpendo.1978.235.2.E165
22. Burd NA, Pennings B, Groen BB, Gijsen AP, Senden JM, van Loon LJ. The single biopsy approach is reliable for the measurement of muscle protein synthesis rates *in vivo* in older men. *J Appl Physiol.* (2012) 113:896–902. doi: 10.1152/japplphysiol.00513.2012
23. Burd NA, West DW, Rerecich T, Prior T, Baker SK, Phillips SM. Validation of a single biopsy approach and bolus protein feeding to determine myofibrillar protein synthesis in stable isotope tracer studies in humans. *Nutr Metab.* (2011) 8:15. doi: 10.1186/1743-7075-8-15
24. Smith GI, Patterson BW, Mittendorfer B. Human muscle protein turnover–why is it so variable? *J Appl Physiol.* (1985). (2011) 110:480–91. doi: 10.1152/japplphysiol.00125.2010
25. Trommelen J, Kouw IWK, Holwerda AM, Snijders T, Halson SL, Rollo I, et al. Pre-sleep dietary protein-derived amino acids are incorporated in myofibrillar protein during post-exercise overnight recovery. *Am J Physiol Endocrinol Metab.* (2017) 314:E457–67. doi: 10.1152/ajpendo.00273.2016
26. Wall BT, Burd NA, Franssen R, Gorissen SHM, Snijders T, Senden JM, et al. Presleep protein ingestion does not compromise the muscle protein synthetic response to protein ingested the following morning. *Am J Physiol Endocrinol Metab.* (2016) 311:E964–73. doi: 10.1152/ajpendo.00325.2016
27. Snijders T, Res PT, Smeets JS, van Vliet S, van Kranenburg J, Maase K, et al. Protein ingestion before sleep increases muscle mass and strength gains during prolonged resistance-type exercise training in healthy young men. *J Nutr.* (2015) 145:1178–84. doi: 10.3945/jn.114.208371
28. Holwerda AM, Kouw IW, Trommelen J, Halson SL, Wodzig WK, Verdijk LB, et al. Physical activity performed in the evening increases the overnight muscle protein synthetic response to presleep protein ingestion in older men. *J Nutr.* (2016) 146:1307–14. doi: 10.3945/jn.116.230086
29. Groen BB, Res PT, Pennings B, Hertle E, Senden JM, Saris WH, et al. Intragastric protein administration stimulates overnight muscle protein synthesis in elderly men. *Am J Physiol Endocrinol Metab.* (2012) 302:E52–60. doi: 10.1152/ajpendo.00321.2011

30. Atherton PJ, Etheridge T, Watt PW, Wilkinson D, Selby A, Rankin D, et al. Muscle full effect after oral protein: Time-dependent concordance and discordance between human muscle protein synthesis and mtorc1 signaling. *Am J Clin Nutr.* (2010) 92:1080–8. doi: 10.3945/ajcn.2010.29819
31. Bohe J, Low JF, Wolfe RR, Rennie MJ. Latency and duration of stimulation of human muscle protein synthesis during continuous infusion of amino acids. *J Physiol.* (2001) 532:575–9. doi: 10.1111/j.1469-7793.2001.0575f.x
32. Mitchell WK, Phillips BE, Williams JP, Rankin D, Lund JN, Wilkinson DJ, et al. The impact of delivery profile of essential amino acids upon skeletal muscle protein synthesis in older men: clinical efficacy of pulse vs. Bolus supply. *Am J Physiol Endocrinol Metab.* (2015) 309:E450–7. doi: 10.1152/ajpendo.00112.2015
33. Kinsey AW, Eddy WR, Madzima TA, Panton LB, Arciero PJ, Kim JS, et al. Influence of night-time protein and carbohydrate intake on appetite and cardiometabolic risk in sedentary overweight and obese women. *Br J Nutr.* (2014) 112:320–7. doi: 10.1017/S0007114514001068
34. Ormsbee MJ, Kinsey AW, Eddy WR, Madzima TA, Arciero PJ, Figueroa A, et al. The influence of nighttime feeding of carbohydrate or protein combined with exercise training on appetite and cardiometabolic risk in young obese women. *Appl Physiol Nutr Metab.* (2014) 40:37–45. doi: 10.1139/apnm-2014-0256
35. Madzima TA, Panton LB, Fretti SK, Kinsey AW, Ormsbee MJ. Night-time consumption of protein or carbohydrate results in increased morning resting energy expenditure in active college-aged men. *Br J Nutr.* (2014) 111:71–7. doi: 10.1017/S000711451300192X
36. Hibi M, Masumoto A, Naito Y, Kiuchi K, Yoshimoto Y, Matsumoto M, et al. Nighttime snacking reduces whole body fat oxidation and increases ldl cholesterol in healthy young women. *Am J Physiol Regul Integr Comp Physiol.* (2013) 304:R94–101. doi: 10.1152/ajpregu.00115.2012
37. Morris CJ, Yang JN, Scheer FA. The impact of the circadian timing system on cardiovascular and metabolic function. *Prog Brain Res.* (2012) 199:337–58. doi: 10.1016/B978-0-444-59427-3.00019-8
38. Rüger M, Scheer FJL. Effects of circadian disruption on the cardiometabolic system. *Rev Endocr Metab Disord.* (2009) 10:245–60. doi: 10.1007/s11154-009-9122-8
39. Scheer FA, Hilton MF, Mantzoros CS, Shea SA. Adverse metabolic and cardiovascular consequences of circadian misalignment. *Proc Natl Acad Sci USA.* (2009) 106:4453–8. doi: 10.1073/pnas.0808180106

Permissions

All chapters in this book were first published by Frontiers; hereby published with permission under the Creative Commons Attribution License or equivalent. Every chapter published in this book has been scrutinized by our experts. Their significance has been extensively debated. The topics covered herein carry significant findings which will fuel the growth of the discipline. They may even be implemented as practical applications or may be referred to as a beginning point for another development.

The contributors of this book come from diverse backgrounds, making this book a truly international effort. This book will bring forth new frontiers with its revolutionizing research information and detailed analysis of the nascent developments around the world.

We would like to thank all the contributing authors for lending their expertise to make the book truly unique. They have played a crucial role in the development of this book. Without their invaluable contributions this book wouldn't have been possible. They have made vital efforts to compile up to date information on the varied aspects of this subject to make this book a valuable addition to the collection of many professionals and students.

This book was conceptualized with the vision of imparting up-to-date information and advanced data in this field. To ensure the same, a matchless editorial board was set up. Every individual on the board went through rigorous rounds of assessment to prove their worth. After which they invested a large part of their time researching and compiling the most relevant data for our readers.

The editorial board has been involved in producing this book since its inception. They have spent rigorous hours researching and exploring the diverse topics which have resulted in the successful publishing of this book. They have passed on their knowledge of decades through this book. To expedite this challenging task, the publisher supported the team at every step. A small team of assistant editors was also appointed to further simplify the editing procedure and attain best results for the readers.

Apart from the editorial board, the designing team has also invested a significant amount of their time in understanding the subject and creating the most relevant covers. They scrutinized every image to scout for the most suitable representation of the subject and create an appropriate cover for the book.

The publishing team has been an ardent support to the editorial, designing and production team. Their endless efforts to recruit the best for this project, has resulted in the accomplishment of this book. They are a veteran in the field of academics and their pool of knowledge is as vast as their experience in printing. Their expertise and guidance has proved useful at every step. Their uncompromising quality standards have made this book an exceptional effort. Their encouragement from time to time has been an inspiration for everyone.

The publisher and the editorial board hope that this book will prove to be a valuable piece of knowledge for researchers, students, practitioners and scholars across the globe.

List of Contributors

Jess A. Gwin
Oak Ridge Institute for Science and Education Supporting the Military Nutrition Division of the US Army Research Institute of Environmental Medicine, Natick, MA, United States
Military Nutrition Division of the US Army Research Institute of Environmental Medicine, Natick, MA, United States

J. Philip Karl, James P. McClung and Stefan M. Pasiakos
Military Nutrition Division of the US Army Research Institute of Environmental Medicine, Natick, MA, United States

Laura J. Lutz and Erin Gaffney-Stomberg
Military Performance Division of the US Army Research Institute of Environmental Medicine, Natick, MA, United States

Sucharita Sambashivaiah
Department of Physiology, St. John's Medical College, Bengaluru, India

Stephen D. R. Harridge
Centre for Human and Applied Physiological Sciences, King's College London, London, United Kingdom

Nidhi Sharma
Division of Nutrition, St. John's Research Institute, Bengaluru, India

Sumithra Selvam
Division of Epidemiology and Biostatistics, St. John's Research Institute, Bengaluru, India

Priyanka Rohatgi
Apollo Hospitals, Bengaluru, India

Anura V. Kurpad
Department of Physiology, St. John's Medical College, Bengaluru, India
Division of Nutrition, St. John's Research Institute, Bengaluru, India

Darren G. Candow
Faculty of Kinesiology and Health Studies, University of Regina, Regina, SK, Canada

Scott C. Forbes
Department of Physical Education, Brandon University, Brandon, MB, Canada

Philip D. Chilibeck
College of Kinesiology, University of Saskatchewan, Saskatoon, SK, Canada

Stephen M. Cornish
Faculty of Kinesiology and Recreation Management, University of Manitoba, Winnipeg, MB, Canada

Jose Antonio
Department of Health and Human Performance, Nova Southeastern University, Davie, FL, United States

Richard B. Kreider
Department of Health and Kinesiology, Texas A&M University, College Station, TX, United States

Joseph W. Beals
Center for Human Nutrition, Washington University School of Medicine, St. Louis, MO, United States

Nicholas A. Burd
Department of Kinesiology and Community Health, University of Illinois at Urbana-Champaign, Urbana, IL, United States

Daniel R. Moore
Faculty of Kinesiology and Physical Education, University of Toronto, Toronto, ON, Canada

Stephan van Vliet
Duke Molecular Physiology Institute, Duke University Medical Center, Durham, NC, United States

Jordan D. Philpott, Niels J. Bootsma, Nidia Rodriguez-Sanchez and Stuart D. R. Galloway
Physiology, Exercise and Nutrition Research Group, Faculty of Health Sciences and Sport, University of Stirling, Stirling, United Kingdom

David Lee Hamilton
Physiology, Exercise and Nutrition Research Group, Faculty of Health Sciences and Sport, University of Stirling, Stirling, United Kingdom
Institute for Physical Activity and Nutrition (IPAN), School of Exercise and Nutrition Sciences, Deakin University, Geelong, VIC, Australia

Elizabeth MacKinlay and James Dick
Institute of Aquaculture, University of Stirling, Stirling, United Kingdom

Samuel Mettler
Department of Health Sciences and Technology, ETH Zurich, Zurich, Switzerland

Kevin D. Tipton
Department of Sport and Exercise Sciences, Faculty of Social Sciences and Health, Durham University, Durham, United Kingdom

Oliver C. Witard
Physiology, Exercise and Nutrition Research Group, Faculty of Health Sciences and Sport, University of Stirling, Stirling, United Kingdom
Centre for Human and Applied Physiological Sciences, School of Basic and Medical Biosciences, Faculty of Life Sciences and Medicine, King's College London, London, United Kingdom

Brenan Durainayagam
Liggins Institute, University of Auckland, Auckland, New Zealand
Division of Systems Medicine and Digestive Medicine, Department of Metabolism, Digestion and Reproduction, Imperial College London, London, United Kingdom

Cameron J. Mitchell
Liggins Institute, University of Auckland, Auckland, New Zealand
School of Kinesiology, The University of British Columbia, Vancouver, BC, Canada

Amber M. Milan
Liggins Institute, University of Auckland, Auckland, New Zealand
Food Nutrition & Health Team, AgResearch, Palmerston North, New Zealand

Nina Zeng, Pankaja Sharma, Sarah M. Mitchell and Farha Ramzan
Liggins Institute, University of Auckland, Auckland, New Zealand

Scott O. Knowles
Food Nutrition & Health Team, AgResearch, Palmerston North, New Zealand

Karl-Heinz Wagner
Department of Nutritional Sciences and Research Platform Active Ageing, University of Vienna, Vienna, Austria

Nicole C. Roy and Karl Fraser
The High-Value Nutrition National Science Challenge, Auckland, New Zealand
Food & Bio-based Products Group, AgResearch, Palmerston North, New Zealand
Riddet Institute, Massey University, Palmerston North, New Zealand

David Cameron-Smith
Liggins Institute, University of Auckland, Auckland, New Zealand
Riddet Institute, Massey University, Palmerston North, New Zealand
Clinical Nutrition Research Centre, Singapore Institute for Clinical Sciences, Agency for Science, Technology, and Research, Singapore, Singapore

Anders Sjödin
Department of Nutrition, Exercise and Sport, Copenhagen University, Copenhagen, Denmark

Kayleigh M. Beaudry and Michaela C. Devries
Department of Kinesiology, Faculty of Applied Health Sciences, University of Waterloo, Waterloo, ON, Canada

Gommaar D'Hulst, Evi Masschelein and Katrien De Bock
Laboratory of Exercise and Health, Department of Health Sciences and Technology, Swiss Federal Institute of Technology (ETH) Zurich, Zurich, Switzerland

Andrew S. Palmer and Ori Bar-Nur
Laboratory of Regenerative and Movement Biology, Department of Health Sciences and Technology, Swiss Federal Institute of Technology (ETH) Zurich, Zurich, Switzerland

Randall F. D'Souza
Liggins Institute, The University of Auckland, Auckland, New Zealand
Discipline of Nutrition, The University of Auckland, Auckland, New Zealand

James F. Markworth
Liggins Institute, The University of Auckland, Auckland, New Zealand
Department of Molecular and Integrative Physiology, University of Michigan, Ann Arbor, MI, United States

Nina Zeng
Liggins Institute, The University of Auckland, Auckland, New Zealand

Vandre C. Figueiredo
Liggins Institute, The University of Auckland, Auckland, New Zealand
College of Health Sciences, University of Kentucky, Lexington, KY, United States

Christopher P. Hedges
Applied Surgery and Metabolism Laboratory, School of Biological Sciences, University of Auckland, Auckland, New Zealand

Aaron C. Petersen
Institute for Health and Sport (iHeS), Victoria University, Melbourne, VIC, Australia

Paul A. Della Gatta
Institute for Physical Activity and Nutrition (IPAN), School of Exercise and Nutrition Sciences, Deakin University, Geelong, VIC, Australia

David Cameron-Smith
Liggins Institute, The University of Auckland, Auckland, New Zealand
Food and Bio-based Products, AgResearch Grasslands, Palmerston North, New Zealand
The Riddet Institute, Massey University, Palmerston North, New Zealand

Cameron J. Mitchell
Liggins Institute, The University of Auckland, Auckland, New Zealand
School of Kinesiology, University of British Colombia, Vancouver, BC, Canada

Tim Snijders, Jorn Trommelen, Imre W. K. Kouw, Andrew M. Holwerda, Lex B. Verdijk and Luc J. C. van Loon
Department of Human Biology, NUTRIM School of Nutrition and Translational Research in Metabolism, Maastricht University Medical Centre, Maastricht, Netherlands

Chris McGlory
School of Kinesiology and Health Studies, Queen's University, Kingston, ON, Canada

Philip C. Calder
Human Development and Health, Faculty of Medicine, University of Southampton, Southampton, United Kingdom
NIHR Southampton Biomedical Research Centre, University Hospital Southampton NHS Foundation Trust and University of Southampton, Southampton, United Kingdom

Everson A. Nunes
Department of Physiological Sciences, Federal University of Santa Catarina, Florianópolis

Marissa K. Caldow, Daniel J. Ham, Jennifer Trieu, Jin Dylan Chung, Gordon S. Lynch and René Koopman
Centre for Muscle Research, Department of Physiology, The University of Melbourne, Melbourne, VIC, Australia

Sebastian Edman, Karin Söderlund, Marcus Moberg and William Apró
The Åstrand Laboratory, the Swedish School of Sport and Health Sciences, Stockholm, Sweden

Eva Blomstrand
The Åstrand Laboratory, the Swedish School of Sport and Health Sciences, Stockholm, Sweden
Department of Physiology and Pharmacology, Karolinska Institutet, Stockholm, Sweden

Aaron Bridge, Joseph Brown and Matthew Nasato
Department of Kinesiology, Faculty of Applied Health Sciences, Brock University, St. Catharines, ON, Canada

Hayden Snider
School of Kinesiology and Health Science, Faculty of Health, York University, Toronto, ON, Canada

Wendy E. Ward and Brian D. Roy
Department of Kinesiology, Faculty of Applied Health Sciences, Brock University, St. Catharines, ON, Canada
Centre for Bone and Muscle Health, Faculty of Applied Health Sciences, Brock University, St. Catharines, ON, Canada

Andrea R. Josse
Department of Kinesiology, Faculty of Applied Health Sciences, Brock University, St. Catharines, ON, Canada
School of Kinesiology and Health Science, Faculty of Health, York University, Toronto, ON, Canada
Centre for Bone and Muscle Health, Faculty of Applied Health Sciences, Brock University, St. Catharines, ON, Canada

Cody T. Haun, Christopher G. Vann, Christopher B. Mobley, Paul A. Roberson, Shelby C. Osburn, Hudson M. Holmes, Petey M. Mumford, Matthew A. Romero and L. Bruce Gladden
School of Kinesiology, Auburn University, Auburn, AL, United States

Kaelin C. Young and Michael D. Roberts
School of Kinesiology, Auburn University, Auburn, AL, United States
Department of Cell Biology and Physiology, Edward Via College of Osteopathic Medicine-Auburn Campus, Auburn, AL, United States

Jordan R. Moon
Impedimed Inc., Carlsbad, CA, United States

Robert D. Arnold
Harrison School of Pharmacy, Auburn University, Auburn, AL, United States

Michael A. Israetel
Renaissance Periodization, Charlotte, NC, United States

Annie N. Kirby
Department of Cell Biology and Physiology, Edward Via College of Osteopathic Medicine-Auburn Campus, Auburn, AL, United States

Gary John Slater
School of Health and Sport Sciences, University of the Sunshine Coast, Maroochydore, QLD, Australia
Australian Institute of Sport, Canberra, ACT, Australia

Brad P. Dieter
Department of Pharmaceutical Sciences, Washington State University, WA Spokane, WA, United States

Damian James Marsh
Fiji Rugby Union, Suva, Fiji

Eric Russell Helms
Auckland University of Technology, Sports Performance Research Institute New Zealand, Auckland, New Zealand

Gregory Shaw
Swimming Australia, Brisbane, QLD, Australia

Juma Iraki
Iraki Nutrition AS, Fjerdingby, Norway

Sara Y. Oikawa, Tanya M. Holloway and Stuart M. Phillips
Exercise Metabolism Research Group, Department of Kinesiology, McMaster University, Hamilton, ON, Canada

Kirsten E. Bell
Department of Kinesiology, University of Waterloo, Waterloo, ON, Canada

Matthew S. Brook
School of Life Sciences, University of Nottingham, Nottingham, United Kingdom

Dinesh Kumbhare
Department of Medicine, University of Toronto, Toronto, ON, Canada

Gianni Parise
Exercise Metabolism Research Group, Department of Kinesiology, McMaster University, Hamilton, ON, Canada

Ken Smith and Philip J. Atherton
School of Graduate Entry Medicine and Health, University of Nottingham, Derby, United Kingdom

Benoit Smeuninx
School of Sport, Exercise and Rehabilitation Sciences, University of Birmingham, Birmingham, United Kingdom
MRC-Arthritis Research UK Centre for Musculoskeletal Ageing, Birmingham, United Kingdom

Carolyn A. Greig and Leigh Breen
School of Sport, Exercise and Rehabilitation Sciences, University of Birmingham, Birmingham, United Kingdom
MRC-Arthritis Research UK Centre for Musculoskeletal Ageing, Birmingham, United Kingdom
NIHR Birmingham Biomedical Research Centre, Birmingham, United Kingdom

Leonidas G. Karagounis
Nestlé Research, Lausanne, Switzerland Institute of Social and Preventive Medicine, University of Bern, Bern, Switzerland
Translation Research, Nestlé Health Science, Lausanne, Switzerland

Maurice Beaumont, Laurence Donato-Capel, Jean-Philippe Godin, Anne-France Kapp, Dimitrios Draganidis, Stéphane Pinaud, Jacques Vuichoud, Maya Shevlyakova, Koraljka Rade-Kukic and Denis Breuillé
Nestlé Research, Lausanne, Switzerland

Index

www.ingramcontent.com/pod-product-compliance
Lightning Source LLC
LaVergne TN
LVHW082155200926
848484LV00008B/2162